FIRST AID THE®

USMLE STEP 1 2025

TAO LE, MD, MHS

Founder, ScholarRx
Associate Clinical Professor, Department of Medicine
University of Louisville School of Medicine

ANUP CHALISE, MBBS, MS, MRCSEd

Registrar, General and Colorectal Surgery
North Middlesex University Hospital, London

CAROLINA CABAN RIVERA

MD/PhD Candidate, Class of 2025
Lewis Katz School of Medicine at Temple University

KIMBERLY KALLIANOS, MD

Assistant Professor, Department of Radiology and Biomedical Imaging
University of California, San Francisco School of Medicine

VIKAS BHUSHAN, MD

Founder, *First Aid for the USMLE Step 1*
Boracay, Philippines

JAIMIE ROGNER, MD, MPH

Resident, Department of Psychiatry
NewYork-Presbyterian/Weill Cornell Medical Center

CAROLINE COLEMAN, MD

Adjunct Professor, Department of Medicine
Emory University School of Medicine

SEAN EVANS, MD

Resident, Department of Medicine
Emory University School of Medicine

McGraw Hill

First Aid for the® USMLE Step 1 2025: A Student-to-Student Guide

Photo and line art credits for this book begin on page 755 and are considered an extension of this copyright page. Portions of this book identified with the symbol ℞ are copyright © USMLE-Rx.com (MedIQ Learning, LLC). Portions of this book identified with the symbol 🆁🆄 are copyright © Dr. Richard Usatine. Portions of this book identified with the symbol ✳ are under license from other third parties. Please refer to page 755 for a complete list of those image source attribution notices.

First Aid for the® is a registered trademark of McGraw Hill.

1 2 3 4 5 LBC 28 27 26 25

ISBN 978-1-266-34646-0
MHID 1-266-34646-5
ISSN 1532-6020

Notice

Medicine is an ever-changing science. As new research and clinical experience broaden our knowledge, changes in treatment and drug therapy are required. The authors and the publisher of this work have checked with sources believed to be reliable in their efforts to provide information that is complete and generally in accord with the standards accepted at the time of publication. However, in view of the possibility of human error or changes in medical sciences, neither the authors nor the publisher nor any other party who has been involved in the preparation or publication of this work warrants that the information contained herein is in every respect accurate or complete, and they disclaim all responsibility for any errors or omissions or for the results obtained from use of the information contained in this work. Readers are encouraged to confirm the information contained herein with other sources. For example and in particular, readers are advised to check the product information sheet included in the package of each drug they plan to administer to be certain that the information contained in this work is accurate and that changes have not been made in the recommended dose or in the contraindications for administration. This recommendation is of particular importance in connection with new or infrequently used drugs.

This book was set in Electra LT Std by GW Inc.
The editors were Bob Boehringer and Peter J. Boyle.
Project management was provided by GW Inc.
The production supervisor was Jeffrey Herzich.
LSC Communications was printer and binder.

This book is printed on acid-free paper.

International Edition ISBN 1-266-25125-2; MHID 1-266-25125-1.

McGraw Hill books are available at special quantity discounts to use as premiums and sales promotions, or for use in corporate training programs. To contact a representative please visit the Contact Us pages at www.mhprofessional.com.

Dedication

To medical students and physicians worldwide for
collaborating to improve medical education and practice.

Contents

▶ SECTION I — GUIDE TO EFFICIENT EXAM PREPARATION — 1

▶ SECTION I SUPPLEMENT — SPECIAL SITUATIONS — 25

▶ SECTION II — HIGH-YIELD GENERAL PRINCIPLES — 27

Contributing Authors

MARIAM ATOBILOYE
University of Utah School of Medicine
Class of 2026

MORGAN BUCHANAN, MPH
Emory University School of Medicine
Class of 2025

ANTHONY G. CHESEBRO
Renaissance School of Medicine, Stony Brook University
MD/PhD candidate

MURTAZA GANDHI, MBBS
Terna Medical College & Hospital

EMILY HAND, MD
Resident, Department of Obstetrics & Gynecology
New York Presbyterian–Brooklyn Methodist Hospital

KATHERINE LEBLANC, MSc
University of Washington School of Medicine
MD/PhD Candidate

ANNA LIGOCKI, MD, MS
Resident, Department of Medicine
Ascension Saint Agnes Hospital

DANUSHA SANCHEZ, MD, MSIS, PMP
Resident, Department of Emergency Medicine
Poznań University of Medical Sciences, Poland

GEORGIOS M. STERGIOPOULOS, MD
Research Fellow, Department of Molecular Medicine
Mayo Clinic, Minnesota

IMAGE AND ILLUSTRATION TEAM

YOOREE GRACE CHUNG
Emory University School of Medicine
MD/PhD Candidate

TANYA KONDOLAY, MPH
Windsor University School of Medicine
MD Candidate

NOAH NEWMAN, MD
Resident, Department of Internal Medicine
Emory University School of Medicine

AUBREY REED
Emory University School of Medicine
MD/PhD Candidate

Associate Authors

MAKENNA ASH
Emory University School of Medicine
Class of 2025

LISA MARIE BABIAK
Saint James School of Medicine
Class of 2025

SHAROON DAVID, MBBS, BSc
Allama Iqbal Medical College, Lahore, Pakistan

MARGARET GINOZA, MD, MPH
Resident, Internal Medicine–Pediatrics
Baylor College of Medicine

MOKI T. M HEIN, MS
Herbert Wertheim College of Medicine at Florida International
    University
Class of 2025

TALEAH KHAN, MBBS
CMH Lahore Medical College and Institute of Dentistry, Pakistan

ALYSSA D. MILBEE
Marshall University Joan C. Edwards School of Medicine
Class of 2026

DIKACHI OSAJI, MSc
Southern Illinois University School of Medicine
Class of 2027

NICHOLAS J. SIRHAN
Central Michigan University College of Medicine
Class of 2025

IMAGE AND ILLUSTRATION TEAM

HILARY LIU
University of Pittsburgh School of Medicine
Class of 2027

ANNABEL LU
Emory University School of Medicine
Class of 2024

Faculty Advisors

RITU AMATYA

FHI 360, Nepal

MARK A.W. ANDREWS, PhD

Professor and Founding Chairman, Department of Physiology
Duquesne University College of Osteopathic Medicine

MARIA ANTONELLI, MD

Assistant Professor, Division of Rheumatology
Case Western Reserve University at MetroHealth Medical Center, Cleveland

HERMAN S. BAGGA, MD, FACS

Physician, Urology, Genitourinary Reconstruction, Men's Health
Advanced Urology, Atlanta

SAMAN BENTOTA, MD

Physician and Microbiologist
Sri Lanka

JOE B. BLUMER, PhD

Associate Professor, Department of Pharmacology
Medical University of South Carolina College of Medicine

BRADLEY J. BRUGGEMAN, MD

Assistant Professor, Obstetrics and Gynecology
University of Florida College of Medicine

CHRISTOPHER M. BURNS, PhD

Professor of Basic Medical Sciences
University of Arizona College of Medicine, Phoenix

BROOKS D. CASH, MD

Chief, Gastroenterology, Hepatology, and Nutrition
University of Texas Health Science Center at Houston

DIMITRI CASSIMATIS, MD

Associate Professor, Department of Medicine
Emory University School of Medicine

CATHERINE CHILES, MD

Associate Clinical Professor of Psychiatry
Yale School of Medicine

BRADLEY COLE, MD

Assistant Professor of Neurology
Loma Linda University School of Medicine

CAROLINE COLEMAN, MD

Assistant Professor, Department of Medicine
Emory University School of Medicine

RAHUL DAMANIA, MD, MS Ed

Assistant Professor of Pediatrics, Division of Pediatric Critical Care Medicine
Cleveland Clinic Lerner College of Medicine at Case Western Reserve
  University

MARTHA FANER, PhD

Associate Professor of Biochemistry and Molecular Biology
Michigan State University College of Osteopathic Medicine

RAYUDU GOPALAKRISHNA, PhD

Professor, Department of Integrative Anatomical Sciences
Keck School of Medicine of University of Southern California

MEREDITH K. GREER, MD

Assistant Professor, Division of Pulmonary, Allergy, Critical Care, and Sleep
  Medicine
Emory University School of Medicine

AMBER J. HECK, PhD

Associate Professor, Department of Microbiology, Immunology, and
  Genetics
University of North Texas Health Science Center, Fort Worth

VASUDEVA G. KAMATH, MSc, PhD

Assistant Professor of Biochemistry
The University of Arizona College of Medicine, Phoenix

CLARK KEBODEAUX, PharmD

Clinical Associate Professor, Pharmacy Practice and Science
University of Kentucky College of Pharmacy

MATTHEW KRAYBILL, PhD

Clinical Neuropsychologist
Cottage Health, Santa Barbara, California

GERALD LEE, MD

Associate Professor, Departments of Pediatrics and Medicine
Emory University School of Medicine

KACHIU C. LEE, MD, MPH

Assistant Professor (Adjunct), Department of Dermatology
Lewis Katz School of Medicine at Temple University

JAMES LYONS, MD

Associate Dean, Professor of Pathology and Family Medicine
Alabama College of Osteopathic Medicine

NILADRI KUMAR MAHATO, MBBS, MS, PhD

Assistant Professor of Anatomy
Marian University–Tom and Julie Wood College of Osteopathic Medicine, Indianapolis

CARL MARFURT, PhD

Professor Emeritus, Department of Anatomy, Cell Biology and Physiology
Indiana University School of Medicine–Northwest, Gary

PETER MARKS, MD, PhD

Center for Biologics Evaluation and Research
US Food and Drug Administration

DOUGLAS A. MATA, MD, MPH

Senior Director of Molecular Pathology
Foundation Medicine, Boston

SOROUSH RAIS-BAHRAMI, MD, MBA

Professor of Urology and Radiology
University of Alabama at Birmingham Heersink School of Medicine

RICHARD P. RAMONELL, MD

Assistant Professor of Medicine, Division of Pulmonary, Allergy, Critical Care, and Sleep Medicine
University of Pittsburgh School of Medicine

KEISHA RAY, PhD

Associate Professor, McGovern Center for Humanities and Ethics
University of Texas Health Science Center at Houston

SASAN SAKIANI, MD

Assistant Professor of Medicine, Department of Medicine
University of Maryland School of Medicine

SARAH SCHIMANSKY, MB BCh BAO

Fellow, Department of Ophthalmology
Bristol Eye Hospital

SHIREEN MADANI SIMS, MD

Professor, Obstetrics and Gynecology
University of Florida College of Medicine

NATHAN WM. SKELLEY, MD

Associate Professor, Medical Director of Orthopaedic Surgery
Sanford Health–University of South Dakota School of Medicine

TONY SLIEMAN, PhD, MSc

Director of Academic Affairs and Associate Professor, Department of Biomedical and Anatomical Sciences
New York Institute of Technology College of Osteopathic Medicine at Arkansas State University

MATTHEW SOCHAT, MD

Physician, Hematology/Oncology
Southeastern Medical Oncology Center

HOWARD M. STEINMAN, PhD

Assistant Dean, Biomedical Science Education
Albert Einstein College of Medicine

RICHARD P. USATINE, MD

Professor, Dermatology and Cutaneous Surgery
University of Texas Health Science Center San Antonio

SYLVIA WASSERTHEIL-SMOLLER, PhD

Professor Emerita, Department of Epidemiology and Population Health
Albert Einstein College of Medicine

ADAM WEINSTEIN, MD

Professor of Medical Sciences and Pediatrics
Frank H. Netter MD School of Medicine at Quinnipiac University

ABHISHEK YADAV, MBBS, MSc

Associate Professor, Department of Medicine
Rutgers New Jersey Medical School

DONG ZHANG, PhD

Professor of Cancer Biology
New York Institute of Technology, College of Osteopathic Medicine at Old Westbury

Preface

With the 35th edition of *First Aid for the USMLE Step 1* we continue our commitment to providing students with the most useful and up-to-date preparation guide for this exam. This edition represents an outstanding revision in many ways, including:

- 24 entirely new or heavily revised high-yield topics reflecting evolving trends in the USMLE Step 1.

- Extensive text revisions, new mnemonics, clarifications, and corrections curated by a team of 18 medical student and resident physician authors who excelled on their Step 1 examinations, and verified by a team of expert faculty advisors and nationally recognized USMLE instructors.

- Updated with 101 new and revised diagrams and illustrations as part of our ongoing collaboration with USMLE-Rx and ScholarRx (MedIQ Learning, LLC).

- Updated with 30 new and revised photos to help visualize various disorders, descriptive findings, and basic science concepts. Additionally, revised imaging photos have been labeled and optimized to show both normal anatomy and pathologic findings.

- Updated exam preparation advice, tailored for the current pass/fail scoring system and Step 1 blueprint changes.

- Advice on how to utilize emerging AI tools to increase studying efficiency.

- Updated photos of patients and pathologies to include a variety of skin colors to better depict real-world presentations.

- Improved organization and integration of text, illustrations, clinical images, and tables throughout for focused review of high-yield topics.

- Revised ratings of current, high-yield review resources, with clear explanations of their relevance to USMLE review. Updated review resources with new recommendations by recent Step 1 examinees.

- Real-time Step 1 updates and corrections can be found exclusively on our blog, www.firstaidteam.com.

We invite students and faculty to share their thoughts and ideas to help us continually improve *First Aid for the USMLE Step 1* through our blog and collaborative editorial platform. (See How to Contribute, p. xv.)

Louisville	Tao Le
Boracay	Vikas Bhushan
London	Anup Chalise
Philadelphia	Carolina Caban Rivera
New York	Jaimie Rogner
Atlanta	Caroline Coleman
Atlanta	Sean Evans
San Francisco	Kimberly Kallianos

Special Acknowledgments

This has been a collaborative project from the start. We gratefully acknowledge the thousands of thoughtful comments, corrections, and advice of the many medical students, international medical graduates, and faculty who have supported the authors in our continuing development of *First Aid for the USMLE Step 1*.

We provide special acknowledgment and thanks to the following individuals who made exemplary contributions to this edition through our voting, proofreading, and crowdsourcing platform: Alameen Alsabbah, Edward Blanco, Emmy Coffey, Verónica Davila Parrilla, Mohammad Hossein Zamani, Sathvika Karne, Yoshita Rao, and Victoria Wong Murray.

For support and encouragement throughout the process, we are grateful to Thao Pham, Jinky Flang, and Jonathan Kirsch, Esq. Thanks to Louise Petersen for organizing and supporting the project. Thanks to our publisher, McGraw Hill, for the valuable assistance of its staff, including Bob Boehringer, Jeffrey Herzich, Kristian Sanford, and Don Goyette.

Thanks to Dr. Richard Usatine and Dr. Kristine Krafts for their outstanding image contributions. Thanks also to Jean-Christophe Fournet (www.humpath.com), Dr. Ed Uthman, and Dr. Frank Gaillard (www.radiopaedia.org) for generously allowing us to access some of their striking photographs.

For exceptional editorial leadership, enormous thanks to Megan Chandler. Special thanks to our indexer, Dr. Anne Fifer. We are also grateful to our illustrators, Stephanie Jones and Rachael Joy, for their creative work on the new and updated illustrations. Lastly, tremendous thanks to our compositor, GW Inc., especially Anne Banning, Gary Clark, Cindy Geiss, Debra Clark, Abby Ermer, and Gabby Sullivan.

Louisville	Tao Le
Boracay	Vikas Bhushan
London	Anup Chalise
Philadelphia	Carolina Caban Rivera
New York	Jaimie Rogner
Atlanta	Caroline Coleman
Atlanta	Sean Evans
San Francisco	Kimberly Kallianos

General Acknowledgments

Each year we are fortunate to receive the input of thousands of medical students and graduates who provide new material, clarifications, and potential corrections through our website and our collaborative editing platform. This has been a tremendous help in clarifying difficult concepts, correcting errata from the previous edition, and minimizing new errata during the revision of the current edition. This reflects our long-standing vision of a true, student-to-student publication. We have done our best to thank each person individually below, but we recognize that errors and omissions are likely. Therefore, we will post an updated list of acknowledgments at our website, www.firstaidteam.com/bonus/. We will gladly make corrections if they are brought to our attention.

For submitting contributions and corrections, many thanks to Suhaib Abusara, Shruti Agarwal, Eman Nayaz Ahmed, Ahmed Alhassan, Stamatios Anagnostou, Jackner Antigua, Karun Bhattarai, Stephanie Brown, Urvashi Chavda, Edgar Chavez Contreras, Vamsi Chekuri, Christopher Crudele, Tamilla Dikinova, Melissa Frangie Machado, Michael Gabriel Johnson, Andrea Gangi, Sondas Gargum, Laura Hepple, Hussein Hisham, Ruzan Jamaleddin, Ujjwal Kumar Jha, Karanvir Jhajj, Saywala Karsor, Sarah Kenney, Siddhi Khushalani, Ruturaj Maniklal Kolhapure, Anuja Konda, Yuliya Kos, Omer Lateef, Phuoc-Hanh Le, Sortirios Manganas, Ioannis Markopoulos, Thalía Medina-Rodríguez, Conrado Montes de Oca, Ezra Nadler, Mohammad Nafeli Shahrestani, Thanh Ngoc Le, Martin Nguyen, Sameer Noor, Odi Odi, Monique Ortiz, Sirwa Padash, Nikhil Parail, Mark Parker, Abigail Poe, Victoria Potter, Khaled Rafeh, Sakshi Rao, Alex Rosiejka, Hasan Saghir, Zouina Sarfraz, Rahul Sarkar, Beck Schur, Karun Dev Sharma, Utsav Sitaula, Grace Sloan, Suman Supratik, Isaac Thorman, Jennifer Vorobej, and Abhiraj Yadav.

How to Contribute

This edition of *First Aid for the USMLE Step 1* incorporates thousands of contributions and improvements suggested by student and faculty advisors. We invite you to participate in this process. Please send us your suggestions for:

- Study and test-taking strategies for the USMLE Step 1

- New facts, mnemonics, diagrams, and clinical images

- High-yield topics that may appear on future Step 1 exams

- Low-yield content that should be deleted

- Personal ratings and comments on review books, question banks, apps, videos, and courses

- Pathology and radiology images (high resolution) relevant to the facts in the book

For each new entry incorporated into the next edition, you will receive **up to a $20 Amazon.com gift card** as well as personal acknowledgment in the next edition. Significant contributions will be compensated at the discretion of the authors. Also, let us know about material in this edition that you feel is low yield and should be deleted.

All submissions including potential errata should ideally be supported with hyperlinks to a dynamically updated Web resource such as UpToDate, AccessMedicine, and ClinicalKey.

We welcome potential errata on grammar and style if the change improves readability. Please note that *First Aid* style is somewhat unique; for example, we have fully adopted the *AMA Manual of Style* recommendations on eponyms ("We recommend that the possessive form be omitted in eponymous terms") and on abbreviations (no periods with eg, ie, etc). We also avoid periods in tables unless required for full sentences. Kindly refrain from submitting "style errata" unless you find specific inconsistencies with the *AMA Manual of Style*.

The preferred way to submit new entries, clarifications, mnemonics, or potential corrections with a valid, authoritative reference is via our website: **www.firstaidteam.com**.

This website will be continuously updated with validated errata, new high-yield content, and a new online platform to contribute suggestions, mnemonics, diagrams, clinical images, and potential errata.

Alternatively, you can email us at: **firstaid@scholarrx.com**.

Contributions submitted by **May 15, 2025**, receive priority consideration for the 2026 edition of *First Aid for the USMLE Step 1*. We thank you for taking the time to share your experience and apologize in advance that we cannot individually respond to all contributors as we receive thousands of contributions each year.

▶ NOTE TO CONTRIBUTORS

All contributions become property of the authors and are subject to editing and reviewing. Please verify all data and spellings carefully. Contributions should be supported by at least two high-quality references.

Check our website first to avoid duplicate submissions. In the event that similar or duplicate entries are received, only the first complete entry received with valid, authoritative references will be credited. Please follow the style, punctuation, and format of this edition as much as possible.

▶ JOIN THE FIRST AID TEAM

The *First Aid*/ScholarRx team is pleased to offer paid editorial and coaching positions. We are looking for passionate, experienced, and dedicated medical students and recent graduates. Participants will have an opportunity to work on a wide variety of projects, including the popular *First Aid* series and the growing line of USMLE-Rx/ScholarRx products, including Rx Bricks. Please use our webform at https://www.usmle-rx.com/join-the-first-aid-team/ to apply, and include a CV and writing examples.

For 2025, we are actively seeking passionate medical students and graduates with a specific interest in improving our medical illustrations, expanding our database of photographs (including clinical images depicting diverse skin types), and developing the software that supports our crowdsourcing platform. We welcome people with prior experience and talent in these areas. Relevant skills include clinical imaging, digital photography, digital asset management, information design, medical illustration, graphic design, tutoring, and software development.

How to Use This Book

CONGRATULATIONS: You now possess the book that has guided nearly two million students to USMLE success for over 30 years. With appropriate care, the binding should last the useful life of the book. Keep in mind that putting excessive flattening pressure on any binding will accelerate its failure. If you purchased a book that you believe is defective, please **immediately** return it to the place of purchase. If you encounter ongoing issues, you can also contact Customer Service at our publisher, McGraw Hill.

START EARLY: Use this book as early as possible while learning the basic medical sciences. The first semester of your first year is not too early! Devise a study plan by reading Section I: Guide to Efficient Exam Preparation, and make an early decision on resources to use by checking Section IV: Top-Rated Review Resources. Note that *First Aid* is neither a textbook nor a comprehensive review book, and it is not a panacea for inadequate preparation.

CONSIDER *FIRST AID* YOUR ANNOTATION HUB: Annotate this book with material from other resources, such as class notes or comprehensive textbooks. This will keep all the high-yield information you need in one place. Other tips on keeping yourself organized:

- For best results, use fine-tipped ballpoint pens (eg, BIC Pro+, Uni-Ball Jetstream Sport, Pilot Drawing Pen, Zebra F-301). If you like gel pens, try Pentel Slicci, and for markers that dry almost immediately, consider Staedtler Triplus Fineliner, Pilot Drawing Pen, and Sharpie.

- Consider using pens with different colors of ink to indicate different sources of information (eg, blue for USMLE-Rx Step 1 Qmax, green for UWorld Step 1 Qbank, red for Rx Bricks).

- Choose highlighters that are bright and dry quickly to minimize smudging and bleeding through the page (eg, Tombow Kei Coat, Sharpie Gel).

- Many students de-spine their book and get it 3-hole-punched. This will allow you to insert materials from other sources, including curricular materials.

INTEGRATE STUDY WITH CASES, FLASH CARDS, AND QUESTIONS: To broaden your learning strategy, consider integrating your *First Aid* study with case-based reviews (eg, *First Aid Cases for the USMLE Step 1*), flash cards (eg, USMLE-Rx Step 1 Flash Facts), and practice questions (eg, the USMLE-Rx Step 1 Qmax). Read the chapter in the book, then test your comprehension by using cases, flash cards, and questions that cover the same topics. Maintain access to more comprehensive resources (eg, ScholarRx Bricks and USMLE-Rx Step 1 Express videos) for deeper review as needed.

PRIME YOUR MEMORY: Return to your annotated Sections II and III several days before taking the USMLE Step 1. The book can serve as a useful way of retaining key associations and keeping high-yield facts fresh in your memory just prior to the exam. The Rapid Review section includes high-yield topics to help guide your studying.

CONTRIBUTE TO FIRST AID: Reviewing the book immediately after your exam can help us improve the next edition. Decide what was truly high and low yield and send us your comments. Feel free to send us scanned images from your annotated *First Aid* book as additional support. Of course, always remember that **all examinees are under agreement with the NBME to not disclose the specific details of copyrighted test material.**

Selected USMLE Laboratory Values

* = Included in the Biochemical Profile (SMA-12)

Blood, Plasma, Serum	Reference Range	SI Reference Intervals
*Alanine aminotransferase (ALT, GPT at 30°C)	10–40 U/L	10–40 U/L
*Alkaline phosphatase	25–100 U/L	25–100 U/L
Amylase, serum	25–125 U/L	25–125 U/L
*Aspartate aminotransferase (AST, GOT at 30°C)	12–38 U/L	12–38 U/L
Bilirubin, serum (adult)		
Total // Direct	0.1–1.0 mg/dL // 0.0–0.3 mg/dL	2–17 μmol/L // 0–5 μmol/L
*Calcium, serum (Total)	8.4–10.2 mg/dL	2.1–2.6 mmol/L
*Cholesterol, serum (Total)	Rec: < 200 mg/dL	< 5.2 mmol/L
*Creatinine, serum (Total)	0.6–1.2 mg/dL	53–106 μmol/L
Electrolytes, serum		
Sodium (Na^+)	136–146 mEq/L	136–146 mmol/L
Chloride (Cl^-)	95–105 mEq/L	95–105 mmol/L
* Potassium (K^+)	3.5–5.0 mEq/L	3.5–5.0 mmol/L
Bicarbonate (HCO_3^-)	22–28 mEq/L	22–28 mmol/L
Magnesium (Mg^{2+})	1.5–2 mEq/L	0.75–1.0 mmol/L
Gases, arterial blood (room air)		
P_{O_2}	75–105 mm Hg	10.0–14.0 kPa
P_{CO_2}	33–45 mm Hg	4.4–5.9 kPa
pH	7.35–7.45	[H^+] 36–44 nmol/L
*Glucose, serum	Fasting: 70–100 mg/dL	3.8–6.1 mmol/L
Growth hormone – arginine stimulation	Fasting: < 5 ng/mL	< 5 μg/L
	Provocative stimuli: > 7 ng/mL	> 7 μg/L
Osmolality, serum	275–295 mOsmol/kg H_2O	275–295 mOsmol/kg H_2O
*Phosphorus (inorganic), serum	3.0–4.5 mg/dL	1.0–1.5 mmol/L
Prolactin, serum (hPRL)	Male: < 17 ng/mL	< 17 μg/L
	Female: < 25 ng/mL	< 25 μg/L
*Proteins, serum		
Total (recumbent)	6.0–7.8 g/dL	60–78 g/L
Albumin	3.5–5.5 g/dL	35–55 g/L
Globulins	2.3–3.5 g/dL	23–35 g/L
Thyroid-stimulating hormone, serum or plasma	0.4–4.0 μU/mL	0.4–4.0 mIU/L
*Urea nitrogen, serum (BUN)	7–18 mg/dL	25–64 nmol/L
*Uric acid, serum	3.0–8.2 mg/dL	0.18–0.48 mmol/L

(continues)

Cerebrospinal Fluid	Reference Range	SI Reference Intervals
Cell count	0–5/mm^3	0–5 × 10^6/L
Glucose	40–70 mg/dL	2.2–3.9 mmol/L
Proteins, total	< 40 mg/dL	< 0.40 g/L

Hematologic		
Erythrocyte count	Male: 4.3–5.9 million/mm^3 Female: 3.5–5.5 million/mm^3	4.3–5.9 × 10^{12}/L 3.5–5.5 × 10^{12}/L
Erythrocyte sedimentation rate (Westergen)	Male: 0–15 mm/hr Female: 0–20 mm/hr	0–15 mm/hr 0–20 mm/hr
Hematocrit	Male: 41–53% Female: 36–46%	0.41–0.53 0.36–0.46
Hemoglobin, blood	Male: 13.5–17.5 g/dL Female: 12.0–16.0 g/dL	135–175 g/L 120–160 g/L
Hemoglobin, plasma	< 4 mg/dL	< 0.62 µmol/L
Leukocyte count and differential		
Leukocyte count	4,500–11,000/mm^3	4.5–11.0 × 10^9/L
Segmented neutrophils	54–62%	0.54–0.62
Band forms	3–5%	0.03–0.05
Eosinophils	1–3%	0.01–0.03
Basophils	0–0.75%	0–0.0075
Lymphocytes	25–33%	0.25–0.33
Monocytes	3–7%	0.03–0.07
Mean corpuscular hemoglobin	25–35 pg/cell	0.39–0.54 fmol/cell
Mean corpuscular hemoglobin concentration	31%–36% Hb/cell	4.8–5.6 mmol Hb/L
Mean corpuscular volume	80–100 µm^3	80–100 fL
Partial thromboplastin time (activated)	25–40 sec	25–40 sec
Platelet count	150,000–400,000/mm^3	150–400 × 10^9/L
Prothrombin time	11–15 sec	11–15 sec
Reticulocyte count	0.5–1.5% of RBCs	0.005–0.015

Urine		
Creatinine clearance	Male: 97–137 mL/min Female: 88–128 mL/min	97–137 mL/min 88–128 mL/min
Osmolality	50–1200 mOsmol/kg H$_2$O	50–1200 mOsmol/kg H$_2$O
Proteins, total	< 150 mg/24 hr	< 0.15 g/24 hr

Other		
Body mass index	Adult: 19–25 kg/m^2	19–25 kg/m^2

First Aid Checklist for the USMLE Step 1

This is an example of how you might use the information in Section I to prepare for the USMLE Step 1. Refer to corresponding topics in Section I for more details.

Years Prior
- ☐ Use top-rated review resources for first-year medical school courses.
- ☐ Ask for advice from those who have recently taken the USMLE Step 1.

Months Prior
- ☐ Review computer test format and registration information.
- ☐ Register six months in advance.
- ☐ Carefully verify name and address printed on scheduling permit. Make sure the name on scheduling permit matches the name printed on your photo ID.
- ☐ Go online for test date ASAP.
- ☐ Set up a realistic timeline for study. Cover less crammable subjects first.
- ☐ Evaluate and choose study materials (review books, question banks).
- ☐ Use a question bank to simulate the USMLE Step 1 to pinpoint strengths and weaknesses in knowledge and test-taking skills from early on.

Weeks Prior
- ☐ Do test simulations in question banks.
- ☐ Assess how close you are to your goal.
- ☐ Pinpoint remaining weaknesses. Stay healthy (eg, exercise, sleep).
- ☐ Verify information on admission ticket (eg, location, date).

One Week Prior
- ☐ Remember comfort measures (eg, loose clothing, earplugs).
- ☐ Work out test site logistics (eg, location, transportation, parking, lunch).
- ☐ Print or download your Scheduling Permit and Scheduling Confirmation to your phone.

One Day Prior
- ☐ Relax.
- ☐ Lightly review short-term material if necessary. Skim high-yield facts.
- ☐ Get a good night's sleep.

Day of Exam
- ☐ Relax.
- ☐ Eat breakfast.
- ☐ Minimize bathroom breaks during exam by avoiding excessive morning caffeine.

After Exam
- ☐ Celebrate, regardless of how well you feel you did.
- ☐ Send feedback to us on our website at **www.firstaidteam.com** or at **firstaid@scholarrx.com**.

Guide to Efficient Exam Preparation

"One important key to success is self-confidence. An important key to self-confidence is preparation."

—Arthur Ashe

"Wisdom is not a product of schooling but of the lifelong attempt to acquire it."

—Albert Einstein

"Finally, from so little sleeping and so much reading, his brain dried up and he went completely out of his mind."

—Miguel de Cervantes Saavedra, *Don Quixote*

"Sometimes the questions are complicated and the answers are simple."

—Dr. Seuss

"He who knows all the answers has not been asked all the questions."

—Confucius

"The expert in anything was once a beginner."

—Helen Hayes

"It always seems impossible until it's done."

—Nelson Mandela

▶ INTRODUCTION

Relax.

This section is intended to make your exam preparation easier, not harder. Our goal is to reduce your level of anxiety and help you make the most of your efforts by helping you understand more about the United States Medical Licensing Examination, Step 1 (USMLE Step 1). As a medical student, you are no doubt familiar with taking standardized examinations and quickly absorbing large amounts of material. When you first confront the USMLE Step 1, however, you may find it all too easy to become sidetracked from your goal of studying with maximal effectiveness. Common mistakes that students make when studying for Step 1 include the following:

- Starting to study (including *First Aid*) too late
- Starting to study intensely too early and burning out
- Starting to prepare for boards before creating a knowledge foundation
- Using inefficient or inappropriate study methods
- Buying the wrong resources or buying too many resources
- Not using question banks early in examination preparation
- Not using practice examinations to maximum benefit
- Not understanding how scoring is performed or what the result means
- Not using review books along with your classes
- Not analyzing and improving your test-taking strategies
- Getting bogged down by reviewing difficult topics excessively
- Studying material that is rarely tested on the USMLE Step 1
- Failing to master certain high-yield subjects owing to overconfidence
- Using *First Aid* as your sole study resource
- Trying to prepare for it all alone

In this section, we offer advice to help you avoid these pitfalls and be more productive in your studies.

▶ USMLE STEP 1—THE BASICS

▶ *The test at a glance:*
- *8-hour exam*
- *Up to a total of 280 multiple choice items*
- *7 test blocks (60 min/block)*
- *Up to 40 test items per block*
- *45 minutes of break time, plus another 15 if you skip the tutorial*

The USMLE Step 1 is the first of three examinations that you would normally pass in order to become a licensed physician in the United States. The USMLE is a joint endeavor of the National Board of Medical Examiners (NBME) and the Federation of State Medical Boards (FSMB). The USMLE serves as the single examination system domestically and internationally for those seeking medical licensure in the United States.

The Step 1 exam includes test items that can be grouped by the organizational constructs outlined in Table 1 (in order of tested frequency). In late 2020, the USMLE increased the number of items assessing communication skills. While pharmacology is still tested, they are focusing on drug mechanisms rather than on pharmacotherapy. You will not be required to identify the specific medications indicated for a specific condition. Instead, you will be asked more about drug mechanisms and side effects.

TABLE 1. Frequency of Various Constructs Tested on the USMLE Step 1.[1]*

Competency	Range, %	System	Range, %
Medical knowledge: applying foundational science concepts	60–70	Reproductive & endocrine systems	12–16
Patient care: diagnosis	20–25	Respiratory & renal/urinary systems	11–15
Communication and interpersonal skills	6–9	Behavioral health & nervous systems/special senses	10–14
Practice-based learning & improvement	4–6	Blood & lymphoreticular/immune systems	9–13
Discipline	**Range, %**	Multisystem processes & disorders	8–12
Pathology	44–52	Musculoskeletal, skin & subcutaneous tissue	8–12
Physiology	25–35	Cardiovascular system	7–11
Pharmacology	15–22	Gastrointestinal system	6–10
Biochemistry & nutrition	14–24	Social sciences: communication & interpersonal skills	6–9
Microbiology	10–15	Biostatistics & epidemiology/population health	4–6
Immunology	6–11	Human development	1–3
Gross anatomy & embryology	11–15		
Histology & cell biology	8–13		
Behavioral sciences	8–13		
Genetics	5–9		

*Percentages are subject to change at any time. www.usmle.org

How Is the Computer-Based Test (CBT) Structured?

The CBT Step 1 exam consists of one "optional" tutorial/simulation block and seven "real" question blocks of up to 40 questions per block with no more than 280 questions in total, timed at 60 minutes per block. A short 11-question survey follows the last question block. The computer begins the survey with a prompt to proceed to the next block of questions.

Once an examinee finishes a particular question block on the CBT, he or she must click on a screen icon to continue to the next block. Examinees **cannot** go back and change their answers to questions from any previously completed block. However, changing answers is allowed **within** a block of questions as long as the block has not been ended and if time permits.

What Is the CBT Like?

Given the unique environment of the CBT, it's important that you become familiar ahead of time with what your test-day conditions will be like. You can access a 15-minute tutorial and practice blocks at http://orientation. nbme.org/Launch/USMLE/STPF1. This tutorial interface is the same as the one you will use in the exam; learn it now and you can skip taking it during the exam, giving you up to 15 extra minutes of break time. You can gain experience with the CBT format by taking the 120 practice questions (3 blocks with 40 questions each) available online for free (https://www.usmle. org/prepare-your-exam) or by signing up for a practice session at a test center for a fee. The practice session is available for $75 ($155 if taken outside of the US and Canada) and is divided into a short tutorial and three 1-hour blocks of ~40 test items each.

▶ *You can take a shortened CBT practice test at a Prometric center.*

For security reasons, examinees are not allowed to bring any personal electronic equipment into the testing area. This includes both digital and analog watches, cell phones, tablets, and calculators. Examinees are also prohibited from carrying in their books, notes, pens/pencils, and scratch paper (laminated note boards and fine-tip dry erase pens will be provided for use within the testing area). Food and beverages are also prohibited in the testing area. The testing centers are monitored by audio and video surveillance equipment. However, most testing centers allot each examinee a small locker outside the testing area in which he or she can store snacks, beverages, and personal items.

> ▶ Keyboard shortcuts:
>   ▪ A, B, etc—letter choices
>   ▪ Esc—exit pop-up Calculator and Notes windows

Questions are typically presented in multiple choice format, with 4 or more possible answer options. There is a countdown timer on the lower left corner of the screen as well. There is also a button that allows the examinee to mark a question for review. If a given question happens to be longer than the screen, a scroll bar will appear on the right, allowing the examinee to see the rest of the question. Regardless of whether the examinee clicks on an answer choice or leaves it blank, he or she must click the "Next" button to advance to the next question.

> ▶ Heart sounds are tested via media questions. Make sure you know how different heart diseases sound on auscultation.

The USMLE features a small number of media clips in the form of audio and/or video. There may even be a question with a multimedia heart sound simulation. In these questions, a digital image of a torso appears on the screen, and the examinee directs a digital stethoscope to various auscultation points to listen for heart and breath sounds. The USMLE orientation materials include several practice questions in these formats. During the exam tutorial, examinees are given an opportunity to ensure that both the audio headphones and the volume are functioning properly. If you are already familiar with the tutorial and planning on skipping it, first skip ahead to the section where you can test your headphones. After you are sure the headphones are working properly, proceed to the exam.

> ▶ Be sure to test your headphones during the tutorial.

The examinee can call up a window displaying normal laboratory values. In order to do so, he or she must click the "Lab" icon on the top part of the screen. Afterward, the examinee will have the option to choose between "Blood," "Cerebrospinal," "Hematologic," or "Sweat and Urine." The normal values screen may obscure the question if it is expanded. The examinee may have to scroll down to search for the needed lab values. You might want to memorize some common lab values so you spend less time on questions that require you to analyze these.

> ▶ Familiarize yourself with the commonly tested lab values (eg, Hb, WBC, Ca^{2+}, Na^+, K^+).

> ▶ Illustrations on the test include:
>   ▪ Gross specimen photos
>   ▪ Histology slides
>   ▪ Medical imaging (eg, x-ray, CT, MRI)
>   ▪ Electron micrographs
>   ▪ Line drawings

The CBT interface provides a running list of questions on the left part of the screen at all times. The software also permits examinees to highlight or cross out information by using their mouse. There is a "Notes" icon on the top part of the screen that allows students to write notes to themselves for review at a later time. Finally, the USMLE has recently added new functionality including text magnification and reverse color (white text on black background). Being familiar with these features can save time and may help you better view and organize the information you need to answer a question.

For those who feel they might benefit, the USMLE offers an opportunity to take a simulated test, or "CBT Practice Session" at a Prometric center. Students are eligible to register for this three-and-one-half-hour practice session after they have received their scheduling permit.

You may register for a practice session online at www.usmle.org. A separate scheduling permit is issued for the practice session. Students should allow two weeks for receipt of this permit.

How Do I Register to Take the Exam?

Prometric test centers offer Step 1 on a year-round basis, except for the first two weeks in January and major holidays. Check with the test center you want to use before making your exam plans.

▶ *The Prometric website will display a calendar with open test dates.*

US students can apply to take Step 1 at the NBME website. This application allows you to select one of 12 overlapping three-month blocks in which to be tested (eg, April–May–June, June–July–August). Choose your three-month eligibility period wisely. If you need to reschedule outside your initial three-month period, you can request a one-time extension of eligibility for the next contiguous three-month period, and pay a rescheduling fee. The application also includes a photo ID form that must be certified by an official at your medical school to verify your enrollment. After the NBME processes your application, it will send you a scheduling permit.

The scheduling permit you receive from the NBME will contain your USMLE identification number, the eligibility period in which you may take the exam, and two additional numbers. The first of these is known as your "scheduling number." You must have this number in order to make your exam appointment with Prometric. The second number is known as the "candidate identification number," or CIN. Examinees must enter their CINs at the Prometric workstation in order to access their exams. However, you will not be allowed to bring your permit into the exam and will be asked to copy your CIN onto your scratch paper. Prometric has no access to the codes. **Make sure to bring a paper or electronic copy of your permit with you to the exam!** Also bring an unexpired, government-issued photo ID that includes your signature (such as a driver's license or passport). Make sure the name on your photo ID exactly matches the name that appears on your scheduling permit.

▶ *Be familiar with Prometric's policies for cancellation and rescheduling due to COVID-19.*

Once you receive your scheduling permit, you may access the Prometric website or call Prometric's toll-free number to arrange a time to take the exam. You may contact Prometric two weeks before the test date if you want to confirm identification requirements. Be aware that your exam may be canceled because of circumstances related to COVID-19 or other unforeseen events. If that were to happen, you should receive an email from Prometric containing notice of the cancellation and instructions on rescheduling.

Although requests for taking the exam may be completed more than six months before the test date, examinees will not receive their scheduling permits earlier than six months before the eligibility period. The eligibility period is the three-month period you have chosen to take the exam. Most US medical students attending a school which uses the two-year preclerkship curriculum choose the April–June or June–August period. Most US medical students attending a school which uses the 18-month preclerkship curriculum choose the December–February or January–March period.

> Test scheduling is done on a "first-come, first-served" basis. It's important to schedule an exam date as soon as you receive your scheduling permit.

What If I Need to Reschedule the Exam?

You can change your test date and/or center by contacting Prometric at 1-800-MED-EXAM (1-800-633-3926) or www.prometric.com. Make sure to have your CIN when rescheduling. If you are rescheduling by phone, you must speak with a Prometric representative; leaving a voicemail message will not suffice. To avoid a rescheduling fee, you will need to request a change at least 46 calendar days before your appointment. Please note that your rescheduled test date must fall within your assigned three-month eligibility period.

> Register six months in advance for seating and scheduling preference.

When Should I Register for the Exam?

You should plan to register as far in advance as possible ahead of your desired test date (eg, six months), but, depending on your particular test center, new dates and times may open closer to the date. Scheduling early will guarantee that you will get either your test center of choice or one within a 50-mile radius of your first choice. For most US medical students, the desired testing window correlates with the end of the preclerkship curriculum, which is around June for schools on a two-year preclerkship schedule, and around January for schools on an 18-month schedule. Thus US medical students should plan to register before January in anticipation of a June test date, or before August in anticipation of a January test date. The timing of the exam is more flexible for IMGs, as it is related only to when they finish exam preparation. Talk with upperclassmen who have already taken the test so you have real-life experience from students who went through a similar curriculum, then formulate your own strategy.

Where Can I Take the Exam?

Your testing location is arranged with Prometric when you book your test date (after you receive your scheduling permit). For a list of Prometric locations nearest you, visit www.prometric.com.

How Long Will I Have to Wait Before I Get My Result?

The USMLE reports results in three to four weeks, unless there are delays in processing. Examinees will be notified via email when their results are available. By following the online instructions, examinees will be able to view, download, and print their exam report online for ~365 days after notification, after which results can only be obtained through requesting an official USMLE transcript. Additional information about results reporting timetables and accessibility is available on the official USMLE website. Between 2021 and 2022, Step 1 pass rates dropped from 95% to 91% across US/Canadian schools and from 77% to 71% across non-US/Canadian schools (see Table 2), following the transition to pass/fail scoring in January 2022.

▶ Step 1 pass rates dropped significantly amongst both US/Canadian students and IMGs in 2022.

What About Time?

Time is of special interest on the CBT exam. Here's a breakdown of the exam schedule:

▶ Gain extra break time by skipping the tutorial, or utilize the tutorial time to add personal notes to your scratch paper.

15 minutes	Tutorial (skip if familiar with test format and features)
7 hours	Seven 60-minute question blocks
45 minutes	Break time (includes time for lunch)

The computer will keep track of how much time has elapsed on the exam. However, the computer will show you only how much time you have remaining in a given block. Therefore, it is up to you to determine if you are pacing yourself properly (at a rate of approximately one question per 90 seconds).

The computer does not warn you if you are spending more than your allotted time for a break. You should therefore budget your time so that you can take a short break when you need one and have time to eat. You must be especially careful not to spend too much time in between blocks (you should keep track of how much time elapses from the time you finish a block of questions to the time you start the next block). After you finish one question block, you'll need to click to proceed to the next block of questions. If you do not click within 30 seconds, you will automatically be entered into a break period.

Break time for the day is 45 minutes, but you are not required to use all of it, nor are you required to use any of it. You can gain extra break time (but not extra time for the question blocks) by skipping the tutorial or by finishing a block ahead of the allotted time. Any time remaining on the clock when you finish a block gets added to your remaining break time. Once a new question block has been started, you may not take a break until you have reached the end of that block. If you do so, this will be recorded as an "unauthorized break" and will be reported on your final exam report.

▶ Be careful to watch the clock on your break time.

Finally, be aware that it may take a few minutes of your break time to "check out" of the secure resting room and then "check in" again to resume testing, so plan accordingly. The "check-in" process may include fingerprints, pocket checks, and metal detector scanning. Some students recommend pocketless clothing on exam day to streamline the process.

If I Freak Out and Leave, What Happens to My Exam?

Your scheduling permit shows a CIN that you will need to enter to start your exam. Entering the CIN is the same as breaking the seal on a test book, and you are considered to have started the exam when you do so. However, no result will be reported if you do not complete the exam. If you leave at any time after starting the test, or do not open every block of your test, your test will not be scored and will be reported as incomplete. Incomplete results count toward the maximum of four attempts for each Step exam. Although a pass or fail result is not posted for incomplete tests, examinees may still be offered an option to request that their scores be calculated and reported if they desire; unanswered questions will be scored as incorrect.

The exam ends when all question blocks have been completed or when their time has expired. As you leave the testing center, you will receive a printed test-completion notice to document your completion of the exam. To receive an official score, you must finish the entire exam.

What Types of Questions Are Asked?

▶ *Nearly three fourths of Step 1 questions begin with a description of a patient.*

All questions on the exam are **one-best-answer multiple choice items.** Most questions consist of a clinical scenario or a direct question followed by a list of four or more options. You are required to select the single best answer among the options given. There are no "except," "not," or matching questions on the exam. A number of options may be partially correct, in which case you must select the option that best answers the question or completes the statement. Additionally, keep in mind that certain questions in the exam are experimental, but you won't know which ones, and they won't impact your final score.

TABLE 2. Passing Rates for the 2022-2023 USMLE Step 1.[2]

	2022		2023	
	No. Tested	% Passing	No. Tested	% Passing
Allopathic 1st takers	22,828	93%	23,100	92%
Repeaters	1,489	71%	2,046	70%
Allopathic total	24,317	91%	25,146	9%
Osteopathic 1st takers	4,659	89%	4,913	87%
Repeaters	63	67%	115	60%
Osteopathic total	4,722	89%	4,913	86%
Total US/Canadian	**29,039**	**91%**	**30,059**	**90%**
IMG 1st takers	22,030	74%	22,611	72%
Repeaters	2,926	45%	3,530	47%
IMG total	24,956	71%	26,141	68%
Total Step 1 examinees	**53,995**	**82%**	**56,200**	**80%**

How Is the Test Scored?

The USMLE transitioned to a pass/fail scoring system for Step 1 on January 26, 2022. Examinees now receive an electronic report that will display the outcome of either "Pass" or "Fail." Failing reports include a graphic depiction of the distance between the examinee's score and the minimum passing standard as well as content area feedback. Feedback for the content area shows the examinee's performance relative to examinees with a low pass (lower, same, or higher) and should be used to guide future study plans. Passing exam reports only displays the outcome of "Pass," along with a breakdown of topics covered on that individual examination (which will closely mirror the frequencies listed in Table 1).

Examinees who took the test before the transition to pass/fail reporting received an electronic report that includes the examinee's pass/fail status, a three-digit test score, a bar chart comparing the examinee's performance in each content area with their overall Step 1 performance, and a graphic depiction of the examinee's performance by physician task, discipline, and organ system. Changes will not be made to transcripts containing three-digit test scores.

The USMLE does not report the minimum number of correct responses needed to pass, but estimates that it is approximately 60%. The USMLE may update exam result reporting in the future, so please check the USMLE website or www.firstaidteam.com for updates.

▶ Depending on the resource used, practice questions may be easier than the actual exam.

Official NBME/USMLE Resources

The NBME offers a Comprehensive Basic Science Examination (CBSE) for practice that is a shorter version of the Step 1. The CBSE contains four blocks of 50 questions each and covers material that is typically learned during the basic science years. CBSE scores represent the percent of content mastered and show an estimated probability of passing Step 1. Many schools use this test to gauge whether a student is expected to pass Step 1. If this test is offered by your school, it is usually conducted at the end of regular didactic time before any dedicated Step 1 preparation. If you do not encounter the CBSE before your dedicated study time, you need not worry about taking it. Use the information to help set realistic goals and timetables for your success.

The NBME also offers six forms of Comprehensive Basic Science Self-Assessment (CBSSA). Students who prepared for the exam using this web-based tool reported that they found the format and content highly indicative of questions tested on the actual exam. In addition, the CBSSA is a fair predictor of historical USMLE performance. The test interface, however, does not match the actual USMLE test interface, so practicing with these forms alone is not advised.

The CBSSA exists in two formats: standard-paced and self-paced, both of which consist of four sections of 50 questions each (for a total of 200 multiple choice items). The standard-paced format allows the user up to 75 minutes to complete each section, reflecting time limits similar to the actual exam. By contrast, the self-paced format places a 5-hour time limit on answering all multiple choice questions. Every few years, new forms are released and older ones are retired, reflecting changes in exam content. Therefore, the newer exams tend to be more similar to the actual Step 1, and scores from these exams tend to provide a better estimation of exam day performance.

Keep in mind that this bank of questions is available only on the web. The NBME requires that users start and complete the exam within 90 days of purchase. Once the assessment has begun, users are required to complete the sections within 20 days. Following completion of the questions, the CBSSA provides a performance profile indicating the user's relative strengths and weaknesses, much like the report profile for the USMLE Step 1 exam. In addition to the performance profile, examinees will be informed of the number of questions answered incorrectly. You will have the ability to review the text of all questions with detailed explanations. The NBME charges $62 for each assessment, payable by credit card or money order. For more information regarding the CBSE and the CBSSA, visit the NBME's website at www.nbme.org.

The NBME scoring system is weighted for each assessment exam. While some exams seem more difficult than others, the equated percent correct reported takes into account these inter-test differences. Also, while many students report seeing Step 1 questions "word-for-word" out of the assessments, the NBME makes special note that no live USMLE questions are shown on any NBME assessment.

Lastly, the International Foundations of Medicine (IFOM) offers a Basic Science Examination (BSE) practice exam at participating Prometric test centers for $200. Students may also take the self-assessment test online for $35 through the NBME's website. The IFOM BSE is intended to determine an examinee's relative areas of strength and weakness in general areas of basic science—not to predict performance on the USMLE Step 1 exam— and the content covered by the two examinations is somewhat different. However, because there is substantial overlap in content coverage and many IFOM items were previously used on the USMLE Step 1, it is possible to roughly project IFOM performance onto the historical USMLE Step 1 score scale. More information is available at http://www.nbme.org/ifom/.

▶ LEARNING STRATEGIES

Many students feel overwhelmed during the preclinical years and struggle to find an effective learning strategy. Table 3 lists several learning strategies you can try and their estimated effectiveness for Step 1 preparation based on the literature (see References). These are merely suggestions, and it's important to take your learning preferences into account. Your comprehensive learning approach will contain a combination of strategies (eg, elaborative interrogation followed by practice testing, mnemonics review using spaced repetition, etc). Regardless of your choice, the foundation of knowledge you build during your basic science years is the most important resource for success on the USMLE Step 1.

HIGH EFFICACY

Practice Testing

Also called "retrieval practice," practice testing has both direct and indirect benefits to the learner.[4] Effortful retrieval of answers does not only identify weak spots—it directly strengthens long-term retention of material.[5] The more effortful the recall, the better the long-term retention. This advantage has been shown to result in higher test scores and GPAs.[6] In fact, research has shown a positive correlation between the number of boards-style practice questions completed and Step 1 performance among medical students.[7]

Practice testing should be done with "interleaving" (mixing of questions from different topics in a single session). Question banks often allow you to intermingle topics. Interleaved practice helps learners develop their ability to

> ▶ The foundation of knowledge you build during your basic science years is the most important resource for success on the USMLE Step 1.

> ▶ Research has shown a positive correlation between the number of boards-style practice questions completed and Step 1 performance among medical students.

TABLE 3. Effective Learning Strategies.

Efficacy	Strategy	Example Resources
High efficacy	Practice testing (retrieval practice)	UWorld Qbank NBME Self-Assessments USMLE-Rx QMax Amboss Qbank
	Distributed practice	USMLE-Rx Flash Facts Anki Firecracker Memorang Osmosis
Moderate efficacy	Mnemonics	*Pre-made:* SketchyMedical Picmonic *Self-made:* Mullen Memory
	Elaborative interrogation/self-explanation	
	Concept mapping	Coggle FreeMind XMind MindNode
Low efficacy	Rereading	
	Highlighting/underlining	
	Summarization	

focus on the relevant concept when faced with many possibilities. Practicing topics in massed fashion (eg, all cardiology, then all dermatology) may seem intuitive, but there is strong evidence that interleaving correlates with longer-term retention and increased student achievement, especially on tasks that involve problem solving.[5]

In addition to using question banks, you can test yourself by arranging your notes in a question-answer format (eg, via flash cards). Testing these Q&As in random order allows you to reap the benefit of interleaved practice. Bear in mind that the utility of practice testing comes from the practice of information retrieval, so simply reading through Q&As will attenuate this benefit.

Distributed Practice

Also called "spaced repetition," distributed practice is the opposite of massed practice or "cramming." Learners review material at increasingly spaced out intervals (days to weeks to months). Massed learning may produce more short-term gains and satisfaction, but learners who use distributed practice have better mastery and retention over the long term.[5,9]

> Studies have linked spaced repetition learning with flash cards to improved long-term knowledge retention and higher exam scores.

Flash cards are a simple way to incorporate both distributed practice and practice testing. Studies have linked spaced repetition learning with flash cards to improved long-term knowledge retention and higher exam scores.[6,8,10] Apps with automated spaced-repetition software (SRS) for flash cards exist for smartphones and tablets, so the cards are accessible anywhere. Proceed with caution: there is an art to making and reviewing cards. The ease of quickly downloading or creating digital cards can lead to flash card overload (it is unsustainable to make 50 flash cards per lecture!). Even at a modest pace, the thousands upon thousands of cards are too overwhelming for Step 1 preparation. Unless you have specific high-yield cards (and have checked the content with high-yield resources), stick to pre-made cards by reputable sources that curate the vast amount of knowledge for you.

If you prefer pen and paper, consider using a planner or spreadsheet to organize your study material over time. Distributed practice allows for some forgetting of information, and the added effort of recall over time strengthens the learning.

MODERATE EFFICACY

Mnemonics

A "mnemonic" refers to any device that assists memory, such as acronyms, mental imagery (eg, keywords with or without memory palaces), etc. Keyword mnemonics have been shown to produce superior knowledge retention when compared with rote memorization in many scenarios. However, they are generally more effective when applied to memorization-heavy, keyword-friendly topics and may not be broadly suitable.[5] Keyword mnemonics may not produce long-term retention, so consider combining mnemonics with distributed, retrieval-based practice (eg, via flash cards with SRS).

Self-made mnemonics may have an advantage when material is simple and keyword friendly. If you can create your own mnemonic that accurately represents the material, this will be more memorable. When topics are complex and accurate mnemonics are challenging to create, pre-made mnemonics may be more effective, especially if you are inexperienced at creating mnemonics.[11]

Elaborative Interrogation/Self-Explanation

Elaborative interrogation ("why" questions) and self-explanation (general questioning) prompt learners to generate explanations for facts. When reading passages of discrete facts, consider using these techniques, which have been shown to be more effective than rereading (eg, improved recall and better problem-solving/diagnostic performance).[5,12,13]

> ▶ Elaborative interrogation and self-explanation prompt learners to generate explanations for facts, which improves recall and problem solving.

Concept Mapping

Concept mapping is a method for graphically organizing knowledge, with concepts enclosed in boxes and lines drawn between related concepts. Creating or studying concept maps may be more effective than other activities (eg, writing or reading summaries/outlines). However, studies have reached mixed conclusions about its utility, and the small size of this effect raises doubts about its authenticity and pedagogic significance.[14]

LOW EFFICACY

Rereading

While the most commonly used method among surveyed students, rereading has not been shown to correlate with grade point average.[9] Due to its popularity, rereading is often a comparator in studies on learning. Other strategies that we have discussed (eg, practice testing) have been shown to be significantly more effective than rereading.

Highlighting/Underlining

Because this method is passive, it tends to be of minimal value for learning and recall. In fact, lower-performing students are more likely to use these techniques.[9] Students who highlight and underline do not learn how to actively recall learned information and thus find it difficult to apply knowledge to exam questions.

Summarization

While more useful for improving performance on generative measures (eg, free recall or essays), summarization is less useful for exams that depend on recognition (eg, multiple choice). Findings on the overall efficacy of this method have been mixed.[5]

▶ TIMELINE FOR STUDY

Before Starting

Your preparation for the USMLE Step 1 should begin when you enter medical school. Organize and commit to studying from the beginning so that when the time comes to prepare for the USMLE, you will be ready with a strong foundation.

Make a Schedule

> ▶ *Customize your schedule. Tackle your weakest section first.*

After you have defined your goals, map out a study schedule that is consistent with your objectives, your vacation time, the difficulty of your ongoing coursework, and your family and social commitments. Determine whether you want to spread out your study time or concentrate it into 10-hour study days in the final weeks. Then factor in your own history in preparing for standardized examinations (eg, SAT, MCAT). Talk to students at your school who have recently taken Step 1. Ask them for their study schedules, especially those who have study habits and goals similar to yours. Sample schedules can be found at https://firstaidteam.com/schedules/.

Typically, US medical schools allot between four and eight weeks for dedicated Step 1 preparation. The time you dedicate to exam preparation will depend on your confidence in comfortably achieving a passing score as well as your success in preparing yourself during the first two years of medical school. Some students reserve about a week at the end of their study period for final review; others save just a few days. When you have scheduled your exam date, do your best to adhere to it.

Make your schedule realistic, and set achievable goals. Many students make the mistake of studying at a level of detail that requires too much time for a comprehensive review—reading *Gray's Anatomy* in a couple of days is not a realistic goal! Have one catch-up day per week of studying. No matter how well you stick to your schedule, unexpected events happen. But don't let yourself procrastinate because you have catch-up days; stick to your schedule as closely as possible and revise it regularly on the basis of your actual progress. Be careful not to lose focus. Beware of feelings of inadequacy when comparing study schedules and progress with your peers. **Avoid others who stress you out.** Focus on a few top-rated resources that suit your learning style—not on some obscure resource your friends may pass down to you. Accept the fact that you cannot learn it all.

> ▶ *Avoid burnout. Maintain proper diet, exercise, and sleep habits.*

You will need time for uninterrupted and focused study. Plan your personal affairs to minimize crisis situations near the date of the test. Allot an adequate number of breaks in your study schedule to avoid burnout. Maintain a healthy lifestyle with proper diet, exercise, and sleep.

Another important aspect of your preparation is your studying environment. **Study where you have always been comfortable studying.** Be sure to include everything you need close by (review books, notes, coffee, snacks, etc). If you're the kind of person who cannot study alone, form a study group with other students taking the exam. The main point here is to create a comfortable environment with minimal distractions.

Year(s) Prior

The knowledge you gained during your first two years of medical school and even during your undergraduate years should provide the groundwork on which to base your test preparation. Student scores on NBME subject tests (commonly known as "shelf exams") have been shown to be highly correlated with subsequent Step 1 performance.[15] Moreover, undergraduate science GPAs as well as MCAT scores are strong predictors of performance on the Step 1 exam.[16]

We also recommend that you buy highly rated review books early in your first year of medical school and use them as you study throughout the two years. When Step 1 comes along, these books will be familiar and personalized to the way in which you learn. It is risky and intimidating to use unfamiliar review books in the final two or three weeks preceding the exam. Some students find it helpful to personalize and annotate *First Aid* throughout the curriculum.

▶ *Buy review resources early (first year) and use while studying for courses.*

Months Prior

Review test dates and the application procedure. Testing for the USMLE Step 1 is done on a year-round basis. If you have disabilities or special circumstances, contact the NBME as early as possible to discuss test accommodations (see the Section I Supplement at www.firstaidteam.com/bonus).

Use this time to finalize your ideal schedule. Consider upcoming breaks and whether you want to relax or study. Work backward from your test date to make sure you finish at least one question bank. Also add time to redo missed or flagged questions (which may be half the bank). This is the time to build a structured plan with enough flexibility for the realities of life.

▶ *Simulate the USMLE Step 1 under "real" conditions before beginning your studies.*

Begin doing blocks of questions from reputable question banks under "real" conditions. Don't use tutor mode until you're sure you can finish blocks in the allotted time. It is important to continue balancing success in your normal studies with the Step 1 test preparation process.

Weeks Prior (Dedicated Preparation)

Your dedicated prep time may be one week or two months. You should have a working plan as you go into this period. Finish your schoolwork strong, take a day off, and then get to work. Start by simulating a full-length USMLE Step 1 if you haven't yet done so. Consider doing one NBME CBSSA and the free questions from the NBME website. Alternatively, you could choose 7 blocks of randomized questions from a commercial question bank. Make sure you get feedback on your strengths and weaknesses and adjust your studying accordingly. Many students study from review sources or comprehensive

▶ In the final two weeks, focus on review, practice questions, and endurance. Stay confident!

programs for part of the day, then do question blocks. Also, keep in mind that reviewing a question block can take upward of two hours. Feedback from CBSSA exams and question banks will help you focus on your weaknesses.

One Week Prior

▶ One week before the test:
- Sleep according to the same schedule you'll use on test day
- Review the CBT tutorial one last time
- Call Prometric to confirm test date and time

Make sure you have your CIN (found on your scheduling permit) as well as other items necessary for the day of the examination, including a current driver's license or another form of photo ID with your signature (make sure the name on your **ID exactly** matches that on your scheduling permit). Confirm the Prometric testing center location and test time. Work out how you will get to the testing center and what parking, traffic, and public transportation problems you might encounter. Exchange cell phone numbers with other students taking the test on the same day in case of emergencies. Check www.prometric.com/closures for test site closures due to unforeseen events. Determine what you will do for lunch. Make sure you have everything you need to ensure that you will be comfortable and alert at the test site. It may be beneficial to adjust your schedule to start waking up at the same time that you will on your test day. And of course, make sure to maintain a healthy lifestyle and get enough sleep.

One Day Prior

Try your best to relax and rest the night before the test. Double-check your admissions and test-taking materials as well as the comfort measures discussed earlier so that you will not have to deal with such details on the morning of the exam. At this point it will be more effective to review short-term memory material that you're already familiar with than to try to learn new material. The Rapid Review section at the end of this book is high yield for last-minute studying. Remember that regardless of how hard you have studied, you cannot (and need not!) know everything. There will be things on the exam that you have never even seen before, so do not panic. Do not underestimate your abilities.

Many students report difficulty sleeping the night prior to the exam. This is often exacerbated by going to bed much earlier than usual. Do whatever it takes to ensure a good night's sleep (eg, massage, exercise, warm milk, no screens at night). Do not change your daily routine prior to the exam. Exam day is not the day for a caffeine-withdrawal headache.

Morning of the Exam

▶ No notes, books, calculators, pagers, cell phones, recording devices, or watches of any kind are allowed in the testing area, but they are allowed in lockers and may be accessed during authorized breaks.

On the morning of the Step 1 exam, wake up at your regular time and eat a normal breakfast. If you think it will help you, have a close friend or family member check to make sure you get out of bed. Make sure you have your scheduling permit admission ticket, test-taking materials, and comfort measures as discussed earlier. Wear loose, comfortable clothing. Limiting the number of pockets in your outfit may save time during security screening. Plan for a variable temperature in the testing center. Arrive at the test site 30 minutes before the time designated on the admission ticket; however, do not come too early, as doing so may intensify your anxiety. When you arrive at the test site, the proctor should give you a USMLE information sheet that will explain critical factors such as the proper use of break time. Seating may be assigned, but ask to be reseated if necessary; you need to be seated in an area that will allow you to remain comfortable and to concentrate. Get to know your testing station, especially if you have never been in a Prometric testing center before. Listen to your proctors regarding any changes in instructions or testing procedures that may apply to your test site.

If you are experiencing symptoms of illness on the day of your exam, we strongly recommend you reschedule. If you become ill or show signs of illness (eg, persistent cough) during the exam, the test center may prohibit you from completing the exam due to health and safety risks for test center staff and other examinees.

Finally, remember that it is natural (and even beneficial) to be a little nervous. Focus on being mentally clear and alert. Avoid panic. When you are asked to begin the exam, take a deep breath, focus on the screen, and then begin. Keep an eye on the timer. Take advantage of breaks between blocks to stretch, maybe do some jumping jacks, and relax for a moment with deep breathing or stretching.

> ▶ Arrive at the testing center 30 minutes before your scheduled exam time. If you arrive more than half an hour late, you will not be allowed to take the test.

After the Test

After you have completed the exam, be sure to have fun and relax regardless of how you may feel. Taking the test is an achievement in itself. Remember, you are much more likely to have passed than not. Enjoy the free time you have before your clerkships. Expect to experience some "reentry" phenomena as you try to regain a real life. Once you have recovered sufficiently from the test (or from partying), we invite you to send us your feedback, corrections, and suggestions for entries, facts, mnemonics, strategies, resource ratings, and the like (see p. xvii, How to Contribute). Sharing your experience will benefit fellow medical students.

▶ STUDY MATERIALS

Quality Considerations

Although an ever-increasing number of review books and software are now available on the market, the quality of such material is highly variable. Some common problems are as follows:

- Certain review books are too detailed to allow for review in a reasonable amount of time or cover subtopics that are not emphasized on the exam.
- Many sample question books were originally written years ago and have not been adequately updated to reflect recent trends.
- Some question banks test to a level of detail that you will not find on the exam.

Review Books

> ▶ *If a given review book is not working for you, stop using it no matter how highly rated it may be or how much it costs.*

In selecting review books, be sure to weigh different opinions against each other, read the reviews and ratings in Section IV of this guide, examine the books closely in the bookstore, and choose carefully. You are investing not only money but also your limited study time. Do not worry about finding the "perfect" book, as many subjects simply do not have one, and different students prefer different formats. Supplement your chosen books with personal notes from other sources, including what you learn from question banks.

There are two types of review books: those that are stand-alone titles and those that are part of a series. Books in a series generally have the same style, and you must decide if that style works for you. However, a given style is not optimal for every subject.

> ▶ *Charts and diagrams may be the best approach for physiology and biochemistry, whereas tables and outlines may be preferable for microbiology.*

You should also find out which books are up to date. Some recent editions reflect major improvements, whereas others contain only cursory changes. Take into consideration how a book reflects the format of the USMLE Step 1.

Apps

With the explosion of smartphones and tablets, apps are an increasingly popular way to review for the Step 1 exam. The majority of apps are compatible with both iOS and Android. Many popular Step 1 review resources (eg, UWorld, USMLE-Rx) have apps that are compatible with their software. Many popular web references (eg, UpToDate) also now offer app versions. All of these apps offer flexibility, allowing you to study while away from a computer (eg, while traveling).

Practice Tests

> ▶ *Most practice exams are shorter and less clinical than the real thing.*

Taking practice tests provides valuable information about potential strengths and weaknesses in your fund of knowledge and test-taking skills. Some students use practice examinations simply as a means of breaking up the monotony of studying and adding variety to their study schedule, whereas other students rely almost solely on practice. You should also subscribe to one or more high-quality question banks.

Additionally, some students preparing for the Step 1 exam have started to incorporate case-based books intended primarily for clinical students on the wards or studying for the Step 2 CK exam. *First Aid Cases for the USMLE Step 1* aims to directly address this need.

> ▶ *Use practice tests to identify concepts and areas of weakness, not just facts that you missed.*

After taking a practice test, spend time on each question and each answer choice whether you were right or wrong. There are important teaching points in each explanation. Knowing why a wrong answer choice is incorrect is just as important as knowing why the right answer is correct. Do not panic if your practice scores are low as many questions try to trick or distract you to highlight a certain point. Use the questions you missed or were unsure about to develop focused plans during your scheduled catch-up time.

Textbooks and Course Syllabi

Limit your use of textbooks and course syllabi for Step 1 review. Many textbooks are too detailed for high-yield review and include material that is generally not tested on the USMLE Step 1 (eg, drug dosages, complex chemical structures). Syllabi, although familiar, are inconsistent across medical schools and frequently reflect the emphasis of individual faculty, which often does not correspond to that of the USMLE Step 1. Syllabi also tend to be less organized than top-rated books and generally contain fewer diagrams and study questions.

Integration of AI in Medical Education: Transforming USMLE Preparation

The integration of AI into education signals a paradigm shift in the acquisition and application of medical knowledge. AI's increasing ability to process extensive data sets and adapt to various learning styles makes it an attractive tool in medical training and practice.[17] Studies have demonstrated that AI language models are capable of achieving high accuracy rates when answering USMLE-style questions, underscoring its potential in supporting medical education.[18]

Although undeniably powerful, effectively utilizing AI as a study tool requires both practice and individual trial and error. We suggest the following approaches and prompts that might help learners more effectively harness AI for exam preparation:

Tailored Mnemonic Creation: Devise unique mnemonics to aid in memorizing complex medical terms efficiently. AI models can be highly creative in generating new ones, although feedback and iteration will likely be needed to produce mnemonics that are both accurate and memorable.

Example prompt: Create a food-related mnemonic for remembering adverse effects 1, 2, and 3 of Drug A.

Custom Summarization of Medical Texts: Efficiently condense extensive medical literature into concise summaries, facilitating efficient and rapid topic reviews.

Example prompt: Summarize this medical school lecture into bullet points. Decrease length by 80%.

AI-Generated Custom Quizzes: Create focused practice questions.

Example Prompt: Create three vignette-style multiple choice questions testing presentations of lysosomal storage disorders.

Clinical Case Simulations: Utilize AI-powered simulations of realistic clinical scenarios to practice decision-making skills and application of medical knowledge.

Example prompt: Create an exercise to practice analyzing acid-base disorders requiring Winter's formula with step-by-step explanations.

Personalized Learning Schedules: Create customized study schedules, adjusting time allocation based on challenging subjects. Modify schedules daily based on progress.

Example prompt: Prepare a schedule to review this book over 4 weeks.

Though both exciting and promising, pitfalls of using AI models for studying include the potential for outdated information or reliance on data that are not validated, resulting in a potential source of misinformation. AI can become unintentionally trained with human biases, and thus produce results that further reinforce or perpetuate potentially harmful biases. When using AI for personal studying, always validate information and maintain a critical eye when creating prompts.

AI is clearly a rapidly evolving study tool, however, how it can be best integrated with proven study methods remains to be seen. For the most recent updates on effectively leveraging AI in medical education, we encourage you to explore our blog at firstaidteam.com and scan a variety of student-centered discussion forums.

▶ TEST-TAKING STRATEGIES

▶ *Practice! Develop your test-taking skills and strategies well before the test date.*

Your test performance will be influenced by both your knowledge and your test-taking skills. You can strengthen your performance by considering each of these factors. Test-taking skills and strategies should be developed and perfected well in advance of the test date so that you can concentrate on the test itself. We suggest that you try the following strategies to see if they might work for you.

Pacing

▶ *Time management is an important skill for exam success.*

You have seven hours to complete up to 280 questions. Note that each one-hour block contains up to 40 questions. This works out to approximately 90 seconds per question. We recommend following the "1 minute rule" to pace yourself. Spend no more than 1 minute on each question. If you are still unsure about the answer after this time, mark the question, make an educated guess, and move on. Following this rule, you should have approximately 20 minutes left after all questions are answered, which you can use to revisit all of your marked questions. Remember that some questions may be experimental and do not count for points (and reassure yourself that these experimental questions are the ones that are stumping you). In the past, pacing errors have been detrimental to the performance of even highly prepared examinees. The bottom line is to keep one eye on the clock at all times!

Dealing with Each Question

There are several established techniques for efficiently approaching multiple choice questions; find what works for you. One technique begins with identifying each question as easy, workable, or impossible. Your goal should be to answer all easy questions, resolve all workable questions in a reasonable amount of time, and make quick and intelligent guesses on all impossible questions. Most students read the stem, think of the answer, and turn immediately to the choices. A second technique is to first skim the answer choices to get a context, then read the last sentence of the question (the lead-in), and then read through the passage quickly, extracting only information relevant to answering the question. This can be particularly helpful for questions with long clinical vignettes. Try a variety of techniques on practice exams and see what works best for you. If you get overwhelmed, remember that a 30-second time out to refocus may get you back on track.

Guessing

There is **no penalty** for wrong answers. Thus **no test block should be left with unanswered questions.** If you don't know the answer, first eliminate incorrect choices, then guess among the remaining options. **Note that dozens of questions are unscored experimental questions** meant to obtain statistics for future exams. Therefore, some questions may seem unusual or unreasonably difficult simply because they are part of the development process for future exams.

Changing Your Answer

The conventional wisdom is not to second-guess your initial answers. However, studies have consistently shown that test takers are more likely to change from a wrong answer to the correct answer than the other way around. Many question banks tell you how many questions you changed from right to wrong, wrong to wrong, and wrong to right. Use this feedback to judge how good a second-guesser you are. If you have extra time, reread the question stem and make sure you didn't misinterpret the question.

▶ *Go with your first hunch, unless you are certain that you are a good second-guesser.*

▶ CLINICAL VIGNETTE STRATEGIES

In recent years, the USMLE Step 1 has become increasingly clinically oriented. This change mirrors the trend in medical education toward introducing students to clinical problem solving during the basic science years. The increasing clinical emphasis on Step 1 may be challenging to those students who attend schools with a more traditional curriculum.

▶ *Be prepared to read fast and think on your feet!*

What Is a Clinical Vignette?

A clinical vignette is a short (usually paragraph-long) description of a patient, including demographics, presenting symptoms, signs, and other information concerning the patient. Sometimes this paragraph is followed by a brief listing of important physical findings and/or laboratory results. The task of assimilating all this information and answering the associated question in the span of one minute can be intimidating. So be prepared to read quickly and think on your feet. Remember that the question is often indirectly asking something you already know.

> ▶ Practice questions that include case histories or descriptive vignettes are critical for Step 1 preparation.

A pseudovignette is a question that includes a description of a case similar to that of a clinical vignette, but it ends with a declarative recall question; thus the material presented in the pseudovignette is not necessary to answer the question. Question writers strive to avoid pseudovignettes on the USMLE Step 1. Be prepared to tackle each vignette as if the information presented is important to answer the associated question correctly.

Strategy

Remember that Step 1 vignettes usually describe diseases or disorders in their most classic presentation. So look for cardinal signs (eg, malar rash for lupus or nuchal rigidity for meningitis) in the narrative history. Be aware that the question will contain classic signs and symptoms instead of buzzwords. Sometimes the data from labs and the physical exam will help you confirm or reject possible diagnoses, thereby helping you rule answer choices in or out. In some cases, they will be a dead giveaway for the diagnosis.

> ▶ Step 1 vignettes usually describe diseases or disorders in their most classic presentation.

Making a diagnosis from the history and data is often not the final answer. Not infrequently, the diagnosis is divulged at the end of the vignette, after you have just struggled through the narrative to come up with a diagnosis of your own. The question might then ask about a related aspect of the diagnosed disease. Consider skimming the answer choices and lead-in before diving into a long stem. However, be careful with skimming the answer choices; going too fast may warp your perception of what the vignette is asking.

▶ IF YOU THINK YOU FAILED

After taking the test, it is normal for many examinees to feel unsure about their performance, despite the majority of them achieving a passing score. Historical pass data are in Table 2. If you remain quite concerned, it may be wise to prepare a course of action should you need to retest. There are several sensible steps you can take to plan for the future in the event that you do not achieve a passing score. First, save and organize all your study materials, including review books, practice tests, and notes. Familiarize yourself with the reapplication procedures for Step 1, including application deadlines and upcoming test dates.

Make sure you know both your school's and the NBME's policies regarding retakes. The total number of attempts an examinee may take per Step examination is four.[18] You may take Step 1 no more than three times within a 12-month period. Your fourth attempt must be at least 12 months after your first attempt at that exam, and at least 6 months after your most recent attempt at that exam.

If you failed, the performance profiles in your score report provide valuable feedback concerning your relative strengths and weaknesses. Study these profiles closely. Set up a study timeline to strengthen gaps in your knowledge as well as to maintain and improve what you already know. Do not neglect high-yield subjects. It is normal to feel somewhat anxious about retaking the test, but if anxiety becomes a problem, seek appropriate counseling.

> ▸ *If you pass Step 1, you are not allowed to retake the exam.*

▸ TESTING AGENCIES

- **National Board of Medical Examiners (NBME) / USMLE Secretariat**
  Department of Licensing Examination Services
  3750 Market Street
  Philadelphia, PA 19104-3102
  (215) 590-9500 (operator) or
  (215) 590-9700 (automated information line)
  Email: webmail@nbme.org
  www.nbme.org

- **Educational Commission for Foreign Medical Graduates (ECFMG)**
  3624 Market Street
  Philadelphia, PA 19104-2685
  (215) 386-5900
  Email: info@ecfmg.org
  www.ecfmg.org

▸ REFERENCES

1. United States Medical Licensing Examination. Available from: https://www.usmle.org/prepare-your-exam/step-1-materials/step-1-content-outline-and-specifications. Accessed October 2024.
2. United States Medical Licensing Examination. Performance Data. Available from: https://www.usmle.org/performance-data. Accessed October 2024.
3. Prober CG, Kolars JC, First LR, et al. A plea to reassess the role of United States Medical Licensing Examination Step 1 scores in residency selection. *Acad Med.* 2016;91(1):12–15.
4. Roediger HL, Butler AC. The critical role of retrieval practice in long-term retention. *Trends Cogn Sci.* 2011;15(1):20–27.
5. Dunlosky J, Rawson KA, Marsh EJ, et al. Improving students' learning with effective learning techniques: promising directions from cognitive and educational psychology. *Psychol Sci Publ Int.* 2013;14(1):4–58.

6. Larsen DP, Butler AC, Lawson AL, et al. The importance of seeing the patient: test-enhanced learning with standardized patients and written tests improves clinical application of knowledge. *Adv Health Sci Educ.* 2013;18(3):409–425.

7. Panus PC, Stewart DW, Hagemeier NE, et al. A subgroup analysis of the impact of self-testing frequency on examination scores in a pathophysiology course. *Am J Pharm Educ.* 2014;78(9):165.

8. Deng F, Gluckstein JA, Larsen DP. Student-directed retrieval practice is a predictor of medical licensing examination performance. *Perspect Med Educ.* 2015;4(6):308–313.

9. McAndrew M, Morrow CS, Atiyeh L, et al. Dental student study strategies: are self-testing and scheduling related to academic performance? *J Dent Educ.* 2016;80(5):542–552.

10. Augustin M. How to learn effectively in medical school: test yourself, learn actively, and repeat in intervals. *Yale J Biol Med.* 2014;87(2):207–212.

11. Bellezza FS. Mnemonic devices: classification, characteristics, and criteria. *Rev Educ Res.* 1981;51(2):247–275.

12. Dyer J-O, Hudon A, Montpetit-Tourangeau K, et al. Example-based learning: comparing the effects of additionally providing three different integrative learning activities on physiotherapy intervention knowledge. *BMC Med Educ.* 2015;15:37.

13. Chamberland M, Mamede S, St-Onge C, et al. Self-explanation in learning clinical reasoning: the added value of examples and prompts. *Med Educ.* 2015;49(2):193–202.

14. Nesbit JC, Adesope OO. Learning with concept and knowledge maps: a meta-analysis. *Rev Educ Res.* 2006;76(3):413–448.

15. Holtman MC, Swanson DB, Ripkey DR, et al. Using basic science subject tests to identify students at risk for failing Step 1. *Acad Med.* 2001;76(10):S48–S51.

16. Basco WT, Way DP, Gilbert GE, et al. Undergraduate institutional MCAT scores as predictors of USMLE Step 1 performance. *Acad Med.* 2002;77(10):S13–S16.

17. Patino GA, Amiel JM, Brown M, et al. The promise and perils of artificial intelligence in health professions education practice and scholarship. *Acad Med.* 2024. doi: 10.1097/ACM.0000000000005636.

18. Kung TH, Cheatham M, Medenilla A, et al. Performance of ChatGPT on USMLE: potential for AI-assisted medical education using large language models. *PLOS Dig Health.* 2023. doi: 10.1371/journal.pdig.0000198.

19. United States Medical Licensing Examination. Number of attempts and time limits. Available from: https://www.usmle.org/bulletin-information/eligibility. Accessed October 2024.

Special Situations

Please visit **www.firstaidteam.com/bonus/** to view this section.

▶ First Aid for the International Medical Graduate

▶ First Aid for the Osteopathic Medical Student

▶ First Aid for the Podiatric Medical Student

▶ First Aid for the Student Requiring Test Accommodations

▶ NOTES

SECTION II

High-Yield
General Principles

"I've learned that I still have a lot to learn."

—Maya Angelou

"Never regard study as a duty, but as the enviable opportunity to learn."

—Albert Einstein

"Live as if you were to die tomorrow. Learn as if you were to live forever."

—Gandhi

"Success is the maximum utilization of the ability that you have."

—Zig Ziglar

"I didn't want to just know names of things. I remember really wanting to know how it all worked."

—Elizabeth Blackburn

"If you do not have time to do it right, how are you going to have time to do it again?"

—Diana Downs

▶ HOW TO USE THE DATABASE

The 2025 edition of *First Aid for the USMLE Step 1* contains a revised and expanded database of basic science material that students, student authors, and faculty authors have identified as high yield for board review. The information is presented in a partially organ-based format. Hence, Section II is devoted to the foundational principles of biochemistry, microbiology, immunology, basic pathology, basic pharmacology, and public health sciences. Section III focuses on organ systems, with subsections covering the embryology, anatomy and histology, physiology, clinical pathology, and clinical pharmacology relevant to each. Each subsection is then divided into smaller topic areas containing related facts. Individual facts are generally presented in a three-column format, with the **Title** of the fact in the first column, the **Description** of the fact in the second column, and the **Mnemonic** or **Special Note** in the third column. Some facts do not have a mnemonic and are presented in a two-column format. Others are presented in list or tabular form in order to emphasize key associations.

The database structure used in Sections II and III is useful for reviewing material already learned. These sections are **not** ideal for learning complex or highly conceptual material for the first time.

The database of high-yield facts is not comprehensive. Use it to complement your core study material and not as your primary study source. The facts and notes have been condensed and edited to emphasize the high-yield material, and as a result, each entry is "incomplete" and arguably "over-simplified." Often, the more you research a topic, the more complex it becomes, with certain topics resisting simplification. Determine your most efficient methods for learning the material, and do not be afraid to abandon a strategy if it is not working for you.

Our database of high-yield facts is updated annually to keep current with new trends in boards emphasis, including clinical relevance. However, we must note that inevitably many other high-yield topics are not yet included in our database.

We actively encourage medical students and faculty to submit high-yield topics, well-written entries, diagrams, clinical images, and useful mnemonics so that we may enhance the database for future students. We also solicit recommendations of alternate tools for study that may be useful in preparing for the examination, such as charts, flash cards, apps, and online resources (see How to Contribute, p. xv).

Image Acknowledgments

All images and diagrams marked with ℞ are © USMLE-Rx.com (MedIQ Learning, LLC) and reproduced here by special permission. All images marked with ℞ʋ are © Dr. Richard P. Usatine, author of *The Color Atlas of Family Medicine*, *The Color Atlas of Internal Medicine*, and *The Color Atlas of Pediatrics*, and are reproduced here by special permission (www.usatinemedia.com). Images and diagrams marked with ✴ are adapted or reproduced with permission of other sources as listed on page 755. Images and diagrams with no acknowledgment are part of this book.

Disclaimer

The entries in this section reflect student opinions on what is high yield. Because of the diverse sources of material, no attempt has been made to trace or reference the origins of entries individually. We have regarded mnemonics as essentially in the public domain. Errata will gladly be corrected if brought to the attention of the authors, either through our online errata submission form at www.firstaidteam.com or directly by email to firstaid@scholarrx.com.

▶ NOTES

Biochemistry

"The nitrogen in our DNA, the calcium in our teeth, the iron in our blood, the carbon in our apple pies were made in the interiors of collapsing stars. We are made of starstuff."

—Carl Sagan

"Biochemistry is the study of carbon compounds that crawl."

—Mike Adams

"The power to control our species' genetic future is awesome and terrifying."

—A Crack in Creation

"Nothing in this world is to be feared, it is only to be understood."

—Marie Curie

This high-yield material includes molecular biology, genetics, cell biology, and principles of metabolism (especially vitamins, cofactors, minerals, and single-enzyme-deficiency diseases). When studying metabolic pathways, emphasize important regulatory steps and enzyme deficiencies that result in disease, as well as reactions targeted by pharmacologic interventions. For example, understanding the defect in Lesch-Nyhan syndrome and its clinical implications (from presentation to management) is higher yield than memorizing every intermediate in the purine salvage pathway.

Do not spend time learning details of organic chemistry, mechanisms, or physical chemistry. Detailed chemical structures are infrequently tested; however, many structures have been included here to help students learn reactions and the important enzymes involved. Familiarity with the biochemical techniques that have medical relevance—such as ELISA, immunoelectrophoresis, Southern blotting, and PCR—is useful. Review the related biochemistry when studying pharmacology or genetic diseases as a way to reinforce and integrate the material.

▶ BIOCHEMISTRY—MOLECULAR

Chromatin structure

DNA exists in the condensed, chromatin form to fit into the nucleus. DNA loops twice around a histone octamer to form a nucleosome ("beads on a string"). H1 binds to the nucleosome and to "linker DNA," thereby stabilizing the chromatin fiber.

DNA has ⊖ charge from phosphate groups. Histones are **large** and have ⊕ charge from **lys**ine and **arg**inine.

DNA and histone synthesis occurs during S phase.

Mitochondria have their own DNA, which is circular and does not bind histones.

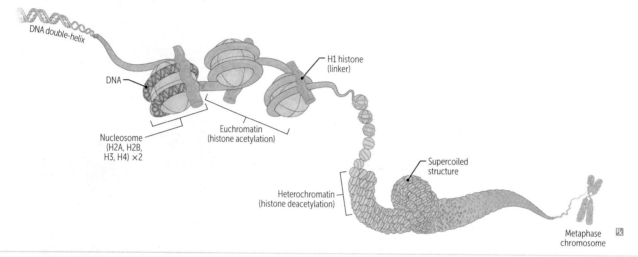

DNA double-helix

DNA

H1 histone (linker)

Nucleosome (H2A, H2B, H3, H4) ×2

Euchromatin (histone acetylation)

Supercoiled structure

Heterochromatin (histone deacetylation)

Metaphase chromosome

Heterochromatin 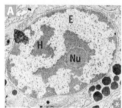	Condensed, appears darker on EM (labeled H in Ⓐ; Nu, nucleolus). Sterically inaccessible, thus transcriptionally inactive. ↑ methylation, ↓ acetylation.	Heterochromatin = **h**ighly **c**ondensed (**h**idden chromatin). Barr bodies (inactive X chromosomes) may be visible on the periphery of nucleus.
Euchromatin	Less condensed, appears lighter on EM (labeled E in Ⓐ). Transcriptionally active, sterically accessible.	*Eu* = true, "truly transcribed." **Eu**chromatin is **e**xpressed.
DNA methylation	Reversibly changes the expression of a DNA segment without changing its sequence. Involved with aging, carcinogenesis, epigenetics, genomic imprinting, transposable element repression, and X chromosome inactivation (lyonization).	DNA is methylated in imprinting. Methylation within gene promoter (CpG islands) typically represses (silences) gene transcription. CpG **m**ethylation **m**akes DNA **m**ute. Dysregulated DNA methylation is implicated in fragile X syndrome.
Histone methylation	Usually causes reversible transcriptional suppression, but can also cause activation depending on location of methyl groups.	Histone **m**ethylation **m**ostly **m**akes DNA **m**ute. Lysine and arginine residues of histones can be methylated.
Histone acetylation	Removal of histone's ⊕ charge → relaxed DNA coiling → ↑ transcription.	Thyroid hormone synthesis is altered by acetylation of thyroid hormone receptor. Histone **a**cetylation makes DNA **a**ctive.
Histone deacetylation	Removal of acetyl groups → tightened DNA coiling → ↓ transcription.	Histone **de**acetylation may be responsible for altered gene expression in Huntington disease. Histone **de**acetylation **de**activates DNA.

Nucleotides

Nucleoside = base + (deoxy)ribose (**s**ugar).

Nucleotide = base + (deoxy)ribose + **p**hosphate; linked by 3′-5′ phosphodiester bond.

Nucleo-"**tri**"-des have **three** components.

Purines (**A,G**)—2 rings.
Pyrimidines (**C,U,T**)—1 ring.

Deamination reactions:
Cytosine → uracil
Adenine → hypoxanthine
Guanine → xanthine
5-methylcytosine → thymine

Uracil found in RNA; thymine in DNA.
Methylation of uracil makes thymine.

5′ end of incoming nucleotide bears the triphosphate (energy source for the bond).

Pure **As** **G**old.
CUT the **pyr**amid.
Thymine has a me**thyl**.
C-G bond (3 H bonds) stronger than A-T bond (2 H bonds). ↑ C-G content → ↑ melting temperature of DNA. "**C-G** bonds are like **C**razy **G**lue."

Amino acids necessary for **pur**ine synthesis (cats **pur**r until they **GAG**):
Glycine
Aspartate
Glutamine

Purine (A, G)

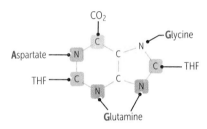

Pyrimidine (C, U, T)

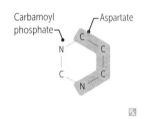

De novo pyrimidine and purine synthesis

Various immunosuppressive, antineoplastic, and antibiotic drugs function by interfering with nucleotide synthesis:

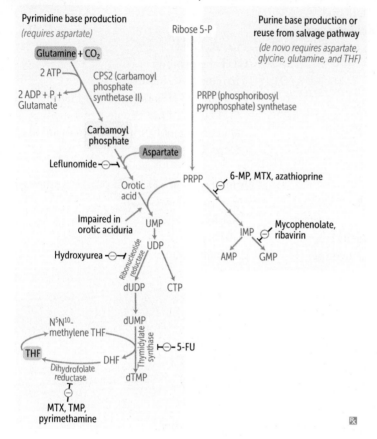

Pyrimidine synthesis:
- Leflunomide: inhibits dihydroorotate dehydrogenase
- 5-fluorouracil (5-FU) and its prodrug capecitabine: form 5-F-dUMP, which inhibits thymidylate synthase (↓ dTMP)

Purine synthesis:
- 6-mercaptopurine (6-MP) and its prodrug azathioprine: inhibit de novo purine synthesis (guanine phosphoribosyltransferase); azathioprine is metabolized via purine degradation pathway and can lead to immunosuppression when administered with xanthine oxidase inhibitor
- Mycophenolate and ribavirin: inhibit inosine monophosphate dehydrogenase

Purine and pyrimidine synthesis:
- Hydroxyurea: inhibits ribonucleotide reductase
- Methotrexate (MTX), trimethoprim (TMP), and pyrimethamine: inhibit dihydrofolate reductase (↓ deoxythymidine monophosphate [dTMP]) in humans (**m**ethotrexate), bacteria (**t**rimethoprim), and **p**rotozoa (**p**yrimethamine)

CPS1 = m**1**tochondria, urea cycle, found in liver
CPS2 = cyt**w**osol, pyrimidine synthesis, found in most cells

Purine salvage deficiencies

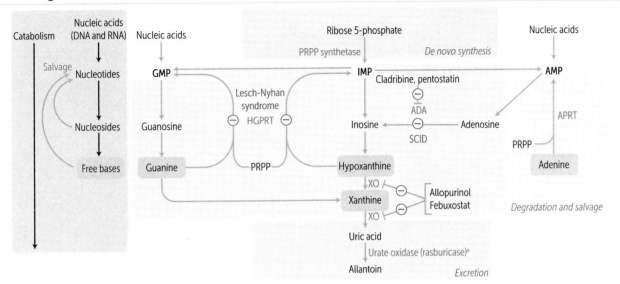

[a]Absent in humans.
ADA, adenosine deaminase; APRT, adenine phosphoribosyltransferase; HGPRT, hypoxanthine guanine phosphoribosyltransferase, XO, xanthine oxidase; SCID, severe combined immune deficiency (autosomal recessive inheritance)

Adenosine deaminase deficiency	ADA is required for degradation of adenosine and deoxyadenosine. ↓ ADA → ↑ dATP → ↓ ribonucleotide reductase activity → ↓ DNA precursors in cells → ↓ lymphocytes.	One of the major causes of autosomal recessive SCID.

Lesch-Nyhan syndrome	Defective purine salvage. Deficient or mutated **HGPRT** → ↓ GMP (from guanine) and ↓ IMP (from hypoxanthine) formation. Compensatory ↑ in purine synthesis (↑ PRPP amidotransferase activity) → excess uric acid production. X-linked recessive.
	Findings: intellectual disability, self-mutilation, aggression, hyperuricemia (red/orange "sand" [sodium urate crystals] in diaper), gout, dystonia, macrocytosis.
		HGPRT:
		   Hyperuricemia
		   Gout
		   Pissed off (aggression, self-mutilation)
		   Red/orange crystals in urine
		   Tense muscles (dystonia)
		Treatment: allopurinol, febuxostat.

Genetic code features

Unambiguous	Each codon specifies only 1 amino acid.	
Degenerate/ redundant	Most amino acids are coded by multiple codons. Wobble hypothesis—first 2 nucleotides of codon are essential for anticodon recognition while the 3rd nucleotide can differ ("wobble").	Exceptions: methionine (AUG) and tryptophan (UGG) are encoded by only 1 codon.
Commaless, nonoverlapping	Read from a fixed starting point as a continuous sequence of bases.	Exceptions: some viruses.
Universal	Genetic code is conserved throughout evolution.	Exception (in animals): mitochondria (some codons specify different amino acids than in non-mitochondrial DNA).

DNA replication	Occurs in 5′ → 3′ direction ("5ynth3sis") in continuous and discontinuous (Okazaki fragment) fashion. Semiconservative. More complex in eukaryotes than in prokaryotes, but shares analogous enzymes.	
Origin of replication A	Particular consensus sequence in genome where DNA replication begins. May be single (prokaryotes) or multiple (eukaryotes).	AT-rich sequences (eg, TATA box regions) are found in promoters (often upstream) and origins of replication (ori).
Replication fork B	Y-shaped region along DNA template where leading and lagging strands are synthesized.	
Helicase C	Unwinds DNA template at replication fork.	Helicase halves DNA. Deficient in **Bloom** syndrome (***BLM*** gene mutation).
Single-stranded binding proteins D	Prevent strands from reannealing or degradation by nucleases.	
DNA topoisomerases E	Creates a **single-** (topoisomerase I) or **double-** (topoisomerase II) stranded break in the helix to add or remove supercoils (as needed due to underwinding or overwinding of DNA).	In eukaryotes: irinotecan/topotecan inhibit topoisomerase (TOP) I, etoposide/teniposide inhibit TOP II. In prokaryotes: fluoroquinolones inhibit TOP II (DNA gyrase) and TOP IV.
Primase F	Makes RNA primer for DNA polymerase III to initiate replication.	
DNA polymerase III G	Prokaryotes only. Elongates leading strand by adding deoxynucleotides to the 3′ end. Elongates lagging strand until it reaches primer of preceding fragment.	DNA polymerase III has 5′ → 3′ synthesis and proofreads with 3′ → 5′ exonuclease. Drugs blocking DNA replication often have a modified 3′ OH, thereby preventing addition of the next nucleotide ("chain termination").
DNA polymerase I H	Prokaryotes only. Degrades RNA primer; replaces it with DNA.	Same functions as DNA polymerase III, also excises RNA primer with 5′ → 3′ exonuclease.
DNA ligase I	Catalyzes the formation of a phosphodiester bond within a strand of double-stranded DNA.	Joins Okazaki fragments. Ligase links DNA.
Telomerase	Eukaryotes only. A reverse transcriptase (RNA-dependent DNA polymerase) that adds DNA (**TTAGGG**) to 3′ ends of chromosomes to avoid loss of genetic material with every duplication.	Upregulated in progenitor cells and also often in cancer; downregulated in aging and progeria. Telomerase **TAG**s for Greatness and Glory.

DNA repair

Double strand

Nonhomologous end joining	Brings together 2 ends of DNA fragments to repair double-stranded breaks. Homology not required. Part of the DNA may be lost or translocated.	
Homologous recombination	Requires 2 homologous DNA duplexes. A strand from damaged dsDNA is repaired using a complementary strand from intact homologous dsDNA as a template. Defective in breast/ovarian cancers with *BRCA1* or *BRCA2* mutations and in certain types of Fanconi anemia. Restores duplexes accurately without loss of nucleotides.	

Single strand

Nucleotide excision repair	Specific endonucleases remove the oligonucleotides containing damaged bases; DNA polymerase and ligase fill and reseal the gap, respectively. Repairs bulky helix-distorting lesions (eg, pyrimidine dimers).	Occurs in G_1 phase of cell cycle. Defective in xeroderma pigmentosum (inability to repair DNA pyrimidine dimers caused by UV exposure). Presents with dry skin, photosensitivity, skin cancer.
Base excision repair	Base-specific Glycosylase removes altered base and creates AP (apurinic/apyrimidinic) site. AP-Endonuclease cleaves 5' end, removing one or more nucleotides. AP-Lyase cleaves 3' end. DNA Polymerase-β fills the gap. DNA ligase seals it.	Occurs throughout cell cycle. Important in repair of spontaneous/toxic deamination. "GEL Please."
Mismatch repair	Mismatched nucleotides in newly synthesized strand are removed and gap is filled and resealed.	Occurs predominantly in S phase of cell cycle. Defective in Lynch syndrome (hereditary nonpolyposis colorectal cancer [HNPCC]).

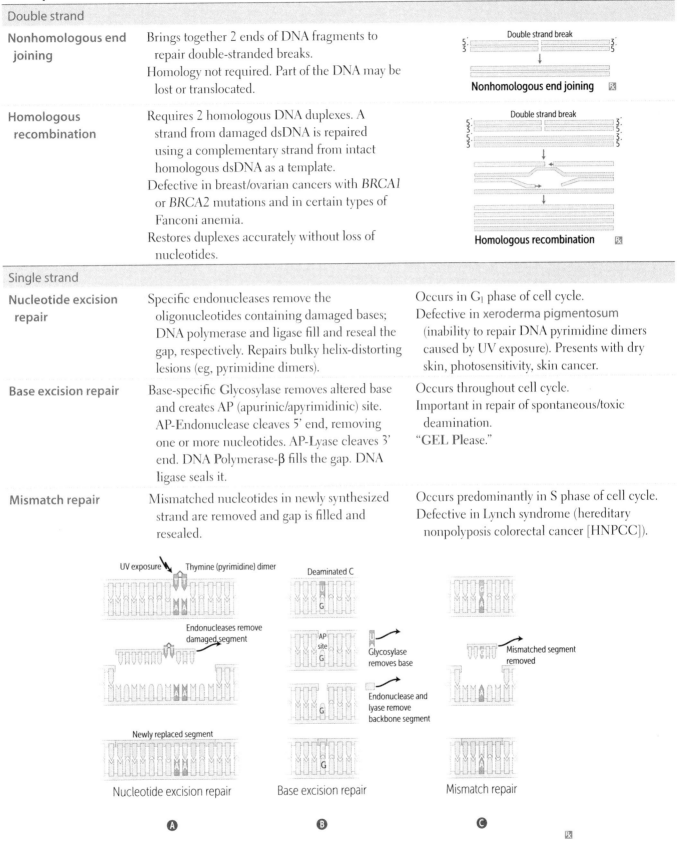

Nucleotide excision repair · Base excision repair · Mismatch repair

Ⓐ Ⓑ Ⓒ

Mutations in DNA	Degree of change: silent ≪ missense < nonsense < frameshift. Single nucleotide substitutions are repaired by DNA polymerase and DNA ligase. Types of single nucleotide (point) mutations: ▪ Transition—purine to purine (eg, A to G) or pyrimidine to pyrimidine (eg, C to T). ▪ Transversion—purine to pyrimidine (eg, A to T) or pyrimidine to purine (eg, C to G).

Single nucleotide substitutions

Silent mutation	Codes for same (synonymous) amino acid; often involves 3rd position of codon (tRNA wobble).
Missense mutation	Results in changed amino acid (called conservative if new amino acid has similar chemical structure). Examples: sickle cell disease (substitution of glutamic acid with valine).
Nonsense mutation	Results in early **stop** codon (UGA, UAA, UAG). Usually generates nonfunctional protein. **Stop** the **nonsense!**

Other mutations

Frameshift mutation	Deletion or insertion of any number of nucleotides not divisible by 3 (or if divisible by 3 split across adjacent codons) → misreading of all nucleotides downstream. Protein may be shorter or longer, and its function may be disrupted or altered. May occur due to slippage of DNA polymerase during replication at repetitive nucleotide regions. Examples: Duchenne muscular dystrophy, Tay-Sachs disease, cystic fibrosis.
Splice site mutation	Retained intron in mRNA → protein with impaired or altered function. Examples: rare causes of cancers, dementia, epilepsy, some types of β-thalassemia, Gaucher disease, Marfan syndrome.
Slipped strand mispairing	Occurs when DNA polymerase slips and either inserts or removes one or more additional nucleotides by mistake in an area of repetitive nucleotides. Anticipation occurs secondary to insertion of increased repeats across generations. Example: CAG repeat expansion in Huntington disease.

***Lac* operon**	Classic example of a genetic response to an environmental change. Glucose is the preferred metabolic substrate in *E coli*, but when glucose is absent and lactose is available, the *lac* operon is activated to switch to lactose metabolism. Mechanism of shift:

- Low glucose → ↑ adenylate cyclase activity → ↑ generation of cAMP from ATP → activation of catabolite activator protein (CAP) → ↑ transcription.
- High lactose → unbinds repressor protein from repressor/operator site → ↑ transcription.

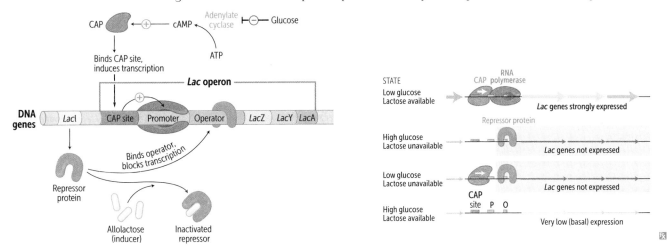

Functional organization of a eukaryotic gene

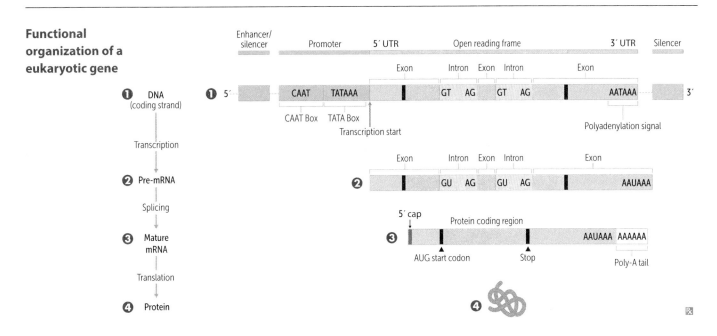

Regulation of gene expression

Promoter	Site where RNA polymerase II and multiple other transcription factors bind to DNA upstream from gene locus (AT-rich upstream sequence with TATA and CAAT boxes, which differ between eukaryotes and prokaryotes).	Promoters increase initiation of transcription. Promoter mutation commonly results in dramatic ↓ in level of gene transcription.
Enhancer	DNA locus where regulatory proteins ("**activators**") bind, **increasing** expression of a gene on the same chromosome.	Enhancers and silencers may be located close to, far from, or even within (in an intron) the gene whose expression they regulate.
Silencer	DNA locus where regulatory proteins ("**repressors**") bind, **decreasing** expression of a gene on the same chromosome.	
Epigenetics	Changes made to gene expression (heritable mitotically/meiotically) without a change in underlying DNA sequence.	Primary mechanisms of epigenetic change include DNA methylation, histone modification, and noncoding RNA.

RNA processing (eukaryotes)

RNA processing (eukaryotes)
 	
	Initial transcript is called heterogeneous nuclear RNA (hnRNA). hnRNA is then modified and becomes mRNA.
	The following processes occur in the nucleus:
	  ▪ Capping of 5′ end (addition of 7-methylguanosine cap; cotranscriptional)
	  ▪ Polyadenylation of 3′ end (~200 A's → poly-A tail; posttranscriptional)
	  ▪ Splicing out of introns (posttranscriptional)
	Capped, tailed, and spliced transcript is called mRNA.
	mRNA is transported out of nucleus to be translated in cytosol.
		mRNA quality control occurs at cytoplasmic processing bodies (P-bodies), which contain exonucleases, decapping enzymes, and microRNAs; mRNAs may be degraded or stored in P-bodies for future translation.
		Poly-A polymerase does not require a template.
		AAUAAA = polyadenylation signal. Mutation in polyadenylation signal → early degradation prior to translation.
		Kozak sequence—initiation site in most eukaryotic mRNA. Facilitates binding of small subunit of ribosome to mRNA. Mutations in sequence → impairment of initiation of translation → ↓ protein synthesis.

RNA polymerases

Eukaryotes	RNA polymerase I makes **r**RNA, the most common (**r**ampant) type; present only in nucleolus. RNA polymerase II makes **m**RNA (**m**assive), **mi**croRNA (**mi**RNA), and **s**mall **n**uclear RNA (**sn**RNA). RNA polymerase III makes 5S rRNA, **t**RNA (**t**iny). No proofreading function, but can initiate chains. RNA polymerase II opens DNA at promoter site.	I, II, and III are numbered in the same order that their products are used in protein synthesis: rRNA, mRNA, then tRNA. α-amanitin, found in *Amanita phalloides* (death cap mushrooms), inhibits RNA polymerase II. Causes dysentery and severe hepatotoxicity if ingested. Dactinomycin inhibits RNA polymerase in both prokaryotes and eukaryotes.
Prokaryotes	1 RNA polymerase (multisubunit complex) makes all 3 kinds of RNA.	Rifamycins (rifampin, rifabutin) inhibit DNA-dependent RNA polymerase in prokaryotes.

Introns vs exons

Exons contain the actual genetic information coding for protein or functional RNA.

Introns do not code for protein, but are important in regulation of gene expression.

Different exons are frequently combined by alternative splicing to produce a larger number of unique proteins.

Introns are intervening sequences and stay in the nucleus, whereas exons exit and are expressed.

Alternative splicing—can produce a variety of protein products from a single hnRNA (heterogenous nuclear RNA) sequence (eg, transmembrane vs secreted Ig, tropomyosin variants in muscle, dopamine receptors in the brain, host defense evasion by tumor cells).

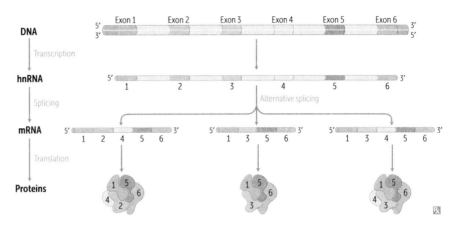

Splicing of pre-mRNA

Part of process by which precursor mRNA (pre-mRNA) is transformed into mature mRNA. Introns typically begin with GU and end with AG. Alterations in snRNP assembly can cause clinical disease; eg, in spinal muscular atrophy, snRNP assembly is affected due to ↓ SMN protein → congenital degeneration of anterior horns of spinal cord → symmetric weakness (hypotonia, or "floppy baby syndrome").

snRNPs are snRNA bound to proteins (eg, Smith [Sm]) to form a spliceosome that cleaves pre-mRNA. Anti-U1 snRNP antibodies are associated with SLE, mixed connective tissue disease, other rheumatic diseases.

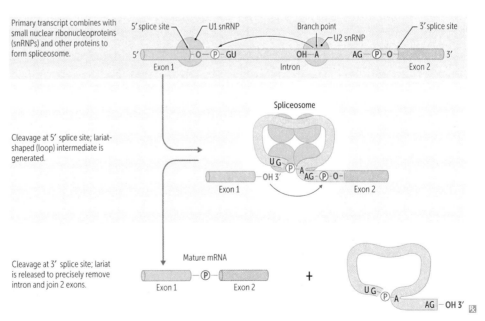

tRNA

Structure	75–90 nucleotides, 2° structure, cloverleaf form, anticodon end is opposite 3′ aminoacyl end. All tRNAs, both eukaryotic and prokaryotic, have CCA at 3′ end along with a high percentage of chemically modified bases. The amino acid is covalently bound to the 3′ end of the tRNA. **CCA Can Carry Amino** acids. T-arm: contains the TΨC (ribothymidine, pseudouridine, cytidine) sequence necessary for tRNA-ribosome binding. **T-arm Tethers** tRNA molecule to ribosome. D-arm: contains **Di**hydrouridine residues necessary for tRNA recognition by the correct aminoacyl-tRNA synthetase. **D-arm** allows **Detection** of the tRNA by aminoacyl-tRNA synthetase. Attachment site: 3′-ACC-5′ is the amino acid **ACC**eptor site.
Charging	Aminoacyl-tRNA synthetase (uses ATP; 1 unique enzyme per respective amino acid) and binding of charged tRNA to the codon are responsible for the accuracy of amino acid selection. Aminoacyl-tRNA synthetase matches an amino acid to the tRNA by scrutinizing the amino acid before and after it binds to tRNA. If an incorrect amino acid is attached, the bond is hydrolyzed. A mischarged tRNA reads the usual codon but inserts the wrong amino acid.

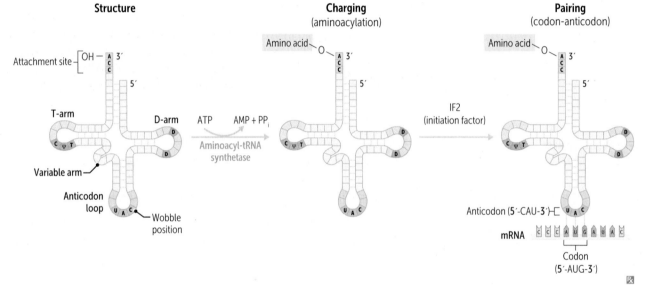

Start and stop codons

mRNA start codon	AUG.	AUG in**AUG**urates protein synthesis.
Eukaryotes	Codes for methionine, which may be removed before translation is completed.	
Prokaryotes	Codes for N-formylmethionine (fMet).	fMet stimulates neutrophil chemotaxis.
mRNA stop codons	UGA, UAA, UAG. Recognized by release factors.	UGA = U Go Away. UAA = U Are Away. UAG = U Are Gone.

Protein synthesis

Initiation	1. Eukaryotic initiation factors (eIFs) identify the 5′ cap. 2. eIFs help assemble the 40S ribosomal subunit with the initiator tRNA. 3. eIFs released when the mRNA and the ribosomal 60S subunit assemble with the complex. Requires GTP.	Eukaryotes: 40S + 60S → 80S (even). Prokaryotes: 30S + 50S → 70S (prime). Synthesis occurs from N-terminus to C-terminus. ATP—tRNA Activation (charging). GTP—tRNA Gripping and Going places (translocation).

Elongation	❶ Aminoacyl-tRNA binds to A site (except for initiator methionine, which binds the P site), requires an elongation factor and GTP.
	❷ rRNA ("ribozyme") catalyzes peptide bond formation, transfers growing polypeptide to amino acid in A site.
	❸ Ribosome advances 3 nucleotides toward 3′ end of mRNA, moving peptidyl tRNA to P site (translocation).
		Think of "going **APE**":
		  A site = incoming Aminoacyl-tRNA.
		  P site = accommodates growing Peptide.
		  E site = holds Empty tRNA as it Exits.
		
		Elongation factors are targets of bacterial toxins (eg, *Diphtheria*, *Pseudomonas*).

Termination	Eukaryotic release factors (eRFs) recognize the stop codon and halt translation → completed polypeptide is released from ribosome. Requires GTP.	Shine-Dalgarno sequence—ribosomal binding site in prokaryotic mRNA. Recognized by 16S RNA in ribosomal subunit. Enables protein synthesis initiation by aligning ribosome with start codon so that code is read correctly.

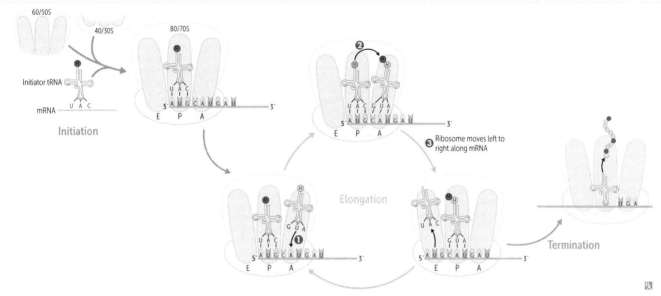

Posttranslational modifications

Trimming	Removal of N- or C-terminal propeptides from zymogen to generate mature protein (eg, trypsinogen to trypsin).
Covalent alterations	Phosphorylation, glycosylation, hydroxylation, methylation, acetylation, and ubiquitination.

Chaperone protein	Intracellular protein involved in facilitating and maintaining protein folding. In yeast, heat shock proteins (eg, HSP60) are constitutively expressed, but expression may increase with high temperatures, acidic pH, and hypoxia to prevent protein denaturing/misfolding.

▶ BIOCHEMISTRY—CELLULAR

Cell cycle phases	Checkpoints control transitions between phases of cell cycle. This process is regulated by cyclins, cyclin-dependent kinases (CDKs), and tumor suppressors. M phase (shortest phase of cell cycle) includes mitosis (prophase, prometaphase, metaphase, anaphase, telophase) and cytokinesis (cytoplasm splits in two). G_1 is of variable duration.

REGULATION OF CELL CYCLE

Cyclin-dependent kinases	Constitutively expressed but inactive when not bound to cyclin.
Cyclin-CDK complexes	Cyclins are phase-specific regulatory proteins that activate CDKs when stimulated by growth factors. The cyclin-CDK complex can then phosphorylate other proteins (eg, Rb) to coordinate cell cycle progression. This complex must be activated/inactivated at appropriate times for cell cycle to progress.
Tumor suppressors	p53 → p21 induction → CDK inhibition → Rb hypophosphorylation (activation) → G_1-S progression inhibition. Mutations in tumor suppressor genes can result in unrestrained cell division (eg, Li-Fraumeni syndrome). Growth factors (eg, insulin, PDGF, EPO, EGF) bind tyrosine kinase receptors to transition the cell from G_1 to S phase.

CELL TYPES

Permanent	Remain in G_0, regenerate from stem cells.	Neurons, skeletal and cardiac muscle, RBCs.
Stable (quiescent)	Enter G_1 from G_0 when stimulated.	Hepatocytes, lymphocytes, PCT, periosteal cells.
Labile	Never go to G_0, divide rapidly with a short G_1. Most affected by chemotherapy.	Bone marrow, gut epithelium, skin, hair follicles, germ cells.

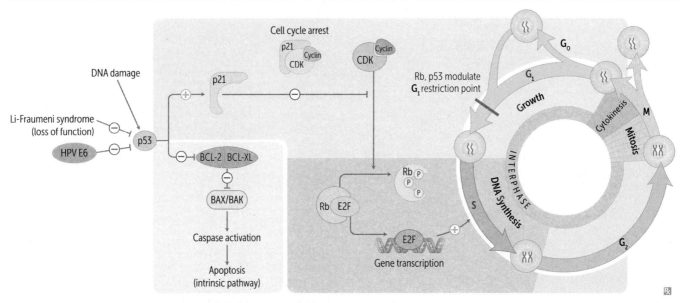

Rough endoplasmic reticulum	Site of synthesis of secretory (exported) proteins and of N-linked oligosaccharide addition to lysosomal and other proteins. Nissl bodies (RER in neurons)—synthesize peptide neurotransmitters for secretion. Free ribosomes—unattached to any membrane; site of synthesis of cytosolic, peroxisomal, and mitochondrial proteins.	N-linked glycosylation occurs in the eNdoplasmic reticulum. Mucus-secreting goblet cells of small intestine and antibody-secreting plasma cells are rich in RER. Proteins within organelles (eg, ER, Golgi bodies, lysosomes) are formed in RER.
Smooth endoplasmic reticulum	Site of steroid synthesis and detoxification of drugs and poisons. Lacks surface ribosomes. Location of glucose-6-phosphatase (last step in both glycogenolysis and gluconeogenesis).	Hepatocytes and steroid hormone–producing cells of the adrenal cortex and gonads are rich in SER.

Cell trafficking

Golgi is distribution center for proteins and lipids from ER to vesicles and plasma membrane. Posttranslational events in GOlgi include modifying N-oligosaccharides on asparagine, adding O-oligosaccharides on serine and threonine, and adding mannose-6-phosphate to proteins for targeting to lysosomes (usually for degradation).

Endosomes are sorting centers for material from outside the cell or from the Golgi, sending it to lysosomes for destruction or back to the membrane/Golgi for further use.

I-cell disease (inclusion cell disease/mucolipidosis type II)—inherited lysosomal storage disorder (autosomal recessive); defect in N-acetylglucosaminyl-1-phosphotransferase → failure of the Golgi to phosphorylate mannose residues (↓ mannose-6-phosphate) on glycoproteins → enzymes secreted extracellularly rather than delivered to lysosomes → lysosomes deficient in digestive enzymes → buildup of cellular debris in lysosomes (inclusion bodies). Results in coarse facial features, gingival hyperplasia, corneal clouding, restricted joint movements, claw hand deformities, kyphoscoliosis, and ↑ plasma levels of lysosomal enzymes. Symptoms similar to but more severe than Hurler syndrome. Often fatal in childhood.

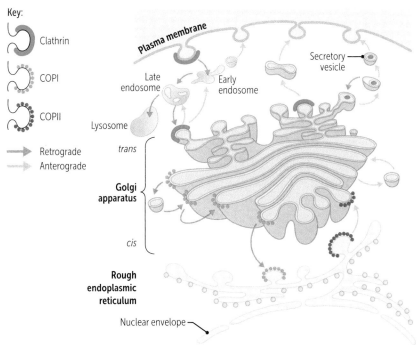

Key:
Clathrin
COPI
COPII
Retrograde
Anterograde
Plasma membrane
Late endosome
Early endosome
Secretory vesicle
Lysosome
trans
Golgi apparatus
cis
Rough endoplasmic reticulum
Nuclear envelope

Signal recognition particle (SRP)—abundant, cytosolic ribonucleoprotein that traffics polypeptide-ribosome complex from the cytosol to the RER. Absent or dysfunctional SRP → accumulation of protein in cytosol.

Vesicular trafficking proteins
- COPI: Golgi → Golgi (retrograde); *cis*-Golgi → ER.
- COPII: ER → *cis*-Golgi (anterograde). "Two (COPII) steps forward (anterograde); one (COPI) step back (retrograde)."
- Clathrin: *trans*-Golgi → lysosomes; plasma membrane → endosomes (receptor-mediated endocytosis [eg, LDL receptor activity]).

Peroxisome

Membrane-enclosed organelle involved in:
- β-oxidation of very-long-chain fatty acids (VLCFA) (strictly peroxisomal process)
- α-oxidation of branched-chain fatty acids (strictly peroxisomal process)
- Catabolism of amino acids and ethanol
- Synthesis of bile acids and plasmalogens (important membrane phospholipid, especially in white matter of brain)

Zellweger syndrome—autosomal recessive disorder of peroxisome biogenesis due to mutated *PEX* genes (accumulation of pipecolic acid in peroxisomes). Hypotonia, seizures, jaundice, craniofacial dysmorphia, hepatomegaly, early death.

Refsum disease—autosomal recessive disorder of α-oxidation → buildup of phytanic acid due to inability to degrade it. Vision loss (retinitis pigmentosa), anosmia, hearing loss, ataxia, peripheral neuropathy, ichthyosis, and cardiac conduction defects. Treatment: diet, plasmapheresis.

Adrenoleukodystrophy—X-linked recessive disorder of β-oxidation due to mutation in *ABCD1* gene → VLCFA buildup in **adrenal** glands, white (**leuko**) matter of brain, testes. Progressive disease that can lead to adrenal gland crisis, progressive loss of neurologic function, death.

Proteasome

Barrel-shaped protein complex that degrades polyubiquitin-tagged proteins. Plays a role in many cellular processes, including immune response (MHC I–mediated). Defects in ubiquitin-proteasome system also implicated in diverse human diseases including neurodegenerative diseases.

Cytoskeletal elements

A network of protein fibers within the cytoplasm that supports cell structure, cell and organelle movement, and cell division.

TYPE OF FILAMENT	PREDOMINANT FUNCTION	EXAMPLES
Microfilaments	Muscle contraction, cytokinesis, phagocytosis	Actin, microvilli
Intermediate filaments	Maintain cell structure	Vimentin, desmin, cytokeratin, lamins, glial fibrillary acidic protein (GFAP), neurofilaments
Microtubules	Movement, cell division	Cilia, flagella, mitotic spindle, axonal trafficking, centrioles

---

Microtubule

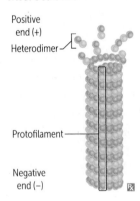

Positive end (+)
Heterodimer
Protofilament
Negative end (–)

Cylindrical outer structure composed of a helical array of polymerized heterodimers of α- and β-tubulin. Each dimer has 2 GTP bound. Incorporated into flagella, cilia, mitotic spindles. Also involved in slow axoplasmic transport in neurons.

Molecular motor proteins—transport cellular cargo toward opposite ends of microtubule.
- Retrograde to microtubule (+ → –)—dynein.
- Anterograde to microtubule (– → +)—kinesin.

Clostridium tetani toxin, poliovirus, rabies virus, and herpes simplex virus (HSV) use dynein for retrograde transport to the neuronal cell body. HSV reactivation occurs via anterograde transport from cell body (kinesin mediated).

Slow anterograde transport rate limiting step of peripheral nerve regeneration after injury.

Drugs that act on microtubules (**m**icrotubules **g**et **c**onstructed **v**ery **t**erribly):
- **M**ebendazole (antihelminthic)
- **G**riseofulvin (antifungal)
- **C**olchicine (antigout)
- **V**inca alkaloids (anticancer)
- **T**axanes (anticancer)

Negative end **near n**ucleus.
Positive end **p**oints to **p**eriphery.

Ready? Attack!

Cilia structure

Motile cilia consist of 9 doublet + 2 singlet arrangement of microtubules (axoneme) 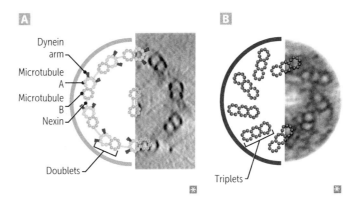.

Basal body (base of cilium below cell membrane) consists of 9 microtubule triplets B with no central microtubules.

Nonmotile (primary) cilia work as chemical signal sensors and have a role in signal transduction and cell growth control. Dysgenesis may lead to polycystic kidney disease, mitral valve prolapse, or retinal degeneration.

Axonemal dynein—ATPase that links peripheral 9 doublets and causes bending of cilium by differential sliding of doublets.

Gap junctions enable coordinated ciliary movement.

Primary ciliary dyskinesia

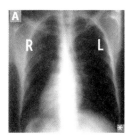

Autosomal recessive. Dynein arm defect → immotile cilia → dysfunctional ciliated epithelia. Most common type is Kartagener syndrome (PCD with situs inversus).

Developmental abnormalities due to impaired migration and orientation (eg, situs inversus A, hearing loss due to dysfunctional eustachian tube cilia); recurrent infections (eg, sinusitis, ear infections, bronchiectasis due to impaired ciliary clearance of debris/pathogens); infertility (↑ risk of ectopic pregnancy due to dysfunctional fallopian tube cilia, immotile spermatozoa).

Lab findings: ↓ nasal nitric oxide (used as screening test).

Sodium-potassium pump

Na^+/K^+-ATPase is located in the plasma membrane with ATP site on cytosolic side. For each ATP consumed, **2 K^+** go **in** to the cell (pump dephosphorylated) and **3 Na^+** go **out** of the cell (pump phosphorylated).

2 strikes? **K**, you're still **in**. 3 strikes? **Nah**, you're **out**!

Digoxin directly inhibits Na^+/K^+-ATPase → indirect inhibition of Na^+/Ca^{2+} exchange → ↑ $[Ca^{2+}]_i$ → ↑ cardiac contractility.

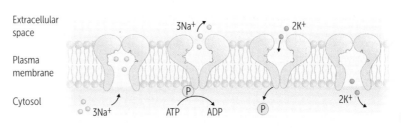

Collagen	Most abundant protein in the human body. Extensively modified by posttranslational modification. Organizes and strengthens extracellular matrix. Types I to IV are the most common types in humans.	Type I: Skeleton Type II: Cartilage Type III: Arteries Type IV: Basement membrane **SCAB**
Type I	Most common (90%)—bone (made by osteoblasts), skin, tendon, dentin, fascia, cornea, **late** wound repair.	Type **I**: **bone**, tend**one**. ↓ production in osteogenesis imperfecta type I.
Type II	Cartilage (including hyaline), vitreous body, nucleus pulposus.	Type **II**: car**two**lage.
Type III	Reticulin—skin, **blood vessels**, uterus, fetal tissue, **early** wound repair.	Type **III**: deficient in **vascular** type of Ehlers-Danlos syndrome (**threE D**). Myofibroblasts are responsible for secretion (proliferative stage) and wound contraction.
Type IV	Basement membrane/basal lamina (glomerulus, cochlea), lens.	Type **IV**: under the **floor** (basement membrane). Defective in Alport syndrome; targeted by autoantibodies in Goodpasture syndrome.

Collagen synthesis and structure

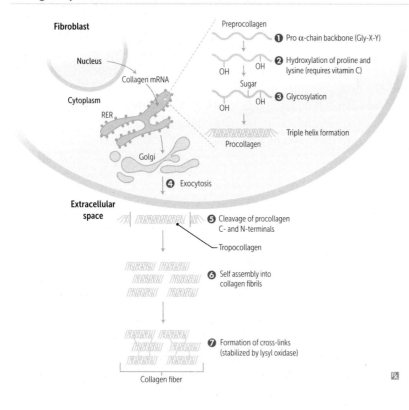

❶ Synthesis—translation of collagen α chains (preprocollagen)—usually Gly-X-Y (X is often proline or lysine and Y is often hydroxyproline or hydroxylysine). Collagen is 1/3 glycine; glycine content of collagen is less variable than that of lysine and proline.

❷ Hydroxylation—hydroxylation ("hydroxCylation") of specific proline and lysine residues. Requires vitamin C; deficiency → scurvy.

❸ Glycosylation—glycosylation of pro-α-chain hydroxylysine residues and formation of procollagen via hydrogen and disulfide bonds (triple helix of 3 collagen α chains). Problems forming triple helix → osteogenesis imperfecta.

❹ Exocytosis—exocytosis of procollagen into extracellular space.

❺ Proteolytic processing—cleavage of disulfide-rich terminal regions of procollagen → insoluble tropocollagen.

❻ Assembly and alignment—collagen assembles in fibrils and aligns for cross-linking.

❼ Cross-linking—reinforcement of staggered tropocollagen molecules by covalent lysine-hydroxylysine cross-linkage (by copper-containing lysyl oxidase) to make collagen fibers. Cross-linking of collagen ↑ with age. Problems with cross-linking → Menkes disease.

Osteogenesis imperfecta

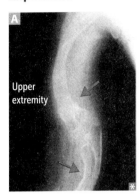

Upper extremity

Genetic bone disorder (brittle bone disease) caused by a variety of gene defects (most commonly *COL1A1* and *COL1A2*).

Most common form is autosomal dominant with ↓ production of otherwise normal type I collagen (altered triple helix formation). Manifestations include:

- Multiple fractures and bone deformities (arrows in A) after minimal trauma (eg, during birth)
- Blue sclerae B due to thin, translucent scleral collagen revealing choroidal veins
- Some forms have tooth abnormalities, including opalescent teeth that wear easily due to lack of dentin (dentinogenesis imperfecta)
- Hearing loss (abnormal ossicles)

May be confused with child abuse.

Treat with bisphosphonates to ↓ fracture risk.

Patients can't **BITE**:
  Bones = multiple fractures
  I (eye) = blue sclerae
  Teeth = dental imperfections
  Ear = hearing loss

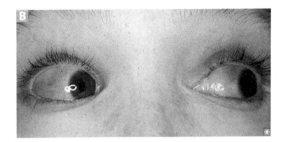

Ehlers-Danlos syndrome

Faulty collagen synthesis causes skin to be hyperextensible and often thin or transparent A, joints to be hypermobile B, and tendency to bleed (easy bruising).

Multiple types. Inheritance and severity vary. Can be autosomal dominant or recessive. May be associated with joint dislocation, berry and aortic aneurysms, organ rupture.

Hypermobility type (joint instability): most common type.

Classical type (joint and skin symptoms): caused by a mutation in type V collagen (eg, *COL5A1*, *COL5A2*).

Vascular type (fragile tissues including vessels [eg, aorta], muscles, and organs that are prone to rupture [eg, gravid uterus]): mutations in type III procollagen (eg, *COL3A1*).

Can be caused by procollagen peptidase deficiency.

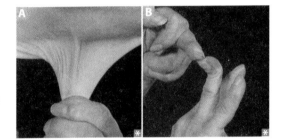

Menkes disease

X-linked recessive connective tissue disease caused by impaired copper absorption and transport due to defective Menkes protein *ATP7A* (**A**bsent copper), vs *ATP7B* in Wilson disease (copper **B**uildup). Leads to ↓ activity of lysyl oxidase (copper is a necessary cofactor) → defective collagen cross-linking. Results in brittle, "kinky" hair, growth and developmental delay, hypotonia, ↑ risk of cerebral aneurysms.

Elastin

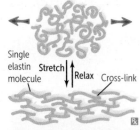

Single
elastic
molecule Stretch ↕ Relax Cross-link

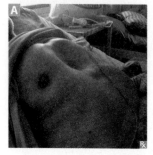

Stretchy protein within skin, lungs, large arteries, elastic ligaments, vocal cords, epiglottis, ligamenta flava (connect vertebrae → relaxed and stretched conformations).

Rich in nonhydroxylated proline, glycine, and lysine residues, vs the hydroxylated residues of collagen.

Tropoelastin with fibrillin scaffolding.

Cross-linking occurs extracellularly via lysyl oxidase and gives elastin its elastic properties.

Broken down by elastase, which is normally inhibited by α_1-antitrypsin.

α_1-Antitrypsin deficiency results in unopposed elastase activity, which can cause COPD.

Marfan syndrome—autosomal dominant (with variable expression and symptoms due to pleiotropy) connective tissue disorder affecting skeleton, heart, and eyes. *FBN1* gene mutation on chromosome 15 (fifteen) results in defective fibrillin-1, a glycoprotein that forms a sheath around elastin and sequesters TGF-β. Findings: tall with long extremities; chest wall deformity (pectus carinatum [pigeon chest] or pectus excavatum A); hypermobile joints; long, tapering fingers and toes (arachnodactyly); cystic medial necrosis of aorta; aortic root aneurysm rupture or dissection (most common cause of death); mitral valve prolapse; ↑ risk of spontaneous pneumothorax.

Homocystinuria—most commonly due to cystathionine synthase deficiency leading to homocysteine buildup. Presentation similar to Marfan syndrome with pectus deformity, tall stature, ↑ arm:height ratio, ↓ upper:lower body segment ratio, arachnodactyly, joint hyperlaxity, skin hyperelasticity, scoliosis, fair complexion (vs Marfan syndrome).

	Marfan syndrome	Homocystinuria
INHERITANCE	Autosomal dominant	Autosomal recessive
INTELLECT	Normal	Decreased
VASCULAR COMPLICATIONS	Aortic root dilatation	Thrombosis
LENS DISLOCATION	Upward/temporal (**Mar**fan **fan**s out)	Downward/nasal

▶ BIOCHEMISTRY—LABORATORY TECHNIQUES

Polymerase chain reaction

Molecular biology lab procedure used to amplify a desired fragment of DNA. Useful as a diagnostic tool (eg, neonatal HIV, herpes encephalitis).

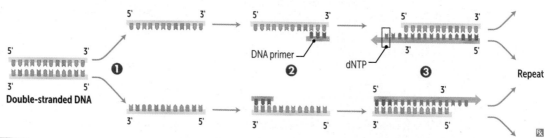

❶ **Denaturation**—DNA template, DNA primers, a heat-stable DNA polymerase, and deoxynucleotide triphosphates (dNTPs) are heated to separate the DNA strands.

❷ **Annealing**—sample is cooled. DNA primers anneal to the specific sequence to be amplified on the DNA template.

❸ **Elongation**—temperature is increased. DNA polymerase adds dNTPs to the strand to replicate the sequence after each primer.

Heating and cooling cycles continue until the amount of DNA is sufficient.

CRISPR/Cas9

A genome editing tool derived from bacteria. Consists of a guide RNA (gRNA), which is complementary to a target DNA sequence, and an endonuclease (Cas9), which makes a single- or double-strand break at the target site.

Applications include removing virulence factors from pathogens, replacing disease-causing alleles of genes with healthy variants (eg, sickle cell disease), and specifically targeting tumor cells.

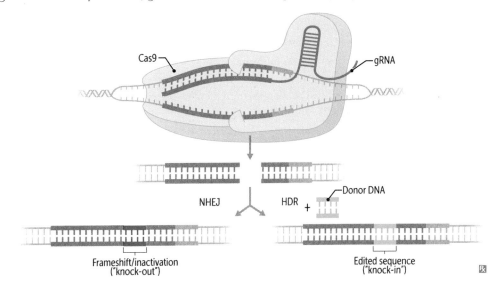

Blotting procedures

Southern blot

1. DNA sample is enzymatically cleaved into smaller pieces, which are separated by gel electrophoresis, and then transferred to a membrane.
2. Membrane is exposed to labeled DNA probe that anneals to its complementary strand.
3. Resulting double-stranded, labeled piece of DNA is visualized when membrane is exposed to film or digital imager.

Useful to identify size of specific sequences (eg, determination of heterozygosity [as seen in image], # of CGG repeats in *FMR1* to diagnose fragile X syndrome).

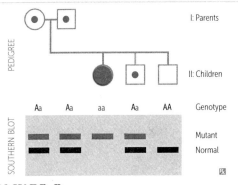

SNoW DRoP:
  Southern = DNA
  Northern = RNA
  Western = Protein

Northern blot

Similar to Southern blot, except that an RNA sample is electrophoresed. Useful for studying mRNA levels and size, which are reflective of gene expression. Detects splicing errors.

Western blot

Sample protein is separated via gel electrophoresis and transferred to a membrane. Labeled antibody is used to bind relevant protein. This helps identify specific protein and determines quantity.

Flow cytometry

Laboratory technique to assess size, granularity, and protein expression (immunophenotype) of individual cells in a sample.

Cells are tagged with antibodies specific to surface or intracellular proteins. Antibodies are then tagged with a unique fluorescent dye. Sample is analyzed one cell at a time by focusing a laser on the cell and measuring light scatter and intensity of fluorescence.

Data are plotted either as histogram (one measure) or scatter plot (any two measures, as shown). In illustration:

- Cells in left lower quadrant ⊖ for both CD8 and CD3.
- Cells in right lower quadrant ⊕ for CD8 and ⊖ for CD3. In this example, right lower quadrant is empty because all CD8-expressing cells also express CD3.
- Cells in left upper quadrant ⊕ for CD3 and ⊖ for CD8.
- Cells in right upper quadrant ⊕ for both CD8 and CD3.

Commonly used in workup of hematologic abnormalities (eg, leukemia, paroxysmal nocturnal hemoglobinuria, fetal RBCs in pregnant person's blood) and immunodeficiencies (eg, CD4+ cell count in HIV).

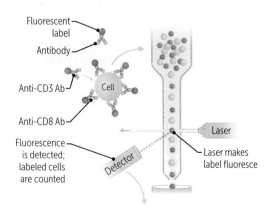

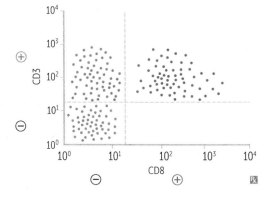

Microarrays

Used to compare the relative transcription of genes in two RNA samples. Can detect single nucleotide polymorphisms (SNPs) and copy number variants (CNVs) for genotyping, clinical genetic testing, forensic analysis, and cancer mutation and genetic linkage analysis when DNA is used.

Enzyme-linked immunosorbent assay

Immunologic test used to detect the presence of either a specific antigen (in direct ELISA) or antibody (in indirect ELISA) in a patient's blood sample. Detection involves the use of an antibody linked to an enzyme. Added substrate reacts with the enzyme, producing a detectable signal. Can have high sensitivity and specificity, but is less specific than Western blot. Often used to screen for HIV infection.

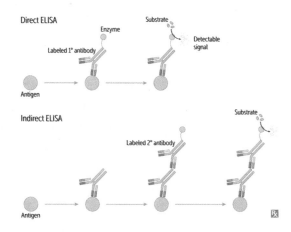

Karyotyping

Colchicine is added to cultured cells to disrupt the assembly of mitotic spindles and arrest cells at mitosis. Chromosomes are stained, ordered, and numbered according to morphology, size, arm-length ratio, and banding pattern (arrows in 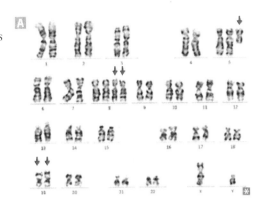 point to extensive abnormalities in a cancer cell).

Can be performed on a sample of blood, bone marrow, amniotic fluid, or placental tissue.

Used to diagnose chromosomal imbalances (eg, autosomal trisomies, sex chromosome disorders).

Fluorescence in situ hybridization

Fluorescent DNA or RNA probe binds to specific gene or other site of interest on chromosomes.

Used for specific localization of genes and direct visualization of chromosomal anomalies.

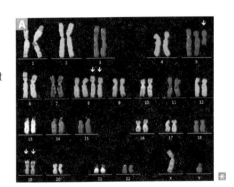

- Microdeletion—no fluorescence on a chromosome compared to fluorescence at the same locus on the second copy of that chromosome.
- Translocation— fluorescence signal that corresponds to tetrasomy (chromosome 8), gain of chromosome (chromosome 5), and unbalanced translocation (between chromosomes 17 and 19).
- Duplication—a second copy of a chromosome, resulting in a trisomy or tetrasomy (eg, chromosome 8 in).

Molecular cloning

Production of a recombinant DNA molecule in a bacterial or eukaryotic cell line host. Useful for production of human proteins in bacteria (eg, human growth hormone, insulin).

Gene expression modifications	Transgenic strategies in mice involve: ▪ Random insertion of gene into mouse genome ▪ Targeted insertion or deletion of gene through homologous recombination with mouse gene	Knock-**out** = removing a gene, taking it **out**. Knock-**in** = inserting a gene. Random insertion—constitutive expression. Targeted insertion—conditional expression.
RNA interference	Process whereby small non-coding RNA molecules target mRNAs to inhibit gene expression.	
MicroRNA	Naturally produced by cell as hairpin structures. Loose nucleotide pairing allows broad targeting of related mRNAs. When miRNA binds to mRNA, it blocks translation of mRNA and sometimes facilitates its degradation.	Abnormal expression of miRNAs contributes to certain malignancies (eg, by silencing an mRNA from a tumor suppressor gene).
Small interfering RNA	Usually derived from exogenous dsRNA source (eg, virus). Once inside a cell, siRNA requires complete nucleotide pairing, leading to highly specific mRNA targeting. Results in mRNA cleavage prior to translation.	Can be produced by transcription or chemically synthesized for gene "knockdown" experiments.

▶ BIOCHEMISTRY—GENETICS

Genetic terms

TERM	DEFINITION	EXAMPLE
Codominance	Both alleles contribute to the phenotype of the heterozygote.	Blood groups A, B, AB; α_1-antitrypsin deficiency; HLA groups.
Variable expressivity	Patients with the same genotype have varying phenotypes.	Two patients with neurofibromatosis type 1 (NF1) may have varying disease severity.
Incomplete penetrance	Not all individuals with a pathogenic gene variant show the disease. % penetrance × probability of inheriting genotype = risk of expressing phenotype.	*BRCA1* gene mutations do not always result in breast or ovarian cancer.
Pleiotropy	One gene contributes to multiple phenotypic effects.	Cystic fibrosis manifests with thick mucus in the lungs and GI tract, pancreatic insufficiency, male infertility.
Anticipation	Increased severity or earlier onset of disease in succeeding generations.	Trinucleotide repeat diseases (eg, Huntington disease).
Loss of heterozygosity	If a patient inherits or develops a mutation in a tumor suppressor gene, the wild type allele must be deleted/mutated/eliminated before cancer develops. This is not true of oncogenes.	Retinoblastoma and the "two-hit hypothesis," Lynch syndrome (HNPCC), Li-Fraumeni syndrome.
Epistasis	The allele of one gene affects the phenotypic expression of alleles in another gene.	Albinism, alopecia.
Aneuploidy	An abnormal number of chromosomes; due to chromosomal nondisjunction during mitosis or meiosis.	Down syndrome (trisomy 21), Turner syndrome (45,XO), oncogenesis.

Genetic terms (continued)

TERM	DEFINITION	EXAMPLE
Dominant negative mutation	Exerts a dominant effect. A heterozygote produces a nonfunctional altered protein that also prevents the normal gene product from functioning.	A single mutated $p53$ tumor suppressor gene results in a protein that is able to bind DNA and block the wild type p53 from binding to the promoter.
Linkage disequilibrium	Tendency for certain alleles to occur in close proximity on the same chromosome more or less often than expected by chance. Measured in a population, not in a family, and often varies in different populations.	HLA gene, CFTR gene.
Mosaicism	Presence of genetically distinct cell lines in the same individual. Somatic mosaicism—mutation arises from mitotic errors after fertilization and propagates through multiple tissues or organs. Germline (gonadal) mosaicism—mutation only in egg or sperm cells. If parents and relatives do not have the disease, suspect gonadal (or germline) mosaicism.	McCune-Albright syndrome—due to G_s-protein (GNAS) activating mutation. Presents with unilateral café-au-lait spots A with ragged edges, polyostotic fibrous dysplasia (bone is replaced by collagen and fibroblasts), and at least one endocrinopathy (eg, precocious puberty). Lethal if mutation occurs before fertilization (affecting all cells), but survivable in patients with mosaicism.
Locus heterogeneity	Mutations at different loci result in the same disease.	Albinism, retinitis pigmentosa, familial hypercholesteremia.
Allelic heterogeneity	Different mutations in the same locus result in the same disease.	β-thalassemia.
Heteroplasmy	Presence of both normal and mutated mtDNA, resulting in variable expression in mitochondrially inherited disease.	mtDNA passed from mother to all children. Example: Leber hereditary optic neuropathy.
Uniparental disomy	Offspring receives 2 copies of a chromosome from 1 parent and no copies from the other parent. HeterodIsomy (heterozygous) indicates a meiosis I error. IsodIsomy (homozygous) indicates a meiosis II error or postzygotic chromosomal duplication of one of a pair of chromosomes, and loss of the other of the original pair.	Uniparental is euploid (correct number of chromosomes). Most occurrences of uniparental disomy (UPD) → normal phenotype. Consider isodisomy in an individual manifesting a recessive disorder when only one parent is a carrier. Examples: Prader-Willi and Angelman syndromes.

Population genetics

CONCEPT	DESCRIPTION	EXAMPLE
Bottleneck effect	Fitness equal across alleles → natural disaster that removes certain alleles by chance → new allelic frequency (by chance, not naturally selected).	The founder effect is a type of bottleneck when cause is due to calamitous population separation.
Natural selection	Alleles that increase species fitness are more likely to be passed down to offspring and vice versa.	Human evolution.
Genetic drift	Also called allelic drift or Wright effect. A dramatic shift in allelic frequency that occurs by chance (not by natural selection).	Founder effect and bottleneck effect are both examples of genetic drift.

Hardy-Weinberg principle

	A (p)	a (q)
A (p)	AA (p²)	Aa (pq)
a (q)	Aa (pq)	aa (q²)

In a given population where mating is at random, allele and genotype frequencies will be constant. If p and q represent the frequencies of alleles A and a in a population, respectively, then $p + q = 1$, where:

- p^2 = frequency of homozygosity for allele A
- q^2 = frequency of homozygosity for allele a
- $2pq$ = frequency of heterozygosity (carrier frequency, if an autosomal recessive disease)

Therefore the sum of the frequencies of these genotypes is $p^2 + 2pq + q^2 = 1$.

The frequency of an X-linked recessive disease in males = q and in females = q^2.

Hardy-Weinberg law assumptions include:
- No mutation occurring at the locus
- Natural selection is not occurring
- Completely random mating
- No net migration
- Large population

If a population is in Hardy-Weinberg equilibrium, then the values of p and q remain constant from generation to generation. In rare autosomal recessive diseases, $p \approx 1$. Example: The prevalence of cystic fibrosis (an autosomal recessive disease) in the US is approximately 1/3200, which tells us that $q^2 = 1/3200$, with $q \approx 0.017$ or 1.7% of the population. Since $p + q = 1$, we know that $p = 1 - \sqrt{1/3200} \approx 0.982$, which gives us a heterozygous carrier frequency of $2pq = 0.035$ or 3.5% of the population. Notice that since the disease is relatively rare, we could have approximated $p \approx 1$ and obtained a similar result.

Disorders of imprinting

One gene copy is silenced by methylation, and only the other copy is expressed → parent-of-origin effects. The expressed copy may be mutated, may not be expressed, or may be deleted altogether.

	Prader-Willi syndrome	Angelman syndrome
WHICH GENE IS SILENT?	Maternally derived genes are silenced (except *UBE3A*) Disease occurs when the paternal allele is deleted or mutated	Paternally derived *UBE3A* is silenced Disease occurs when the maternal allele is deleted or mutated
SIGNS AND SYMPTOMS	Hyperphagia, obesity, intellectual disability, hypogonadism, hypotonia	Hand-flapping, Ataxia, severe Intellectual disability, inappropriate Laughter, Seizures. **HAILS** the Angels.
CHROMOSOMES INVOLVED	Chromosome 15 of paternal origin	*UBE3A* on maternal copy of chromosome 15
NOTES	25% of cases are due to maternal uniparental disomy	5% of cases are due to paternal uniparental disomy
	POP: Prader-Willi, Obesity/overeating, Paternal allele deleted	**MAMAS:** Maternal allele deleted, Angelman syndrome, Mood, Ataxia, Seizures

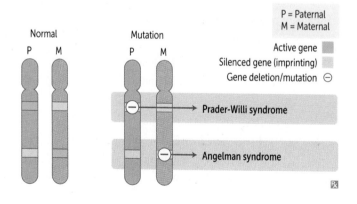

P = Paternal
M = Maternal

Active gene ▮
Silenced gene (imprinting) ▮
Gene deletion/mutation ⊖

Modes of inheritance

Autosomal dominant

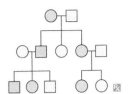

Often due to defects in structural genes. Many generations, both males and females are affected.

	A	a
a	Aa	aa
a	Aa	aa

Often pleiotropic (multiple apparently unrelated effects) and variably expressive (different between individuals). Family history crucial to diagnosis. With one affected (heterozygous) parent, each child has a 50% chance of being affected.

Autosomal recessive

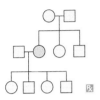

With 2 carrier (heterozygous) parents, on average: each child has a 25% chance of being affected, 50% chance of being a carrier, and 25% chance of not being affected nor a carrier.

	A	a
A	AA	Aa
a	Aa	aa

Often due to enzyme deficiencies. Usually seen in only 1 generation. Commonly more severe than dominant disorders; patients often present in childhood.
↑ risk in consanguineous families.
Unaffected individual with affected sibling has 2/3 probability of being a carrier.

X-linked recessive

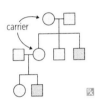

Sons of heterozygous mothers have a 50% chance of being affected. No male-to-male transmission. Skips generations.

	X	X		X	X
X	XX	XX	X	XX	XX
Y	XY	XY	Y	XY	XY

Commonly more severe in males. Females usually must be homozygous to be affected.

X-linked dominant

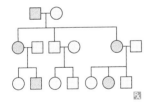

Transmitted through both parents. Children of affected mothers each have a 50% chance of being affected. 100% of daughters and 0% of sons of affected fathers will be affected.

	X	X		X	X
X	XX	XX	X	XX	XX
Y	XY	XY	Y	XY	XY

Examples: fragile X syndrome, Alport syndrome, hypophosphatemic rickets (also called X-linked hypophosphatemia)—phosphate wasting at proximal tubule → ricketslike presentation.

Mitochondrial inheritance

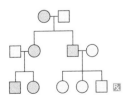

Transmitted only through the mother. All offspring of affected females may show signs of disease.
Variable expression in a population or even within a family due to heteroplasmy.

Caused by mutations in mtDNA.
Examples: mitochondrial myopathies, Leber hereditary optic neuropathy.

□ = unaffected male; ▨ = affected male; ◯ = unaffected female; ⬤ = affected female.

Autosomal dominant diseases	Achondroplasia, autosomal dominant polycystic kidney disease, familial adenomatous polyposis, familial hypercholesterolemia, hereditary hemorrhagic telangiectasia (Osler-Weber-Rendu syndrome), hereditary spherocytosis, Huntington disease, Li-Fraumeni syndrome, Marfan syndrome, multiple endocrine neoplasias, myotonic muscular dystrophy, neurofibromatosis type 1 (von Recklinghausen disease), neurofibromatosis type 2, tuberous sclerosis, von Hippel-Lindau disease.
Autosomal recessive diseases	Mostly consist of enzyme defects. Oculocutaneous albinism, phenylketonuria, cystic fibrosis, sickle cell disease, Wilson disease, sphingolipidoses (except Fabry disease), hemochromatosis, glycogen storage diseases, thalassemia, mucopolysaccharidoses (except Hunter syndrome), Friedreich ataxia, Kartagener syndrome, **ARPKD**. Oh, please! Can students who score high grades tell me features of the kidney disorder **Autosomal Recessive Polycystic Kidney Disease**?

Cystic fibrosis

GENETICS	Autosomal recessive; defect in CFTR gene on chromosome 7 (deletion; ΔF508). Most common lethal genetic disease in patients with European ancestry.
PATHOPHYSIOLOGY	CFTR encodes an ATP-gated Cl^- channel (secretes Cl^- in lungs/GI tract, reabsorbs Cl^- in sweat glands). Phe508 deletion → misfolded protein → improper protein trafficking → protein absent from cell membrane → ↓ Cl^- (and H_2O and HCO_3^-) secretion → compensatory ↑ Na^+ reabsorption via epithelial Na^+ channels (ENaC) → ↑ H_2O reabsorption → abnormally thick mucus secreted into lungs/GI tract. ↑ Na^+ reabsorption → more negative transepithelial potential difference.
DIAGNOSIS	↑ Cl^- concentration in pilocarpine-induced sweat test. Can present with contraction alkalosis and hypokalemia (ECF effects analogous to loop diuretic effect) due to ECF H_2O/Na^+ losses via sweating and concomitant renal K^+/H^+ wasting. ↑ immunoreactive trypsinogen (newborn screening) due to clogging of pancreatic duct.
COMPLICATIONS	Recurrent pulmonary infections (eg, S aureus [infancy and early childhood], P aeruginosa [adulthood], allergic bronchopulmonary aspergillosis [ABPA]), chronic bronchitis and bronchiectasis → reticulonodular pattern on CXR, opacification of sinuses. Nasal polyps, nail clubbing. Pancreatic insufficiency, malabsorption with steatorrhea, and fat-soluble vitamin deficiencies (A, D, E, K) progressing to endocrine dysfunction (CF-related diabetes), biliary cirrhosis, liver disease. Meconium ileus in newborns. Infertility in males (absence of vas deferens, spermatogenesis may be unaffected) and subfertility in females (amenorrhea, abnormally thick cervical mucus).
TREATMENT	Multifactorial: chest physiotherapy, aerosolized dornase alfa (DNase), and inhaled hypertonic saline → mucus clearance. Azithromycin prevents acute exacerbations. Ibuprofen for anti-inflammatory effect. Pancreatic enzyme replacement therapy (pancrelipase) for pancreatic insufficiency. CFTR modulators can be used alone or in combination. Efficacy varies by different genetic mutations (pharmacogenomics). Are either potentiators (hold gate of CFTR channel open → Cl^- flows through cell membrane; eg, ivacaftor) or correctors (help **CFTR** protein to form right 3-D shape → moves to the cell surface; eg, lumaCaFToR, tezaCaFToR).

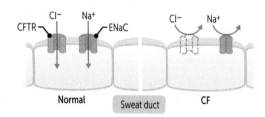

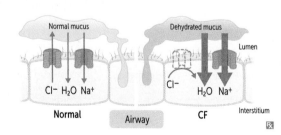

X-linked recessive diseases	Bruton agammaglobulinemia, Duchenne and Becker muscular dystrophies, Fabry disease, G6PD deficiency, hemophilia A and B, Hunter syndrome, Lesch-Nyhan syndrome, ocular albinism, ornithine transcarbamylase (OTC) deficiency, Wiskott-Aldrich syndrome. Females with Turner syndrome (45,XO) are more likely to have an X-linked recessive disorder. X-inactivation (lyonization)—during development, one of the X chromosomes in each XX cell is randomly deactivated and condensed into a Barr body (methylated heterochromatin). If skewed inactivation occurs, XX individuals may express X-linked recessive diseases (eg, G6PD); penetrance and severity of X-linked dominant diseases in XX individuals may also be impacted.

Muscular dystrophies

Duchenne	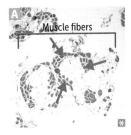 X-linked recessive disorder typically due to **frameshift** deletions or nonsense mutations → truncated or absent dystrophin protein → progressive myofiber damage. Can also result from splicing errors. Weakness begins in pelvic girdle muscles and progresses superiorly. Pseudohypertrophy of calf muscles due to fibrofatty replacement of muscle A. Waddling gait. Onset before 5 years of age. Dilated cardiomyopathy is common cause of death. **Gowers sign**—patient uses upper extremities to help stand up. Classically seen in Duchenne muscular dystrophy, but also seen in other muscular dystrophies and inflammatory myopathies (eg, polymyositis).	Duchenne = deleted dystrophin. Dystrophin gene (*DMD*) is the largest protein-coding human gene → ↑ chance of spontaneous mutation. Dystrophin helps to anchor muscle fibers to the extracellular matrix, primarily in skeletal and cardiac muscles. Loss of dystrophin → myonecrosis. ↑ CK and aldolase; genetic testing confirms diagnosis. 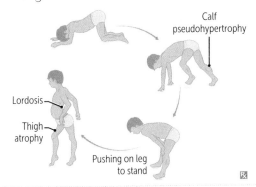
Becker	X-linked recessive disorder typically due to **non-frameshift** deletions in dystrophin gene (partially functional instead of truncated). Less severe than Duchenne (**B**ecker is **b**etter). Onset in adolescence or early adulthood.	Deletions can cause both Duchenne and Becker muscular dystrophies. ⅔ of cases have large deletions spanning one or more exons.
Myotonic dystrophy	Autosomal dominant. Onset 20–30 years. CTG trinucleotide repeat expansion in the *DMPK* gene → abnormal expression of myotonin protein kinase → percussion myotonia (eg, difficulty releasing hand from handshake), muscle wasting, cataracts, testicular atrophy, frontal balding, arrhythmia.	**C**ataracts, **T**oupee (early balding in males), **G**onadal atrophy. Muscle biopsy shows ring fibers and central nuclei.

Mitochondrial diseases

Rare disorders arising 2° to failure in oxidative phosphorylation. Tissues with ↑ energy requirements are preferentially affected (eg, CNS, skeletal muscle).

Mitochondrial myopathies—include **MELAS** (mitochondrial encephalomyopathy with lactic acidosis and strokelike episodes) and **MERRF** (myoclonic epilepsy with ragged red fibers). Light microscopy with stain: ragged red fibers due to compensatory proliferation of mitochondria. Electron microscopy: mitochondrial crystalline inclusions.

Leber hereditary optic neuropathy—mutations in complex I of ETC → neuronal death in retina and optic nerve → subacute bilateral vision loss in teens/young adults (males > females). Usually permanent. May be accompanied by neurologic dysfunction (eg, tremors, multiple sclerosis–like illness).

Rett syndrome

Sporadic disorder caused by de novo mutation of *MECP2* on X chromosome. Seen mostly in females. Embryonically lethal in males. Individuals with **Rett** syndrome experience initial normal development (6–18 months) followed by regression ("**retturn**") in motor, verbal, and cognitive abilities; ataxia; seizures; scoliosis; and stereotypic hand-wringing.

Fragile X syndrome

X-linked (atypical) inheritance. Trinucleotide repeats in *FMR1* → hypermethylation of cytosine residues → ↓ expression.

Most common inherited cause of intellectual disability (Down syndrome is most common genetic cause, but most cases occur sporadically).

Trinucleotide repeat expansion [$(CGG)_n$] occurs during oogenesis.

Premutation (50–200 repeats) → tremor, ataxia, 1° ovarian insufficiency.

Full mutation (>200 repeats) → postpubertal macroorchidism (enlarged testes), long face with large jaw, large everted ears, autism, mitral valve prolapse, hypermobile joints. Self-mutilation is common and can be confused with Lesch-Nyhan syndrome.

Trinucleotide repeat expansion diseases

May show genetic anticipation (disease severity ↑ and age of onset ↓ in successive generations).

DISEASE	TRINUCLEOTIDE REPEAT	MODE OF INHERITANCE	MNEMONIC
Huntington disease	$(CAG)_n$	AD	Caudate has ↓ ACh and GABA
Myotonic dystrophy	$(CTG)_n$	AD	Cataracts, Toupee (early balding in males), Gonadal atrophy in males, reduced fertility in females
Fragile X syndrome	$(CGG)_n$	XD	Chin (protruding), Giant Gonads
Friedreich ataxia	$(GAA)_n$	AR	Ataxic GAAit

Autosomal trisomies	Autosomal trisomies are screened in first and second trimesters with noninvasive prenatal tests. Incidence of trisomies: Down (21) > Edwards (18) > Patau (13). Autosomal monosomies are incompatible with life (high chance of recessive trait expression).	

Down syndrome (trisomy 21)

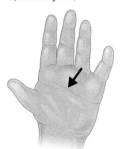

Single palmar crease

Findings: intellectual disability, flat facies, prominent epicanthal folds, single palmar crease, incurved 5th finger, gap between 1st 2 toes, duodenal atresia, Hirschsprung disease, congenital heart disease (eg, AVSD), Brushfield spots (whitish spots at the periphery of the iris). Associated with early-onset Alzheimer disease (chromosome 21 codes for amyloid precursor protein), ↑ risk of AML/ALL.

95% of cases due to meiotic nondisjunction, most commonly during meiosis I (↑ with advanced maternal age: from 1:1500 in females < 20 to 1:25 in females > 45). 4% of cases due to unbalanced Robertsonian translocation, most typically between chromosomes 14 and 21. 1% of cases due to postfertilization mitotic error.

Drinking age (21).

Most common viable chromosomal disorder and most common cause of genetic intellectual disability.

First-trimester ultrasound commonly shows ↑ nuchal translucency and hypoplastic nasal bone. Markers are hi up: ↑ hCG, ↑ inhibin.

↑ risk of umbilical hernia (incomplete closure of umbilical ring).

The 6 As of Down syndrome:
- Atlantoaxial instability
- Advanced maternal age
- Atresia (duodenal)
- Atrioventricular septal defect
- Alzheimer disease (early onset)
- AML (<5 years of age)/ALL (>5 years of age)

Edwards syndrome (trisomy 18)

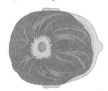

Findings: PRINCE Edward—Prominent occiput, Rocker-bottom feet, Intellectual disability, Nondisjunction, Clenched fists with overlapping fingers, low-set Ears, micrognathia (small jaw), congenital heart disease (eg, VSD), omphalocele, myelomeningocele. Death usually occurs by age 1.

Election age (18).

2nd most common autosomal trisomy resulting in live birth (most common is Down syndrome). In Edwards syndrome, every prenatal screening marker decreases.

Patau syndrome (trisomy 13)

Cutis aplasia

Findings: severe intellectual disability, rocker-bottom feet, microphthalmia, microcephaly, cleft lip/palate, holoprosencephaly, polydactyly, cutis aplasia, congenital heart (pump) disease, polycystic kidney disease, omphalocele. Death usually occurs by age 1.

Puberty at age 13.

Defect in fusion of prechordal mesoderm → midline defects.

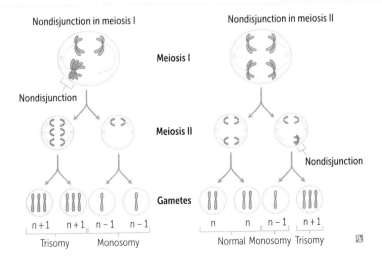

1st trimester screening

Trisomy	β-hCG	PAPP-A
21	↑	↓
18	↓	↓
13	↓	↓

2nd trimester (quadruple) screening

Trisomy	hCG	Inhibin A	Estriol	AFP
21	↑	↑	↓	↓
18	↓	— or ↓	↓	↓
13	—	—	—	—

Genetic disorders by chromosome

CHROMOSOME	SELECTED EXAMPLES
3	von Hippel-Lindau disease, renal cell carcinoma
4	ADPKD (*PKD2*), achondroplasia, Huntington disease
5	Cri-du-chat syndrome, familial adenomatous polyposis
6	Hemochromatosis (*HFE*)
7	Williams syndrome, cystic fibrosis
9	Friedreich ataxia, tuberous sclerosis (*TSC1*)
11	Wilms tumor, β-globin gene defects (eg, sickle cell disease, β-thalassemia), MEN1
13	Patau syndrome, Wilson disease, retinoblastoma (*RB1*), BRCA2
15	Prader-Willi syndrome, Angelman syndrome, Marfan syndrome
16	ADPKD (*PKD1*), α-globin gene defects (eg, α-thalassemia), tuberous sclerosis (*TSC2*)
17	Neurofibromatosis type 1, *BRCA1*, *TP53* (Li-Fraumeni syndrome)
18	Edwards syndrome
21	Down syndrome
22	Neurofibromatosis type 2, DiGeorge syndrome (22q11)
X	Fragile X syndrome, Turner syndrome (XO), XLA, Klinefelter syndrome (XXY)

Robertsonian translocation

Chromosomal translocation that commonly involves chromosome pairs 21, 22, 13, 14, and 15. One of the most common types of translocation. Occurs when the long arms of 2 acrocentric chromosomes (chromosomes with centromeres near their ends) fuse at the centromere and the 2 short arms are lost.

Balanced translocations (no gain or loss of significant genetic material) normally do not cause abnormal phenotype. Unbalanced translocations (missing or extra genes) can result in miscarriage, stillbirth, and chromosomal imbalance (eg, Down syndrome, Patau syndrome).

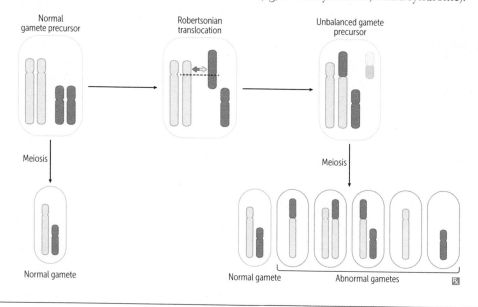

Cri-du-chat syndrome

Cri du chat = cry of the cat. Congenital deletion on short arm of chromosome 5 (46,XX or XY, 5p−). Findings: microcephaly, moderate to severe intellectual disability, high-pitched crying, epicanthal folds, cardiac abnormalities (VSD). I **cry** when I am Very SaD.

Williams syndrome	Congenital microdeletion of long arm of chromosome 7 (deleted region includes elastin gene). Findings: distinctive "elfin" facies, intellectual disability, hypercalcemia, well-developed verbal skills, extreme friendliness with strangers, cardiovascular problems (eg, supravalvular aortic stenosis, pulmonary artery stenosis, renal artery stenosis).

▶ BIOCHEMISTRY—NUTRITION

Essential fatty acids	Polyunsaturated fatty acids that cannot be synthesized in the body and must be provided in the diet (eg, nuts/seeds, plant oils, seafood). Linoleic acid (omega-6) is metabolized to arachidonic acid, which serves as the precursor to leukotrienes and prostaglandins. Linolenic acid (omega-3) and its metabolites have cardioprotective and antihyperlipidemic effects.	In contrast, consumption of *trans*-unsaturated fatty acids (found in fast food) promotes cardiovascular disease by ↑ LDL and ↓ HDL.
Vitamins: fat soluble	A, D, E, K. Absorption dependent on bile emulsification, pancreatic secretions, and intact ileum. Toxicity more common than for water-soluble vitamins because fat-soluble vitamins accumulate in fat.	Malabsorption syndromes with steatorrhea (eg, cystic fibrosis and celiac disease) or mineral oil intake can cause fat-soluble vitamin deficiencies.
Vitamins: water soluble	B_1 (thiamine: TPP) B_2 (riboflavin: FAD, FMN) B_3 (niacin: NAD^+) B_5 (pantothenic acid: CoA) B_6 (pyridoxine: PLP) B_7 (biotin) B_9 (folate) B_{12} (cobalamin) C (ascorbic acid)	Wash out easily from body except B_{12} and B_9. B_{12} stored in liver for ~ 3–4 years. B_9 stored in liver for ~ 3–4 months. B-complex deficiencies often result in dermatitis, glossitis, and diarrhea. Can be coenzymes (eg, ascorbic acid) or precursors to coenzymes (eg, FAD, NAD^+).

Dietary supplementation	DIET	SUPPLEMENTATION REQUIRED
	Vegetarian/vegan	Vitamin B_{12} Iron Vitamin B_2 Frequently, vitamin D (although this is commonly deficient in many diets)
	High egg white (raw)	Vitamin B_7 (avidin in egg whites binds biotin and prevents absorption)
	Untreated corn	Vitamin B_3 (deficiency is common in resource-limited areas)

Vitamin A	Includes retinal, retinol, retinoic acid.	
FUNCTION	Antioxidant; constituent of visual pigments (**retinal**); essential for normal differentiation of epithelial cells into specialized tissue (pancreatic cells, mucus-secreting cells); prevents squamous metaplasia.	**Retinol** is vitamin A, so think **retin-A** (used topically for wrinkles and Acne). Found in liver and leafy vegetables. Supplementation in vitamin A-deficient measles patients may improve outcomes. Use oral isotretinoin to treat severe cystic acne. Use *all*-trans retinoic acid to treat acute promyelocytic leukemia.
DEFICIENCY	Night blindness (nyctalopia); dry, scaly skin (xerosis cutis); dry eyes (xerophthalmia); conjunctival squamous metaplasia → Bitot spots (keratin debris; foamy appearance on conjunctiva A); corneal degeneration (keratomalacia); immunosuppression.	
EXCESS	Acute toxicity—nausea, vomiting, ↑ ICP (eg, vertigo, blurred vision). Chronic toxicity—alopecia, dry skin (eg, scaliness), hepatic toxicity and enlargement, arthralgias, and idiopathic intracranial hypertension.	Teratogenic (interferes with homeobox gene; cleft palate, cardiac abnormalities), therefore a ⊖ pregnancy test and two forms of contraception are required before isotretinoin (vitamin A derivative) is prescribed. **Isotretinoin is terat**ogenic.

Vitamin B₁	Also called thiamine.
FUNCTION	In thiamine pyrophosphate (TPP), a cofactor for several dehydrogenase enzyme reactions (**Be APT**): ▪ Branched-chain ketoacid dehydrogenase ▪ α-Ketoglutarate dehydrogenase (TCA cycle) ▪ Pyruvate dehydrogenase (links glycolysis to TCA cycle) ▪ Transketolase (HMP shunt)
DEFICIENCY	Impaired glucose breakdown → ATP depletion worsened by glucose infusion; highly aerobic tissues (eg, brain, heart) are affected first. In patients with chronic alcohol overuse or malnutrition, give thiamine before dextrose to ↓ risk of precipitating Wernicke encephalopathy. Diagnosis made by ↑ in RBC transketolase activity following vitamin B₁ administration.

DISORDER	CHARACTERISTICS	
Wernicke encephalopathy	Acute, reversible, life-threatening neurologic condition. Symptoms: Confusion, Ophthalmoplegia/ Nystagmus, Ataxia (Cor**ONA** beer).	
Korsakoff syndrome	Amnestic disorder due to chronic alcohol overuse; presents with confabulation, personality changes, memory loss (permanent).	
Wernicke-Korsakoff syndrome	Damage to medial dorsal nucleus of thalamus, mammillary bodies. Presentation is combination of Wernicke encephalopathy and Korsakoff syndrome.	
Dry beriberi	Polyneuropathy, symmetric muscle wasting.	Spell beriberi as **Ber1Ber1** to remember vitamin B₁.
Wet beriberi	High-output cardiac failure (due to systemic vasodilation).	

Vitamin B$_2$ Also called riboflavin.

FUNCTION	Component of flavins FAD and FMN, used as cofactors in redox reactions, eg, the succinate dehydrogenase reaction in the TCA cycle.	FAD and FMN are derived from riboFlavin (B$_2$ ≈ 2 ATP).
DEFICIENCY	Cheilosis **A** (inflammation of lips, scaling and fissures at the corners of the mouth), "magenta" tongue, corneal vascularization.	The 2 C's of B$_2$.

Vitamin B$_3$ Also called niacin, nicotinic acid.

FUNCTION	Constituent of NAD$^+$, NADP$^+$ (used in redox reactions and as cofactor by dehydrogenases). Derived from tryptophan. Synthesis requires vitamins B$_2$ and B$_6$. Used to treat dyslipidemia (↓ VLDL, ↑ HDL).	NAD derived from Niacin (B$_3$ ≈ 3 ATP).
DEFICIENCY	Glossitis. Severe deficiency of B$_3$ leads to pellagra, which can also be caused by Hartnup disease, malignant carcinoid syndrome (↑ tryptophan metabolism → ↑ serotonin synthesis), and isoniazid (↓ vitamin B$_6$). Symptoms of B$_3$ deficiency (pellagra) (the 3 D's): diarrhea, dementia (also hallucinations), dermatitis (C3/C4 dermatome circumferential "broad collar" rash [Casal necklace], hyperpigmentation of sun-exposed limbs **A**).	**Hartnup disease**—autosomal recessive. Deficiency of neutral amino acid (eg, tryptophan) transporters in proximal renal tubular cells and on enterocytes → neutral aminoaciduria and ↓ absorption from the gut → ↓ tryptophan for conversion to niacin → pellagra-like symptoms. Treat with high-protein diet and nicotinic acid. Pellagra = vitamin B$_3$ levels fell.
EXCESS	Facial flushing (induced by prostaglandin, not histamine; can avoid by taking aspirin before niacin), pruritus, hyperglycemia, hyperuricemia.	Podagra = vitamin B$_3$ OD (overdose).

Vitamin B$_5$ Also called pantothenic acid. B$_5$ is "pento"thenic acid.

FUNCTION	Component of coenzyme A (CoA, a cofactor for acyl transfers) and fatty acid synthase.
DEFICIENCY	Dermatitis, enteritis, alopecia, adrenal insufficiency may lead to burning sensation of feet ("burning feet syndrome"; distal paresthesias, dysesthesia).

Vitamin B$_6$	Also called pyridoxine.
FUNCTION	Converted to pyridoxal phosphate (PLP), a cofactor used in transamination (eg, ALT and AST), decarboxylation reactions, glycogen phosphorylase. Synthesis of glutathione, cystathionine, heme, niacin, histamine, and neurotransmitters including serotonin, epinephrine, norepinephrine (NE), dopamine, and GABA.
DEFICIENCY	Convulsions, hyperirritability, peripheral neuropathy (deficiency inducible by isoniazid and oral contraceptives), sideroblastic anemia (due to impaired hemoglobin synthesis and iron excess).

Vitamin B$_7$	Also called biotin.
FUNCTION	Cofactor for carboxylation enzymes (which add a 1-carbon group): ▪ Pyruvate carboxylase (gluconeogenesis): pyruvate (3C) → oxaloacetate (4C) ▪ Acetyl-CoA carboxylase (fatty acid synthesis): acetyl-CoA (2C) → malonyl-CoA (3C) ▪ Propionyl-CoA carboxylase (fatty acid oxidation and branched-chain amino acid breakdown): propionyl-CoA (3C) → methylmalonyl-CoA (4C)
DEFICIENCY	Relatively rare. Dermatitis, enteritis, alopecia. Caused by long-term antibiotic use or excessive ingestion of raw egg whites. "**Avid**in in egg whites **avid**ly binds biotin."

Vitamin B$_9$	Also called folate.
FUNCTION	Converted to tetrahydrofolic acid (THF), a coenzyme for 1-carbon transfer/methylation reactions. Important for the synthesis of nitrogenous bases in DNA and RNA.	Found in leafy green vegetables. Also produced by gut microbiota. Folate absorbed in jejunum (think foliage in the "jejun"gle). Small reserve pool stored primarily in the liver.
DEFICIENCY	Macrocytic, megaloblastic anemia; hypersegmented polymorphonuclear cells (PMNs); glossitis; no neurologic symptoms (as opposed to vitamin B$_{12}$ deficiency). Labs: ↑ homocysteine, normal methylmalonic acid levels. Seen in chronic alcohol overuse and in pregnancy.	Deficiency can be caused by several drugs (eg, phenytoin, trimethoprim, methotrexate). Supplemental folic acid at least 1 month prior to conception and during pregnancy to ↓ risk of neural tube defects. Give vitamin B$_9$ for the 9 months of pregnancy, and 1 month prior to conception.

Vitamin B$_{12}$	Also called cobalamin.	
FUNCTION	Cofactor for methionine synthase (transfers CH$_3$ groups as methylcobalamin) and methylmalonyl-CoA mutase. Important for DNA synthesis.	Found in animal products. Synthesized only by intestinal microbiota. Site of synthesis in humans is distal to site of absorption; thus B$_{12}$ must be consumed via animal products.
DEFICIENCY	Macrocytic, megaloblastic anemia; hypersegmented PMNs; paresthesias and subacute combined degeneration (degeneration of dorsal columns, lateral corticospinal tracts, and spinocerebellar tracts) due to abnormal myelin. Associated with ↑ serum homocysteine and methylmalonic acid levels, along with 2° folate deficiency. Prolonged deficiency → irreversible nerve damage.	Very large reserve pool (several years) stored primarily in the liver. Deficiency caused by malabsorption (eg, sprue, enteritis, *Diphyllobothrium latum*, achlorhydria, bacterial overgrowth, alcohol overuse), lack of intrinsic factor (eg, pernicious anemia, gastric bypass surgery), absence of terminal ileum (surgical resection, eg, for Crohn disease), certain drugs (eg, metformin), or insufficient intake (eg, veganism). B$_9$ (folate) supplementation can mask the hematologic symptoms of B$_{12}$ deficiency, but not the neurologic symptoms.

Vitamin C	Also called ascorbic acid.	
FUNCTION	Antioxidant; also facilitates iron absorption by reducing it to Fe^{2+} state. Necessary for hydroxylation of proline and lysine in collagen synthesis. Necessary for dopamine β-hydroxylase (converts dopamine to NE).	Found in fruits and vegetables. Pronounce "absorbic" acid. Ancillary treatment for methemoglobinemia by reducing Fe^{3+} to Fe^{2+}.
DEFICIENCY	**Scurvy**—swollen gums, easy bruising, petechiae, hemarthrosis, anemia, poor wound healing, perifollicular and subperiosteal hemorrhages, "corkscrew" hair. Weakened immune response.	Deficiency may be precipitated by tea and toast diet. Vitamin C deficiency causes sCurvy due to a Collagen hydroCylation defect.
EXCESS	Nausea, vomiting, diarrhea, fatigue, calcium oxalate nephrolithiasis (excess oxalate from vitamin C metabolism). Can ↑ iron toxicity in predisposed individuals by increasing dietary iron absorption (ie, can worsen hemochromatosis or transfusion-related iron overload).	

Vitamin D

D_3 (cholecalciferol) from exposure of skin (stratum basale) to sun, ingestion of fish, milk, plants.
D_2 (ergocalciferol) from ingestion of plants, fungi, yeasts.
Both converted to 25-OH D_3 (storage form) in liver and to the active form 1,25-$(OH)_2$ D_3 (calcitriol) in kidney.

FUNCTION	↑ intestinal absorption of Ca^{2+} and PO_4^{3-}. ↑ bone mineralization at low levels. ↑ bone resorption at higher levels.
REGULATION	↑ PTH, ↓ Ca^{2+}, ↓ PO_4^{3-} → ↑ 1,25-$(OH)_2D_3$ production. 1,25-$(OH)_2D_3$ feedback inhibits its own production. ↑ PTH → ↑ Ca^{2+} reabsorption and ↓ PO_4^{3-} reabsorption in the kidney.
DEFICIENCY	Rickets in children (deformity, such as genu varum "bowlegs" A), osteomalacia in adults (bone pain and muscle weakness), hypocalcemic tetany. Caused by malabsorption, ↓ sun exposure, poor diet, chronic kidney disease (CKD), advanced liver disease. Give oral vitamin D to breastfed infants. Darker skin and prematurity predispose to deficiency.
EXCESS	Hypercalcemia, hypercalciuria, loss of appetite, stupor. Seen in granulomatous diseases (↑ activation of vitamin D by epithelioid macrophages).

Diet   Cholesterol →
7-dehydrocholesterol
Sun/UV exposure
D_2 (Ergocalciferol) D_3 (Cholecalciferol)
25-hydroxylase
25-OH D_3
↓ Ca^{2+}, ↓ PO_4^{3-}
⊕
1α-hydroxylase
⊖
1,25-$(OH)_2$ D_3

Bone   Intestines   Renal tubular cells

↑ Ca^{2+} and ↑ PO_4^{3-} released from bone   ↑ absorption of Ca^{2+} and PO_4^{3-} Reabsorption: ↑ Ca^{2+}, ↑ PO_4^{3-}
 Urine: ↓ Ca^{2+}, ↓ PO_4^{3-}

↑ Ca^{2+} and ↑ PO_4^{3-}

Vitamin E

Includes tocopherol, tocotrienol.

FUNCTION	Antioxidant (protects RBCs and neuronal membranes from free radical damage).	
DEFICIENCY	Hemolytic anemia, acanthocytosis, muscle weakness, demyelination of posterior columns (↓ proprioception and vibration sensation) and spinocerebellar tract (ataxia). Closely mimics Friedreich ataxia.	Neurologic presentation may appear similar to vitamin B_{12} deficiency, but without megaloblastic anemia, hypersegmented neutrophils, or ↑ serum methylmalonic acid levels.
EXCESS	Risk of enterocolitis in enfants (infants) with excess of vitamin E.	High-dose supplementation may alter metabolism of vitamin K–dependent proteins (factors II, VII, IX, X; protein C/S) → enhanced anticoagulant effects of warfarin.

Vitamin K	Includes phytomenadione, phylloquinone, phytonadione, menaquinone.	
FUNCTION	Activated by epoxide reductase to the reduced form, which is a cofactor for the γ-carboxylation of glutamic acid residues on various proteins required for blood clotting. Synthesized by intestinal microbiota; dietary sources include leafy greens.	**K** is for **K**oagulation. Necessary for the maturation of clotting factors II, VII, IX, X, and proteins C and S. Warfarin inhibits vitamin K–dependent synthesis of these factors and proteins.
DEFICIENCY	Neonatal hemorrhage with ↑ PT and ↑ aPTT but normal bleeding time (neonates have sterile intestines and are unable to synthesize vitamin K). Can also occur after prolonged use of broad-spectrum antibiotics or hepatocellular disease.	Not in breast milk; "breast-fed infants **D**on't **K**now about vitamins **D** and **K**". Neonates are given vitamin K injection at birth to prevent hemorrhagic disease of the newborn.

Zinc		
FUNCTION	Mineral essential for the activity of 100+ enzymes. Important in the formation of zinc fingers (transcription factor motif).	
DEFICIENCY	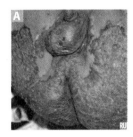 Delayed wound healing, suppressed immunity, male hypogonadism, ↓ adult hair (axillary, facial, pubic), dysgeusia, anosmia. Associated with **acrodermatitis enteropathica** 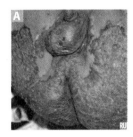—congenital defect in intestinal zinc absorption manifesting with triad of hair loss, diarrhea, and inflammatory skin rash around body openings (periorificial) and tips of fingers/toes (acral). May predispose to alcoholic cirrhosis.	

Protein-energy malnutrition		
Kwashiorkor	Protein malnutrition resulting in skin lesions, edema due to ↓ plasma oncotic pressure (arising from ↓ serum albumin and ↓ antidiuretic hormone), liver malfunction (fatty change due to ↓ apolipoprotein synthesis and deposition). Clinical picture is small child with swollen abdomen 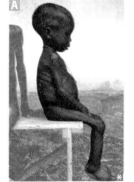. Kwashiorkor results from protein-deficient **MEALS**: **M**alnutrition **E**dema **A**nemia **L**iver (fatty) **S**kin lesions (eg, hyperkeratosis, dyspigmentation)	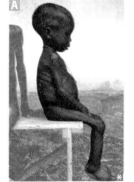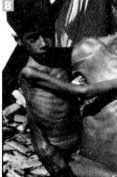
Marasmus	Malnutrition not causing edema. Diet is deficient in calories but no nutrients are entirely absent.	Marasmus results in muscle wasting 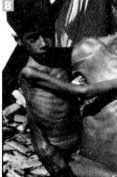. Linear growth maintained in acute protein-energy malnutrition (vs chronic malnutrition).

Ethanol metabolism

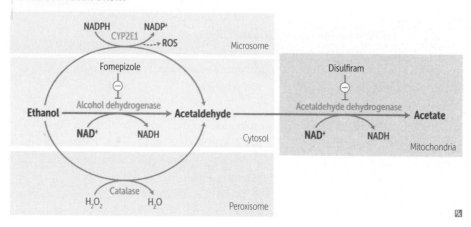

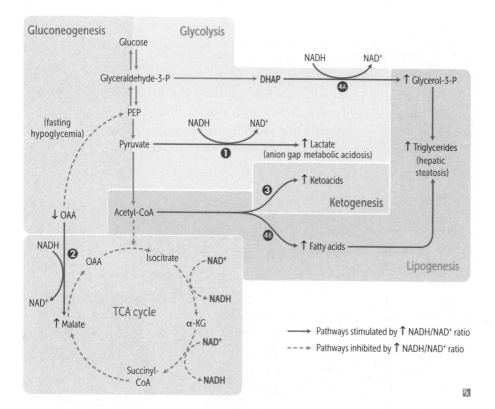

Pathways stimulated by ↑ NADH/NAD⁺ ratio
Pathways inhibited by ↑ NADH/NAD⁺ ratio

↑ NADH/NAD⁺ ratio inhibits TCA cycle → ↑ acetyl-CoA used in ketogenesis (→ ketoacidosis), lipogenesis (→ hepatosteatosis). Females are more susceptible than males to effects of alcohol due to ↓ activity of gastric alcohol dehydrogenase, ↓ body size, ↓ percentage of water in body weight.

NAD⁺ is the limiting reagent. Alcohol dehydrogenase operates via zero-order kinetics.

Ethanol metabolism ↑ NADH/NAD⁺ ratio in liver, causing:
❶ Lactic acidosis—↑ pyruvate conversion to lactate
❷ Fasting hypoglycemia— ↓ gluconeogenesis due to ↑ conversion of OAA to malate
❸ Ketoacidosis—diversion of acetyl-CoA into ketogenesis rather than TCA cycle
❹ Hepatosteatosis— ↑ conversion of DHAP to glycerol-3-P ❹ⓐ; acetyl-CoA diverges into fatty acid synthesis ❹ⓑ, which combines with glycerol-3-P to synthesize triglycerides

Fomepizole—competitive inhibitor of alcohol dehydrogenase; preferred antidote for overdoses of methanol or ethylene glycol. Alcohol dehydrogenase has higher affinity for ethanol than for methanol or ethylene glycol → ethanol can be used as competitive inhibitor of alcohol dehydrogenase to treat methanol or ethylene glycol poisoning.

Disulfiram—blocks acetaldehyde dehydrogenase → ↑ acetaldehyde → ↑ hangover symptoms → discouraging drinking.

▶ BIOCHEMISTRY—METABOLISM

Enzyme terminology	An enzyme's name often describes its function. For example, glucokinase is an enzyme that catalyzes the phosphorylation of glucose using a molecule of ATP. The following are commonly used enzyme descriptors.
Kinase	Catalyzes transfer of a phosphate group from a high-energy molecule (usually ATP) to a substrate (eg, phosphofructokinase).
Phosphorylase	Adds inorganic phosphate onto substrate without using ATP (eg, glycogen phosphorylase).
Phosphatase	Removes phosphate group from substrate (eg, fructose-1,6-bisphosphatase 1).
Dehydrogenase	Catalyzes oxidation-reduction reactions (eg, pyruvate dehydrogenase).
Hydroxylase	Adds hydroxyl group (–OH) onto substrate (eg, tyrosine hydroxylase).
Carboxylase	Transfers carboxyl groups (–COOH) with the help of biotin (eg, pyruvate carboxylase).
Mutase	Relocates a functional group within a molecule (eg, vitamin B_{12}–dependent methylmalonyl-CoA mutase).
Synthase	Catalyzes synthesis reactions without using ATP as a source of energy.

Rate-determining enzymes of metabolic processes

PROCESS	ENZYME	REGULATORS
Glycolysis	Phosphofructokinase-1 (PFK-1)	AMP ⊕, fructose-2,6-bisphosphate ⊕ ATP ⊖, citrate ⊖
Gluconeogenesis	Fructose-1,6-bisphosphatase 1	AMP ⊖, fructose-2,6-bisphosphate ⊖
TCA cycle	Isocitrate dehydrogenase	ADP ⊕ ATP ⊖, NADH ⊖
Glycogenesis	Glycogen synthase	Glucose-6-phosphate ⊕, insulin ⊕, cortisol ⊕ Epinephrine ⊖, glucagon ⊖
Glycogenolysis	Glycogen phosphorylase	Epinephrine ⊕, glucagon ⊕, AMP ⊕ Glucose-6-phosphate ⊖, insulin ⊖, ATP ⊖
HMP shunt	Glucose-6-phosphate dehydrogenase (G6PD)	$NADP^+$ ⊕ NADPH ⊖
De novo pyrimidine synthesis	Carbamoyl phosphate synthetase II	ATP ⊕, PRPP ⊕ UTP ⊖
De novo purine synthesis	Glutamine-phosphoribosylpyrophosphate (PRPP) amidotransferase	PRPP ⊕, AMP ⊖, inosine monophosphate (IMP) ⊖, GMP ⊖
Urea cycle	Carbamoyl phosphate synthetase I	N-acetylglutamate ⊕
Fatty acid synthesis	Acetyl-CoA carboxylase (ACC)	Insulin ⊕, citrate ⊕ Glucagon ⊖, palmitoyl-CoA ⊖
Fatty acid oxidation	Carnitine acyltransferase I	Malonyl-CoA ⊖
Ketogenesis	HMG-CoA synthase (HOMG! I'm starving!)	
Cholesterol synthesis	HMG-CoA reductase	Insulin ⊕, thyroxine ⊕, estrogen ⊕ Glucagon ⊖, cholesterol ⊖

Metabolic compartmentation

Mitochondria	Fatty acid oxidation (β-oxidation), acetyl-CoA production, TCA cycle, oxidative phosphorylation, ketogenesis.
Cytoplasm	Glycolysis, HMP shunt, and synthesis of cholesterol (SER), proteins (ribosomes, RER), fatty acids, and nucleotides.
Both	Heme synthesis, urea cycle, gluconeogenesis. Hugs take two (both).

Summary of pathways

1. Galactokinase *(mild galactosemia)*
2. Galactose-1-phosphate uridyltransferase *(severe galactosemia)*
3. Hexokinase/glucokinase
4. Glucose-6-phosphatase *(von Gierke disease)*
5. Glucose-6-phosphate dehydrogenase
6. Transketolase
7. Phosphofructokinase-1
8. Fructose-1,6-bisphosphatase 1
9. Fructokinase *(essential fructosuria)*
10. Aldolase B *(fructose intolerance)*
11. Aldolase B *(liver)*, A *(muscle)*
12. Triose phosphate isomerase
13. Pyruvate kinase
14. Pyruvate dehydrogenase
15. Pyruvate carboxylase
16. PEP carboxykinase
17. Citrate synthase
18. Isocitrate dehydrogenase
19. α-ketoglutarate dehydrogenase
20. Carbamoyl phosphate synthetase I
21. Ornithine transcarbamylase
22. Propionyl-CoA carboxylase
23. HMG-CoA reductase

- B Requires biotin cofactor
- T Requires thiamine cofactor *(TPP)*
- # Irreversible, important point of regulation

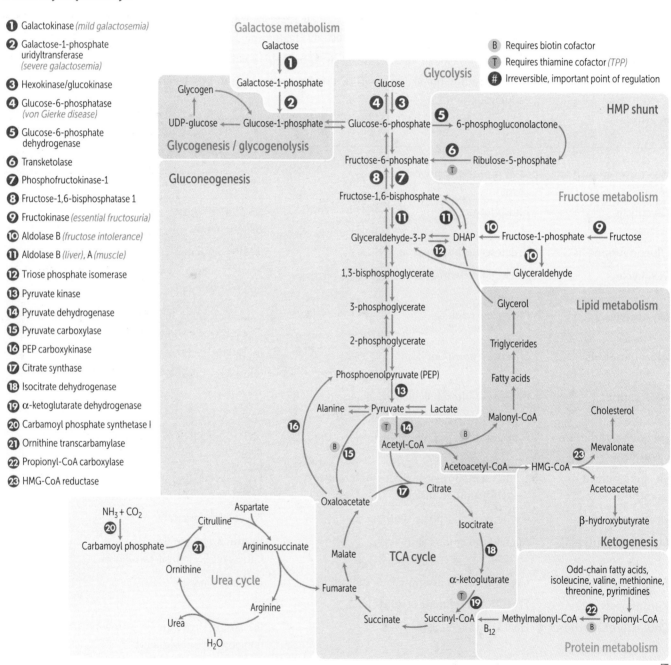

Activated carriers

CARRIER MOLECULE	CARRIED IN ACTIVATED FORM
ATP	Phosphoryl groups
NADH, NADPH, $FADH_2$	Electrons
CoA, lipoamide	Acyl groups
Biotin	CO_2
Tetrahydrofolates	1-carbon units
S-adenosylmethionine (SAM)	CH_3 groups
TPP	Aldehydes

Universal electron acceptors

Nicotinamides (NAD^+, $NADP^+$ from vitamin B_3) and flavin nucleotides (FAD from vitamin B_2). NAD^+ is generally used in **catabolic** processes to carry reducing equivalents away as NADH. NADPH is used in **anabolic** processes (eg, steroid and fatty acid synthesis) as a supply of reducing equivalents.

NADPH is a product of the HMP shunt.
NADPH is used in:
- Anabolic processes
- Respiratory burst
- Cytochrome P-450 system
- Glutathione reductase

Hexokinase vs glucokinase

Phosphorylation of glucose to yield glucose-6-phosphate is catalyzed by glucokinase in the liver and hexokinase in other tissues. Hexokinase sequesters glucose in tissues, where it is used even when glucose concentrations are low. At high glucose concentrations, glucokinase helps to store glucose in liver. Glucokinase deficiency (→ ↑↑ glucose needed for activation → impaired insulin release [vs. diabetes mellitus]) is a cause of maturity onset diabetes of the young (MODY) and gestational diabetes.

	Hexokinase	Glucokinase
Location	Most tissues, except liver and pancreatic β cells	Liver, β cells of pancreas
K_m	Lower (↑ affinity)	Higher (↓ affinity)
V_{max}	Lower (↓ capacity)	Higher (↑ capacity)
Induced by insulin	No	Yes
Feedback inhibition by	Glucose-6-phosphate	Fructose-6-phosphate

Glycolysis regulation, key enzymes	Net glycolysis (cytoplasm): Glucose + 2 P_i + 2 ADP + 2 NAD^+ → 2 pyruvate + 2 ATP + 2 NADH + 2 H^+ + 2 H_2O. Equation not balanced chemically, and exact balanced equation depends on ionization state of reactants and products.

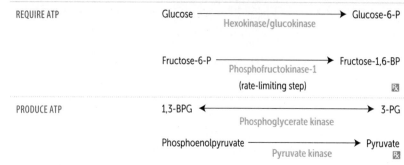

REQUIRE ATP	Glucose-6-P ⊖ hexokinase. Fructose-6-P ⊖ glucokinase.
	AMP ⊕, fructose-2,6-bisphosphate ⊕. ATP ⊖, citrate ⊖.
PRODUCE ATP	
	Fructose-1,6-bisphosphate ⊕. ATP ⊖, alanine ⊖, glucagon ⊖, epinephrine ⊖.

Regulation by fructose-2,6-bisphosphate	Fructose bisphosphatase-2 (FBPase-2) and phosphofructokinase-2 (PFK-2) are the same bifunctional enzyme whose function is reversed by phosphorylation by protein kinase A.

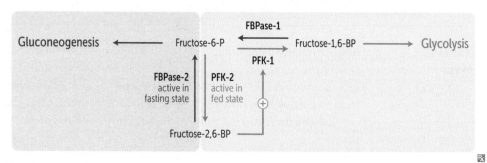

Fasting state: ↑ glucagon → ↑ cAMP → ↑ protein kinase A → ↑ FBPase-2, ↓ PFK-2, less glycolysis, more gluconeogenesis.	Fa**B**ian the **P**easant (**FBP**) has to work hard when starving.
Fed state: ↑ insulin → ↑ PFK-2 → more glycolysis, less gluconeogenesis.	Prince Frederic**K** (**PFK**) works only when fed.

Pyruvate dehydrogenase complex	Mitochondrial enzyme complex linking glycolysis and TCA cycle. Differentially regulated in fed (active)/fasting (inactive) states. Reaction: pyruvate + NAD^+ + CoA → acetyl-CoA + CO_2 + NADH. Contains 3 enzymes requiring 5 cofactors: 　1. Thiamine pyrophosphate (B_1) 　2. Lipoic acid 　3. CoA (B_5, pantothenic acid) 　4. FAD (B_2, riboflavin) 　5. NAD^+ (B_3, niacin) Activated by: ↑ NAD^+/NADH ratio, ↑ ADP ↑ Ca^{2+}.	The complex is similar to the α-ketoglutarate dehydrogenase complex (same cofactors, similar substrate and action), which converts α-ketoglutarate → succinyl-CoA (TCA cycle). **T**he **l**ovely **c**oenzymes **f**or **n**erds. Arsenic inhibits lipoic acid. Arsenic poisoning clinical findings: imagine a vampire (pigmentary skin changes, skin cancer), vomiting and having diarrhea, running away from a cutie (QT prolongation) with garlic breath.

Pyruvate dehydrogenase complex deficiency	Causes a buildup of pyruvate that gets shunted to lactate (via LDH) and alanine (via ALT). X-linked.
FINDINGS	Neurologic defects, lactic acidosis, ↑ serum alanine starting in infancy.
TREATMENT	↑ intake of ketogenic nutrients (eg, high fat content or ↑ lysine and leucine), B_1 and lipoic acid.

Pyruvate metabolism

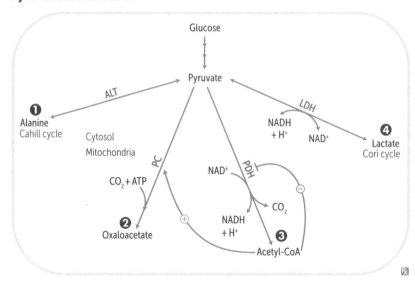

Functions of different pyruvate metabolic pathways (and their associated cofactors):

❶ Alanine aminotransferase (B_6): alanine carries amino groups to the liver from muscle

❷ Pyruvate carboxylase (B_7): oxaloacetate can replenish TCA cycle or be used in gluconeogenesis

❸ Pyruvate dehydrogenase (B_1, B_2, B_3, B_5, lipoic acid): transition from glycolysis to the TCA cycle

❹ Lactic acid dehydrogenase (B_3): end of anaerobic glycolysis (major pathway in RBCs, WBCs, kidney medulla, lens, cornea, and Sertoli cells in testes)

TCA cycle

Pyruvate (3C)
CO_2 + **NADH**
PDH — ⊖ — ATP / Acetyl-CoA / NADH
Acetyl-CoA (2C)
⊖ — ATP
Citrate synthase
Oxaloacetate (4C)
Citrate (6C)
cis-Aconitate
NADH
Isocitrate (6C)
Malate (4C)
CO_2 + **NADH**
Isocitrate dehydrogenase — ⊖ — ATP / NADH — ⊕ — ADP
Fumarate (4C)
α-KG (5C)
FADH₂
Succinate (4C)
α-KG dehydrogenase
CO_2 + **NADH**
GTP + CoA
Succinyl-CoA (4C)
⊖ — Succinyl-CoA / NADH / ATP

* Enzymes are irreversible

Also called Krebs cycle. Pyruvate → acetyl-CoA produces 1 NADH, 1 CO_2.

The TCA cycle produces 3 NADH, 1 $FADH_2$, 2 CO_2, 1 GTP per acetyl-CoA = 10 ATP/ acetyl-CoA (2× everything per glucose). TCA cycle reactions occur in the mitochondria.

α-ketoglutarate dehydrogenase complex requires the same cofactors as the pyruvate dehydrogenase complex (vitamins B_1, B_2, B_3, B_5, lipoic acid).

Citrate is Krebs' starting substrate for making oxaloacetate.

Electron transport chain and oxidative phosphorylation	NADH electrons are transferred to complex I. FADH$_2$ electrons are transferred to complex II (at a lower energy level than NADH). Oxygen acts as an electron acceptor to provide energy. The passage of electrons results in the formation of a proton gradient that, coupled to oxidative phosphorylation, drives ATP production. ATP hydrolysis can be coupled to energetically unfavorable reactions. Uncoupling proteins (found in brown fat, which has more mitochondria than white fat) produce heat by ↑ inner mitochondrial membrane permeability → ↓ proton gradient. ATP synthesis stops, but electron transport continues.	1 NADH → 2.5 ATP; 1 FADH$_2$ → 1.5 ATP NADH electrons from glycolysis enter mitochondria via the malate-aspartate or glycerol-3-phosphate shuttle. Aerobic metabolism of one glucose molecule produces 32 net ATP via malate-aspartate shuttle (heart and liver), 30 net ATP via glycerol-3-phosphate shuttle (muscle). Anaerobic glycolysis produces only 2 net ATP per glucose molecule. Aspirin overdose can also cause uncoupling of oxidative phosphorylation resulting in hyperthermia.

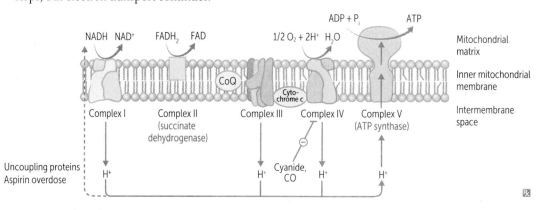

Gluconeogenesis, irreversible enzymes	All enzymes may be subject to activation by glucagon in fasting state.	Pathway produces fresh glucose.
Pyruvate carboxylase	In mitochondria. Pyruvate → oxaloacetate.	Requires biotin, ATP. Activated by acetyl-CoA.
Phosphoenolpyruvate carboxykinase	In cytosol. Oxaloacetate → phosphoenolpyruvate (PEP).	Requires GTP.
Fructose-1,6-bisphosphatase 1	In cytosol. Fructose-1,6-bisphosphate → fructose-6-phosphate.	Citrate ⊕, AMP ⊖, fructose 2,6-bisphosphate ⊖.
Glucose-6-phosphatase	In ER. Glucose-6-phosphate → glucose.	

Occurs primarily in liver; serves to maintain euglycemia during fasting. Enzymes also found in kidney, intestinal epithelium. Deficiency of the key gluconeogenic enzymes causes hypoglycemia. (Muscle cannot participate in gluconeogenesis because it lacks glucose-6-phosphatase).

Odd-chain **fatty acids** yield 1 propionyl-CoA during metabolism, which can enter the TCA cycle (as succinyl-CoA), undergo gluconeogenesis, and serve as a **glucose** source (It's **odd** for **fatty acids** to make **glucose**). Even-chain fatty acids cannot produce new glucose, since they yield only acetyl-CoA equivalents.

Pentose phosphate pathway	Also called HMP shunt. Provides a source of NADPH from abundantly available glucose-6-P (NADPH is required for reductive reactions, eg, glutathione reduction inside RBCs, fatty acid and cholesterol biosynthesis). Additionally, this pathway yields ribose for nucleotide synthesis. Two distinct phases (oxidative and nonoxidative), both of which occur in the cytoplasm. No ATP is used or produced. Sites: lactating mammary glands, liver, adrenal cortex (sites of fatty acid or steroid synthesis), RBCs.

REACTIONS

Oxidative (irreversible)

Nonoxidative (reversible)

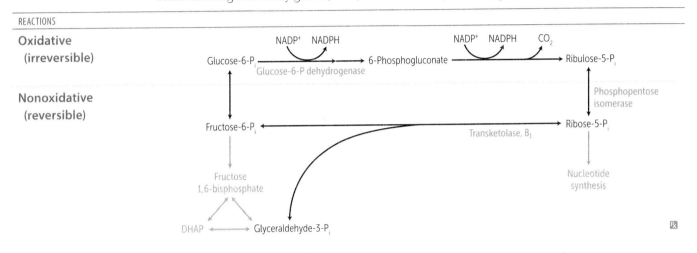

Glucose-6-phosphate dehydrogenase deficiency	NADPH is necessary to keep glutathione reduced, which in turn detoxifies free radicals and peroxides. ↓ NADPH in RBCs leads to hemolytic anemia due to poor RBC defense against oxidizing agents (eg, fava beans, sulfonamides, nitrofurantoin, primaquine). Infection (most common cause) can also precipitate hemolysis; inflammatory response produces free radicals that diffuse into RBCs, causing oxidative damage.

X-linked recessive disorder; most common human enzyme deficiency; more prevalent among descendants of populations in malaria-endemic regions (eg, sub-Saharan Africa, Southeast Asia).

Heinz bodies—denatured globin chains precipitate within RBCs due to oxidative stress.

Bite cells—result from the phagocytic removal of **Heinz** bodies by splenic macrophages. Think, "**Bite** into some **Heinz** ketchup."

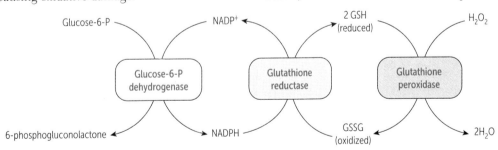

Disorders of fructose metabolism

	Essential fructosuria	Hereditary fructose intolerance
ENZYME DEFICIENCY	Fructokinase (autosomal recessive)	Aldolase B (autosomal recessive)
PATHOPHYSIOLOGY	Fructose is not trapped into cells. Hexokinase becomes 1° pathway for converting fructose to fructose-1-phosphate.	Fructose-1-phosphate accumulates → ↓ available phosphate → inhibition of glycogenolysis and gluconeogenesis.
PRESENTATION (SIGNS/SYMPTOMS)	Asymptomatic, benign. Fructose appears in blood and urine (fructo**kin**ase deficiency is **kinder**).	Hypoglycemia, jaundice, cirrhosis, vomiting. Symptoms only present following consumption of fruit, juice, or honey.
ADDITIONAL REMARKS	Urine dipstick will be ⊖ (tests for glucose only); reducing sugar can be detected in the urine (nonspecific test for inborn errors of carbohydrate metabolism).	
TREATMENT	–	↓ intake of fructose, sucrose (glucose + fructose), and sorbitol (metabolized to fructose).

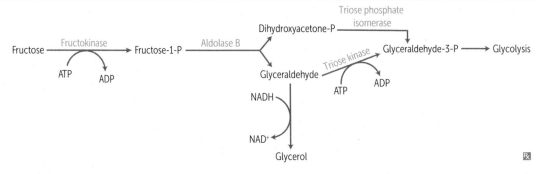

Disorders of galactose metabolism

	Galactokinase deficiency	Classic galactosemia
ENZYME DEFICIENCY	Galactokinase (autosomal recessive).	Galactose-1-phosphate uridyltransferase (autosomal recessive).
PATHOPHYSIOLOGY	Galactitol accumulates if diet has galactose.	Damage caused by accumulation of toxic substances (eg, galactitol).
PRESENTATION (SIGNS/SYMPTOMS)	Relatively mild/benign condition (galacto**kin**ase deficiency is **kinder**). Galactose appears in blood (galactosemia) and urine (galactosuria); infantile cataracts. May present as failure to track objects or develop social smile.	Symptoms start when infant is fed formula or breast milk → failure to thrive, jaundice, hepatomegaly, infantile cataracts (galacitol deposition in eye lens), intellectual disability. Can predispose neonates to *E coli* sepsis.
TREATMENT	–	Exclude galactose and lactose (galactose + glucose) from diet.

Galactose → (Galactokinase, ATP → ADP) → Galactose-1-P → (Uridylyltransferase) → Glucose-1-P

Galactose → (Aldose reductase) → Galactitol

Galactose-1-P ↔ (UDP-Glu UDP-Gal, 4-Epimerase) → Glucose-1-P → Glycolysis/glycogenesis

Sorbitol	An alternative method of trapping glucose in the cell is to convert it to its alcohol counterpart, sorbitol, via aldose reductase. Some tissues then convert sorbitol to fructose using sorbitol dehydrogenase; tissues with an insufficient amount/activity of this enzyme are at risk of intracellular sorbitol accumulation, causing osmotic damage (eg, cataracts, retinopathy, and peripheral neuropathy seen with chronic hyperglycemia in diabetes).

High blood levels of galactose also result in conversion to the osmotically active galactitol via aldose reductase.

Liver, ovaries, and seminal vesicles have both enzymes (they **lose** sorbitol).

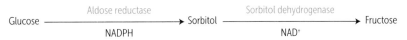

Lens has primarily Aldose reductase. Retina, Kidneys, and Schwann cells have only aldose reductase (**LARKS**).

Lactase deficiency	Insufficient lactase enzyme → dietary lactose intolerance. Lactase functions on the intestinal brush border to digest lactose (in milk and milk products) into glucose and galactose. Primary: age-dependent decline after childhood (absence of lactase-persistent allele), common in people of Asian, African, or Native American descent. Secondary: loss of intestinal brush border due to gastroenteritis (eg, rotavirus), autoimmune disease. Congenital lactase deficiency: rare, due to defective gene. Stool demonstrates ↓ pH and breath shows ↑ hydrogen content with lactose hydrogen breath test (H^+ is produced when colonic bacteria ferment undigested lactose). Intestinal biopsy reveals normal mucosa in patients with hereditary lactose intolerance.
FINDINGS	Bloating, cramps, flatulence (all due to fermentation of lactose by colonic bacteria → gas), and osmotic diarrhea (undigested lactose).
TREATMENT	Avoid dairy products or add lactase pills to diet; lactose-free milk.

Amino acids	Only L-amino acids are found in proteins.
Essential	**PVT TIM HaLL**: Phenylalanine, Valine, Tryptophan, Threonine, Isoleucine, Methionine, Histidine, Leucine, Lysine. Glucogenic: Methionine, histidine, valine. We **met his valentine**, who is so **sweet** (**glucogenic**). Glucogenic/ketogenic: Isoleucine, phenylalanine, threonine, tryptophan. Ketogenic: leucine, lysine. The only purely ketogenic amino acids.
Acidic	Aspartic **acid**, glutamic **acid**. Negatively charged at body pH.
Basic	Histidine, lysine, arginine. Arginine is most **basic**. Histidine has no charge at body pH. Arginine and histidine are required during periods of growth. Arginine and lysine are ↑ in histones which bind negatively charged DNA. **His lys** (lies) **are** basic.

Urea cycle

Amino acid catabolism generates common metabolites (eg, pyruvate, acetyl-CoA), which serve as metabolic fuels. Excess nitrogen is converted to urea and excreted by the kidneys.

Ordinarily, Careless Crappers Are Also Frivolous About Urination.

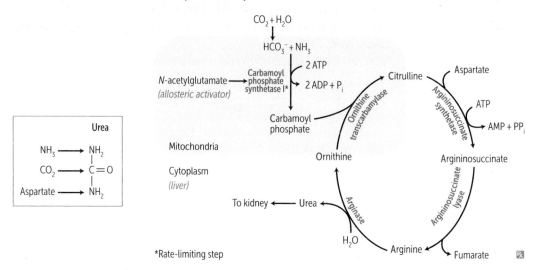

*Rate-limiting step

Transport of ammonia by alanine

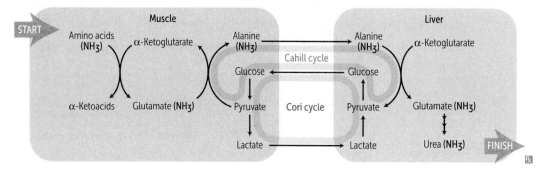

Hyperammonemia

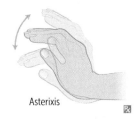

Asterixis

Can be acquired (eg, liver disease) or hereditary (eg, urea cycle enzyme deficiencies).

Presents with flapping tremor (asterixis), slurring of speech, somnolence, vomiting, cerebral edema, blurring of vision.

↑ NH_3 causes CNS toxicity, involving:
- TCA cycle inhibition (↓ α-ketoglutarate)
- ↓ glutamate
- ↑ GABAergic tone (↑ GABA)
- ↑ glutamine
- Cerebral edema (glutamine induced osmotic shifts)

Treatment: limit protein in diet.

May be given to ↓ ammonia levels:
- Lactulose to acidify GI tract and trap NH_4^+ for excretion.
- Antibiotics (eg, rifaximin) to ↓ ammoniagenic bacteria.
- Benzoate, phenylacetate, or phenylbutyrate react with glycine or glutamine, forming products that are excreted renally.

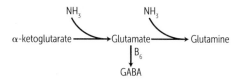

Ornithine transcarbamylase deficiency

Most common urea cycle disorder. X-linked recessive (vs other urea cycle enzyme deficiencies, which are autosomal recessive). Interferes with the body's ability to eliminate ammonia. Often evident in the first few days of life, but may present later. Excess carbamoyl phosphate is converted to orotic acid (part of the pyrimidine synthesis pathway; vs. carbamoyl phosphate synthetase I deficiency).

Findings: ↑ orotic acid in blood and urine, ↓ BUN, symptoms of hyperammonemia. No megaloblastic anemia (vs orotic aciduria).

Amino acid derivatives

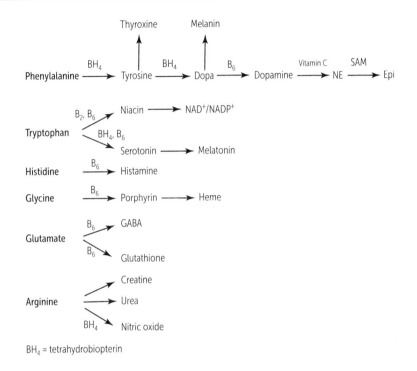

BH_4 = tetrahydrobiopterin

Catecholamine synthesis/tyrosine catabolism

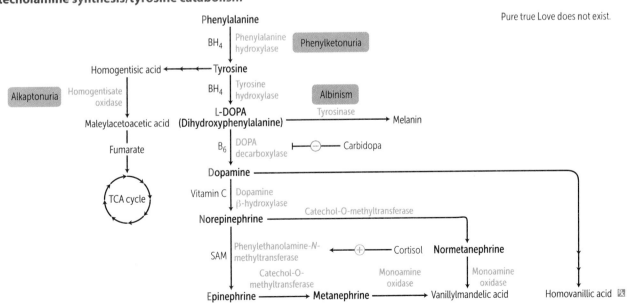

Pure true Love does not exist.

Phenylketonuria

Caused by ↓ phenylalanine hydroxylase (PAH). Tyrosine becomes essential. ↑ phenylalanine → ↑ phenyl ketones in urine.

Tetrahydrobiopterin (BH_4) deficiency—BH_4 essential cofactor for PAH. BH_4 deficiency → ↑ phenylalanine. Varying degrees of clinical severity. Untreated patients typically die in infancy.

Phenylalanine embryopathy—↑ phenylalanine levels in pregnant patients with untreated phenylketonuria (PKU) can cause fetal growth restriction, microcephaly, intellectual disability, congenital heart defects. Can be prevented with dietary measures.

Autosomal recessive.

Screening occurs 2–3 days after birth (normal at birth because of maternal enzyme during fetal life).

Findings: intellectual disability, microcephaly, seizures, hypopigmented skin, eczema, musty body odor. Findings are rare due to neonatal screening.

Treatment: ↓ phenylalanine and ↑ tyrosine in diet (eg, soy products, chicken, fish, milk), tetrahydrobiopterin supplementation.

Phenyl ketones—phenylacetate, phenyllactate, and phenylpyruvate.

Disorder of **aromatic** amino acid metabolism → musty body **odor**.

Patients with PKU must avoid the artificial sweetener aspartame, which is converted to phenylalanine.

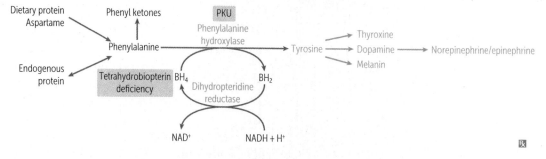

Maple syrup urine disease

Blocked degradation of **branched** amino acids (isoleucine, leucine, valine) due to ↓ branched-chain α-ketoacid dehydrogenase (B_1). Causes ↑ α-ketoacids in the blood, especially those of leucine.

Treatment: restriction of isoleucine, leucine, valine in diet, and thiamine supplementation.

Autosomal recessive.

Presentation: vomiting, poor feeding, secretions (urine, sweat, ear wax) smell like maple syrup/burnt sugar. Causes progressive neurologic decline, including seizures and dystonia.

I love Vermont **maple syrup** from maple trees (with **B_1ranches**).

Alkaptonuria

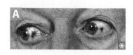

Congenital deficiency of homogentisate oxidase in the degradative pathway of tyrosine to fumarate → pigment-forming homogentisic acid builds up in tissue. Autosomal recessive. Usually benign.

Findings: bluish-black connective tissue, ear cartilage, and sclerae (ochronosis **A**); urine turns black on prolonged exposure to air. May have debilitating arthralgias (homogentisic acid toxic to cartilage).

Homocystinuria	Causes (all autosomal recessive): ▪ Cystathionine synthase deficiency (treatment: ↓ methionine, ↑ cysteine, ↑ B_6, B_{12}, and folate in diet) ▪ ↓ affinity of cystathionine synthase for pyridoxal phosphate (treatment: ↑↑ B_6 and ↑ cysteine in diet) ▪ Methionine synthase (homocysteine methyltransferase) deficiency (treatment: ↑ methionine in diet) ▪ Methylenetetrahydrofolate reductase (MTHFR) deficiency (treatment: ↑ folate in diet)	All forms result in excess homocysteine. HOMOCYstinuria: ↑↑ Homocysteine in urine, Osteoporosis, Marfanoid habitus, Ocular changes (downward and inward lens subluxation), Cardiovascular effects (thrombosis and atherosclerosis → stroke and MI), kYphosis, intellectual disability, hypopigmented skin. In homocystinuria, lens subluxes "down and in" (vs Marfan, "up and fans out").

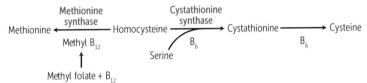

Cystinuria	Hereditary defect of renal PCT and intestinal amino acid transporter that prevents reabsorption of Cystine, Ornithine, Lysine, and Arginine (COLA). Cystine is made of 2 cysteines connected by a disulfide bond. Excess cystine in the urine can lead to recurrent precipitation of hexagonal cystine stones. Treatment: urinary alkalinization (eg, potassium citrate, acetazolamide) and chelating agents (eg, penicillamine) ↑ solubility of cystine stones; good hydration; diet low in methionine.	Autosomal recessive. Common (1:7000). Cystinuria detected with urinary sodium-cyanide nitroprusside test and proton nuclear magnetic resonance spectroscopy of urine.

Organic acidemias	Most commonly present in infancy with poor feeding, vomiting, hypotonia, high anion gap metabolic acidosis, hepatomegaly, seizures. Organic acid accumulation: ▪ Inhibits gluconeogenesis → ↓ fasting blood glucose levels, ↑ ketoacidosis → high anion gap metabolic acidosis ▪ Inhibits urea cycle → hyperammonemia	
Propionic acidemia	Deficiency of propionyl-CoA carboxylase → ↑ propionyl-CoA, ↓ methylmalonic acid.	Treatment: low-protein diet limited in substances that metabolize into propionyl-CoA: Valine, Odd-chain fatty acids, Methionine, Isoleucine, Threonine (VOMIT).
Methylmalonic acidemia	Deficiency of methylmalonyl-CoA mutase or vitamin B_{12}.	

Protein metabolism

TCA cycle

Valine
Odd-chain fatty acids
Methionine
Isoleucine
Threonine

→ Propionate → Propionyl-CoA $\xrightarrow[\text{Biotin}]{\text{Propionyl-CoA carboxylase}}$ Methylmalonyl-CoA $\xrightarrow[B_{12}]{\text{Methylmalonyl-CoA mutase}}$ Succinyl-CoA → Intermediates of citric acid cycle

Glycogen regulation by insulin and glucagon/epinephrine

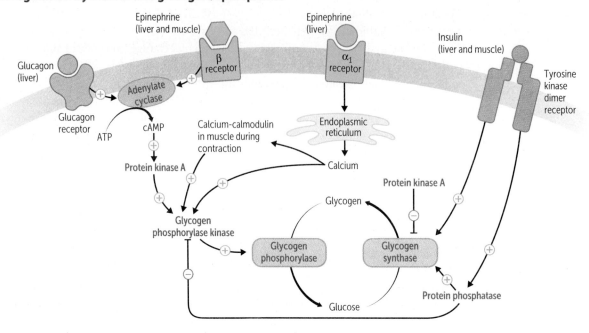

Glycogen	Branches have α-(1,6) bonds; linear linkages have α-(1,4) bonds.
Skeletal muscle	Glycogen undergoes glycogenolysis → glucose-1-phosphate → glucose-6-phosphate, which is rapidly metabolized during exercise.
Hepatocytes	Glycogen is stored and undergoes glycogenolysis to maintain blood sugar at appropriate levels. Glycogen phosphorylase ❺ liberates glucose-1-phosphate residues off branched glycogen until 4 glucose units remain on a branch. Then 4-α-D-glucanotransferase (debranching enzyme ❻) moves 3 of the 4 glucose units from the branch to the linear linkage. Then α-1,6-glucosidase (debranching enzyme ❼) cleaves off the last residue, liberating a free glucose. Limit dextrin—2–4 residues remaining on a branch after glycogen phosphorylase has shortened it.

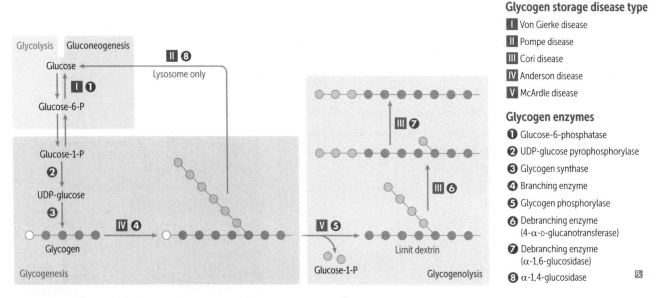

Glycogen storage disease type

I Von Gierke disease
II Pompe disease
III Cori disease
IV Anderson disease
V McArdle disease

Glycogen enzymes

❶ Glucose-6-phosphatase
❷ UDP-glucose pyrophosphorylase
❸ Glycogen synthase
❹ Branching enzyme
❺ Glycogen phosphorylase
❻ Debranching enzyme (4-α-D-glucanotransferase)
❼ Debranching enzyme (α-1,6-glucosidase)
❽ α-1,4-glucosidase

Note: A small amount of glycogen is degraded in lysosomes by ❽ α-1,4-glucosidase (acid maltase).

Glycogen storage diseases	At least 15 types have been identified, all resulting in abnormal glycogen metabolism and an accumulation of glycogen within cells. Periodic acid–Schiff stain identifies glycogen and is useful in identifying these diseases.	Vice president can't accept money. Types I-V are autosomal recessive. Andersen: Branching. Cori: Debranching. (ABCD)

DISEASE	FINDINGS	DEFICIENT ENZYME	COMMENTS
Von Gierke disease (type I)	Severe fasting hypoglycemia, ↑↑ Glycogen in liver and kidneys, ↑ blood lactate, ↑ triglycerides, ↑ uric acid (Gout), and hepatomegaly, renomegaly. Liver does not regulate blood glucose.	Glucose-6-phosphatase.	Treatment: frequent oral glucose/cornstarch; avoidance of fructose and galactose. Impaired gluconeogenesis and glycogenolysis.
Pompe disease (type II)	Cardiomyopathy, hypotonia, exercise intolerance, enlarged tongue, and systemic findings lead to early death.	Lysosomal acid α-1,4-glucosidase (acid maltase).	Pompe trashes the pump (1st and 4th letter; heart, liver, and muscle).
Cori disease (type III)	Similar to von Gierke disease, but milder symptoms and normal blood lactate levels. Can lead to cardiomyopathy. Limit dextrin–like structures accumulate in cytosol; can lead to hepatomegaly, cirrhosis, and hepatic adenomas.	Debranching enzymes (α-1,6-glucosidase and 4-α-D-glucanotransferase).	Gluconeogenesis is intact.
Andersen disease (type IV)	Most commonly presents with hepatosplenomegaly and failure to thrive in early infancy. Other findings include infantile cirrhosis, muscular weakness, hypotonia, cardiomyopathy early childhood death.	Branching enzyme. Neuromuscular form can present at any age.	Hypoglycemia occurs late in the disease.
McArdle disease (type V)	↑ glycogen in muscle, but muscle cannot break it down → painful muscle cramps, myoglobinuria (red urine) with strenuous exercise, and arrhythmia from electrolyte abnormalities. Second-wind phenomenon noted during exercise due to ↑ muscular blood flow.	Skeletal muscle glycogen phosphorylase (myophosphorylase). Characterized by a flat venous lactate curve with normal rise in ammonia levels during exercise.	Blood glucose levels typically unaffected. McArdle = muscle.

Lysosomal storage diseases

Lysosomal enzyme deficiency → accumulation of abnormal metabolic products. ↑ incidence of Tay-Sachs, Niemann-Pick, and some forms of Gaucher disease in Ashkenazi Jews.

DISEASE	FINDINGS	DEFICIENT ENZYME	ACCUMULATED SUBSTRATE	INHERITANCE
Sphingolipidoses				
Tay-Sachs disease	Progressive neurodegeneration, developmental delay/regression, hyperreflexia, hyperacusis, "cherry-red"* spot on macula A (lipid accumulation in ganglion cell layer), lysosomes with onion skin, no hepatosplenomegaly.	❶ Hexosaminidase A ("TAy-Sax").	GM$_2$ ganglioside.	AR
Fabry disease	Early: triad of episodic peripheral neuropathy, angiokeratomas B, hypohidrosis. Late: progressive renal failure, cardiovascular disease.	❷ α-galactosidase A; treat with recombinant α-galactosidase.	Ceramide trihexoside (globotriaosylce-ramide).	XR
Metachromatic leukodystrophy	Central and peripheral demyelination with ataxia, dementia.	❸ Arylsulfatase A.	Cerebroside sulfate.	AR
Krabbe disease	Peripheral neuropathy, destruction of oligodendrocytes, developmental delay, CN II atrophy, globoid cells.	❹ Galactocerebrosi-dase (galactosylce-ramidase).	Galactocerebroside, psychosine.	AR
Gaucher disease	Most common. Hepatosplenomegaly, pancytopenia, osteoporosis, avascular necrosis of femur, bone crises, Gaucher cells (lipid-laden macrophages resembling crumpled tissue paper C).	❺ Glucocerebrosidase (β-glucosidase); treat with recombinant glucocerebrosidase.	Glucocerebroside.	AR
Niemann-Pick disease	Progressive neurodegeneration, hepatosplenomegaly (vs Tay-Sachs disease), foam cells (lipid-laden macrophages) D, "cherry-red"* spot on macula A.	❻ Sphingomyelinase.	Sphingomyelin, cholesterol.	AR
Mucopolysaccharidoses				
Hurler syndrome	Developmental delay, hirsutism, skeletal anomalies, airway obstruction, clouded cornea, hepatosplenomegaly.	α-L-iduronidase.	Heparan sulfate, dermatan sulfate.	AR
Hunter syndrome	Mild Hurler + aggressive behavior, no corneal clouding.	Iduronate-2 (two)-sulfatase.		XR

GM$_2$ Ceramide trihexoside
❶ ↓ ❷ ↓
GM$_3$ Glucocerebroside

Sulfatide (cerebroside sulfate)
❸ ↓
Galactocerebroside → ❹ → Ceramide ← ❺ / ← ❻ ← Sphingomyelin

Hunters see clearly (no corneal clouding) and aggressively aim for the **X** (**X**-linked recessive).

*Red-tinted region at the center of the macula surrounded by retinal opacification.

Fatty acid metabolism

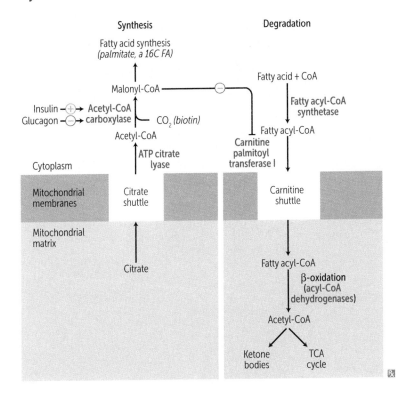

Fatty acid synthesis requires transport of citrate from mitochondria to cytosol. Predominantly occurs in liver, lactating mammary glands, and adipose tissue.

Long-chain fatty acid (LCFA) degradation requires carnitine-dependent transport into the mitochondrial matrix.

"**Sy**trate" = **sy**nthesis.

Carnitine = **carn**age of fatty acids.

Systemic 1° carnitine deficiency—no cellular uptake of carnitine → no transport of LCFAs into mitochondria → toxic accumulation of LCFAs in the cytosol. Causes weakness, hypotonia, hypoketotic hypoglycemia, dilated cardiomyopathy.

Medium-chain acyl-CoA dehydrogenase deficiency—↓ ability to break down fatty acids into acetyl-CoA → accumulation of fatty acyl carnitines and dicarboxylic acids in the blood with hypoketotic hypoglycemia. Causes vomiting, lethargy, seizures, coma, liver dysfunction, hyperammonemia. Can lead to sudden death in infants or children. Treat by avoiding fasting.

Ketone bodies

In the liver, fatty acids and amino acids are metabolized to acetoacetate and β-hydroxybutyrate (to be used in muscle and brain).

In prolonged starvation and diabetic ketoacidosis, oxaloacetate is depleted for gluconeogenesis. With chronic alcohol overuse, high NADH state leads to accumulation of oxaloacetate (downregulated TCA cycle), shunting it to malate.

Ketone bodies: acetone (ketone), acetoacetate (ketoacid), β-hydroxybutyrate (ketoacid).
Breath smells like acetone (fruity odor).
Urine test for ketones can detect acetoacetate, but not β-hydroxybutyrate.
RBCs cannot utilize ketone bodies; they strictly use glucose. Liver cells lack β ketoacyl-CoA transferase → cannot use ketone bodies as fuel.
HMG-CoA lyase for ketone body production.
HMG-CoA reductase for cholesterol synthesis.

	Hyperammonemia	Hypoketosis	Ketosis
KETONE LEVELS	Normal	↓	↑
GLUCOSE LEVELS	Normal	↓	↓
DEFICIENCY	OTC (urea cycle)	MCAD deficiency	Methylmalonic acidemia, propionic acidemia

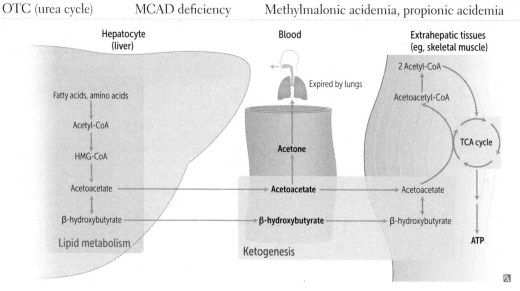

Fasted vs fed state

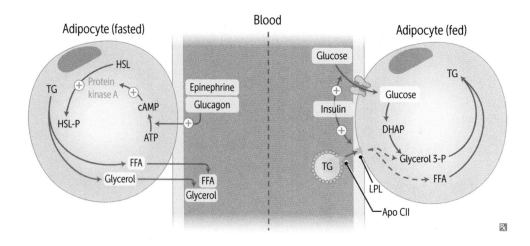

Metabolic fuel use

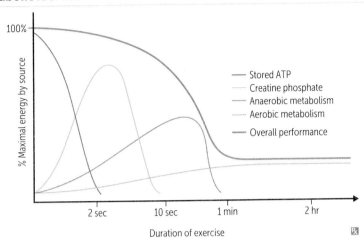

1g carb/protein = 4 kcal
1g alcohol = 7 kcal
1g fatty acid = 9 kcal
(# letters = # kcal)

Fasting and starvation	Priorities are to supply sufficient glucose to the brain and RBCs and to preserve protein.	
Fed state (after meals)	Glycolysis and aerobic respiration.	Insulin stimulates triglyceride (lipid) and glycogen (carbohydrate) storage alongside protein synthesis.
Fasting (between meals)	Hepatic glycogenolysis (major); hepatic gluconeogenesis, adipose release of FFA (minor).	Glucagon and epinephrine stimulate use of fuel reserves.
Starvation days 1–3	Blood glucose levels maintained by: <ul><li>Hepatic glycogenolysis</li><li>Adipose release of FFA</li><li>Muscle and liver, which shift fuel use from glucose to FFA</li><li>Hepatic gluconeogenesis from peripheral tissue lactate and alanine, and from adipose tissue glycerol and propionyl-CoA (from odd-chain FFA—the only triacylglycerol component that contributes to gluconeogenesis)</li></ul>	Glycogen reserves depleted after day 1. RBCs lack mitochondria and therefore cannot use ketone bodies. 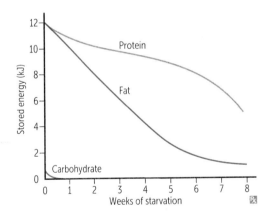
Starvation after day 3	Adipose stores (ketone bodies become the main source of energy for the brain). After these are depleted, vital protein degradation accelerates, leading to organ failure and death. Amount of excess stores determines survival time.	

Lipid transport

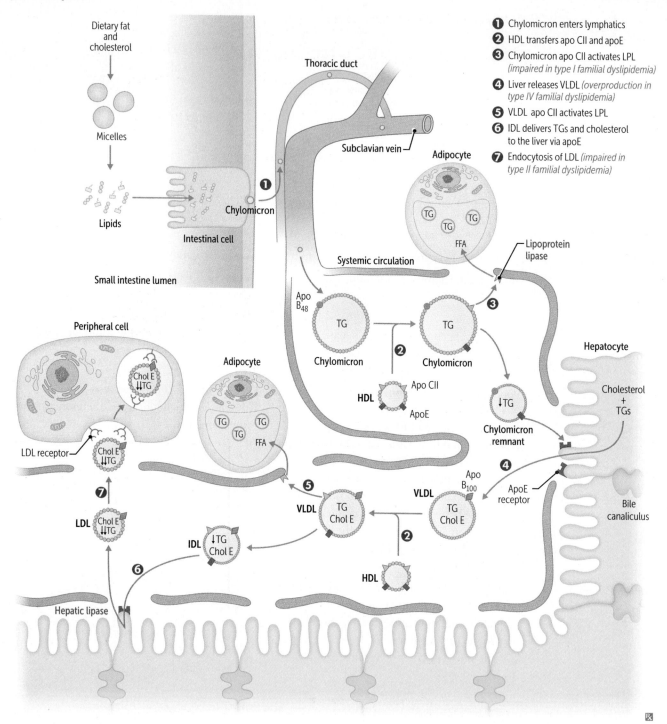

Dietary fat and cholesterol
Micelles
Lipids
Intestinal cell
Small intestine lumen
Thoracic duct
Subclavian vein
Chylomicron
Systemic circulation
Adipocyte
TG TG
TG
FFA
Lipoprotein lipase
Apo B₄₈
TG
Chylomicron
HDL
Apo CII
ApoE
Chylomicron
TG
↓TG
Chylomicron remnant
Hepatocyte
Cholesterol + TGs
Peripheral cell
Chol E ↓↓TG
LDL receptor
Chol E ↓↓TG
Adipocyte
TG TG
TG
FFA
VLDL
TG Chol E
VLDL
Apo B₁₀₀
TG Chol E
ApoE receptor
Bile canaliculus
LDL
Chol E ↓↓TG
IDL
↓TG Chol E
HDL
Hepatic lipase

1. Chylomicron enters lymphatics
2. HDL transfers apo CII and apoE
3. Chylomicron apo CII activates LPL *(impaired in type I familial dyslipidemia)*
4. Liver releases VLDL *(overproduction in type IV familial dyslipidemia)*
5. VLDL apo CII activates LPL
6. IDL delivers TGs and cholesterol to the liver via apoE
7. Endocytosis of LDL *(impaired in type II familial dyslipidemia)*

Key enzymes in lipid transport

Cholesteryl ester transfer protein	Mediates transfer of cholesteryl esters to other lipoprotein particles.
Hepatic lipase	Degrades TGs remaining in IDL and chylomicron remnants.
Hormone-sensitive lipase	Degrades TGs stored in adipocytes. Promotes gluconeogenesis by releasing glycerol.
Lecithin-cholesterol acyltransferase	Catalyzes esterification of ⅔ of plasma cholesterol (ie, required for HDL maturation).
Lipoprotein lipase	Degrades TGs in circulating chylomicrons and VLDL.
Pancreatic lipase	Degrades dietary TGs in small intestine.
PCSK9	Degrades LDL receptor → ↑ serum LDL. Inhibition → ↑ LDL receptor recycling → ↓ serum LDL.

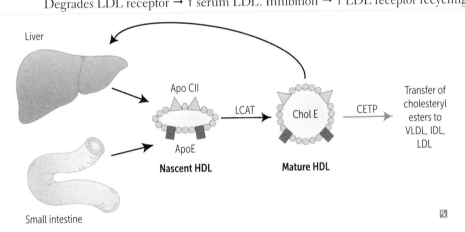

Major apolipoproteins

APOLIPOPROTEIN	FUNCTION	CHYLOMICRON	CHYLOMICRON REMNANT	VLDL	IDL	LDL	HDL
E	Mediates remnant uptake (everything except LDL)	✓	✓	✓	✓		✓
AI	Found only on alpha-lipoproteins (HDL), activates LCAT						✓
CII	Lipoprotein lipase cofactor that catalyzes cleavage	✓		✓	✓		✓
B_{48}	Mediates chylomicron secretion into lymphatics. Only on particles originating from the intestines	✓	✓				
B_{100}	Binds LDL receptor. Only on particles originating from the liver (I hope I live to Be 100)			✓	✓	✓	

Lipoprotein functions	Lipoproteins are composed of varying proportions of proteins, cholesterol, TGs, and phospholipids. LDL and HDL carry the most cholesterol. Cholesterol is needed to maintain cell membrane integrity and synthesize bile acids, steroids, and vitamin D.
Chylomicron	Delivers dietary TGs to peripheral tissues. Delivers cholesterol to liver in the form of chylomicron remnants, which are mostly depleted of their TGs. Secreted by intestinal epithelial cells.
VLDL	Delivers hepatic TGs to peripheral tissue. Secreted by liver.
IDL	Delivers TGs and cholesterol to liver. Formed from degradation of VLDL.
LDL	Delivers hepatic cholesterol to peripheral tissues. Formed by hepatic lipase modification of IDL in the liver and peripheral tissue. Taken up by target cells via receptor-mediated endocytosis. LDL is **L**ethal.
HDL	Mediates reverse cholesterol transport from peripheral tissues to liver. Acts as a repository for apoC and apoE (which are needed for chylomicron and VLDL metabolism). Secreted from both liver and intestine. Alcohol ↑ synthesis. HDL is **H**ealthy.

Abetalipoproteinemia 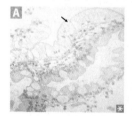	Autosomal recessive. Mutation in gene that encodes microsomal transfer protein (*MTP*). Chylomicrons, VLDL, LDL absent. Deficiency in apo B_{48}– and apo B_{100}–containing lipoproteins. Affected infants present with severe fat malabsorption, steatorrhea, failure to thrive. Later manifestations include retinitis pigmentosa, spinocerebellar degeneration due to vitamin E deficiency, progressive ataxia, acanthocytosis. Intestinal biopsy shows lipid-laden enterocytes (arrow in **A**). Treatment: restriction of long-chain fatty acids, large doses of oral vitamin E.

Familial dyslipidemias

TYPE	INHERITANCE	PATHOGENESIS	↑ BLOOD LEVEL	CLINICAL
I—Hyper-chylomicronemia	AR	Lipoprotein lipase or apo CII deficiency	Chylomicrons, TG, cholesterol	Pancreatitis, hepatosplenomegaly, and eruptive/pruritic xanthomas (no ↑ risk for atherosclerosis). Creamy layer in supernatant.
II—Hyper-cholesterolemia	AD	Absent or defective LDL receptors, or defective apo B_{100}	IIa: LDL, cholesterol IIb: LDL, cholesterol, VLDL	Heterozygotes (1:500) have cholesterol ≈ 300 mg/dL; homozygotes (very rare) have cholesterol ≥ 700 mg/dL. Accelerated atherosclerosis (may have MI before age 20), tendon (Achilles) xanthomas, and corneal arcus.
III—Dysbeta-lipoproteinemia	AR	ApoE (defective in type thr**EE**)	Chylomicrons, VLDL, TG	Premature atherosclerosis, tuberoeruptive and palmar xanthomas.
IV—Hyper-triglyceridemia	AD	Hepatic overproduction of VLDL	VLDL, TG	Hypertriglyceridemia (> 1000 mg/dL) can cause acute pancreatitis. Related to insulin resistance.

Immunology

"I hate to disappoint you, but my rubber lips are immune to your charms."
—*Batman & Robin*

"Imagine the action of a vaccine not just in terms of how it affects a single body, but also in terms of how it affects the collective body of a community."
—*Eula Biss*

"Some people are immune to good advice."
—Saul Goodman, *Breaking Bad*

Learning the components of the immune system and their roles in host defense at the cellular level is essential for both the understanding of disease pathophysiology and clinical practice. Know the immune mechanisms of responses to vaccines. Both congenital and acquired immunodeficiencies are very testable. Cell surface markers are high yield for understanding immune cell interactions and for laboratory diagnosis. Know the roles and functions of major cytokines and chemokines.

▶ IMMUNOLOGY—LYMPHOID STRUCTURES

Immune system organs	1° organs: ▪ **B**one marrow—immune cell production, **B** cell maturation ▪ **T**hymus—**T** cell maturation 2° organs: ▪ Spleen, lymph nodes, tonsils, adenoids, appendix, Peyer patches ▪ Allow immune cells to interact with antigen
Lymph node	A 2° lymphoid organ that has many afferents, 1 or more efferents. Encapsulated, with trabeculae 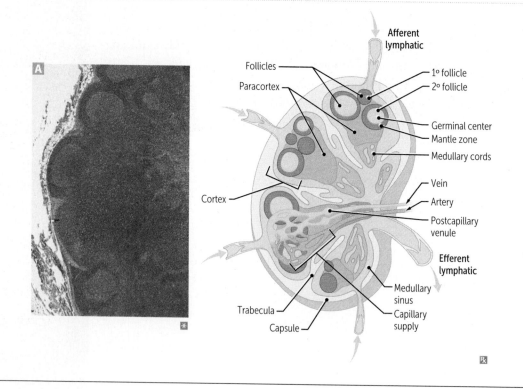. Functions are nonspecific filtration by macrophages, circulation of B and T cells, and immune response activation.
Follicle	Located in outer cortex; site of B-cell localization and proliferation. 1° follicles are dense and quiescent. 2° follicles have pale central germinal centers and are active.
Medulla	Consists of medullary cords (closely packed lymphocytes and plasma cells) and medullary sinuses (contain reticular cells and macrophages). Medullary sinuses communicate with efferent lymphatics.
Paracortex	Contains T cells. Region of cortex between follicles and medulla. Contains high endothelial venules through which T and B cells enter from blood. Underdeveloped in patients with DiGeorge syndrome. Paracortex enlarges in an extreme cellular immune response (eg, EBV and other viral infections → paracortical hyperplasia → lymphadenopathy).

Lymphatic drainage associations

Lymph node cluster	Area of body drained	Associated pathology
Submandibular, submental	Oral cavity, anterior tongue, lower lip	Malignancy of and metastasis to the oral cavity
Deep cervical	Head, neck, oropharynx	Upper respiratory tract infection Infectious mononucleosis Kawasaki disease Malignancy of head, neck, oropharynx
Supraclavicular	Right: right hemithorax Left (Virchow node): left hemithorax, abdomen, pelvis	Malignancies of thorax, abdomen, pelvis
Mediastinal	Trachea, esophagus	Pulmonary TB (unilateral hilar) Sarcoidosis (bilateral hilar) Lung cancer Granulomatous disease
Hilar	Lungs	
Axillary	Upper limb, breast, skin above umbilicus	Mastitis Metastasis (especially breast cancer)
Epitrochlear	Hand, forearm	Secondary syphilis
Celiac	Liver, stomach, spleen, pancreas, upper duodenum	Mesenteric lymphadenitis Inflammatory bowel disease Celiac disease
Superior mesenteric	Lower duodenum, jejunum, ileum, colon to splenic flexure	
Inferior mesenteric	Colon from splenic flexure to upper rectum	
Periumbilical (Sister Mary Joseph node)	Abdomen, pelvis	Gastric cancer
Para-aortic	**Pair** of testes, ovaries, kidneys, fallopian tubes, fundus of uterus	Metastasis
External iliac	Body of uterus, cervix, superior bladder	Sexually transmitted infections Medial foot/leg cellulitis (superficial inguinal)
Internal iliac	Cervix, proximal vagina, corpus cavernosum, prostate, inferior bladder, lower rectum to anal canal (above pectinate line)	
Superficial inguinal	Distal vagina, vulva, scrotum, urethra, anal canal (below pectinate line), skin below umbilicus (except popliteal area)	
Popliteal ("pop-**lateral**")	**Dorsolateral** foot, posterior calf	Lateral foot/leg cellulitis

○ Palpable lymph node

◎ Nonpalpable lymph node

▪ Right lymphatic duct drains right side of body above diaphragm into junction of the right subclavian and internal jugular vein

▪ Thoracic duct drains below the diaphragm and left thorax and upper limb into junction of left subclavian and internal jugular veins (rupture of thoracic duct can cause chylothorax)

Spleen

Capsule
Trabecula

Red pulp (RBCs)
Sinusoid
Reticular fibrous framework

White pulp (WBCs)
Follicle (B cells)
  Mantle zone
  Germinal center
Marginal zone
Periarteriolar lymphoid sheath (T cells)

Open circulation

Closed circulation

Pulp vein

Artery

Vein

Located in LUQ of abdomen, anterolateral to left kidney, protected by 9th-11th ribs. Splenic dysfunction (eg, postsplenectomy, sickle cell disease autosplenectomy) → ↓ IgM → ↓ complement activation → ↓ C3b opsonization → ↑ susceptibility to encapsulated organisms, against which patients should be vaccinated (from most to least common: pneumococci, meningococci, *Haemophilus influenzae* type b [Hib]).

Postsplenectomy findings:

- Howell-Jolly bodies (nuclear remnants)
- Target cells
- Thrombocytosis (loss of sequestration and removal)
- Lymphocytosis (loss of sequestration)

Periarteriolar lymphatic sheath	Contains T cells. Located within white pulp.
Follicle	Contains B cells. Located within white pulp.
Marginal zone	Contains macrophages and specialized B cells. Site where antigen-presenting cells (APCs) capture blood-borne antigens for recognition by lymphocytes. Located between red pulp and white pulp.

Thymus

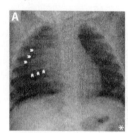

Located in the anterosuperior mediastinum. Site of T-cell differentiation and maturation. Encapsulated. Thymus epithelium is derived from third pharyngeal pouch (endoderm), whereas thymic lymphocytes are of mesodermal origin. Cortex is dense with immature T cells; medulla is pale with mature T cells and Hassall corpuscles containing epithelial reticular cells.

Normal neonatal thymus "sail-shaped" on CXR (arrows in A), involutes by age 3 years.

T cells = Thymus
B cells = Bone marrow
Absent thymic shadow or hypoplastic thymus seen in some immunodeficiencies (eg, SCID, DiGeorge syndrome).

Thymoma—neoplasm of thymus. Associated with myasthenia gravis, superior vena cava syndrome, pure red cell aplasia, Good syndrome.

▶ IMMUNOLOGY—CELLULAR COMPONENTS

Innate vs adaptive immunity

	Innate immunity	Adaptive immunity
COMPONENTS	Neutrophils, macrophages, monocytes, dendritic cells, natural killer (NK) cells (lymphoid origin), complement, physical epithelial barriers, secreted enzymes.	T cells, B cells, circulating antibodies.
MECHANISM	Germline encoded.	Variation through V(D)J recombination during lymphocyte development.
RESPONSE TO PATHOGENS	Nonspecific. Occurs rapidly (minutes to hours). No memory response.	Highly specific, refined over time. Develops over long periods; memory response is faster and more robust.
SECRETED PROTEINS	Lysozyme, complement, C-reactive protein (CRP), defensins, cytokines.	Immunoglobulins, cytokines.
KEY FEATURES IN PATHOGEN RECOGNITION	Toll-like receptors (TLRs): pattern recognition receptors that recognize pathogen- and damage-associated molecular patterns (PAMPs and DAMPs) → activation of NF-κB → release of pro-inflammatory cytokines. Examples of PAMPs: LPS (gram ⊖ bacteria), flagellin (bacteria), nucleic acids (viruses). Examples of DAMPs: mitochondrial DNA, histones, heat shock proteins.	Memory cells: activated B and T cells; subsequent exposure to a previously encountered antigen → stronger, quicker immune response. Adaptive immune responses decrease with age (immunosenescence).

Immune privilege

Organs (eg, eye, brain, placenta, testes) and tissues where chemical or physical mechanisms limit immune responses to foreign antigens to avoid damage that would occur from inflammatory sequelae. Allograft rejection at these sites is less likely.

Major histocompatibility complex I and II

MHC encoded by HLA genes. Present antigen fragments to T cells and bind T-cell receptors (TCRs).

	MHC I	MHC II
LOCI	HLA-A, HLA-B, HLA-C MHC I loci have 1 letter	HLA-DP, HLA-DQ, HLA-DR MHC II loci have 2 letters
BINDING	TCR and CD8 (CD8 × MHC 1 = 8)	TCR and CD4 (CD4 × MHC 2 = 8)
STRUCTURE	1 long chain, 1 short chain (3 α, 1 β)	2 equal-length chains (2 α, 2 β)
EXPRESSION	All nucleated cells, APCs, platelets (except RBCs)	APCs
FUNCTION	Present endogenous antigens (eg, viral or cytosolic proteins) to CD8+ cytotoxic T cells	Present exogenous antigens (eg, bacterial proteins) to CD4+ helper T cells
ANTIGEN LOADING	Antigen peptides loaded onto MHC I in RER after delivery via TAP (transporter associated with antigen processing)	Antigen loaded following release of invariant chain in an acidified endosome
ASSOCIATED PROTEINS	β_2-microglobulin	Invariant chain
STRUCTURE		

HLA subtypes associated with diseases

HLA SUBTYPE	DISEASE	MNEMONIC
B27	Psoriatic arthritis, Ankylosing spondylitis, IBD-associated arthritis, Reactive arthritis	PAIR
DR3	DM type 1, SLE, Graves disease, Hashimoto thyroiditis, Addison disease	DM type 1: HLA-3 and -4 (1 + 3 = 4) SL3 (SLE)
DR4	Rheumatoid arthritis, DM type 1, Addison disease	There are 4 walls in 1 "rheum" (room)

Major functions of natural killer cells	Lymphocyte member of innate immune system.
	Use perforin and granzymes to induce apoptosis of virally infected cells and tumor cells.
	Activity enhanced by IL-2, IL-12, IFN-α, and IFN-β. Produce IFN-γ → macrophage activation.
	Induced to kill when exposed to a nonspecific activation signal on target cell and/or to an absence of an inhibitory signal such as MHC I on target cell surface.
	Also kills via antibody-dependent cell-mediated cytotoxicity (CD16 binds Fc region of bound IgG, activating the NK cell).

Major functions of B and T cells

B cells	Humoral immunity.
	Recognize and present antigen—undergo somatic hypermutation to optimize antigen specificity.
	Produce antibody—differentiate into plasma cells to secrete specific immunoglobulins.
	Maintain immunologic memory—memory B cells persist and accelerate future response to antigen.
T cells	Cell-mediated immunity.
	CD4+ T cells help B cells make antibodies and produce cytokines to recruit phagocytes and activate other leukocytes.
	CD8+ T cells directly kill virus-infected and tumor cells via perforin and granzymes (similar to NK cells).
	Type IV hypersensitivity reaction.
	Acute and chronic cellular organ rejection.

Differentiation of T cells

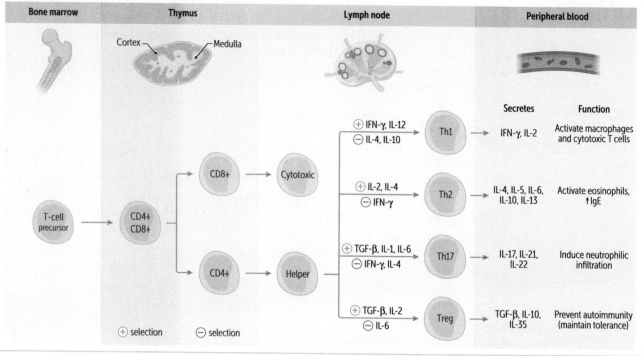

Positive selection

Thymic cortex. Keeps T cells that recognize self-peptides to allow for cooperation in immune responses. Double positive thymocytes expressing TCRs that recognize self-peptide MHC complexes receive a survival signal.

Negative selection

Thymic medulla. Removes T cells that bind too strongly to self-peptides. Thymocytes expressing TCRs with high affinity for self antigens undergo apoptosis or become regulatory T cells. The autoimmune regulator (**AIRE**) protein drives negative selection, and deficiency leads to autoimmune polyendocrine syndrome (**C**hronic mucocutaneous candidiasis, **H**ypoparathyroidism, **A**drenal insufficiency, **R**ecurrent *Candida* infections). "Without **AIRE**, your body will **CHAR**".

Macrophage-lymphocyte interaction

Th1 cells secrete IFN-γ, which enhances the ability of monocytes and macrophages to kill microbes they ingest. This function is also enhanced by interaction of T cell CD40L with CD40 on macrophages. Macrophages also activate lymphocytes via antigen presentation.

Cytotoxic T cells

Kill virus-infected, neoplastic, and donor graft cells by inducing apoptosis.
Release cytotoxic granules containing preformed proteins (eg, perforin, granzyme B).
Cytotoxic T cells have CD8, which binds to MHC I on virus-infected cells.

Regulatory T cells

Help maintain specific immune tolerance by suppressing CD4+ and CD8+ T-cell effector functions.
Identified by expression of CD3, CD4, CD25, and FOXP3.
Activated regulatory T cells (Tregs) produce anti-inflammatory cytokines (eg, IL-10, TGF-β).

IPEX (Immune dysregulation, Polyendocrinopathy, Enteropathy, X-linked) syndrome— genetic deficiency of FOXP3 → autoimmunity. Characterized by enteropathy, endocrinopathy, nail dystrophy, dermatitis, and/or other autoimmune dermatologic conditions. Associated with diabetes in male infants.

T- and B-cell activation	APCs: B cells, dendritic cells, Langerhans cells, macrophages. Two signals are required for T-cell activation, B-cell activation, and class switching.

T-cell activation	❶ APC ingests and processes antigen, then migrates to the draining lymph node. ❷ T-cell activation (signal 1): exogenous antigen is presented on MHC II and recognized by TCR on Th (CD4+) cell. Endogenous or cross-presented antigen is presented on MHC I to Tc (CD8+) cell. ❸ Proliferation and survival (signal 2): costimulatory signal via interaction of B7 protein (CD80/86) on dendritic cell and CD28 on naïve T cell. ❹ Activated Th cell produces cytokines. Tc cell able to recognize and kill virus-infected cell.	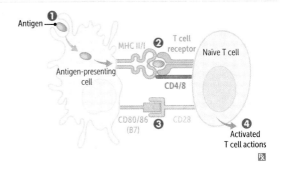
B-cell activation and class switching	❶ Th-cell activation as above. ❷ B-cell receptor–mediated endocytosis. ❸ Exogenous antigen is presented on MHC II and recognized by TCR on Th cell. ❹ CD40 receptor on B cell binds CD40 ligand (CD40L) on Th cell. ❺ Th cells secrete cytokines that determine Ig class switching of B cells. ❻ B cells are activated and produce IgM. They undergo class switching and affinity maturation.	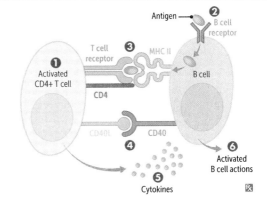

Anergy	State during which a cell cannot become activated by exposure to its antigen. T and B cells become anergic when exposed to their antigen without costimulatory signal (signal 2). Another example of peripheral tolerance mechanism.

▶ IMMUNOLOGY—IMMUNE RESPONSES

Antibody structure and function

Fab fragment consisting of light (L) and heavy (H) chains recognizes antigens. Fc region of IgM and IgG fixes complement. Heavy chain contributes to Fc and Fab regions. Light chain contributes only to Fab region.

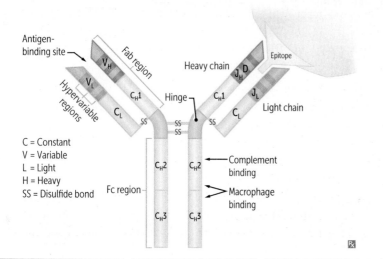

C = Constant
V = Variable
L = Light
H = Heavy
SS = Disulfide bond

Fab:
- Fragment, antigen binding
- Determines idiotype: unique antigen-binding pocket; only 1 antigenic specificity expressed per B cell

Fc (5 C's):
- Constant
- Carboxy terminal
- Complement binding
- Carbohydrate side chains
- Confers (determines) isotype (IgM, IgD, etc)

Generation of antibody diversity (antigen independent)
  1. Random recombination of VJ (light-chain) or V(D)J (heavy-chain) genes by RAG1 and RAG2
  2. Random addition of nucleotides to DNA during recombination by terminal deoxynucleotidyl transferase (TdT)
  3. Random combination of heavy chains with light chains

Generation of antibody specificity (antigen dependent)
  4. Somatic hypermutation and affinity maturation (variable region)
  5. Isotype switching (constant region)

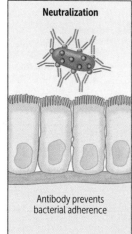

Neutralization

Antibody prevents bacterial adherence

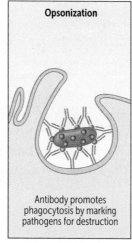

Opsonization

Antibody promotes phagocytosis by marking pathogens for destruction

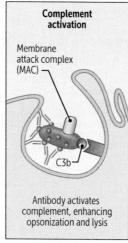

Complement activation

Membrane attack complex (MAC)

C3b

Antibody activates complement, enhancing opsonization and lysis

Immunoglobulin isotypes	All isotypes can exist as monomers. Mature, naïve B cells prior to activation express IgM and IgD on their surfaces. They may differentiate in germinal centers of lymph nodes by isotype switching (gene rearrangement; induced by cytokines and CD40L) into plasma cells that secrete IgA, IgG, or IgE. "For B cells, IgMom and IgDad mature to plasma cells as they **AGE**." Affinity refers to the individual antibody-antigen interaction, while avidity describes the cumulative binding strength of all antibody-antigen interactions in a multivalent molecule.
IgG	Main antibody in 2° response to an antigen. Most abundant isotype in serum. Fixes complement, opsonizes bacteria, neutralizes bacterial toxins and viruses. Only isotype that crosses the placenta (provides infants with passive immunity that starts to wane after birth). "IgG Greets the Growing fetus." Associated with **warm** autoimmune hemolytic anemia ("**warm** weather is Good!").
IgA	Prevents attachment of bacteria and viruses to mucous membranes; does not fix complement. Monomer (in circulation) or dimer (with J chain when secreted). Crosses epithelial cells by transcytosis. Produced in GI tract (eg, by Peyer patches) and protects against gut infections (eg, *Giardia*). Most produced antibody overall, but has lower serum concentrations. Released into secretions (tears, saliva, mucus) and breast milk. Picks up secretory component from epithelial cells, which protects the Fc portion from luminal proteases.
IgM	First antibody to be produced during an immune response. Fixes complement. Antigen receptor on the surface of B cells. Monomer on B cell, pentamer with J chain when secreted. Pentamer enables avid binding to antigen while humoral response evolves. Associated with cold autoimmune hemolytic anemia.
IgD	Expressed on the surface of mature, naïve B cells. Normally, low levels are detectable in serum.
IgE	Binds mast cells and basophils; cross-links when exposed to allergen, mediating immediate (type I) hypersensitivity through release of inflammatory mediators such as histamine. Contributes to immunity to parasites by activating **E**osinophils.

Antigen type and memory

Thymus-independent antigens	Antigens lacking a peptide component (eg, lipopolysaccharides from gram ⊖ bacteria); cannot be presented by MHC to T cells. Weakly immunogenic; vaccines often require boosters and adjuvants (eg, capsular polysaccharide subunit of *Streptococcus pneumoniae* PPSV23 vaccine).
Thymus-dependent antigens	Antigens containing a protein component (eg, diphtheria toxoid). Class switching and immunologic memory occur as a result of direct contact of B cells with Th cells.

Complement	System of hepatically synthesized plasma proteins that play a role in innate immunity and inflammation. Membrane attack complex (MAC) defends against gram ⊖ bacteria. The CH_{50} test is used to screen for activation of the classical complement pathway.	
ACTIVATION PATHWAYS	Classic—IgG or IgM mediated. Alternative—bacterial products. Lectin—mannose or other sugars on microbe surface.	General Motors makes classic cars.
FUNCTIONS	C3b—opsonization. C3a, C4a, C5a—anaphylaxis. C5a—neutrophil chemotaxis. C5b-9 (MAC)—cytolysis.	C3b binds to lipopolysaccharides on bacteria. MAC complex is important for neutralizing *Neisseria* species. Deficiency results in recurrent infection. Get "Neis" (nice) Big MACs from 5-9 pm.
	Opsonins—C3b and IgG are the two 1° opsonins in bacterial defense; enhance phagocytosis. C3b also helps clear immune complexes.	*Opsonin* (Greek) = to prepare for eating.
	Inhibitors—decay-accelerating factor (DAF, also called CD55) and C1 inhibitor (formerly called C1 esterase inhibitor) help prevent complement activation on self cells (eg, RBCs).	

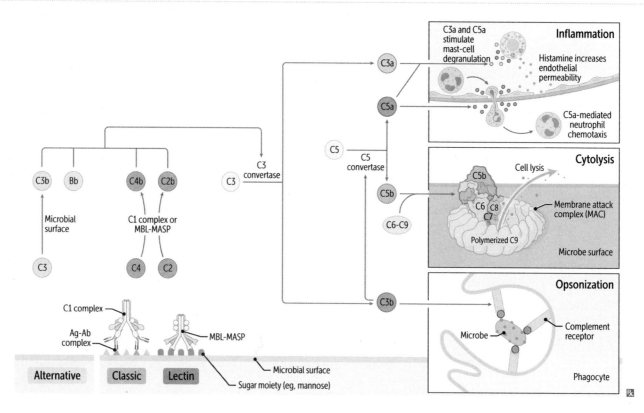

Complement disorders

Complement protein deficiencies

Early complement deficiencies (C1–C4)	↑ risk of severe, recurrent pyogenic sinus and respiratory tract infections. C3b used in clearance of antigen-antibody complexes → ↑ risk of **SLE** (think **SLEarly**).
Terminal complement deficiencies (C5–C9)	↑ susceptibility to recurrent *Neisseria* bacteremia.

Complement regulatory protein deficiencies

C1 inhibitor deficiency	Causes hereditary angioedema due to unregulated activation of kallikrein → ↑ bradykinin. Characterized by ↓ C4 levels. ACE inhibitors are contraindicated (also ↑ bradykinin).
Paroxysmal nocturnal hemoglobinuria 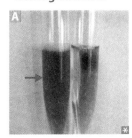	A defect in the *PIGA* gene prevents the formation of glycosylphosphatidylinositol (GPI) anchors for complement inhibitors, such as decay-accelerating factor (DAF/CD55) and membrane inhibitor of reactive lysis (MIRL/CD59). Causes complement-mediated intravascular hemolysis → ↓ haptoglobin, dark urine A. Can cause atypical venous thrombosis (eg, Budd-Chiari syndrome; portal vein, cerebral, or dermal thrombosis). Treatment: eculizumab (anti-C5 antibody; inhibits terminal complement system and MAC formation).

Important cytokines   Acute (IL-1, IL-6, TNF-α), then recruit (IL-8, IL-12).

Secreted by macrophages

Interleukin-1	Causes fever, acute inflammation. Activates endothelium to express adhesion molecules. Induces chemokine secretion to recruit WBCs. Also called osteoclast-activating factor.	"Hot T-bone stEAK": IL-1: fever (hot). IL-2: stimulates T cells. IL-3: stimulates bone marrow. IL-4: stimulates IgE production. IL-5: stimulates IgA production. IL-6: stimulates aKute-phase protein production.
Interleukin-6	Causes fever and stimulates production of acute-phase proteins.	
Tumor necrosis factor-α	Activates endothelium. Causes WBC recruitment, vascular leak.	Causes cachexia in malignancy. Maintains granulomas in TB. IL-1, IL-6, TNF-α can mediate fever and sepsis.
Interleukin-8	Major chemotactic factor for neutrophils.	"Clean up on aisle 8." Neutrophils are recruited by IL-8 to clear infections.
Interleukin-12	Induces differentiation of T cells into Th1 cells. Activates NK cells.	Facilitates granuloma formation in TB.

Secreted by T cells

Interleukin-2	Stimulates growth of helper, cytotoxic, and regulatory T cells, and NK cells.	
Interleukin-3	Supports growth and differentiation of bone marrow stem cells. Functions like GM-CSF.	Stimulates proliferation of eosinophils, basophils, neutrophils, monocytes.

From Th1 cells

Interferon-gamma	Secreted by NK cells and T cells in response to antigen or IL-12 from macrophages; stimulates macrophages to kill phagocytosed pathogens. Inhibits differentiation of Th2 cells. Induces IgG isotype switching in B cells.	Increases MHC expression and antigen presentation by all cells. Activates macrophages to induce granuloma formation.

From Th2 cells

Interleukin-4	Induces differentiation of T cells into Th (helper) 2 cells. Promotes growth of B cells. Enhances class switching to IgE and IgG.	Ain't too proud 2 BEG 4 help.
Interleukin-5	Promotes growth and differentiation of B cells. Enhances class switching to IgA. Stimulates growth and differentiation of Eosinophils.	I have 5 BAEs.
Interleukin-10	Attenuates inflammatory response. Decreases expression of MHC class II and Th1 cytokines. Inhibits activated macrophages and dendritic cells. Also secreted by regulatory T cells.	TGF-β and IL-10 both attenuate the immune response.
Interleukin-13	Promotes IgE production by B cells. Induces alternative macrophage activation.	Interleukin thirtEEn promotes IgE.

Respiratory burst	Also called oxidative burst. Involves the activation of the phagocyte NADPH oxidase complex (eg, in neutrophils, monocytes), which utilizes O_2 as a substrate. Plays an important role in the immune response → rapid release of reactive oxygen species (ROS). NADPH plays a role in both the creation and neutralization of ROS. Myeloperoxidase contains a blue-green, heme-containing pigment that gives sputum its color. **NO Safe Microbe** (**N**ADPH Oxidase → **S**uperoxide dismutase → **M**yeloperoxidase).

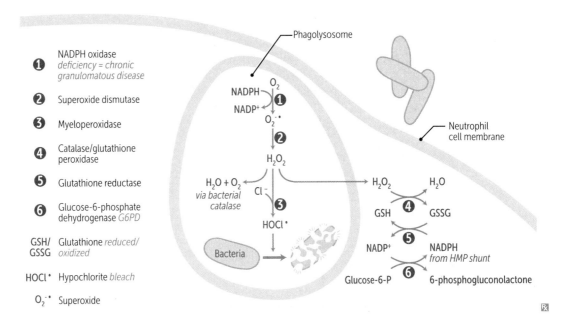

❶	NADPH oxidase *deficiency = chronic granulomatous disease*
❷	Superoxide dismutase
❸	Myeloperoxidase
❹	Catalase/glutathione peroxidase
❺	Glutathione reductase
❻	Glucose-6-phosphate dehydrogenase *G6PD*
GSH/ GSSG	Glutathione *reduced/ oxidized*
HOCl˙	Hypochlorite *bleach*
O_2^-˙	Superoxide

Phagocytes of patients with CGD can utilize H_2O_2 generated by invading organisms and convert it to ROS. Patients are at ↑ risk for infection by catalase ⊕ species (eg, *S aureus, Aspergillus*) capable of neutralizing their own H_2O_2, leaving phagocytes without ROS for fighting infections.

Pyocyanin of *P aeruginosa* generates ROS to kill competing pathogens. Oxidative burst leads to release of lysosomal enzymes.

Type I interferons	IFN-α, IFN-β.
MECHANISM	A part of innate host defense, **interferons interfere** with both RNA and DNA viruses. Cells infected with a virus synthesize these glycoproteins, which act on local cells, priming them for viral defense by downregulating protein synthesis to resist potential viral replication and by upregulating MHC expression to facilitate recognition of infected cells. Also play a major role in activating antitumor immunity.
CLINICAL USE	Chronic HBV, Kaposi sarcoma, hairy cell leukemia, condyloma acuminatum, renal cell carcinoma, malignant melanoma, multiple sclerosis.
ADVERSE EFFECTS	Flulike symptoms, depression, neutropenia, myopathy, interferon-induced autoimmunity.

Cell surface proteins

T cells	TCR (binds antigen-MHC complex), CD3 (associated with TCR for signal transduction), CD28 (binds B7 on APC)	
Helper T cells	CD4, CD40L, CXCR4/CCR5 (coreceptors for HIV)	
Cytotoxic T cells	CD8	
Regulatory T cells	CD4, CD25	
B cells	Ig (binds antigen), CD19, CD20, CD21 (receptor for Epstein-**Barr** virus), CD40, MHC II, B7 (CD80/86)	Must be **21** to drink at a **Barr**
NK cells	CD16 (binds Fc of IgG), CD56 (suggestive marker for NK cells)	
Macrophages	CD14 (receptor for PAMPs [eg, LPS]), CD40, CCR5, MHC II, B7, Fc and C3b receptors (enhanced phagocytosis)	
Hematopoietic stem cells	CD34	

Passive vs active immunity

	Passive	Active
MEANS OF ACQUISITION	Receiving preformed antibodies	Exposure to exogenous antigens
ONSET	Rapid	Slow
DURATION	Short span of antibodies (half-life = 3 weeks)	Long-lasting protection (memory)
EXAMPLES	IgA in breast milk, maternal IgG crossing placenta, antitoxin, humanized monoclonal antibody	Natural infection, vaccines, toxoid
NOTES	IVIG and other immune globulin preparations can be administered to provide temporary but specific passive immunity to a target pathogen	Combined passive and active immunizations can be given for hepatitis B or rabies exposure

Vaccination — Induces an active immune response (humoral and/or cellular) to specific pathogens.

VACCINE TYPE	DESCRIPTION	PROS/CONS	EXAMPLES
Live attenuated vaccine	Microorganism rendered nonpathogenic but retains capacity for transient growth within inoculated host. Certain live vaccines (MMR, varicella) may be given to people living with HIV who have a CD4+ cell count ≥ 200 cells/mm^3 in consultation with a specialist in infectious disease or immunology.	Pros: induces cellular and humoral responses. Induces strong, often lifelong immunity. Cons: may revert to virulent form. Contraindicated in pregnancy and patients with immunodeficiency.	Adenovirus (nonattenuated, given to military recruits), typhoid (Ty21a, oral), polio (Sabin), varicella (chickenpox), **smallpox**, BCG, yellow fever, **influenza** (intranasal), **MMR**, rotavirus. "Attention teachers! Please vaccinate **small**, Beautiful young **infants** with **MMR** routinely!"
Killed or inactivated vaccine	Pathogen is inactivated by heat or chemicals. Maintaining epitope structure on surface antigens is important for immune response. Mainly induces a humoral response.	Pros: safer than live vaccines. Cons: weaker cell-mediated immune response; mainly induces a humoral response. Booster shots usually needed.	Hepatitis **A**, **T**yphoid (Vi polysaccharide, intramuscular), **R**abies, **I**nfluenza (intramuscular), **P**olio (Sal**K**). **A TRIP** could **K**ill you.
Subunit, recombinant, polysaccharide, and conjugate Polysaccharides with conjugate proteins	All use specific antigens that best stimulate the immune system.	Pros: targets specific epitopes of antigen; lower chance of adverse reactions. Cons: expensive; weaker immune response.	HBV (antigen = HBsAg), HPV, acellular pertussis (aP), *Neisseria meningitidis* (various strains), *Streptococcus pneumoniae* (PPSV23 polysaccharide primarily T-cell–independent response; PCV13, PCV15, and PCV20 polysaccharide produces T-cell–dependent response), Hib, herpes zoster.
Toxoid	Denatured bacterial toxin with an intact receptor binding site. Stimulates immune system to make antibodies without potential for causing disease.	Pros: protects against the bacterial toxins. Cons: antitoxin levels decrease with time, thus booster shots may be needed.	*Clostridium tetani*, *Corynebacterium diphtheriae*.
mRNA	A lipid nanoparticle delivers mRNA, causing cells to synthesize foreign protein (eg, spike protein of SARS-CoV-2).	Pros: high efficacy; induces cellular and humoral immunity. Safe in pregnancy. Cons: local and transient systemic (fatigue, headache, myalgia) reactions are common. Rare myocarditis, pericarditis particularly in young males.	SARS-CoV-2.

Hypersensitivity types	Four types: Anaphylactic and atopic (type I), antibody-mediated (type II), immune complex (type III), cell-mediated (type IV). Types I, II, and III are all antibody-mediated.	
Type I hypersensitivity 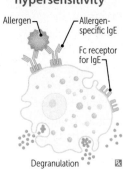 Allergen / Allergen-specific IgE / Fc receptor for IgE / Degranulation ℞	Anaphylactic and atopic—two phases: <ul><li>Immediate (minutes): antigen crosslinks preformed IgE on presensitized mast cells → immediate degranulation → release of histamine (a vasoactive amine), tryptase (marker of mast cell activation), and leukotrienes.</li><li>Late (hours): chemokines (attract inflammatory cells, eg, eosinophils) and other mediators from mast cells → inflammation and tissue damage.</li></ul>	First (type) and Fast (anaphylaxis). Test: skin test or blood test (ELISA) for allergen-specific IgE. Example: <ul><li>Anaphylaxis (eg, food, drug, or bee sting allergies)</li><li>Allergic asthma</li></ul>
Type II hypersensitivity 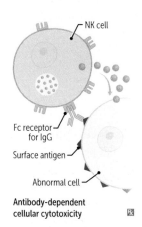 NK cell / Fc receptor for IgG / Surface antigen / Abnormal cell / **Antibody-dependent cellular cytotoxicity** ℞	Antibodies bind to cell-surface antigens or extracellular matrix → cellular destruction, inflammation, and cellular dysfunction. Cellular destruction—cell is opsonized (coated) by antibodies, leading to either: <ul><li>Phagocytosis and/or activation of complement system.</li><li>NK cell killing (antibody-dependent cellular cytotoxicity).</li></ul>Inflammation—binding of antibodies to cell surfaces → activation of complement system and Fc receptor-mediated inflammation. Cellular dysfunction—antibodies bind to cell-surface receptors → abnormal blockade or activation of downstream process.	**Direct** Coombs test—detects antibodies attached **directly** to the RBC surface. Indirect Coombs test—detects presence of unbound antibodies in the serum. Examples: <ul><li>Autoimmune hemolytic anemia (including drug-induced form)</li><li>Immune thrombocytopenia</li><li>Transfusion reactions</li><li>Hemolytic disease of the newborn</li></ul>Examples: <ul><li>Goodpasture syndrome</li><li>Rheumatic fever</li><li>Hyperacute transplant rejection</li></ul>Examples: <ul><li>Myasthenia gravis</li><li>Graves disease</li><li>Pemphigus vulgaris</li></ul>

Hypersensitivity types *(continued)*

Type III hypersensitivity

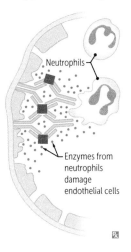

Neutrophils

Enzymes from neutrophils damage endothelial cells

℞

Immune complex—antigen-antibody (mostly IgG) complexes activate complement, which attracts neutrophils; neutrophils release lysosomal enzymes.
Can be associated with vasculitis and systemic manifestations.

In type III reaction, imagine an immune complex as **3** things stuck together: antigen-antibody-complement.
Examples:
- SLE
- Reactive arthritis
- Polyarteritis nodosa
- Poststreptococcal glomerulonephritis
- IgA vasculitis

Serum sickness—the prototypic immune complex disease. Antibodies to foreign proteins are produced and 1–2 weeks later, antibody-antigen complexes form and deposit in tissues → complement activation → inflammation and tissue damage (↓ serum C3, C4).

Fever, urticaria, arthralgia, proteinuria, lymphadenopathy occur 1–2 weeks after antigen exposure. Serum sickness–like reactions are associated with some drugs (may act as haptens, eg, penicillin, monoclonal antibodies) and infections (eg, hepatitis B).

Arthus reaction—a local subacute immune complex-mediated hypersensitivity reaction. Intradermal injection of antigen into a presensitized (has circulating IgG) individual leads to immune complex formation in the skin (eg, enhanced local reaction to a booster vaccination). Characterized by edema, fibrinoid necrosis, activation of complement.

Type IV hypersensitivity

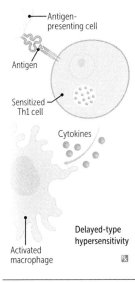

Antigen-presenting cell

Antigen

Sensitized Th1 cell

Cytokines

Activated macrophage

Delayed-type hypersensitivity

℞

Two mechanisms, each involving T cells:
1. Direct cell cytotoxicity: CD8+ cytotoxic T cells kill targeted cells.
2. Inflammatory reaction: effector CD4+ T cells recognize antigen and release inflammation-inducing cytokines (shown in illustration).

Response does not involve antibodies (vs types I, II, and III).
Examples:
- Contact dermatitis (eg, poison ivy, nickel allergy)
- Drug reaction with eosinophilia and systemic symptoms (DRESS)
- Graft-versus-host disease

Tests: PPD for TB infection; patch test for contact dermatitis; *Candida* skin test for T cell immune function.
4T's: **T** cells, **T**ransplant rejections, **T**B skin tests, **T**ouching (contact dermatitis).

Fourth (type) and **last** (delayed).

Immunologic blood transfusion reactions

TYPE	PATHOGENESIS	TIMING	CLINICAL PRESENTATION	DONOR BLOOD	HOST BLOOD
Allergic/ anaphylactic reaction	Type I hypersensitivity reaction against plasma proteins in transfused blood IgA-deficient individuals should receive blood products without IgA	Within minutes to 2–3 hr (due to release of preformed inflammatory mediators in degranulating mast cells)	Allergies: urticaria, pruritus Anaphylaxis: wheezing, hypotension, respiratory arrest, shock	Donor plasma proteins, including IgA	Host mast cell
Acute hemolytic transfusion reaction	Type II hypersensitivity reaction Typically causes intravascular hemolysis (ABO blood group incompatibility)	During transfusion or within 24 hr (due to preformed antibodies)	Fever, hypotension, tachypnea, tachycardia, flank pain, hemoglobinuria (intravascular), jaundice (extravascular)	Donor RBC with A and/ or B group antigens	Host anti-A, anti-B IgG, IgM
Febrile nonhemolytic transfusion reaction	Cytokines created by donor WBCs accumulate during storage of blood products Reactions prevented by leukoreduction of blood products	Within 1–6 hr (due to preformed cytokines)	Fever, headaches, chills, flushing More common in children	Donor WBC releases preformed cytokines	
Transfusion-related acute lung injury	Two-hit mechanism: ▪ Neutrophils are sequestered and primed in pulmonary vasculature due to recipient risk factors ▪ Neutrophils are activated by a product (eg, antileukocyte antibodies) in the transfused blood and release inflammatory mediators → ↑ capillary permeability → pulmonary edema	Within minutes to 6 hr	Respiratory distress, noncardiogenic pulmonary edema	Donor antileukocyte antibody	Host neutrophils
Delayed hemolytic transfusion reaction	Anamnestic response to a foreign antigen on donor RBCs (Rh [D] or other minor blood group antigens) previously encountered by recipient Typically causes extravascular hemolysis	Onset over 24 hr Usually presents within 1–2 wk (due to slow destruction by reticuloendothelial system)	Generally self limited and clinically silent Mild fever, hyperbilirubinemia		

Autoantibodies

AUTOANTIBODY	ASSOCIATED DISORDER
Anti-postsynaptic ACh receptor	Myasthenia gravis
Anti-presynaptic voltage-gated Ca^{2+} channel	Lambert-Eaton myasthenic syndrome
Anti-β_2 glycoprotein I	Antiphospholipid syndrome
Antinuclear (ANA)	Nonspecific screening antibody, often associated with SLE
Anticardiolipin, lupus anticoagulant	SLE, antiphospholipid syndrome
Anti-dsDNA, anti-Smith	SLE
Antihistone	Drug-induced lupus
Anti-U1 RNP (ribonucleoprotein)	Mixed connective tissue disease
Rheumatoid factor (IgM antibody against IgG Fc region), anti-cyclic citrullinated peptide (anti-CCP, more specific)	Rheumatoid arthritis
Anti-Ro/SSA, anti-La/SSB	Sjögren syndrome
Anti-Scl-70 (anti-DNA topoisomerase I)	Scleroderma (diffuse)
Anticentromere	Limited scleroderma (CREST syndrome)
Antisynthetase (eg, anti-Jo-1), anti-SRP, anti-helicase (anti-Mi-2)	Polymyositis, dermatomyositis
Antimitochondrial	1° biliary cholangitis
Anti-smooth muscle, anti-liver/kidney microsomal-1	Autoimmune hepatitis
Myeloperoxidase-antineutrophil cytoplasmic antibody (MPO-ANCA)/perinuclear ANCA (p-ANCA)	Microscopic polyangiitis, eosinophilic granulomatosis with polyangiitis, ulcerative colitis, 1° sclerosing cholangitis
PR3-ANCA/cytoplasmic ANCA (c-ANCA)	Granulomatosis with polyangiitis
Anti-phospholipase A_2 receptor	1° membranous nephropathy
Anti-hemidesmosome	Bullous pemphigoid
Anti-desmoglein (anti-desmosome)	Pemphigus vulgaris
Antithyroglobulin, antithyroid peroxidase (antimicrosomal)	Hashimoto thyroiditis
Anti-TSH receptor	Graves disease
IgA anti-endomysial, IgA anti-tissue transglutaminase, IgA and IgG deamidated gliadin peptide	Celiac disease
Anti-glutamic acid decarboxylase, islet cell cytoplasmic antibodies	Type 1 diabetes mellitus
Antiparietal cell, anti-intrinsic factor	Pernicious anemia
Anti-glomerular basement membrane	Goodpasture syndrome

Immunodeficiencies

DISEASE	DEFECT	PRESENTATION	FINDINGS
B-cell disorders			
X-linked (Bruton) agammaglobulinemia	Defect in *BTK*, a tyrosine kinase gene → no **B**-cell maturation; X-linked recessive (↑ in **B**oys)	Recurrent bacterial and enteroviral infections after 6 months (↓ maternal IgG)	Absent B cells in peripheral blood, ↓ Ig of all classes. Absent/scanty lymph nodes and tonsils (1° follicles and germinal centers absent) → live vaccines contraindicated
Selective IgA deficiency	May be familial or sporadic Most common 1° immunodeficiency May also arise 2° to certain viral infections or medications	Majority **A**symptomatic Can see **A**irway and GI infections, **A**utoimmune disease, **A**topy, **A**naphylaxis to IgA in blood products	↓ IgA with normal IgG, IgM levels ↑ susceptibility to giardiasis Can cause false-negative celiac disease test and false-positive serum pregnancy test
Common variable immunodeficiency	Defect in B-cell differentiation. Cause unknown in most cases	May present in childhood but usually diagnosed after puberty ↑ risk of autoimmune disease, bronchiectasis, lymphoma, sinopulmonary infections	↓ plasma cells, ↓ immunoglobulins
T-cell disorders			
Thymic aplasia	22q11 microdeletion; failure to develop 3rd and 4th pharyngeal pouches → absent thymus and parathyroids DiGeorge syndrome—thymic, parathyroid, cardiac defects Velocardiofacial syndrome—palate, facial, cardiac defects	**CATCH-22**: **C**ardiac defects (conotruncal abnormalities [eg, tetralogy of Fallot, truncus arteriosus]), **A**bnormal facies, **T**hymic hypoplasia → T-cell deficiency (recurrent viral/fungal infections), **C**left palate, **H**ypocalcemia 2° to parathyroid aplasia → tetany	↓ T cells, ↓ PTH, ↓ Ca^{2+} Thymic shadow absent on CXR
IL-12 receptor deficiency	↓ Th1 response; autosomal recessive	Disseminated mycobacterial and fungal infections; may present after administration of BCG vaccine	↓ IFN-γ Most common cause of Mendelian susceptibility to mycobacterial diseases (MSMD)
Autosomal dominant hyper-IgE syndrome (Job syndrome)	Deficiency of Th17 cells due to *STAT3* mutation → impaired recruitment of neutrophils to sites of infection	Cold (noninflamed) staphylococcal **A**bscesses, retained **B**aby teeth, **C**oarse facies, **D**ermatologic problems (eczema), ↑ Ig**E**, bone **F**ractures from minor trauma	↑ IgE ↑ eosinophils Learn the **ABCDEF**'s to get a **Job STAT**!
Chronic mucocutaneous candidiasis	T-cell dysfunction Impaired cell-mediated immunity against *Candida* sp Classic form caused by defects in *AIRE*	Persistent noninvasive *Candida albicans* infections of skin and mucous membranes	Absent in vitro T-cell proliferation in response to *Candida* antigens Absent cutaneous reaction to *Candida* antigens

Immunodeficiencies *(continued)*

DISEASE	DEFECT	PRESENTATION	FINDINGS
B- and T-cell disorders			
Severe combined immunodeficiency	Several types including defective IL-2R gamma chain (most common, X-linked recessive); adenosine deaminase deficiency (autosomal recessive); *RAG* mutation → VDJ recombination defect	Failure to thrive, chronic diarrhea, thrush Recurrent viral, bacterial, fungal, and protozoal infections	↓ T-cell receptor excision circles (TRECs) Part of newborn screening for SCID Absence of thymic shadow (CXR), germinal centers (lymph node biopsy), and T cells (flow cytometry)
Ataxia-telangiectasia 	Defects in *ATM* gene → failure to detect DNA damage → failure to halt progression of cell cycle → mutations accumulate; autosomal recessive	Triad: cerebellar defects (Ataxia), spider Angiomas (telangiectasia A), IgA deficiency ↑↑ sensitivity to radiation (limit x-ray exposure)	↑ AFP ↓ IgA, IgG, and IgE Lymphopenia, cerebellar atrophy ↑ risk of lymphoma and leukemia
Hyper-IgM syndrome	Most commonly due to defective CD40L on Th cells → class switching defect; X-linked recessive	Severe pyogenic infections early in life; opportunistic infection with *Pneumocystis*, *Cryptosporidium*, CMV	Normal or ↑ IgM ↓↓ IgG, IgA, IgE Failure to make germinal centers
Wiskott-Aldrich syndrome	WAS mutation; leukocytes and platelets unable to reorganize actin cytoskeleton → defective antigen presentation; X-linked recessive	WATER: Wiskott-Aldrich: Thrombocytopenia, Eczema, Recurrent (pyogenic) infections ↑ risk of autoimmune disease and malignancy	↓ to normal IgG, IgM ↑ IgE, IgA Fewer and smaller platelets
Phagocyte dysfunction			
Leukocyte adhesion deficiency (type 1)	Autosomal recessive defect in LFA-1 integrin (CD18) protein on phagocytes leads to impaired migration and chemotaxis by C5a, IL-8, and leukotriene B4	Late separation (>30 days) of umbilical cord, absent pus, dysfunctional neutrophils → recurrent skin and mucosal bacterial infections	↑ neutrophils in blood Absence of neutrophils at infection sites → impaired wound healing
Chédiak-Higashi syndrome 	Defect in lysosomal trafficking regulator gene (*LYST*) Microtubule dysfunction in phagosome-lysosome fusion; autosomal recessive	PLAIN: Progressive neurodegeneration, Lymphohistiocytosis, Albinism (partial), recurrent pyogenic Infections, peripheral Neuropathy	Giant granules (B, arrows) in granulocytes and platelets Pancytopenia Mild coagulation defects
Chronic granulomatous disease	Defect of NADPH oxidase → ↓ reactive oxygen species (eg, superoxide) and ↓ respiratory burst in neutrophils; X-linked form most common	↑ susceptibility to catalase ⊕ organisms (**granny's cats keep her positive**) Recurrent infections and granulomas	Abnormal dihydrorhodamine (flow cytometry) test (↓ green fluorescence) Nitroblue tetrazolium dye reduction test (obsolete) fails to turn blue

Infections in immunodeficiency

PATHOGEN	↓ T CELLS	↓ B CELLS	↓ GRANULOCYTES	↓ COMPLEMENT
Bacteria	Sepsis	Encapsulated (Please **SHINE** my **SKiS**): *Pseudomonas aeruginosa, Streptococcus pneumoniae, Haemophilus Influenzae* type b, *Neisseria meningitidis, Escherichia coli, Salmonella, Klebsiella pneumoniae,* group B *Streptococcus*	Some Bacteria Produce No Serious granules: *Staphylococcus, Burkholderia cepacia, Pseudomonas aeruginosa, Nocardia, Serratia*	Encapsulated species with early complement deficiencies *Neisseria* with late complement (C5–C9) deficiencies
Viruses	CMV, EBV, JC virus, VZV, chronic infection with respiratory/GI viruses	Enteroviral encephalitis, poliovirus (live vaccine contraindicated)	N/A	N/A
Fungi/parasites	*Candida* (local), PCP, *Cryptococcus*	GI giardiasis (no IgA)	*Candida* (systemic), *Aspergillus, Mucor*	N/A

Note: B-cell deficiencies tend to produce recurrent bacterial infections, whereas T-cell deficiencies produce more fungal and viral infections.

Transplant rejection

TYPE OF REJECTION	ONSET	PATHOGENESIS	FEATURES
Hyperacute	Within minutes	Pre-existing recipient antibodies react to donor antigen (type II hypersensitivity reaction), activate complement	Widespread thrombosis of graft vessels (arrows within glomerulus A) → ischemia and fibrinoid necrosis Graft must be removed
Acute	Weeks to months	Cellular: CD8+ T cells and/or CD4+ T cells activated against donor MHCs (type IV hypersensitivity reaction) Humoral: similar to hyperacute, except antibodies develop after transplant (associated with C4d deposition)	Vasculitis of graft vessels with dense interstitial lymphocytic infiltrate B Prevent/reverse with immunosuppressants
Chronic	Months to years	CD4+ T cells respond to recipient APCs presenting donor peptides, including allogeneic MHC Both cellular and humoral components (type II and IV hypersensitivity reactions)	Dominated by arteriosclerosis C Recipient T cells react and secrete cytokines → proliferation of vascular smooth muscle, parenchymal atrophy, interstitial fibrosis Organ-specific examples: ▫ Chronic allograft nephropathy ▫ Bronchiolitis obliterans ▫ Accelerated atherosclerosis (heart) ▫ Vanishing bile duct syndrome
Graft-versus-host disease	Varies	Grafted immunocompetent T cells proliferate in the immunocompromised host and reject host cells with "foreign" proteins → severe organ dysfunction HLA mismatches ↑ the risk for GVHD Type IV hypersensitivity reaction	Maculopapular rash, jaundice, diarrhea, hepatosplenomegaly Usually in bone marrow and liver transplants (rich in lymphocytes) Potentially beneficial in bone marrow transplant for leukemia (graft-versus-tumor effect) For patients who are immunocompromised, irradiate blood products prior to transfusion to prevent GVHD

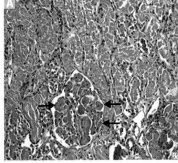
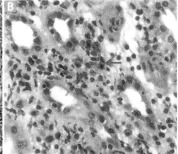
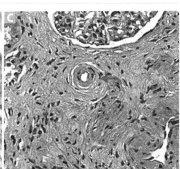

▶ IMMUNOLOGY—IMMUNOSUPPRESSANTS

Immunosuppressants   Agents that block lymphocyte activation and proliferation. Reduce acute transplant rejection by suppressing cellular immunity (used as prophylaxis). Frequently combined to achieve greater efficacy with ↓ toxicity. Chronic suppression ↑ risk of infection and malignancy.

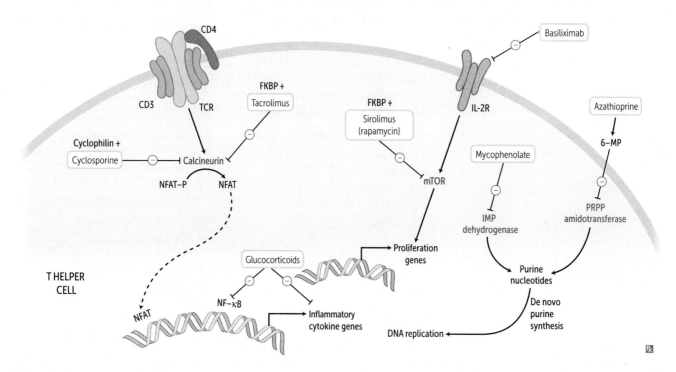

DRUG	MECHANISM	INDICATIONS	TOXICITY	NOTES
Cyclosporine	Calcineurin inhibitor; binds **cyclophilin** Blocks T-cell activation by **preventing IL-2 transcription**	Psoriasis, rheumatoid arthritis	**Nephrotoxicity,** hypertension, hyperlipidemia, neurotoxicity, gingival hyperplasia, hirsutism	Both calcineurin inhibitors are highly nephrotoxic, especially in higher doses or in patients with ↓ renal function
Tacrolimus (FK506)	Calcineurin inhibitor; binds FK506 binding protein (FKBP) Blocks T-cell activation by **preventing IL-2 transcription**	Immunosuppression after solid organ transplant	Similar to cyclosporine, ↑ risk of diabetes and neurotoxicity; no gingival hyperplasia or hirsutism	
Sirolimus (Rapamycin)	mTOR inhibitor; binds FKBP Blocks T-cell activation and B-cell differentiation by **preventing response to IL-2**	Kidney transplant rejection prophylaxis specifically **Sir Basil's** kidney transplant	"Pan**sir**topenia" (pancytopenia), insulin resistance, hyperlipidemia; **not nephrotoxic**	Kidney "**sir**-vives." Synergistic with cyclosporine Also used in drug-eluting stents
Basiliximab	Monoclonal antibody; blocks IL-2R		Edema, hypertension, tremor	

Immunosuppressants (continued)

DRUG	MECHANISM	INDICATIONS	TOXICITY	NOTES
Azathioprine	Antimetabolite precursor of 6-mercaptopurine Inhibits lymphocyte proliferation by blocking nucleotide synthesis	Rheumatoid arthritis, Crohn disease, glomerulonephritis, other autoimmune conditions	Pancytopenia	6-MP degraded by xanthine oxidase; toxicity ↑ by allopurinol Pronounce "azathio-purine"
Mycophenolate mofetil	Reversibly inhibits IMP dehydrogenase, preventing purine synthesis of B and T cells	Glucocorticoid-sparing agent in rheumatic disease	GI upset, pancytopenia, hypertension Less nephrotoxic and neurotoxic	Associated with invasive CMV infection
Glucocorticoids	Inhibit NF-κB Suppress both B- and T-cell function by ↓ transcription of many cytokines Induce T cell apoptosis	Many autoimmune and inflammatory disorders, adrenal insufficiency, asthma, CLL, non-Hodgkin lymphoma	Cushing syndrome, osteoporosis, hyperglycemia, diabetes, amenorrhea, adrenocortical atrophy, peptic ulcers, psychosis, cataracts, avascular necrosis (femoral head)	Demargination of WBCs causes artificial leukocytosis Adrenal insufficiency may develop if drug is stopped abruptly after chronic use

Recombinant cytokines and clinical uses

CYTOKINE	AGENT	CLINICAL USES
Bone marrow stimulation		
Erythropoietin	Epoetin alfa (EPO analog)	Anemias (especially in renal failure) Associated with ↑ risk of hypertension, thromboembolic events
Colony stimulating factors	Filgrastim (G-CSF), sargramostim (**GM-CSF**)	Leukopenia; recovery of granulocyte and monocyte counts
Thrombopoietin	Romiplostim (TPO analog), eltrombopag (think "elthrombopag." TPO receptor agonist)	Autoimmune thrombocytopenia Platelet stimulator
Immunotherapy		
Interleukin-2	Aldesleukin	Renal cell carcinoma, metastatic melanoma
Interferons	IFN-α	Chronic hepatitis C (not preferred) and B, renal cell carcinoma
	IFN-β	Multiple sclerosis
	IFN-γ	Chronic granulomatous disease

▶ NOTES

Microbiology

"Within one linear centimeter of your lower colon there lives and works more bacteria (about 100 billion) than all humans who have ever been born. Yet many people continue to assert that it is we who are in charge of the world."

—Neil deGrasse Tyson

"What lies behind us and what lies ahead of us are tiny matters compared to what lies within us."

—Henry S. Haskins

"Wise and humane management of the patient is the best safeguard against infection."

—Florence Nightingale

"I sing and play the guitar, and I'm a walking, talking bacterial infection."

—Kurt Cobain

Microbiology questions on the Step 1 exam often require two (or more) steps: Given a certain clinical presentation, you will first need to identify the most likely causative organism, and you will then need to provide an answer regarding some features of that organism or relevant antimicrobial agents. For example, a description of a child with fever and a petechial rash will be followed by a question that reads, "From what site does the responsible organism usually enter the blood?"

This section therefore presents organisms in two major ways: in individual microbial "profiles" and in the context of the systems they infect and the clinical presentations they produce. You should become familiar with both formats. When reviewing the systems approach, remind yourself of the features of each microbe by returning to the individual profiles. Also be sure to memorize the laboratory characteristics that allow you to identify microbes.

▶ MICROBIOLOGY—BASIC BACTERIOLOGY

Bacterial structures

STRUCTURE	CHEMICAL COMPOSITION	FUNCTION
Appendages		
Flagellum	Proteins	Motility
Pilus/fimbria	Glycoprotein	Mediate adherence of bacteria to cell surface; sex pilus forms during conjugation
Specialized structures		
Spore	Keratinlike coat, dipicolinic acid, peptidoglycan, DNA	Survival: resist dehydration, heat, chemicals
Cell envelope		
Capsule	Discrete layer usually made of polysaccharides (and rarely proteins)	Protects against phagocytosis
Slime (S) layer	Loose network of polysaccharides	Mediates adherence to surfaces, plays a role in biofilm formation (eg, indwelling catheters)
Outer membrane	Outer leaflet: contains endotoxin (LPS/LOS) Embedded proteins: porins and other outer membrane proteins (OMPs) Inner leaflet: phospholipids	Gram ⊖ only Endotoxin: lipid A induces TNF and IL-1; antigenic O polysaccharide component Most OMPs are antigenic Porins: transport across outer membrane
Periplasm	Space between cytoplasmic membrane and outer membrane in gram ⊖ bacteria (peptidoglycan in middle)	Accumulates components exiting gram ⊖ cells, including hydrolytic enzymes (eg, β-lactamases)
Cell wall	Peptidoglycan is a sugar backbone with peptide side chains cross-linked by transpeptidase	Netlike structure gives rigid support, protects against osmotic pressure damage
Cytoplasmic membrane	Phospholipid bilayer sac with embedded proteins (eg, penicillin-binding proteins [PBPs]) and other enzymes Lipoteichoic acids (gram **positive**) only extend from membrane to exterior	Site of oxidative and transport enzymes; PBPs involved in cell wall synthesis Lipoteichoic acids induce TNF-α and IL-1

Cell envelope

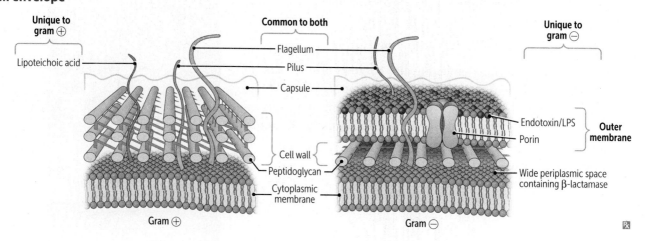

Stains

Gram stain	First-line lab test in bacterial identification. Bacteria with thick peptidoglycan layer retain crystal violet dye (gram ⊕); bacteria with thin peptidoglycan layer turn red or pink (gram ⊖) with counterstain. These bugs do not Gram stain well (These Little Microbes May Unfortunately Lack Real Color But Are Everywhere):	
	Treponema, *Leptospira*	Too thin to be visualized
	Mycobacteria	Cell wall has high lipid content
	Mycoplasma, Ureaplasma	No cell wall
	Legionella, Rickettsia, Chlamydia, Bartonella, Anaplasma, Ehrlichia	Primarily intracellular; also, *Chlamydia* lack classic peptidoglycan because of ↓ muramic acid
Giemsa stain	*H pylori, Chlamydia, Borrelia, Rickettsia,* Trypanosomes 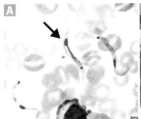, *Plasmodium*	Help! Certain Bugs Really Try my Patience
Periodic acid–Schiff stain	Stains glycogen, mucopolysaccharides; used to diagnose Whipple disease (*Tropheryma whipplei* 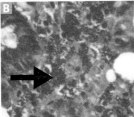)	
Ziehl-Neelsen stain (carbol fuchsin)	Acid-fast bacteria (eg, *Mycobacteria* 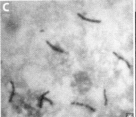, *Nocardia*; stains mycolic acid in cell wall); protozoa (eg, *Cryptosporidium* oocysts)	Auramine-rhodamine stain is more often used for screening (inexpensive, more sensitive)
India ink stain	*Cryptococcus neoformans* 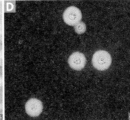; mucicarmine can also be used to stain thick polysaccharide capsule red	
Silver stain	*Helicobacter pylori, Legionella, Bartonella henselae,* and fungi (eg, *Coccidioides* 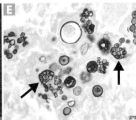, *Pneumocystis jirovecii, Aspergillus fumigatus*)	HeLiCoPters Are silver
Fluorescent antibody stain	Used to identify many bacteria, viruses, *Pneumocystis jirovecii, Giardia,* and *Cryptosporidium*	Example is FTA-ABS for syphilis

Special culture requirements

BUG	MEDIA USED FOR ISOLATION	MEDIA CONTENTS/OTHER
H influenzae	Chocolate agar	Factors V (NAD$^+$) and X (hematin)
N gonorrhoeae, N meningitidis	Thayer-Martin agar	Selectively favors growth of *Neisseria* by inhibiting growth of gram ⊕ organisms with vancomycin, gram ⊖ organisms except *Neisseria* with trimethoprim and colistin, and fungi with nystatin Very typically cultures *Neisseria*
B pertussis	Bordet-Gengou agar (**Bordet** for *Bordetella*) Regan-Lowe medium	Potato extract Charcoal, blood, and antibiotic
C diphtheriae	Tellurite agar, Löffler medium	
M tuberculosis	Löwenstein-Jensen medium, Middlebrook medium, rapid automated broth cultures	
M pneumoniae	Eaton agar	Requires cholesterol
Lactose-fermenting enterics	MacConkey agar	Fermentation produces acid, causing colonies to turn pink
E coli	Eosin–methylene blue (EMB) agar	Colonies with green metallic sheen
Brucella, Francisella, Legionella, Pasteurella	Buffered **charcoal** yeast extract agar with **cysteine** and **iron**	The **Ella** siblings, **Bruce**, **Francis**, a **legion**naire, and a **pasteur** (pastor), built the Sistine (**cysteine**) chapel out of **charcoal** and **iron**
Fungi	Sabouraud agar	"**Sab**'s a **fun** guy!"

Anaerobes	Examples include *Clostridioides, Clostridium, Bacteroides, Fusobacterium,* and *Actinomyces israelii*. They lack catalase and/or superoxide dismutase and are thus susceptible to oxidative damage. Generally foul smelling (short-chain fatty acids), are difficult to culture, and produce gas in tissue (CO_2 and H_2).	Anaerobes Can't Breathe Fresh Air. Anaerobes are normal microbiota in GI tract, typically pathogenic elsewhere (eg, causes aspiration pneumonia). AminO_2glycosides are ineffective against anaerobes because these antibiotics require O_2 to enter into bacterial cell.
Facultative anaerobes	May use O_2 as a terminal electron acceptor to generate ATP, but can also use fermentation and other O_2-independent pathways.	Streptococci, staphylococci, and enteric gram ⊖ bacteria.

Intracellular bacteria

Obligate intracellular	*Rickettsia, Chlamydia, Coxiella* Rely on host ATP	Stay inside (cells) when it is Really Chilly and Cold
Facultative intracellular	*Salmonella, Neisseria, Brucella, Mycobacterium, Listeria, Francisella, Legionella, Yersinia pestis*	Some Nasty Bugs May Live FacultativeLY

Encapsulated bacteria 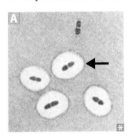	Examples are *Pseudomonas aeruginosa, Streptococcus pneumoniae* 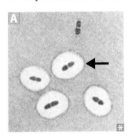, *Haemophilus influenzae* type b, *Neisseria meningitidis, Escherichia coli, Salmonella, Klebsiella pneumoniae,* and group B Strep. Their capsules serve as an antiphagocytic virulence factor. Capsular polysaccharide +/− protein conjugate can serve as an antigen in vaccines. A polysaccharide antigen alone cannot be presented to T cells; immunogenicity can be enhanced by conjugating capsule antigens to a carrier protein.	Please SHiNE my SKiS. Are opsonized, and then cleared by spleen. Asplenics (No Spleen Here) have ↓ opsonizing ability and thus ↑ risk for severe infections; need vaccines to protect against: ▪ *N meningitidis* ▪ *S pneumoniae* ▪ *H influenzae*

Urease-positive organisms	*Proteus, Cryptococcus, H pylori, Ureaplasma, Nocardia, Klebsiella, S epidermidis, S saprophyticus*. Urease hydrolyzes urea to release ammonia and CO_2 → ↑ pH. Predisposes to struvite (magnesium ammonium phosphate) stones, particularly *Proteus*.	Pee CHUNKSS.

Catalase-positive organisms

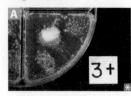

Catalase degrades H_2O_2 into H_2O and bubbles of O_2 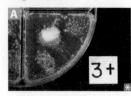 before it can be converted to microbicidal products by the enzyme myeloperoxidase. People with chronic granulomatous disease (NADPH oxidase deficiency) have recurrent infections with certain catalase ⊕ organisms.

Catalase ⊕ organisms include *Candida, Pseudomonas, Nocardia, Bordetella pertussis, Burkholderia cepacia, Helicobacter pylori, Aspergillus, Staphylococci, Serratia, Listeria, E coli.* Catalase Positive: Notoriously Big Bubbling **HASSLE.**

Pigment-producing bacteria

Actinomyces israelii—yellow "sulfur" granules, which are composed of filaments of bacteria	Israel has yellow sand
S aureus—**gold**en yellow pigment	*Aureus* (Latin) = **gold**
P aeruginosa—blue-**green** pigment (pyocyanin and pyoverdin)	Aerugula is **green**
Serratia marcescens—**red** pigment	Think **red Sriracha** hot sauce

---

In vivo biofilm-producing bacteria

S epidermidis	Catheter and prosthetic device infections
Viridans streptococci (*S mutans, S sanguinis*)	Dental plaques, infective endocarditis
P aeruginosa	Respiratory tree colonization in patients with cystic fibrosis, ventilator-associated pneumonia Contact lens–associated keratitis
Nontypeable (unencapsulated) *H influenzae*	Otitis media

| **Spore-forming bacteria** | Some gram ⊕ bacteria can form spores when nutrients are limited. Spores lack metabolic activity and are highly resistant to heat and chemicals. Core contains dipicolinic acid (responsible for heat resistance). Must autoclave to kill spores (as is done to surgical equipment) by steaming at 121°C for 15 minutes at a pressure of 15 psi. Hydrogen peroxide and iodine-based agents are also sporicidal. | Examples: *B anthracis* (anthrax), *B cereus* (food poisoning), *Clostridium botulinum* (botulism), *Clostridioides difficile* (pseudomembranous colitis), *Clostridium perfringens* (gas gangrene), *Clostridium tetani* (tetanus). Autoclave to kill **B**acillus and **C**lostridium (**ABC**). |

Bacterial virulence factors	These promote evasion of host immune response.
Capsular polysaccharide	Highly charged, hydrophilic structure. Acts as barrier to phagocytosis and complement-mediated lysis. Major determinant of virulence.
Protein A	Binds Fc region of IgG. Prevents opsonization and phagocytosis. Expressed by *S aureus*.
IgA protease	Enzyme that cleaves IgA, allowing bacteria to adhere to and colonize mucous membranes. Secreted by *S pneumoniae*, *H influenzae* type b, and *Neisseria* (**SHiN**).
M protein	Helps prevent phagocytosis. Expressed by group A streptococci. Sequence homology with human cardiac myosin (molecular mimicry); possibly underlies the autoimmune response seen in acute rheumatic fever.

Antibiotic resistance mechanisms

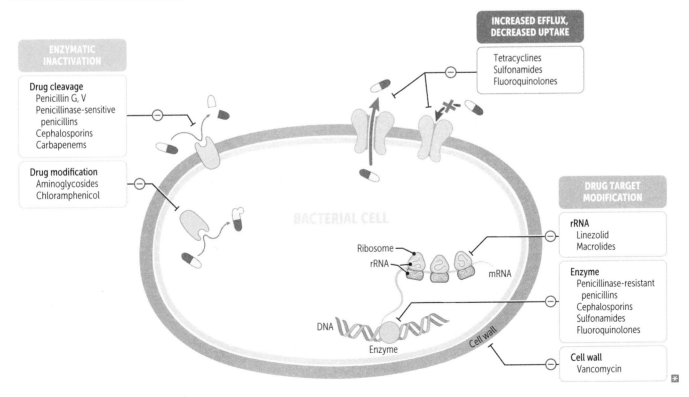

Bacterial genetics	Horizontal gene transfer is the main mechanism for transfer of antibiotic resistance among bacteria.
Transformation	Competent bacteria can bind and import short pieces of environmental naked bacterial chromosomal DNA (from bacterial cell lysis). The transfer and expression of newly transferred genes is called transformation. A feature of many bacteria, especially *S pneumoniae*, *H influenzae* type b, and *Neisseria* (**SHiN**). Adding deoxyribonuclease degrades naked DNA, preventing transformation.

Conjugation	
F⁺ × F⁻	F⁺ (fertility factor) plasmid contains genes required for sex pilus and conjugation. Bacteria without this plasmid are termed F⁻. Sex pilus on F⁺ bacterium contacts F⁻ bacterium. A single strand of plasmid DNA is transferred across the conjugal bridge ("mating bridge"). No transfer of chromosomal DNA.

Hfr × F⁻	F⁺ plasmid can become incorporated into bacterial chromosomal DNA, termed high-frequency recombination (Hfr) cell. Transfer of leading part of plasmid and a few flanking chromosomal genes. High-frequency recombination may integrate some of those bacterial genes. Recipient cell remains F⁻ but now may have new bacterial genes.

Transduction	
Generalized	A "packaging" error. Lytic phage infects bacterium, leading to cleavage of bacterial DNA. Parts of bacterial chromosomal DNA may become packaged in phage capsid. Phage infects another bacterium, transferring these genes.

Specialized	An "excision" event. Lysogenic phage infects bacterium; viral DNA incorporates into bacterial chromosome. When phage DNA is excised, flanking bacterial genes may be excised with it. DNA is packaged into phage capsid and can infect another bacterium. Genes for the following 5 bacterial toxins are encoded in a lysogenic phage (**ABCD'S**): Group A strep erythrogenic toxin, Botulinum toxin, Cholera toxin, Diphtheria toxin, Shiga toxin.

Bacterial genetics (continued)

Transposition	A "jumping" process involving a transposon (specialized segment of DNA), which can copy and excise itself and then insert into the same DNA molecule or an unrelated DNA (eg, plasmid or chromosome). Critical in creating plasmids with multiple drug resistance and transfer across species lines (eg, Tn*1546* with *vanA* from *Enterococcus* to *S aureus*).	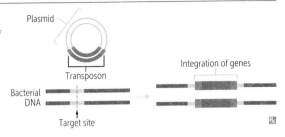

Main features of exotoxins and endotoxins

	Exotoxins	Endotoxins
SOURCE	Certain species of gram ⊕ and gram ⊖ bacteria	Outer cell membrane of most gram ⊖ bacteria
SECRETED FROM CELL	Yes	No
CHEMISTRY	Polypeptide	Lipid A component of LPS (structural part of bacteria; released when lysed)
LOCATION OF GENES	Plasmid or bacteriophage	Bacterial chromosome
TOXICITY	High (fatal dose on the order of 1 μg)	Low (fatal dose on the order of hundreds of micrograms)
CLINICAL EFFECTS	Various effects (see following pages)	Fever, shock (hypotension), DIC
MODE OF ACTION	Various modes (see following pages)	Induces TNF, IL-1, and IL-6
ANTIGENICITY	Induces high-titer antibodies called antitoxins	Poorly antigenic
VACCINES	Toxoids used as vaccines	No toxoids formed and no vaccine available
HEAT STABILITY	Destroyed rapidly at 60°C (except staphylococcal enterotoxin, *E coli* heat-stable toxin, and *B cereus* emetic toxin)	Stable at 100°C for 1 hr
TYPICAL DISEASES	Tetanus, botulism, diphtheria, cholera	Meningococcemia; sepsis by gram ⊖ rods

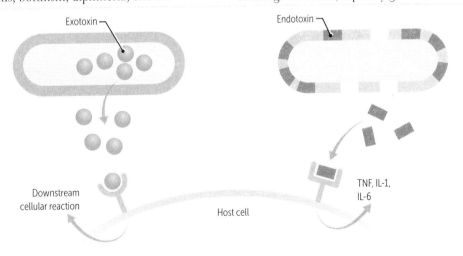

Bacteria with exotoxins

BACTERIA	TOXIN	MECHANISM	MANIFESTATION
Inhibit protein synthesis			
Corynebacterium diphtheriae	Diphtheria toxin[a]	Inactivate elongation factor (EF-2) through ADP-ribosylation	Pharyngitis with pseudomembranes in throat and severe lymphadenopathy (bull neck), myocarditis
Pseudomonas aeruginosa	Exotoxin A[a]		Host cell death
Shigella spp	Shiga toxin[a]	Inactivate 60S ribosome by removing adenine from rRNA	Damages GI mucosa → dysentery
Enterohemorrhagic E coli			Toxin-mediated injury and cytokine release → hemolytic-uremic syndrome (HUS; prototypically in EHEC serotype O157:H7) Unlike *Shigella*, EHEC does not invade host cells
Increase fluid secretion			
Enterotoxigenic E coli	Heat-labile toxin (LT)[a]	Overactivates adenylate cyclase (↑ cAMP) → ↑ Cl⁻ secretion in gut and H_2O efflux	Watery diarrhea: "**labile** in the **Air** (Adenylate cyclase), **stable** on the **Ground** (Guanylate cyclase)"
	Heat-**stable** toxin (ST)	Overactivates guanylate cyclase (↑ cGMP) → ↓ resorption of NaCl and H_2O in gut	Bacteria that ↑ cAMP include *V cholerae*, *B anthracis*, *B pertussis*, *E coli*
Bacillus anthracis	Anthrax toxin[a]	Mimics adenylate cyclase (↑ cAMP)	Likely responsible for characteristic edematous borders of black eschar in cutaneous anthrax
Vibrio cholerae	Cholera toxin[a]	Overactivates adenylate cyclase (↑ cAMP) by permanently activating G_s	Voluminous "rice-water" diarrhea
Inhibit phagocytic ability			
Bordetella pertussis	Pertussis toxin[a]	Activates adenylate cyclase (↑ cAMP) by inactivating inhibitory subunit (G_i).	Whooping cough—child coughs on expiration and "whoops" on inspiration; can cause "100-day cough" in adults; associated with posttussive emesis
Inhibit release of neurotransmitter			
Clostridium tetani	Tetanospasmin[a]	Both are proteases that cleave SNARE (soluble NSF attachment protein receptor), a set of proteins required for neurotransmitter release via vesicular fusion	Toxin prevents release of **inhibitory** (GABA and glycine) neurotransmitters from Renshaw cells in spinal cord → spastic paralysis, risus sardonicus, trismus (lockjaw), opisthotonos
Clostridium botulinum	Botulinum toxin[a]		Infant botulism—caused by ingestion of spores (eg, from soil, raw honey). Toxin produced in vivo Foodborne botulism—caused by ingestion of preformed toxin (eg, from canned foods)

[a]An AB toxin (also called two-component toxin [or three for anthrax]) with **B** enabling **B**inding and triggering uptake (endocytosis) of the **A**ctive **A** component. The A components are usually ADP ribosyltransferases; others have enzymatic activities as listed in chart.

Bacteria with exotoxins (continued)

BACTERIA	TOXIN	MECHANISM	MANIFESTATION
Lyse cell membranes			
Clostridium perfringens	Alpha toxin	Phospholipase (lecithinase) that degrades tissue and cell membranes	Degradation of phospholipids → myonecrosis ("gas gangrene") and hemolysis ("double zone" of hemolysis on blood agar)
Streptococcus pyogenes	Streptolysin O	Protein that degrades cell membrane	Lyses RBCs; contributes to β-hemolysis; host antibodies against toxin (ASO) used to diagnose rheumatic fever (do not confuse with immune complexes of poststreptococcal glomerulonephritis)
Superantigens causing shock			
Staphylococcus aureus	Toxic shock syndrome toxin (TSST-1)	Cross-links β region of TCR to MHC class II on APCs outside of the antigen binding site → overwhelming release of IL-1, IL-2, IFN-γ, and TNF-α → shock	Toxic shock syndrome: fever, rash, shock; other toxins cause scalded skin syndrome (exfoliative toxin) and food poisoning (heat-stable enterotoxin)
Streptococcus pyogenes	Erythrogenic exotoxin A		Toxic shock–like syndrome: fever, rash, shock; scarlet fever

Endotoxin	LPS found in outer membrane of gram ⊖ bacteria (both cocci and rods). Composed of O-antigen + core polysaccharide + lipid A (the toxic component). *Neisseria* have lipooligosaccharide. Released upon cell lysis or by living cells by blebs detaching from outer surface membrane (vs exotoxin, which is actively secreted). Three main effects: macrophage activation (TLR4/CD14), complement activation, and tissue factor activation.	**ENDOTOXINS:** Edema Nitric oxide DIC/Death Outer membrane TNF-α O-antigen + core polysaccharide + lipid A eXtremely heat stable IL-1 and IL-6 Neutrophil chemotaxis Shock

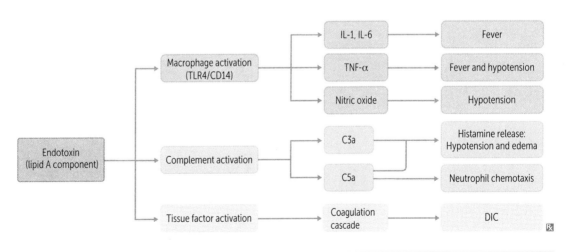

Gram-positive lab algorithm

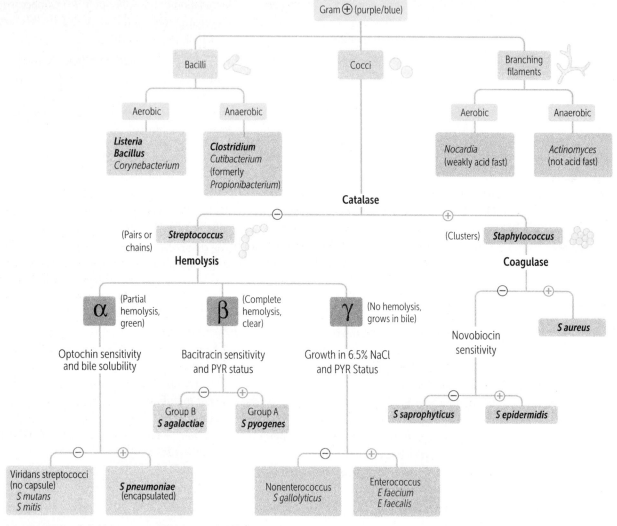

Important **tests** are in **bold.** Important *pathogens* are in *bold italics.*

Note. Enterococcus is either α- or γ-hemolytic.

PYR, Pyrrolidonyl aminopeptidase.

Hemolytic bacteria

α-hemolytic bacteria	Partial oxidation of hemoglobin → greenish or brownish color without clearing around growth on blood agar 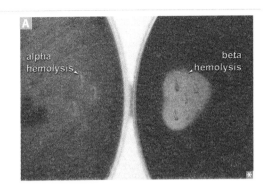. Include *Streptococcus pneumoniae* and viridans streptococci.
β-hemolytic bacteria	Complete lysis of RBCs → pale/clear area surrounding colony on blood agar. Include *Staphylococcus aureus*, *Streptococcus pyogenes* (group A strep), *Streptococcus agalactiae* (group B strep), *Listeria monocytogenes*.

alpha hemolysis · beta hemolysis

Staphylococcus aureus

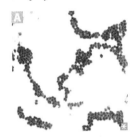

Gram ⊕, β-hemolytic, catalase ⊕, coagulase ⊕ cocci in clusters. Protein A (virulence factor) binds Fc-IgG, inhibiting complement activation and phagocytosis. Commonly colonizes the skin, nares, ears, axilla, and groin.
Causes:
- Inflammatory disease—skin infections, organ abscesses, pneumonia (often after influenza virus infection), infective endocarditis, septic arthritis, and osteomyelitis.
- Toxin-mediated disease—toxic shock syndrome (TSST-1), scalded skin syndrome (exfoliative toxin), rapid-onset food poisoning (enterotoxins).

MRSA (methicillin-resistant *S aureus*)— important cause of serious healthcare-associated and community-acquired infections. Resistance due to altered penicillin-binding proteins (conferred by *mecA* gene). Some strains release Panton-Valentine leukocidin (PVL), which kills leukocytes and causes tissue necrosis.

TSST-1 is a superantigen that binds to MHC II and T-cell receptor, resulting in polyclonal T-cell activation and cytokine release.
Staphylococcal toxic shock syndrome (TSS)— fever, vomiting, diarrhea, rash, desquamation, shock, end-organ failure. TSS results in ↑ AST, ↑ ALT, ↑ bilirubin. Associated with prolonged use of vaginal tampons or nasal packing.
Compare with *Streptococcus pyogenes* TSS (a toxic shock–like syndrome associated with painful skin infection).
S aureus food poisoning due to ingestion of preformed toxin → short incubation period (2–6 hr) followed by nonbloody diarrhea and emesis. Enterotoxin is heat stable → not destroyed by cooking.
S aureus makes coagulase and toxins. Forms fibrin clot around itself → abscess.

Staphylococcus epidermidis

Gram ⊕, catalase ⊕, coagulase ⊖, urease ⊕ cocci in clusters. Novobiocin sensitive. Does not ferment mannitol (vs *S aureus*).
Normal microbiota of skin; contaminates blood cultures.
Infects prosthetic devices (eg, hip implant, heart valve) and IV catheters by producing adherent biofilms.

Staphylococcus saprophyticus

Gram ⊕, catalase ⊕, coagulase ⊖, urease ⊕ cocci in clusters. Novobiocin resistant.
Normal microbiota of female genital tract and perineum.
Second most common cause of uncomplicated UTI in young females (most common is *E coli*).

Streptococcus pneumoniae

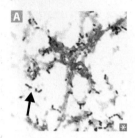

Gram ⊕, α-hemolytic, lancet-shaped diplococci **A**.
Encapsulated. IgA protease. Optochin sensitive and bile soluble.
Most commonly causes **MOPS**:
- Meningitis
- Otitis media (in children)
- Pneumonia
- Sinusitis

Pneumococcal pneumonia is associated with "rusty" sputum.
Patients with anatomic or functional hyposplenia or asplenia are predisposed to infection.
No virulence without capsule.
Pneumococcal vaccines are available in both conjugate (PCV13, PCV15, PCV20) and polysaccharide (PPSV23) formulations.

Viridans group streptococci

Gram ⊕, α-hemolytic cocci. Optochin resistant and bile insoluble. Normal microbiota of the oropharynx.
Streptococcus mutans and *S mitis* cause dental caries.
S sanguinis makes dextrans that bind to fibrin-platelet aggregates on damaged **heart** valves, causing infective endocarditis.

Viridans group strep live in the mouth, because they are not afraid **of-the-chin** (**op-to-chin** resistant).
Sanguinis = **blood**. Think, "there is lots of **blood** in the **heart**" (infective endocarditis).

Streptococcus pyogenes (group A streptococci)

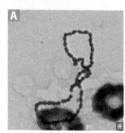

Gram ⊕ cocci in chains **A**. Group A strep cause:
- Pyogenic—pharyngitis, cellulitis, impetigo ("honey-crusted" lesions), erysipelas
- Toxigenic—scarlet fever, toxic shock–like syndrome, necrotizing fasciitis
- Immunologic—rheumatic fever, glomerulonephritis

Bacitracin sensitive, β-hemolytic, pyrrolidonyl arylamidase (PYR) ⊕. Hyaluronic acid capsule and M protein inhibit phagocytosis. Antibodies to M protein enhance host defenses. Structurally similar to host proteins (ie, myosin); can lead to autoimmunity (ie, carditis seen in acute rheumatic fever).
Diagnose strep pharyngitis via throat swab, which can be tested with an antigen detection assay (rapid, in-office results) or cultured on blood agar (results in 48 hours).

"**Ph**"yogenes **ph**aryngitis can result in rheumatic "**ph**ever" and glomerulonephritis.
Strains causing impetigo can induce glomerulonephritis.
Key virulence factors include DNase, erythrogenic exotoxin, streptokinase, streptolysin O. ASO titer or anti-DNase B antibodies indicate recent *S pyogenes* infection.
Scarlet fever—fine, blanching, generalized sandpaperlike rash sparing palms and soles, strawberry tongue, and circumoral pallor in the setting of group A streptococcal pharyngitis (erythrogenic toxin ⊕).

***Streptococcus agalactiae* (group B streptococci)**	Gram ⊕ cocci, bacitracin resistant, β-hemolytic, colonizes vagina; causes pneumonia, meningitis, and sepsis, mainly in **babies**. Polysaccharide capsule confers virulence. Produces CAMP factor, which enlarges the area of hemolysis formed by *S aureus*. (Note: CAMP stands for the authors of the test, not cyclic AMP.) Hippurate test ⊕. PYR ⊖. Screen pregnant patients at 35–37 weeks of gestation with rectal and vaginal swabs. Patients with ⊕ culture receive intrapartum penicillin/ampicillin prophylaxis.	Group B for Babies!
***Streptococcus gallolyticus**	Formerly *S bovis*. Gram ⊕ cocci, colonizes the gut. Can cause bacteremia and infective endocarditis. Patients with *S gallolyticus* endocarditis have ↑ incidence of colon cancer.	Bovis in the blood = cancer in the colon.
Enterococci	Gram ⊕ cocci. Enterococci (*E faecalis* and *E faecium*) are normal colonic microbiota that are intrinsically resistant to penicillin G and cause UTI, biliary tract infections, and infective endocarditis (following GI/GU procedures). Catalase ⊖, PYR ⊕, typically nonhemolytic. VRE (vancomycin-resistant enterococci) are an important cause of healthcare-associated infection.	Enterococci are more resilient than streptococci, can grow in 6.5% NaCl and bile (lab test). *Entero* = intestine, *faecalis* = feces, *strepto* = twisted (chains), *coccus* = berry.

Bacillus anthracis

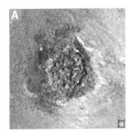

Gram ⊕, spore-forming rod that produces anthrax toxin, exotoxins consisting of protective antigen, lethal factor (inhibits MAP kinase → macrophage apoptosis), and edema factor (acts as adenylyl cyclase → ↑ intracellular cAMP, upsetting homeostasis → edema, necrosis). Has a polypeptide capsule (poly D-glutamate). Colonies show a halo of projections, sometimes called "medusa head" appearance.

Cutaneous anthrax—painless papule surrounded by vesicles → ulcer with black eschar Ⓐ (painless, necrotic) → uncommonly progresses to bacteremia and death.

Pulmonary anthrax—inhalation of spores, most commonly from contaminated animals or animal products, although also a potential bioweapon → flulike symptoms that rapidly progress to fever, pulmonary hemorrhage, mediastinitis (CXR may show widened mediastinum), and shock. Also called woolsorter's disease. Prophylaxis with ciprofloxacin or doxycycline when exposed.

Both cutaneous and pulmonary anthrax may be complicated by hemorrhagic meningitis.

Bacillus cereus	Gram ⊕ rod. Causes food poisoning. Spores survive cooking rice (reheated rice syndrome). Keeping rice warm results in germination of spores and enterotoxin formation. Emetic type causes nausea and vomiting within 1–5 hours. Caused by cereulide, a preformed toxin. Diarrheal type causes watery, nonbloody diarrhea and GI pain within 8–18 hours. Management: supportive care (antibiotics are ineffective against toxins).

Clostridioides difficile

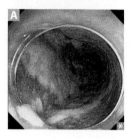

Produces toxins A and B, which damage enterocytes. Both toxins lead to watery diarrhea → pseudomembranous colitis A. Often 2° to antibiotic use, especially clindamycin, ampicillin, cephalosporins, fluoroquinolones; associated with PPIs.

Fulminant infection: toxic megacolon, ileus, shock.

Difficile causes **di**arrhea.

Diagnosed by PCR or antigen detection of one or both toxins in stool.

Treatment: oral vancomycin or fidaxomicin. For recurrent cases, consider repeating prior regimen or fecal microbiota transplant.

Clostridia

Gram ⊕, spore-forming, obligate anaerobic rods. Tetanus toxin and botulinum toxin are proteases that cleave SNARE proteins involved in neurotransmission.

Clostridium tetani

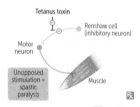

Pathogen is noninvasive and remains localized to wound site. Produces tetanospasmin, an exotoxin causing tetanus. Tetano**spas**min spreads by retrograde axonal transport to CNS and blocks release of GABA and glycine from Renshaw cells in spinal cord.

Causes **spas**tic paralysis, trismus (lockjaw), risus sardonicus (raised eyebrows and open grin), opisthotonos (spasms of spinal extensors).

Tetanus is **tet**anic paralysis.

Prevent with tetanus vaccine. Treat with antitoxin +/– vaccine booster, antibiotics, diazepam (for muscle spasms), and wound debridement.

Clostridium botulinum

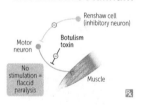

Produces a heat-labile toxin that damages SNARE proteins, thus preventing ACh release at the neuromuscular junction, causing botulism. In babies, ingestion of spores (eg, in honey) leads to disease (**floppy** baby syndrome). In adults, disease is caused by ingestion of preformed toxin (eg, in canned food).

Symptoms of botulism (the **5 D's**): **d**iplopia, **d**ysarthria, **d**ysphagia, **d**yspnea, **d**escending **fl**accid paralysis. Does not present with sensory deficits.

Botulinum is from bad **bot**tles of food, juice, and honey.

Treatment: human botulinum immunoglobulin.

Local botulinum toxin A (Botox) injections used to treat focal dystonia, hyperhidrosis, muscle spasms, and cosmetic reduction of facial wrinkles.

Clostridium perfringens

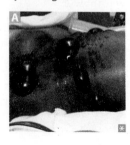

Produces α-toxin (lecithinase, a phospholipase) that can cause myonecrosis (gas gangrene A; presents as soft tissue crepitus) and hemolysis.

If heavily spore-contaminated food is cooked but left standing too long at < 60°C, spore germinate → vegetative bacteria ingested → enterotoxin → late-onset (10–12 hours) food poisoning symptoms, resolution in 24 hours.

Perfringens **perf**orates a gangrenous leg.

Spontaneous gas gangrene (via hematogenous seeding; associated with colonic malignancy) is most commonly caused by *Clostridium septicum*.

Corynebacterium diphtheriae

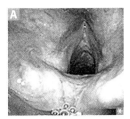

Gram ⊕ rods occurring in angular arrangements; transmitted via respiratory droplets. Causes diphtheria via exotoxin encoded by β-prophage. Potent exotoxin inhibits protein synthesis via ADP-ribosylation of EF-2, leading to possible necrosis in pharynx, cardiac, and CNS tissue.

Symptoms include pseudomembranous pharyngitis (grayish-white membrane) with lymphadenopathy ("bull's neck" appearance). Toxin dissemination may cause myocarditis, arrhythmias, neuropathies.

Lab diagnosis based on gram ⊕ rods with metachromatic (blue and red) granules and ⊕ Elek test for toxin.

Toxoid vaccine prevents diphtheria.

Coryne = club shaped (metachromatic granules on Löffler media).

Black colonies on cystine-tellurite agar.

ABCDEFG:
ADP-ribosylation
β-prophage
Corynebacterium
Diphtheriae
Elongation Factor 2
Granules

Treatment: diphtheria antitoxin +/– erythromycin or penicillin.

Listeria monocytogenes

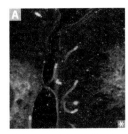

Gram ⊕, facultative intracellular rod; acquired by ingestion of unpasteurized dairy products and cold deli meats, transplacental transmission, and by vaginal transmission during birth. Grows well at refrigeration temperatures ("cold enrichment").

Forms "rocket tails" (red in) via actin polymerization that allow intracellular movement and cell-to-cell spread across cell membranes, thereby avoiding antibody. Listeriolysin generates pores in phagosomes, allowing its escape into cytoplasm. Characteristic tumbling motility in broth.

Can cause amnionitis, sepsis, and spontaneous abortion in pregnant patients; granulomatosis infantiseptica; meningitis in immunocompromised patients, neonates, and older adults; mild, self-limited gastroenteritis in healthy individuals.

Treatment: ampicillin.

Nocardia vs Actinomyces

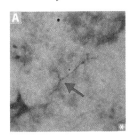

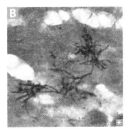

Both are gram ⊕ and form long, branching filaments resembling fungi.

Nocardia	Actinomyces
Aerobe, catalase ⊕	Anaerobe, catalase ⊖
Acid fast (weak)	Not acid fast
Found in soil	Normal oral, reproductive, and GI microbiota
Causes pulmonary infections in immunocompromised (can mimic TB but with ⊖ PPD); cutaneous infections after trauma in immunocompetent; can spread to CNS → cerebral abscess	Causes oral/facial abscesses that drain through sinus tracts; often associated with dental caries/extraction and other maxillofacial trauma; forms yellow "sulfur granules"; can also cause PID with IUDs
Treat with sulfonamides (TMP-SMX)	Treat with penicillin

Treatment is a **SNAP**: Sulfonamides—*Nocardia*; *Actinomyces*—Penicillin

Mycobacteria

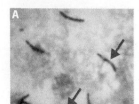

Acid-fast rods (pink rods, arrows in 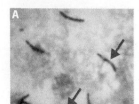). Grows slowly in culture.

Mycobacterium tuberculosis (TB, often resistant to multiple drugs).

M avium–intracellulare (causes disseminated, non-TB disease in AIDS; often resistant to multiple drugs).

M scrofulaceum (cervical lymphadenitis in children).

M marinum (skin infection in aquarium handlers).

TB symptoms include fever, night sweats, weight loss, cough (nonproductive or productive), hemoptysis.

Cord factor creates a "serpentine cord" appearance in virulent *M tuberculosis* strains; activates macrophages (promoting granuloma formation) and induces release of TNF-α. Sulfatides (surface glycolipids) inhibit phagolysosomal fusion.

Tuberculosis

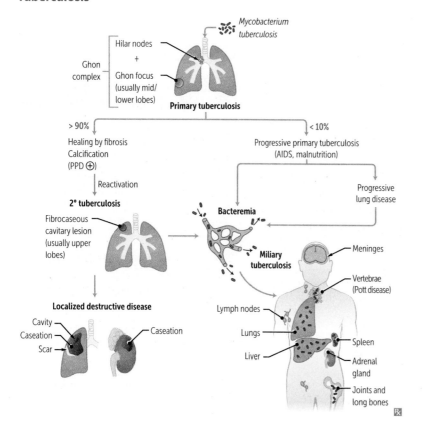

PPD ⊕ if current or past infection.

PPD ⊖ if no infection and in immunocompromised patients (especially with low CD4+ cell count).

Interferon-γ release assay (IGRA) has fewer false positives from BCG vaccination.

Caseating granulomas with central necrosis and Langhans giant cell (single example in 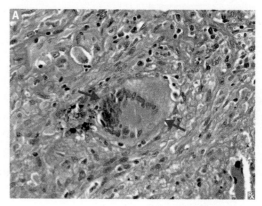) are characteristic of 2° tuberculosis. Do not confuse Langhans giant cell (fused macrophages) with Langerhans cell (dermal APC).

TB reactivation risk highest in immunocompromised individuals (eg, HIV, organ transplant recipients, TNF-α inhibitor use). Reactivation has a predilection for the apices of the lung (due to the bacteria being highly aerobic).

Leprosy

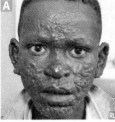
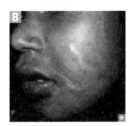

Also called Hansen disease. Caused by *Mycobacterium leprae*, an acid-fast bacillus that likes cool temperatures (infects skin and superficial nerves—"glove and stocking" loss of sensation) and cannot be grown in vitro. Diagnosed via skin biopsy or tissue PCR. Reservoir in United States: armadillos.

Leprosy has 2 forms (many cases fall temporarily between two extremes):

- Lepromatous—presents diffusely over the skin, with leonine (lionlike) facies , and is communicable (high bacterial load); characterized by low cell-mediated immunity with a largely Th2 response. Lepromatous form can be lethal.
- Tuberculoid—limited to a few hypoesthetic, hairless skin plaques **B**; characterized by high cell-mediated immunity with a largely Th1 response and low bacterial load.

Treatment: **d**apsone and **rif**ampin for tuberculoid form; **cl**ofazimine is added for **lep**romatous form. **D**aring **rif**les target **cl**oaked **lep**rechauns.

Gram-negative lab algorithm

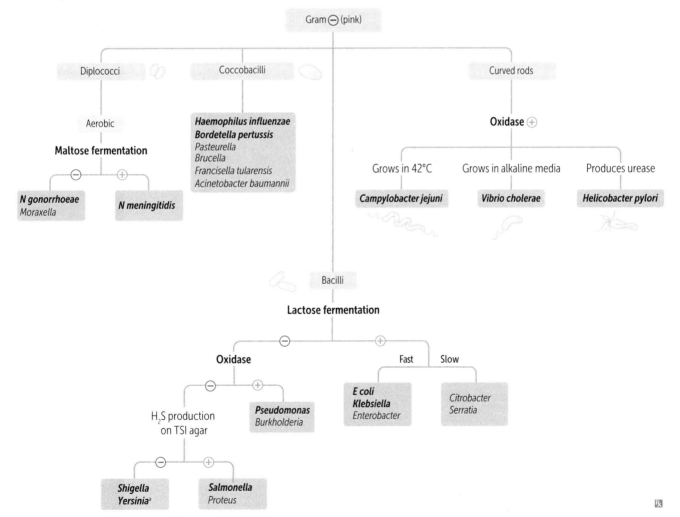

Important **tests** are in bold. Important ***pathogens*** are in **bold italics**.
[a]Pleomorphic rod/coccobacillus

Neisseria

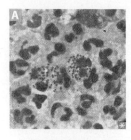

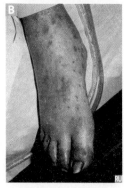

Gram ⊖ diplococci. Metabolize glucose and produce IgA proteases. Contain lipooligosaccharides (LOS) with strong endotoxin activity.

N gonorrhoeae is often intracellular (within neutrophils) .

Acid production: meningococci—maltose and glucose; gonococci—glucose.

Gonococci	Meningococci
No polysaccharide capsule	Polysaccharide capsule
No maltose acid detection	Maltose acid detection
No vaccine due to antigenic variation of pilus proteins	Vaccine (type B vaccine available for at-risk individuals)
Sexually or perinatally transmitted	Transmitted via respiratory and oral secretions. More common among individuals in close quarters (eg, army barracks, college dorms)
Causes gonorrhea, septic arthritis, neonatal conjunctivitis (2–5 days after birth), pelvic inflammatory disease (PID), and Fitz-Hugh–Curtis syndrome	Causes meningococcemia with petechial hemorrhages and gangrene of toes , meningitis, Waterhouse-Friderichsen syndrome (acute hemorrhagic adrenal insufficiency)
Diagnosed with NAAT	Diagnosed via culture-based tests or PCR
Condoms ↓ sexual transmission, erythromycin eye ointment prevents neonatal blindness	Rifampin, ciprofloxacin, or ceftriaxone prophylaxis in close contacts
Treatment: single dose IM ceftriaxone; if chlamydial coinfection not excluded by molecular testing, add doxycycline	Treatment: ceftriaxone or penicillin G

Haemophilus influenzae

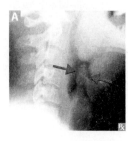

Small gram ⊖ (coccobacillary) rod. Transmitted through respiratory droplets. Nontypeable (unencapsulated) strains are the most common cause of mucosal infections (otitis media, conjunctivitis, bronchitis) as well as invasive infections since the vaccine for capsular type b was introduced. Produces IgA protease.

Culture on chocolate agar, which contains factors V (NAD⁺) and X (hematin) for growth; can also be grown with S aureus, which provides factor V via RBC hemolysis.

Haemophilus causes epiglottitis (endoscopic appearance can be "cherry red" in children; "thumb sign" on lateral neck x-ray), meningitis, otitis media, and pneumonia.

Vaccine contains type b capsular polysaccharide (polyribosylribitol phosphate) conjugated to diphtheria toxoid or other protein. Given between 2 and 18 months of age.

Does not cause the flu (influenza virus does).

Treatment: amoxicillin +/– clavulanate for mucosal infections; ceftriaxone for meningitis; rifampin prophylaxis for close contacts.

Burkholderia cepacia complex

Aerobic, catalase ⊕, gram ⊖ rod. Causes pneumonia in patients with underlying lung disease, such as cystic fibrosis. Often multidrug resistant. Infection is a relative contraindication to undergoing lung transplant due to its association with poor outcomes.

Bordetella pertussis

Gram ⊖, aerobic coccobacillus. Virulence factors include pertussis toxin (disables G_i), adenylate cyclase toxin (↑ cAMP), and tracheal cytotoxin (destroys respiratory ciliated epithelium). Three clinical stages:

- Catarrhal—low-grade fevers, coryza.
- Paroxysmal—paroxysms of intense cough followed by inspiratory "whoop" ("whooping cough"), posttussive vomiting.
- Convalescent—gradual recovery of chronic cough.

Prevented by Tdap, DTaP vaccines (Tdap for preTeens and adulTs, DTaP for chilDren).

Produces lymphocytosis (unlike most acute bacterial infections).

Treatment: macrolides; if allergic use TMP-SMX.

Brucella

Gram ⊖, aerobic coccobacillus. Transmitted via ingestion of contaminated animal products (eg, unpasteurized milk). Survives in macrophages in the reticuloendothelial system. Can form non-caseating granulomas. Typically presents with undulant fever, night sweats, and arthralgia. Treatment: doxycycline + rifampin or streptomycin.

Legionella pneumophila

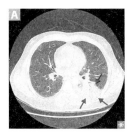

Gram ⊖ rod. Gram stains poorly—use **silver** stain. Grow on **charcoal** yeast extract medium with **iron** and **cysteine**. Detected by presence of antigen in urine. Labs may show hyponatremia and elevated transaminases.

Aerosol transmission from environmental water source (eg, air conditioning systems, hot water tanks). Outbreaks associated with cruise ships, nursing homes. No person-to-person transmission.

Treatment: macrolide or quinolone.

Think of a French **legionnaire** (soldier) with his **silver** helmet, sitting around a campfire (**charcoal**) with his **iron** dagger—he is missing his **sister** (cysteine).

Legionnaires' disease—severe pneumonia (often unilateral and lobar A), fever, GI and CNS symptoms. Risk factors include older age, tobacco smoking, chronic lung disease.

Pontiac fever—mild flulike symptoms.

Pseudomonas aeruginosa

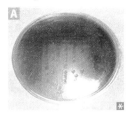

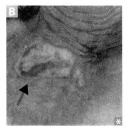

Aeruginosa—aerobic; motile, catalase ⊕, gram ⊖ rod. Non-lactose fermenting. Oxidase ⊕. Frequently found in water. Increased virulence in acidic environments. Has a grapelike odor.

PSEUDOMONAS is associated with: Pneumonia, Sepsis, Ecthyma gangrenosum, UTIs, Diabetes, Osteomyelitis, Mucoid polysaccharide capsule, Otitis externa (swimmer's ear), Nosocomial (healthcare-associated) infections (eg, catheters, equipment), Addiction (injection drug use), Skin infections (eg, hot tub folliculitis, wound infection in burn victims).

Mucoid polysaccharide capsule may contribute to chronic pneumonia in patients with cystic fibrosis due to biofilm formation.

Produces **PEEP**: Phospholipase C (degrades cell membranes); Endotoxin (fever, shock); Exotoxin A (inactivates EF-2); green Pigment A.

Corneal ulcers/keratitis in contact lens wearers/minor eye trauma.

Ecthyma gangrenosum—rapidly progressive, necrotic cutaneous lesion B caused by *Pseudomonas* bacteremia. Typically seen in immunocompromised patients.

Treatments:

- Antipseudomonal penicillins in combination with β-lactamase inhibitor (eg, piperacillin-tazobactam)
- 3rd- and 4th-generation cephalosporins (eg, ceftazidime, cefepime)
- Monobactams
- Fluoroquinolones
- Carbapenems

Despite antipseudomonal activity, aminoglycoside monotherapy is avoided due to poor performance in acidic environments.

Salmonella vs Shigella   Both *Salmonella* and *Shigella* are gram ⊖ rods, non-lactose fermenters, oxidase ⊖, and can invade the GI tract via M cells of Peyer patches.

	Salmonella typhi (ty-Vi)	*Salmonella* spp. except *S typhi*	*Shigella*
RESERVOIRS	Humans only	Humans and animals	Humans only
SPREAD	Hematogenous spread	Hematogenous spread is rare	Cell to cell; no hematogenous spread
H₂S PRODUCTION	Yes	Yes	No
FLAGELLA	Yes (**salmon swim**)	Yes (**salmon swim**)	No
VIRULENCE FACTORS	Endotoxin; **Vi** capsule (pronounce "tyVi")	Endotoxin	Endotoxin; Shiga toxin (enterotoxin)
INFECTIOUS DOSE (ID₅₀)	High—large inoculum required; acid-labile (inactivated by gastric acids)	High	Low—very small inoculum required; acid stable (resistant to gastric acids)
EFFECT OF ANTIBIOTICS ON FECAL EXCRETION	Prolongs duration	Prolongs duration	Shortens duration (shortens *Shigella*)
IMMUNE RESPONSE	Primarily monocytes	PMNs in disseminated disease	Primarily PMN infiltration
GI MANIFESTATIONS	Constipation, followed by diarrhea	Diarrhea (possibly bloody)	Crampy abdominal pain → tenesmus, bloody mucoid stools (bacillary dysentery)
VACCINE	Oral vaccine contains live attenuated *S typhi* IM vaccine contains Vi capsular polysaccharide	No vaccine	No vaccine
UNIQUE PROPERTIES	Causes typhoid fever (salmon-colored truncal macular rash, abdominal pain, fever [pulse-temperature dissociation]; later GI ulceration and hemorrhage); treat with ceftriaxone or fluoroquinolone Carrier state with gallbladder colonization	Poultry, eggs, pets, and turtles are common sources Treatment is supportive; antibiotics are not indicated in immunocompetent individuals	4 F's: fingers, flies, food, feces In order of decreasing severity (less toxin produced): *S dysenteriae*, *S flexneri*, *S boydii*, *S sonnei* Invasion of M cells is key to pathogenicity; infectious dose is low

Yersinia enterocolitica   Gram ⊖ pleomorphic rod/coccobacillus with bipolar staining. Usually transmitted from pet feces (eg, cats, dogs), contaminated milk, or pork. Can cause acute bloody diarrhea, pseudoappendicitis (right lower abdominal pain due to mesenteric adenitis and/or terminal ileitis), reactive arthritis in adults.

Lactose-fermenting enteric bacteria   Fermentation of lactose → pink colonies on MacConkey agar. Examples include *Citrobacter*, *E coli*, *Enterobacter*, *Klebsiella*, *Serratia*.

McCowkey **CEEKS** milk.
EMB agar—lactose fermenters grow as purple/black colonies. *E coli* grows colonies with a green sheen.

Escherichia coli Gram ⊖, indole ⊕ rod. *E coli* virulence factors: fimbriae (ie, P pili)—cystitis and pyelonephritis; K capsule—pneumonia, neonatal meningitis; LPS endotoxin—septic shock.

STRAIN	TOXIN AND MECHANISM	PRESENTATION
Enteroinvasive *E coli*	Microbe invades intestinal mucosa and causes necrosis and inflammation.	EIEC is Invasive; dysentery. Clinical manifestations similar to *Shigella*.
Enterotoxigenic *E coli*	Produces heat-labile and heat-stable enteroToxins. No inflammation or invasion.	ETEC; Traveler's diarrhea (watery).
Enteropathogenic *E coli*	No toxin produced. Adheres to apical surface, flattens villi, prevents absorption.	Diarrhea, usually in children (think EPEC and Pediatrics).
Enterohemorrhagic *E coli*	O157:H7 is most common serotype in US. Often transmitted via undercooked meat, raw leafy vegetables. Shiga toxin causes hemolytic-uremic syndrome—triad of anemia, thrombocytopenia, and acute kidney injury due to microthrombi forming on damaged endothelium → mechanical hemolysis (with schistocytes on peripheral blood smear), platelet consumption → thrombocytopenia, and ↓ renal blood flow.	Dysentery (toxin alone causes necrosis and inflammation). Does not ferment sorbitol (vs other *E coli*). EHEC associated with hemorrhage, hamburgers, hemolytic-uremic syndrome.

Klebsiella

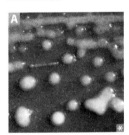

Gram ⊖ rod; intestinal microbiota that causes lobar pneumonia; more common in patients with heavy alcohol use or with impaired host defenses. Very mucoid colonies A caused by abundant polysaccharide capsules. Dark red "currant jelly" sputum (blood/mucus).
Also cause of healthcare-associated UTIs. Associated with evolution of multidrug resistance (MDR).

ABCDE's of Klebsiella:
Aspiration pneumonia
aBscess in lungs and liver
"Currant jelly" sputum
Diabetes mellitus
EtOH overuse

Campylobacter jejuni

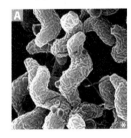

Gram ⊖, comma or S shaped (with polar flagella) A, oxidase ⊕, grows at 42°C ("*Campylobacter* likes the **hot campfire**").
Major cause of bloody diarrhea, especially in children. Fecal-oral transmission through person-to-person contact or via ingestion of undercooked contaminated poultry or meat, unpasteurized milk. Contact with infected animals (dogs, cats, pigs) is also a risk factor.
Common antecedent to Guillain-Barré syndrome and reactive arthritis.

Proteus mirabilis Gram ⊖, urease ⊕, facultative anaerobe, long flagellae with "swarming" motility.
Common cause of UTIs. Urease (virulence factor) hydrolyzes urea to carbon dioxide and ammonia → net increase in pH → promotes formation of struvite stones. Significant blockage of renal calyces results in branched stones called staghorn calculi.

Vibrio cholerae

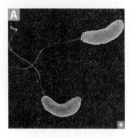

Gram $\ominus$, flagellated, comma shaped , oxidase $\oplus$, grows in alkaline media. Endemic to developing countries. Produces profuse rice-water diarrhea via enterotoxin that permanently activates G_s, ↑ cAMP. Sensitive to stomach acid (acid labile); requires large inoculum (high ID_{50}) unless host has ↓ gastric acidity. Transmitted via ingestion of contaminated water or uncooked food (eg, raw shellfish). Treat promptly with oral rehydration solution.

Vibrio vulnificus—gram $\ominus$ bacillus, usually found in marine environments. Causes severe wound infections or septicemia due to exposure to contaminated sea water. Presents as cellulitis that can progress to necrotizing fasciitis in high-risk patients, especially those with high serum iron (eg, cirrhosis, hemochromatosis). Serious wound infection requires surgical debridement.

Helicobacter pylori

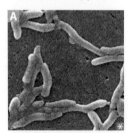

Curved, flagellated (motile), gram $\ominus$ rod that is **triple** $\oplus$: catalase $\oplus$, oxidase $\oplus$, and urease $\oplus$ (can use urea breath test or fecal antigen test for diagnosis). Urease produces ammonia, creating an alkaline environment, which helps *H pylori* survive in acidic mucosa. Colonizes mainly antrum of stomach; causes gastritis and peptic ulcers (especially duodenal). Risk factor for peptic ulcer disease, gastric adenocarcinoma, and MALT lymphoma.

Most common initial treatment is **triple** therapy: amoxicillin (metronidazole if penicillin allergy) + clarithromycin + proton pump inhibitor; antibiotics cure *Pylori*. Bismuth-based quadruple therapy if concerned about macrolide resistance.

Spirochetes

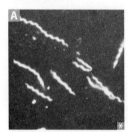

Spiral-shaped bacteria with axial filaments. Includes *Leptospira*, *Treponema*, and *Borrelia*. Only *Borrelia* can be visualized using aniline dyes (Wright or Giemsa stain) in light microscopy due to size. *Treponema* is visualized by dark-field microscopy or direct fluorescent antibody (DFA) microscopy.

Little Twirling Bacteria.

Jarisch-Herxheimer reaction—flulike symptoms (fever, chills, headache, myalgia) after antibiotics are started due to host response to sudden release of bacterial antigens. Usually occurs during treatment of spirochetal infections.

Lyme disease

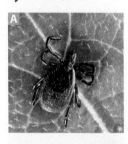

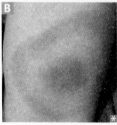

Caused by *Borrelia burgdorferi*, which is transmitted by the *Ixodes* deer tick 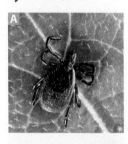 (also vector for *Anaplasma* spp. and protozoa *Babesia*). Natural reservoir is the mouse; deer are essential to tick life cycle but do not harbor *Borrelia*.

Common in northeastern United States.

Stage 1—early localized: erythema migrans (typical "bulls-eye" configuration is pathognomonic but not always present), flulike symptoms.

Stage 2—early disseminated: secondary lesions, carditis, AV block, facial nerve (Bell) palsy, migratory myalgias/transient arthritis.

Stage 3—late disseminated: encephalopathy, chronic arthritis, peripheral neuropathy.

A Key **Lyme** pie to the **FACE**:
Facial nerve palsy (typically bilateral)
Arthritis
Cardiac block
Erythema migrans

Treatment: doxycycline (1st line); amoxicillin (pregnant patients, children < 8 years old); ceftriaxone if IV therapy required

Leptospira interrogans   Spirochete with hook-shaped ends found in water contaminated with animal urine.

Leptospirosis—flulike symptoms, myalgias (classically of calves), jaundice, photophobia with conjunctival suffusion (erythema without exudate). Prevalent among surfers and in the tropics (eg, Hawaii).

Weil disease (icterohemorrhagic leptospirosis)—severe form with jaundice and azotemia from liver and kidney dysfunction, fever, hemorrhage, and anemia.

Syphilis

Caused by spirochete *Treponema pallidum.* Treatment: penicillin G.

Primary syphilis

Localized disease presenting with **painless** chancre. Use fluorescent or dark-field microscopy to visualize treponemes in fluid from chancre **A**. VDRL ⊕ in ~ 80% of patients.

Secondary syphilis

Disseminated disease with constitutional symptoms, maculopapular rash **B** (including palms **C** and soles), condylomata lata **D** (smooth, painless, wartlike white lesions on genitals), lymphadenopathy, patchy hair loss; also confirmable with dark-field microscopy.
Serologic testing: VDRL/RPR (nonspecific), confirm diagnosis with specific test (eg, FTA-ABS).
Secondary syphilis = systemic. Latent syphilis (⊕ serology without symptoms) may follow.

Tertiary syphilis

Gummas **E** (chronic granulomas), aortitis (vasa vasorum destruction), neurosyphilis (tabes dorsalis, "general paresis"), Argyll Robertson pupil (constricts with accommodation but is not reactive to light).
Signs: broad-based ataxia, ⊕ Romberg, Charcot joint, stroke without hypertension.

Congenital syphilis

Presents with facial abnormalities such as rhagades (linear scars at angle of mouth, black arrow in **F**), snuffles (nasal discharge, red arrow in **F**), saddle nose, notched (Hutchinson) teeth **G**, mulberry molars, and short maxilla; saber shins; CN VIII deafness.
To prevent, treat patient early in pregnancy, as placental transmission typically occurs after first trimester.

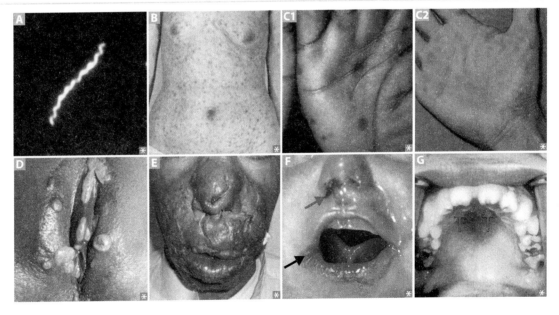

Diagnosing syphilis

VDRL and RPR detects nonspecific antibody that reacts with beef cardiolipin. Quantitative, inexpensive, and widely available test for syphilis (sensitive but not specific). Nontreponemal tests (VDRL, RPR) and direct testing revert to negative after treatment. Antibodies detected by treponemal tests (FTA-ABS, TP-PA) will remain positive.

False-Positive results on **VDRL** with:
Pregnancy
Viral infection (eg, EBV, hepatitis)
Drugs (eg, chlorpromazine, procainamide)
Rheumatic fever (rare)
Lupus (anticardiolipin antibody) and Leprosy

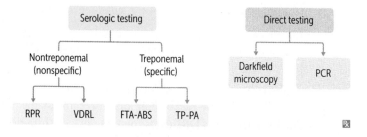

Chlamydiae

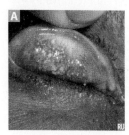

Chlamydiae cannot make their own ATP. They are obligate intracellular organisms that cause mucosal infections. 2 forms:
- Elementary body (small, dense) is "enfectious" and enters cell via endocytosis; transforms into reticulate body.
- Reticulate body replicates in cell by fission; reorganizes into elementary bodies.

Chlamydia trachomatis causes neonatal and follicular adult conjunctivitis , nongonococcal urethritis, PID, and reactive arthritis.

Chlamydophila pneumoniae and *Chlamydophila psittaci* cause atypical pneumonia; transmitted by aerosol.

Chlamydial cell wall lacks classic peptidoglycan (due to reduced muramic acid), rendering β-lactam antibiotics ineffective.
Chlamys = cloak (intracellular).
C psittaci—has an avian reservoir (parrots), causes atypical pneumonia.
Lab diagnosis: PCR, NAAT. Cytoplasmic inclusions (reticulate bodies) seen on Giemsa or fluorescent antibody–stained smear.
Treatment: doxycycline, azithromycin (for pregnant patients). Add ceftriaxone if concurrent gonorrhea testing is positive.

Chlamydia trachomatis serotypes

Types A, B, and C	Chronic infection, cause blindness due to follicular conjunctivitis in resource-limited areas.	ABC = Africa, Blindness, Chronic infection.
Types D–K	Urethritis/PID, ectopic pregnancy, neonatal pneumonia (staccato cough) with eosinophilia, neonatal conjunctivitis (1–2 weeks after birth).	D–K = everything else. Neonatal disease can be acquired during vaginal birth if pregnant patient is infected.
Types L1, L2, and L3	Lymphogranuloma venereum—small, painless ulcers on genitals → swollen, painful inguinal lymph nodes that ulcerate (buboes). Treat with doxycycline.	

Gardnerella vaginalis

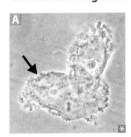

A pleomorphic, gram-variable rod involved in bacterial vaginosis. Presents as a gray vaginal discharge with a fishy smell; nonpainful (vs vaginitis). Associated with sexual activity, but not sexually transmitted. Bacterial vaginosis is also characterized by overgrowth of certain anaerobic bacteria in vagina (due to ↓ lactobacilli). Clue cells (vaginal epithelial cells covered with *Gardnerella*) have stippled appearance along outer margin (arrow in A).

Amine whiff test—mixing discharge with 10% KOH enhances fishy odor.
Vaginal pH >4.5 during infection.
Treatment: metronidazole or clindamycin.

Zoonotic bacteria   Zoonosis—infectious disease transmitted between animals and humans.

SPECIES	DISEASE	TRANSMISSION AND SOURCE
Anaplasma spp	Anaplasmosis	*Ixodes* ticks (live on deer and mice)
Bartonella spp	Cat scratch disease, bacillary angiomatosis	Cat scratch
Borrelia burgdorferi	Lyme disease	*Ixodes* ticks (live on deer and mice)
Borrelia recurrentis	Relapsing fever	Louse (recurrent due to variable surface antigens)
Brucella spp	Brucellosis/undulant fever	Unpasteurized dairy; inhalation of or contact with infected animal tissue or fluids
Campylobacter	Bloody diarrhea	Feces from infected pets/animals; contaminated meats/foods/hands
Chlamydophila psittaci	Psittacosis	Parrots, other birds
Coxiella burnetii	Q fever	Aerosols of cattle/sheep amniotic fluid
Ehrlichia chaffeensis	Ehrlichiosis	*Amblyomma* (Lone Star tick)
Francisella tularensis	Tularemia	Ticks, rabbits, deer flies
Leptospira spp	Leptospirosis	Animal urine in water; recreational water use
Mycobacterium leprae	Leprosy	Humans with lepromatous leprosy; armadillo (rare)
Pasteurella multocida	Cellulitis, osteomyelitis	Animal bite, cats, dogs
Rickettsia prowazekii	Epidemic typhus	Human to human via human body louse
Rickettsia rickettsii	Rocky Mountain spotted fever	*Dermacentor* (dog tick)
Rickettsia typhi	Endemic typhus	Fleas
Salmonella spp (except *S typhi*)	Diarrhea (which may be bloody), vomiting, fever, abdominal cramps	Reptiles and poultry
Yersinia pestis	Plague	Fleas (rats and prairie dogs are reservoirs)

Rickettsial diseases and vector-borne illnesses

Treatment: doxycycline.

RASH COMMON

Rocky Mountain spotted fever	*Rickettsia rickettsii*, vector is tick. Despite its name, disease occurs primarily in the South Atlantic states, especially North Carolina. Rash typically starts at wrists 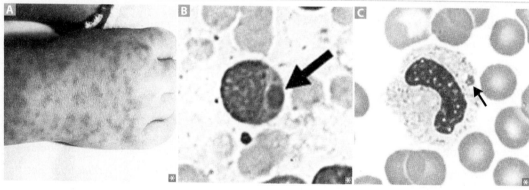 and ankles and then spreads to trunk, palms, and soles.	Classic triad—headache, fever, rash (vasculitis). **Palms** and **soles** rash is seen in Coxsackievirus A infection (hand, foot, and mouth disease), Rocky Mountain spotted fever, and 2° Syphilis (you drive **CARS** using your **palms** and **soles**).
Typhus	Endemic (fleas)—*R typhi*. Epidemic (human body louse)—*R prowazekii*. Rash starts centrally and spreads out, sparing palms and soles.	*Rickettsii* on the wrists, typhus on the trunk.

RASH RARE

Ehrlichiosis	*Ehrlichia*, vector is tick. Monocytes with morulae B (mulberrylike inclusions) in cytoplasm.	**MEGA:** Monocytes = Ehrlichiosis Granulocytes = Anaplasmosis
Anaplasmosis	*Anaplasma*, vector is tick. Granulocytes with morulae C in cytoplasm.	
Q fever	*Coxiella burnetii*, no arthropod vector. Bacterium inhaled as aerosols from cattle/sheep amniotic fluid. Presents with headache, cough, flulike symptoms, pneumonia, possibly in combination with hepatitis. Common cause of culture ⊖ endocarditis.	Q fever is caused by a Quite Complicated bug because it has no rash or vector and its causative organism can survive outside in its endospore form. Not in the *Rickettsia* genus, but closely related.

Mycoplasma pneumoniae

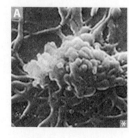

Classic cause of atypical "walking pneumonia" (insidious onset, headache, nonproductive cough, patchy or diffuse interstitial infiltrate, macular rash).

Occurs frequently in those <30 years old; outbreaks in military recruits, prisons, colleges.

Treatment: macrolides, doxycycline, or fluoroquinolone (penicillin ineffective since *Mycoplasma* has no cell wall).

Not seen on Gram stain. Pleomorphic A. Bacterial membrane contains sterols for stability. Grown on Eaton agar.

CXR appears more severe than patient presentation. High titer of **cold** agglutinins (IgM), which can agglutinate RBCs. *Mycoplasma* gets **cold** without a **coat** (no cell wall).

▶ MICROBIOLOGY—MYCOLOGY

Systemic mycoses

All of the following can cause pneumonia and can disseminate.

All are caused by dimorphic fungi: **cold** (20°C) = **mold**; **heat** (37°C) = **yeast**. Only exception is *Coccidioides*, which is a spherule (not yeast) in tissue.

Systemic mycoses can form granulomas (like TB); cannot be transmitted person-to-person (unlike TB).

Treatment: fluconazole or itraconazole for **local** infection; amphotericin B for **systemic** infection.

DISEASE	ENDEMIC LOCATION	PATHOLOGIC FEATURES	UNIQUE SIGNS/SYMPTOMS	NOTES
Histoplasmosis	Mississippi and Ohio River Valleys	Macrophage filled with *Histoplasma* (smaller than RBC) A Tuberculate macroconidia on culture	Palatal/tongue ulcers, splenomegaly, pancytopenia, erythema nodosum	**Histo hides** (within macrophages) Associated with bird or bat droppings (eg, caves) Diagnosis via urine/serum antigen
Blastomycosis	Eastern and Central US, Great Lakes	**Broad**-based budding of *Blastomyces* (same size as RBC) B	Inflammatory lung disease Disseminates to bone/skin (verrucous lesions C, may mimic SCC).	**Blasto buds broadly**
Coccidioidomycosis	Southwestern US, California	Spherule filled with endospores of *Coccidioides* (much larger than RBC) D	Disseminates to bone/skin Erythema nodosum (desert bumps) or multiforme Arthralgias (desert rheumatism) Can cause meningitis	Associated with dust exposure in endemic areas (eg, archeological excavations, earthquakes)
Para-coccidioidomycosis	Latin America	Budding yeast of *Paracoccidioides* with "captain's wheel" formation (much larger than RBC) E	Similar to blastomycosis, males > females	**Paracoccidio parasails** with the **captain's wheel** all the way to **Latin America**

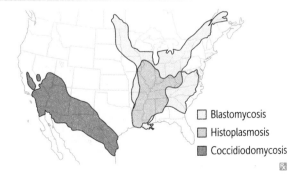

☐ Blastomycosis
☐ Histoplasmosis
☐ Coccidiodomycosis

℞

Opportunistic fungal infections

Candida albicans	*alba* = white. Dimorphic; forms pseudohyphae and budding yeasts at 20°C **A**, germ tubes at 37°C **B**.
	Systemic or superficial fungal infection. Causes oral **C** and esophageal thrush in immunocompromised (neonates, steroids, diabetes, AIDS), vulvovaginitis (diabetes, use of antibiotics), diaper rash, infective endocarditis (people who inject drugs), disseminated candidiasis (especially in neutropenic patients as host defense relies on phagocytes), chronic mucocutaneous candidiasis.
	Treatment: oral fluconazole/topical azoles for vaginal; nystatin, azoles, or, rarely, echinocandins for oral; fluconazole, echinocandins, or amphotericin B for esophageal or systemic disease.
Aspergillus fumigatus	Acute angle (45°) **D** branching of septate hyphae.
	Causes invasive aspergillosis in immunocompromised patients, especially those with neutrophil dysfunction (eg, chronic granulomatous disease) because *Aspergillus* is catalase ⊕.
	Can cause aspergillomas **E** in pre-existing lung cavities, especially after TB infection.
	Some species of Aspergillus produce aflatoxins (induce TP53 mutations leading to hepatocellular carcinoma).
	Treatment: voriconazole or echinocandins (2nd-line).
	Allergic bronchopulmonary aspergillosis (ABPA)—hypersensitivity response to *Aspergillus* growing in lung mucus. Associated with asthma and cystic fibrosis; may cause bronchiectasis and eosinophilia.
Cryptococcus neoformans	5–10 μm with narrow budding. Heavily encapsulated yeast. Not dimorphic. ⊕ PAS staining.
	Found in soil, pigeon droppings. Acquired through inhalation with hematogenous dissemination to meninges. Highlighted with India ink (clear halo **F**) and mucicarmine (red inner capsule **G**). Latex agglutination test detects polysaccharide capsular antigen and is more sensitive and specific.
	Causes cryptococcosis, which can manifest with meningitis, pneumonia, and/or encephalitis ("soap bubble" lesions in brain), primarily in immunocompromised.
	Treatment: amphotericin B + flucytosine followed by fluconazole for cryptococcal meningitis.
Mucor and *Rhizopus* spp	Irregular, broad, nonseptate hyphae branching at wide angles **H**.
	Causes mucormycosis, mostly in patients with DKA and/or neutropenia (eg, leukemia). Inhalation of spores → fungi proliferate in blood vessel walls, penetrate cribriform plate, and enter brain. Rhinocerebral, frontal lobe abscess; cavernous sinus thrombosis. Headache, facial pain, black necrotic eschar on face **I**; may have cranial nerve involvement.
	Treatment: surgical debridement, amphotericin B or isavuconazole.

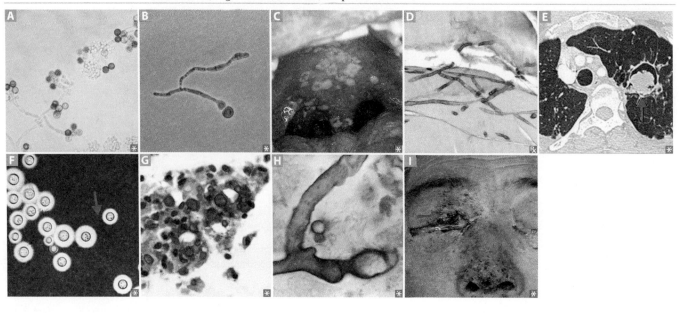

Pneumocystis jirovecii

Yeastlike fungus that causes *Pneumocystis* pneumonia (PCP), a diffuse interstitial pneumonia 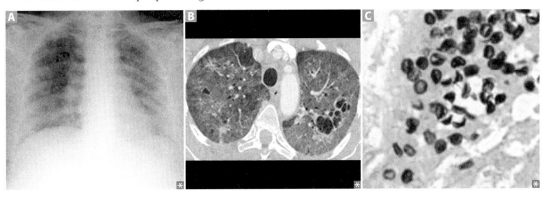. Most infections are asymptomatic. Immunosuppression (eg, AIDS) predisposes to disease. Diffuse, bilateral ground-glass opacities on chest imaging, with pneumatoceles B. Diagnosed by bronchoalveolar lavage or lung biopsy. Disc-shaped yeast seen on methenamine silver stain of lung tissue C or with fluorescent antibody.

Treatment/prophylaxis: TMP-SMX, pentamidine, dapsone (prophylaxis as single agent, or treatment in combination with TMP), atovaquone. Start prophylaxis when CD4+ cell count drops to < 200 cells/mm^3 in people living with HIV.

Sporothrix schenckii

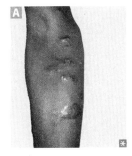

Causes sporotrichosis. Dimorphic fungus. Exists as a **cigar**-shaped yeast at 37 °C in the human body and as hyphae with spores in soil (conidia). Lives on vegetation. When spores are traumatically introduced into the skin, typically by a thorn ("**rose gardener**'s disease"), causes local pustule or ulcer with nodules along draining lymphatics (ascending lymphangitis A). Disseminated disease possible in immunocompromised host.

Treatment: itraconazole or **pot**assium iodide (only for cutaneous/lymphocutaneous).

Think of a **rose gardener** who smokes a **cigar** and **pot**.

▶ MICROBIOLOGY—PARASITOLOGY

Protozoa—gastrointestinal infections

ORGANISM	DISEASE	TRANSMISSION	DIAGNOSIS	TREATMENT
Giardia lamblia	**Giardiasis**—bloating, flatulence, foul-smelling, nonbloody, fatty diarrhea (often seen in campers/hikers)—think **fat**-rich **Ghirardelli** chocolates for **fatty** stools of *Giardia*	Cysts in water	Multinucleated trophozoites **A** or cysts **B** in stool, antigen detection, PCR	Tinidazole, nitazoxanide, or metronidazole
Entamoeba histolytica	**Amebiasis**—bloody diarrhea (dysentery), liver abscess ("anchovy paste" exudate), RUQ pain; histology of colon biopsy shows flask-shaped ulcers **C**	Cysts in water	Serology, antigen testing, PCR, and/ or trophozoites (with engulfed RBCs **D** in the cytoplasm) or cysts with up to 4 nuclei in stool **E**; *Entamoeba* Eats Erythrocytes	Metronidazole; paromomycin for asymptomatic cyst passers
Cryptosporidium	Severe diarrhea in AIDS Mild disease (watery diarrhea) in immunocompetent hosts	Oocysts in water	Oocysts on acid-fast stain **F**, antigen detection, PCR	Prevention (eg, filtering); nitazoxanide (severe disease and/or immuno-compromised)

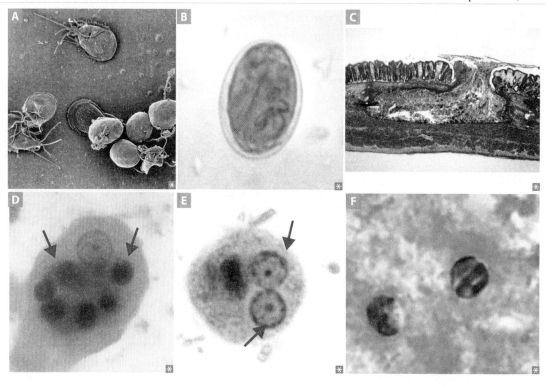

Protozoa—CNS infections

ORGANISM	DISEASE	TRANSMISSION	DIAGNOSIS	TREATMENT
Toxoplasma gondii	Immunocompetent: mononucleosis-like symptoms, ⊖ heterophile antibody test Reactivation in AIDS → brain abscesses usually seen as multiple ring-enhancing lesions on MRI A Congenital toxoplasmosis: classic triad of chorioretinitis, hydrocephalus, and intracranial calcifications	Cysts in meat (most common); oocysts in cat feces; crosses placenta (pregnant patients should avoid cats)	Serology, biopsy (tachyzoite) B; PCR of amniotic fluid for possible intrauterine disease	Sulfadiazine + pyrimethamine Prophylaxis with TMP-SMX when CD4+ cell count < 100 cells/mm^3
Naegleria fowleri	Rapidly fatal meningoencephalitis	Swimming in warm freshwater; enters CNS through olfactory nerve via cribriform plate	Amoebas in CSF C	Amphotericin B has been effective for a few survivors
Trypanosoma brucei	**African sleeping sickness**— enlarged lymph nodes, recurring fever (due to antigenic variation), somnolence, coma	Tsetse fly, a painful bite	Trypomastigote in blood smear D	Suramin for blood-borne disease or melarsoprol for CNS penetration ("I sure am mellow when I'm sleeping")

Protozoa—hematologic infections

ORGANISM	DISEASE	TRANSMISSION	DIAGNOSIS	TREATMENT
Plasmodium	Malaria—cyclic fevers, headache, anemia, splenomegaly; hypoglycemia in severe disease	*Anopheles* mosquito	Peripheral blood smear (also allows for identification of species)	If sensitive, chloroquine; if resistant, mefloquine, doxycycline or atovaquone/proguanil. If life threatening, use intravenous quinine or artesunate (test for G6PD deficiency)
P malariae	72-hr fever cycle (quartan)		Trophozoite ring within RBC	
P vivax/ovale	48-hr fever cycle (tertian); dormant form (hypnozoite) in liver		Trophozoites and Schüffner stippling (small red granules) within RBC cytoplasm A	Add primaquine to target hypnozoites
P falciparum	Severe, irregular fever pattern; parasitized RBCs may occlude capillaries in brain (cerebral malaria), kidneys, lungs		Trophozoite ring (headphone shaped) within RBC B; crescent-shaped gametocytes C	
Babesia	Babesiosis—fever and hemolytic anemia; predominantly in northeastern and north central United States; asplenia ↑ risk of severe disease due to inability to clear infected RBCs	*Ixodes* tick (also vector for *Borrelia burgdorferi* and *Anaplasma* spp)	Ring form D1, "Maltese cross" D2; PCR	Atovaquone + azithromycin

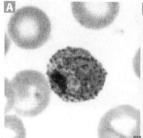
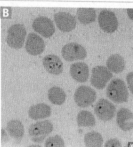
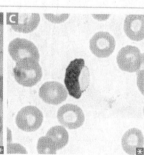
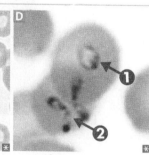

Protozoa—others

ORGANISM	DISEASE	TRANSMISSION	DIAGNOSIS	TREATMENT
Visceral infections				
Trypanosoma cruzi	Chagas disease—dilated cardiomyopathy with apical atrophy, **megacolon**, **megaesophagus**; (*T cruzi* causes **big** problems); predominantly in South America Unilateral periorbital swelling (Romaña sign) characteristic of acute stage	Triatomine insect (kissing bug) bites and defecates around the mouth or eyes → fecal transmission into bite site or mucosa	Trypomastigote in blood smear A	Benznidazole or nifurtimox
Leishmania spp	Visceral leishmaniasis (kala-azar)—spiking fevers, hepatosplenomegaly, pancytopenia Cutaneous leishmaniasis—skin ulcers B	Sandfly	Macrophages containing amastigotes C	Amphotericin B, sodium stibogluconate
Sexually transmitted infections				
Trichomonas vaginalis	Vaginitis—foul-smelling, greenish discharge; itching and burning; do not confuse with *Gardnerella vaginalis*, a gram-variable bacterium associated with bacterial vaginosis	Sexual (cannot exist outside human because it cannot form cysts)	Trophozoites (motile) D on wet mount; punctate cervical hemorrhages ("strawberry cervix")	Metronidazole for patient and partner(s) (prophylaxis; check for STI)

Nematode routes of infection	Ingested—*Enterobius, Ascaris, Toxocara, Trichinella, Trichuris* Cutaneous—*Strongyloides, Ancylostoma, Necator* Bites—*Loa loa, Onchocerca volvulus, Wuchereria bancrofti*	You'll get sick if you **EATTT** these! These get into your feet from the **SAN**d Lay **LOW** to avoid getting bitten

Nematodes (roundworms)

ORGANISM	DISEASE	TRANSMISSION	TREATMENT
Intestinal			
Enterobius vermicularis (pinworm)	Causes anal pruritus, worse at night (eggs 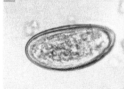 visualized via tape test). Most common in children aged 5–10.	Fecal-oral.	Bendazoles, pyrantel pamoate.
Ascaris lumbricoides (giant roundworm)	May cause obstruction at ileocecal valve, biliary obstruction, intestinal perforation, migrates from nose/mouth. Migration of larvae to alveoli → Löeffler syndrome (pulmonary eosinophilia).	Fecal-oral; knobby-coated, oval eggs seen in feces under microscope 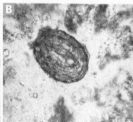.	Bendazoles.
Strongyloides stercoralis (threadworm)	GI (eg, duodenitis), pulmonary (eg, dry cough, hemoptysis), and cutaneous (eg, pruritus) symptoms. Hyperinfection syndrome can be caused by accelerated autoinfection in the immunocompromised.	Larvae in soil penetrate skin; rhabditiform larvae seen in feces under microscope.	Ivermectin or bendazoles.
Ancylostoma spp, *Necator americanus* (hookworms)	Cause microcytic anemia by sucking blood from intestinal wall. Cutaneous larva migrans—pruritic, serpiginous rash 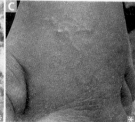.	Larvae penetrate skin from walking barefoot on contaminated beach/soil.	Bendazoles or pyrantel pamoate.
Trichinella spiralis	Larvae enter bloodstream, encyst in striated muscle 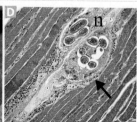 → myositis. Trichinosis—fever, vomiting, nausea, periorbital edema, myalgia.	Undercooked meat (especially pork); fecal-oral (less likely).	Bendazoles.
Trichuris trichiura (whipworm)	Often asymptomatic; loose stools, anemia, rectal prolapse in children.	Fecal-oral.	Bendazoles.
Tissue			
Toxocara canis	Visceral larva migrans—migration into blood → inflammation of liver, eyes (visual impairment), CNS (seizures, coma), heart (myocarditis). Patients often asymptomatic.	Fecal-oral.	Bendazoles.
Onchocerca volvulus	**Black** skin nodules, river blindness ("**black** sight").	Female **black** fly.	Ivermectin (**ivermectin** for **river** blindness).
Loa loa	Swelling in skin, worm in conjunctiva.	Deer fly, horse fly, mango fly.	Diethylcarbamazine.
Wuchereria bancrofti, *Brugia malayi*	Lymphatic filariasis (elephantiasis)— worms invade lymph nodes → inflammation → lymphedema 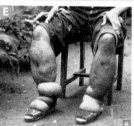; symptom onset after 9 mo–1 yr.	Female mosquito.	Diethylcarbamazine.

Cestodes (tapeworms)

ORGANISM	DISEASE	TRANSMISSION	TREATMENT
Taenia solium 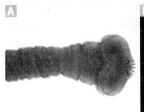	Intestinal tapeworm	Ingestion of larvae encysted in undercooked pork	Praziquantel
	Cysticercosis, neurocysticercosis (cystic CNS lesions, seizures) B	Ingestion of eggs in food contaminated with human feces	Praziquantel; albendazole for neurocysticercosis
Diphyllobothrium latum	Vitamin B_{12} deficiency ("DiphylloB$_{12}$ latum"; tapeworm competes for B_{12} in intestine) → megaloblastic anemia	Ingestion of larvae in raw freshwater fish	Praziquantel, niclosamide
Echinococcus granulosus C	Hydatid cysts D ("eggshell calcification") most commonly in liver E and lungs; cyst rupture can cause anaphylaxis	Ingestion of eggs in food contaminated with dog feces Sheep are an intermediate host	Albendazole; surgery for complicated cysts

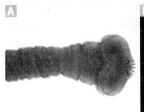 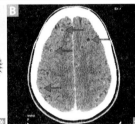 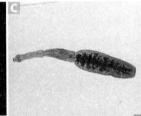 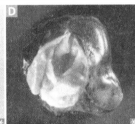 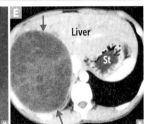

Trematodes (flukes)

ORGANISM	DISEASE	TRANSMISSION	TREATMENT
Schistosoma	Liver and spleen enlargement (A shows *S mansoni* egg with lateral spine), fibrosis, inflammation, portal hypertension; *S mansoni* and *S japonicum* can both also cause intestinal schistosomiasis, presenting with diarrhea, abdominal pain, iron deficiency anemia Chronic infection with *S haematobium* (egg with terminal spine B) can lead to squamous cell carcinoma of the bladder (painless hematuria) and pulmonary hypertension	Snails are intermediate host; cercariae penetrate skin of humans in contact with contaminated fresh water (eg, swimming or bathing)	Praziquantel
Clonorchis sinensis	Biliary tract inflammation → pigmented gallstones Associated with cholangiocarcinoma	Undercooked fish	Praziquantel

Ectoparasites

Sarcoptes scabiei 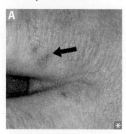	Mites burrow into stratum corneum and cause scabies—pruritus (worse at night) and serpiginous burrows (lines) often between fingers and toes A.	Common in children, crowded populations (jails, nursing homes); transmission through skin-to-skin contact (most common) or via fomites. Treatment: permethrin cream, oral ivermectin, washing/drying all clothing/bedding, treat close contacts.
Pediculus humanus and *Phthirus pubis* 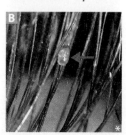	Blood-sucking lice that cause intense pruritus with associated excoriations, commonly on scalp and neck (head lice), waistband and axilla (body lice), or pubic and perianal regions (pubic lice).	Body lice can transmit *Rickettsia prowazekii* (epidemic typhus), *Borrelia recurrentis* (relapsing fever), *Bartonella quintana* (trench fever). Treatment: pyrethroids, malathion, or ivermectin lotion, and nit B combing. Children with head lice can be treated at home without interrupting school attendance.
Cimex lectularius and *Cimex hemipterus*	Bed bugs. Blood-feeding insects that infest dwellings. Painless bites result in a range of skin reactions, typically pruritic, erythematous papules with central hemorrhagic punctum. A clustered or linear pattern of bites seen upon awakening is suggestive. Diagnosis is confirmed by direct identification of bed bugs in patient's dwelling.	Bed bugs can spread among rooms; cohabitants may exhibit similar symptoms. Infestations can also spread via travelers from infested hotels and the use of unwashed, used bedding. Treatment: bites self resolve within 1 week. Eradication of the infestation is critical.

Parasite hints

ASSOCIATIONS	ORGANISM
Biliary tract disease, cholangiocarcinoma	*Clonorchis sinensis*
Brain cysts, seizures	*Taenia solium* (neurocysticercosis)
Hematuria, squamous cell bladder cancer	*Schistosoma haematobium*
Liver (hydatid) cysts, exposure to infected dogs	*Echinococcus granulosus*
Iron deficiency anemia	*Ancylostoma, Necator*
Myalgias, periorbital edema	*Trichinella spiralis*
Nocturnal perianal pruritus	*Enterobius*
Portal hypertension	*Schistosoma mansoni, Schistosoma japonicum*
Vitamin B_{12} deficiency	*Diphyllobothrium latum*

▸ MICROBIOLOGY—VIROLOGY

Viral structure—general features

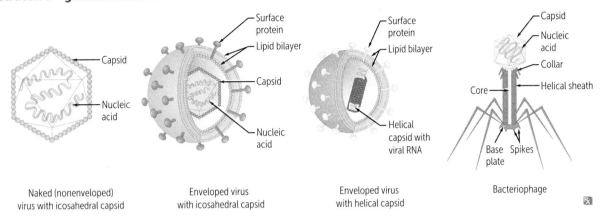

Naked (nonenveloped) virus with icosahedral capsid

Enveloped virus with icosahedral capsid

Enveloped virus with helical capsid

Bacteriophage

Viral genetics

Recombination	Exchange of genes between 2 chromosomes by crossing over within regions of significant base sequence homology.	
Reassortment	When viruses with segmented genomes (eg, influenza virus) exchange genetic material. For example, the 2009 novel H1N1 influenza A pandemic emerged via complex viral reassortment of genes from human, swine, and avian viruses. Has potential to cause antigenic shift. Reassortment of genome segments.	
Complementation	When 1 of 2 viruses that infect the cell has a mutation that results in a nonfunctional protein, the nonmutated virus "complements" the mutated one by making a functional protein that serves both viruses. For example, hepatitis D virus requires the presence of replicating hepatitis B virus to supply HBsAg, the envelope protein for HDV.	Functional Nonfunctional Functional
Phenotypic mixing	Occurs with simultaneous infection of a cell with 2 viruses. For progeny 1, genome of virus A can be partially or completely coated (forming pseudovirion) with the surface proteins of virus B. Type B protein coat determines the tropism (infectivity) of the hybrid virus. Progeny from subsequent infection of a cell by progeny 1 will have a type A coat that is encoded by its type A genetic material.	Virus A Virus B Progeny 1 Progeny 2

Viral genomes	Naked nucleic acids of most dsDNA viruses (except poxviruses and HBV) and ⊕ strand ssRNA viruses are infectious. Naked nucleic acids of ⊖ strand ssRNA and dsRNA viruses are not infectious because they lack the required polymerases to replicate. Virions of ⊖ strand ssRNA viruses carry RNA-dependent RNA polymerases to transcribe ⊖ strand to ⊕.	

	CHARACTERISTICS	MNEMONIC
DNA viruses	All have dsDNA genomes (like our cells) except **Parvoviridae** (ssDNA). All are linear except papilloma-, polyoma-, and hepadnaviruses (circular).	Part of a virus
RNA viruses	All have ssRNA genomes except **Reoviridae** (dsRNA). ⊕ stranded (≈ mRNA): **retro-, toga-, flavi-, corona-, hepe-, calici-,** and **picornaviruses**. ⊖ stranded: arena-, bunya-, paramyxo-, orthomyxo-, filo-, and rhabdoviruses. Segmented: Bunya-, Orthomyxo-, Arena-, and Reoviruses.	Repeato-virus While at a **retro toga** party, I drank flavored **Corona** and ate **hippie California** pickles. Always bring polymerase or fail replication. **BOAR**
Viral envelopes	Generally, enveloped viruses acquire their envelopes from plasma membrane when they exit from cell. Exceptions include herpesviruses, which acquire envelopes from nuclear membrane.	Enveloped DNA viruses (herpesvirus, hepadnavirus, poxvirus) have helpful protection.

DNA viruses

All are icosahedral and replicate in the nucleus (except poxvirus). "**Pox** is out of the **box** (nucleus)."

VIRAL FAMILY	ENVELOPE	DNA STRUCTURE	MEDICAL IMPORTANCE
Herpesviruses	Yes	DS and linear	See Herpesviruses entry
Poxvirus	Yes	DS and linear (largest DNA virus)	Smallpox eradicated world wide by use of the live-attenuated vaccine Cowpox ("milkmaid blisters") **Molluscum contagiosum**—flesh-colored papule with central umbilication; keratinocytes contain molluscum bodies A
Hepadnavirus	Yes	Partially DS and circular	HBV: ▪ Acute or chronic hepatitis ▪ Not a retrovirus but has reverse transcriptase
Adenovirus	No	DS and linear	Febrile pharyngitis B—sore throat Acute hemorrhagic cystitis Pneumonia Conjunctivitis—"pink eye" Gastroenteritis Myocarditis
Papillomavirus	No	DS and circular	HPV—warts, cancer (cervical, anal, penile, or oropharyngeal); serotypes 1, 2, 6, 11 associated with warts; serotypes 16, 18 associated with cancer
Polyomavirus	No	DS and circular	JC virus—progressive multifocal leukoencephalopathy (PML) in immunocompromised patients (eg, HIV) BK virus—transplant patients, commonly targets kidney **JC: Junky Cerebrum; BK: Bad Kidney**
Parvovirus	No	SS and linear (smallest DNA virus; *parvus* = small)	B19 virus—aplastic crises in sickle cell disease, "slapped cheek" rash in children (erythema infectiosum, or fifth disease); infects RBC precursors and endothelial cells → RBC destruction → hydrops fetalis and death in fetus, pure RBC aplasia and rheumatoid arthritis–like symptoms in adults

Herpesviruses Enveloped, DS, and linear viruses. Recent data suggest both HSV-1 and HSV-2 can affect both genital and extragenital areas.

VIRUS	ROUTE OF TRANSMISSION	CLINICAL SIGNIFICANCE	NOTES
Herpes simplex virus-1	Respiratory secretions, saliva	Gingivostomatitis, keratoconjunctivitis **A**, herpes labialis (cold sores) **B**, herpetic whitlow on finger, temporal lobe encephalitis, esophagitis, erythema multiforme. Responsible for a growing percentage of herpes genitalis.	Most commonly latent in trigeminal ganglia Most common cause of sporadic encephalitis, can present as altered mental status, seizures, and/or aphasia
Herpes simplex virus-2	Sexual contact, perinatal	Herpes genitalis, neonatal herpes **C**	Most commonly latent in sacral ganglia Viral meningitis more common with HSV-2 than with HSV-1
Varicella-zoster virus (HHV-3)	Respiratory secretions, contact with fluid from vesicles	Varicella-zoster (chickenpox **D**, shingles **E**), encephalitis, pneumonia Most common complication of shingles is post-herpetic neuralgia	Latent in dorsal root or trigeminal ganglia; CN V_1 branch involvement can cause herpes zoster ophthalmicus
Epstein-Barr virus (HHV-4)	Respiratory secretions, saliva; also called "kissing disease," (common in teens, young adults)	**Mononucleosis**—fever, hepatosplenomegaly **F**, pharyngitis, and lymphadenopathy (especially posterior cervical nodes); avoid contact sports until resolution due to risk of splenic rupture Associated with lymphomas (eg, endemic Burkitt lymphoma), nasopharyngeal carcinoma (especially Asian adults), lymphoproliferative disease in transplant patients	Infects B cells through CD21, "Must be 21 to drink **B**eer in a **Barr**" Atypical lymphocytes on peripheral blood smear **G**—not infected B cells but reactive cytotoxic T cells ⊕ Monospot test—heterophile antibodies detected by agglutination of sheep or horse RBCs Use of amoxicillin (eg, for presumed strep pharyngitis) can cause maculopapular rash
Cytomegalo-virus (HHV-5)	Congenital, transfusion, sexual contact, saliva, urine, transplant	Mononucleosis (⊖ Monospot) in immunocompetent patients; infection in immunocompromised, especially pneumonia in transplant patients; esophagitis; colitis; AIDS **retinitis** ("**sight**omegalovirus"): hemorrhage, cotton-wool exudates, vision loss Congenital CMV	Infected cells have characteristic "owl eye" intranuclear inclusions **H** Latent in mononuclear cells
Human herpes-viruses 6 and 7	Saliva	Roseola infantum (exanthem subitum): high fevers for several days that can cause seizures, followed by diffuse macular rash (starts on trunk then spreads to extremities) **I**; usually seen in children < 2 years old	**Roseola**: fever first, **R**osy (rash) later Self-limited illness HHV-7—less common cause of roseola
Human herpesvirus 8	Sexual contact	Kaposi sarcoma (neoplasm of endothelial cells). Seen in HIV/AIDS and transplant patients. Dark/violaceous plaques or nodules **J** representing vascular proliferations	Can also affect GI tract and lungs

Herpesviruses *(continued)*

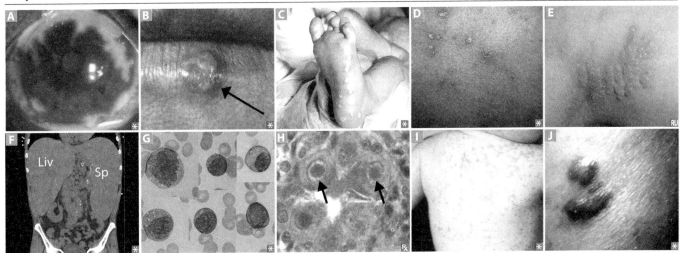

HSV identification	PCR of skin lesions is test of choice. CSF PCR for herpes encephalitis. Tzanck test (outdated)—a smear of an opened skin vesicle to detect multinucleated giant cells Ⓐ commonly seen in HSV-1, HSV-2, and VZV infection. Intranuclear eosinophilic Cowdry A inclusions also seen with HSV-1, HSV-2, VZV.

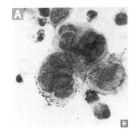

Receptors used by viruses	VIRUS	RECEPTOR(S)
	CMV	Integrins (heparan sulfate)
	EBV	CD21
	HIV	CD4, CXCR4, CCR5
	Parvovirus B19	P antigen on RBCs
	Rabies	Nicotinic AChR
	Rhinovirus	ICAM-1 (I CAMe to see the rhino)
	SARS-CoV-2	ACE2

RNA viruses   All replicate in the **cyt**oplasm (except **retro**virus and in**flu**enza virus). "**Retro flu** is outta **cyt** (sight)."

VIRAL FAMILY	ENVELOPE	RNA STRUCTURE	MEDICAL IMPORTANCE
Reoviruses	No	DS linear Multisegmented	Rotavirus—important cause of diarrhea in young children; may be fatal.
Picornaviruses	No	SS ⊕ linear	**P**oliovirus—polio-Salk/Sabin vaccines—IPV/OPV **E**chovirus—aseptic meningitis **R**hinovirus—"common cold" **C**oxsackievirus—aseptic meningitis; herpangina (mouth blisters, fever); hand, foot, and mouth disease; myocarditis; pericarditis **H**AV—acute viral hepatitis **PERCH**
Hepevirus	No	SS ⊕ linear	HEV
Caliciviruses	No	SS ⊕ linear	Norovirus—viral gastroenteritis
Flaviviruses	Yes	SS ⊕ linear	HCV Yellow fever[a] Dengue[a] West Nile virus[a]—meningoencephalitis, acute asymmetric flaccid paralysis Zika virus[a]
Togaviruses	Yes	SS ⊕ linear	**Toga CREW**—**C**hikungunya virus[a] (co-infection with dengue virus can occur), **R**ubella (formerly a togavirus), **E**astern and **W**estern equine encephalitis[a]
Matonavirus	Yes	SS ⊕ linear	Rubella
Retroviruses	Yes	SS ⊕ linear	Have reverse transcriptase HTLV—T-cell leukemia HIV—AIDS
Coronaviruses	Yes	SS ⊕ linear	"Common cold," SARS, COVID-19, MERS
Orthomyxoviruses	Yes	SS ⊖ linear Multisegmented	Influenza virus
Paramyxoviruses	Yes	SS ⊖ linear	**PaRaM**yxovirus: **Pa**rainfluenza—croup **R**SV—bronchiolitis in babies **M**easles, **M**umps
Pneumoviruses	Yes	SS ⊖ linear	RSV—bronchiolitis in babies
Rhabdoviruses	Yes	SS ⊖ linear	Rabies
Filoviruses	Yes	SS ⊖ linear	Ebola/Marburg virus disease—often fatal.
Arenaviruses	Yes	SS ⊕ and ⊖ circular Multisegmented	LCMV—lymphocytic choriomeningitis virus Lassa fever encephalitis—spread by rodents
Bunyaviruses	Yes	SS ⊖ circular Multisegmented	California encephalitis[a] Sandfly/Rift Valley fevers[a] Crimean-Congo hemorrhagic fever[a] Hantavirus—hemorrhagic fever, pneumonia
Delta virus	Yes	SS ⊖ circular	HDV is "**D**efective"; requires presence of HBV to replicate

SS, single-stranded; DS, double-stranded; ⊕, positive sense; ⊖, negative sense; [a]= **arbo**virus, **arthropod borne** (mosquitoes, ticks).

Picornavirus	Includes Poliovirus, Echovirus, Rhinovirus, Coxsackievirus, and HAV. RNA is translated into 1 large polypeptide that is cleaved by virus-encoded proteases into functional viral proteins. Poliovirus, echovirus, and coxsackievirus are enteroviruses and can cause aseptic (viral) meningitis.	PicoRNAvirus = small RNA virus. PERCH on a "peak" (pico).
Rhinovirus	A picornavirus. Nonenveloped RNA virus. Cause of common cold; > 100 serologic types. Acid labile—destroyed by stomach acid; therefore, does not infect the GI tract (unlike the other picornaviruses).	Rhino has a runny nose.
Rotavirus 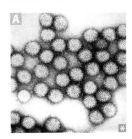	Segmented dsRNA virus (a reovirus) A. Most important global cause of infantile gastroenteritis. Major cause of acute diarrhea in the United States during winter, especially in day care centers, kindergartens. Villous destruction with atrophy leads to ↓ absorption of Na^+ and loss of K^+.	Rotavirus = right out the anus. CDC recommends routine vaccination of all infants except those with a history of intussusception (rare adverse effect of rotavirus vaccination) or SCID.

Influenza viruses	Orthomyxoviruses. Enveloped, ⊖ ssRNA viruses with segmented genome. Contain hemagglutinin (binds sialic acid and promotes viral entry) and neuraminidase (promotes progeny virion release) antigens. Patients at risk for fatal bacterial superinfection, most commonly *S aureus*, *S pneumoniae*, and *H influenzae*. Treatment: supportive +/– neuraminidase inhibitor (eg, oseltamivir, zanamivir).	Hemagglutinin: lets the virus **in** Neuraminid**aways**: sends the virus **away** Reformulated vaccine ("the flu shot") contains viral strains most likely to appear during the flu season, due to the virus' rapid genetic change. Killed viral vaccine is most frequently used. Live attenuated vaccine contains temperature-sensitive mutant that replicates in the nose but not in the lung; administered intranasally. Sudden shift is more deadly than gradual drift.
Genetic/antigenic shift	Infection of 1 cell by 2 different segmented viruses (eg, swine influenza and human influenza viruses) → RNA segment reassortment → dramatically different virus (genetic shift) → major global outbreaks (pandemics).	
Genetic/antigenic drift	Random mutation in hemagglutinin (HA) or neuraminidase (NA) genes → minor changes in HA or NA protein (drift) occur frequently → local seasonal outbreaks (epidemics).	

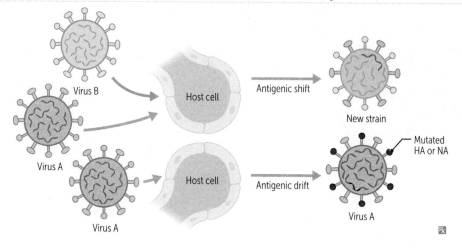

Rubella virus	A matonavirus. Causes rubella, formerly called German (3-day) measles. Fever, postauricular and other lymphadenopathy, arthralgias, and fine, maculopapular rash that starts on face and spreads centrifugally to involve trunk and extremities A. Causes mild disease in children but serious congenital disease (a TORCH infection). Congenital rubella findings include classic triad of sensorineural deafness, cataracts, and patent ductus arteriosus. "Blueberry muffin" appearance may be seen due to dermal extramedullary hematopoiesis.

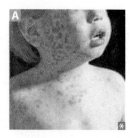

Paramyxoviruses	Paramyxoviruses cause disease in children. They include those that cause parainfluenza (croup), mumps, measles, RSV, and human metapneumovirus. All subtypes can cause respiratory tract infection (bronchiolitis, pneumonia) in infants. All contain surface F (fusion) protein, which causes respiratory epithelial cells to fuse and form multinucleated cells. Palivizumab (monoclonal antibody against F protein) prevents pneumonia caused by RSV infection in premature infants. Palivizumab for paramyxovirus (RSV) prophylaxis in preemies.

Acute laryngotracheobronchitis 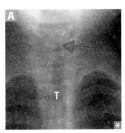	Also called croup. Caused by parainfluenza viruses. Virus membrane contains hemagglutinin (binds sialic acid and promotes viral entry) and neuraminidase (promotes progeny virion release) antigens. Results in a "seal-like" barking cough and inspiratory stridor. Narrowing of upper trachea and subglottis leads to characteristic steeple sign on x-ray 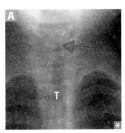.	

Measles (rubeola) virus 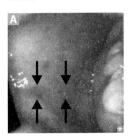	Usual presentation involves prodromal fever with cough, coryza, and conjunctivitis, then eventually Koplik spots (bright red spots with blue-white center on buccal mucosa 🅐), followed 1–2 days later by a maculopapular rash that starts at the head/neck and spreads downward.
	Lymphadenitis with Warthin-Finkeldey giant cells (fused lymphocytes) in a background of paracortical hyperplasia. Possible sequelae:
	▪ Subacute sclerosing panencephalitis (SSPE): personality changes, dementia, autonomic dysfunction, death (occurs years later)
	▪ Encephalitis (1:1000): symptoms appear within few days of rash
	▪ Giant cell pneumonia (rare except in immunosuppressed)
		4 C's of measles:
		  Cough
		  Coryza
		  Conjunctivitis
		  "C"oplik spots
		Vitamin A supplementation can reduce morbidity and mortality from measles, particularly in malnourished children.
		Pneumonia is the most common cause of measles-associated death in children.

Mumps virus 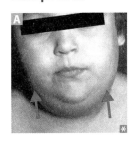	Uncommon due to effectiveness of MMR vaccine. Symptoms: Parotitis 🅐, Orchitis (inflammation of testes), aseptic Meningitis, and Pancreatitis. Can cause sterility (especially after puberty).	Mumps makes your parotid glands and testes as big as POM-Poms.

Arboviruses transmitted by *Aedes* mosquitoes

	Chikungunya virus	Dengue virus
VIRUS TYPE	Alphavirus/togavirus.	Flavivirus.
SYMPTOMS	High fever, maculopapular rash, headache, lymphadenopathy, and inflammatory polyarthritis. Arthralgias are more commonly reported (vs dengue); joint swelling is highly specific for Chikungunya. Thrombocytopenia, leukopenia, and hemorrhagic manifestations are less common.	Dengue fever: fever, rash, headache, myalgias, arthralgias, retro-orbital pain, neutropenia. Dengue hemorrhagic fever: dengue fever + bleeding and plasma leakage due to severe thrombocytopenia and RBC perturbations. Most common if infected with a different serotype after initial infection due to antibody-dependent enhancement of disease. May progress to dengue shock syndrome: plasma leakage → circulatory collapse.
DIAGNOSIS	RT-PCR, serology	
TREATMENT	Supportive. Steroids or disease-modifying antirheumatic drugs for chronic arthritis.	Supportive. Intravascular volume repletion or blood transfusion if severe shock.
PREVENTION	Minimize mosquito exposure. No vaccine currently available.	Live, recombinant vaccine available. Derived from the yellow fever virus backbone with insertion of genes for the envelope and pre-membrane proteins of dengue virus.

Yellow fever virus

A flavivirus (also an arbovirus) transmitted by *Aedes* mosquito bites. Virus has monkey or human reservoir. *Flavi* = yellow, jaundice.

Symptoms: high fever, black vomitus, jaundice, hemorrhage, backache. May see Councilman bodies (eosinophilic apoptotic globules) on liver biopsy.

Live, attenuated vaccine recommended for travelers to endemic countries.

Zika virus

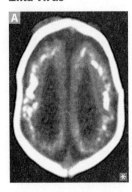

A flavivirus most commonly transmitted by *Aedes* mosquito bites.

Causes conjunctivitis, low-grade pyrexia, and itchy rash in 20% of cases. Outbreaks more common in tropical and subtropical climates. May be complicated by Guillain-Barré syndrome. Supportive care, no definitive treatment.

Diagnose with RT-PCR or serology.

Sexual and vertical transmission occurs.

In pregnancy, can lead to miscarriage or congenital Zika syndrome: brain imaging shows ventriculomegaly, subcortical calcifications A. Clinical features in the affected newborn include
- Microcephaly
- Ocular anomalies
- Motor abnormalities (spasticity, seizures)

Rabies virus

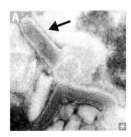

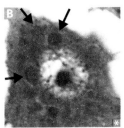

Bullet-shaped virus . Negri bodies (cytoplasmic inclusions) commonly found in Purkinje cells of cerebellum and in hippocampal neurons. Rabies has long incubation period (weeks to months) before symptom onset. Postexposure prophylaxis is wound cleaning plus immunization with killed vaccine and rabies immunoglobulin. Example of passive-active immunity.

Travels to the CNS by migrating in a retrograde fashion (via dynein motors) up nerve axons after binding to ACh receptors.

Progression of disease: fever, malaise → agitation, photophobia, hydrophobia, hypersalivation → paralysis, coma → death.

Infection more commonly from bat, raccoon, and skunk bites than from dog bites in the United States; aerosol transmission (eg, bat caves) also possible.

Ebola virus

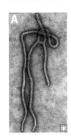

A filovirus 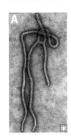. Following an incubation period of up to 21 days, presents with abrupt onset of flulike symptoms, diarrhea/vomiting, high fever, myalgia. Can progress to DIC, diffuse hemorrhage, shock.

Diagnosed with RT-PCR within 48 hr of symptom onset. High mortality rate.

Transmission requires direct contact with bodily fluids, fomites (including dead bodies), infected bats or primates (apes/monkeys); high incidence of healthcare-associated infection.

Supportive care, no definitive treatment. Vaccination of contacts, strict isolation of infected individuals, and barrier practices for healthcare workers are key to preventing transmission.

Severe acute respiratory syndrome coronavirus 2

SARS-CoV-2 is a ⊕ ssRNA virus and the cause of the COVID-19 pandemic. Spread is via respiratory droplets, aerosols and fomites.

Varying symptoms include: fever, myalgia, headache, nasal congestion, sneezing, cough, sore throat, nausea, diarrhea, anosmia, dysgeusia.

Severe cases may lead to complications like: pneumonia, hypercoagulability (DVT, PE, stroke), myocardial injury, neurologic sequelae, shock, organ failure, death.

Diagnosed by:
- NAAT (RT-PCR)
- Viral Antigen Test (RAT) → rapid, accessible, less sensitive than NAAT

Host cell entry occurs by attachment of viral spike protein to ACE2 receptor on cell membranes (highly expressed in the lungs, intestines, heart, and kidneys).

Vaccines: mRNA and viral vector vaccines induce immunity by presenting the spike protein to the immune system leading to anti-spike protein antibodies.

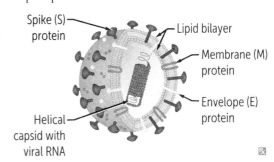

Spike (S) protein — Lipid bilayer — Membrane (M) protein — Envelope (E) protein — Helical capsid with viral RNA

Hepatitis viruses

Signs and symptoms of all hepatitis viruses: episodes of fever, jaundice, ↑ ALT and AST. NAkEd viruses (HAV and HEV) lack an envelope and are not destroyed by the gut: the **vowels** hit your **bowels**.

HBV DNA polymerase has DNA- and RNA-dependent activities. Upon entry into nucleus, the polymerase completes the partial dsDNA. Host RNA polymerase transcribes mRNA from viral DNA to make viral proteins. The DNA polymerase then reverse transcribes viral RNA to DNA, which is the genome of the progeny virus.

HCV lacks 3′-5′ exonuclease activity → no proofreading ability → antigenic variation of HCV envelope proteins. Host antibody production lags behind production of new mutant strains of HCV.

Virus	HAV	HBV	HCV	HDV	HEV
FAMILY	RNA picornavirus	DNA hepadnavirus	RNA flavivirus	RNA deltavirus	RNA hepevirus
TRANSMISSION	Fecal-oral (shellfish, travelers, day care)	Parenteral (**B**lood), sexual (**B**edroom), perinatal (**B**irthing)	Primarily blood (injection drug use, posttransfusion)	Parenteral, sexual, perinatal	Fecal-oral, especially waterborne
INCUBATION	Short (weeks)	Long (months)	Long	Superinfection (HDV after HBV) = short Coinfection (HDV with HBV) = long	Short
CLINICAL COURSE	Acute and self limiting (adults), Asymptomatic (children)	Initially like serum sickness (fever, arthralgias, rash); may progress to carcinoma	May progress to Cirrhosis or Carcinoma	Similar to HBV	Fulminant hepatitis in Expectant (pregnant) patients
PROGNOSIS	Good	Adults → mostly full resolution; neonates → worse prognosis	Majority develop stable, Chronic hepatitis C	Superinfection → worse prognosis	High mortality in pregnant patients
HCC RISK	No	Yes	Yes	Yes	No
LIVER BIOPSY	Hepatocyte swelling, monocyte infiltration, Councilman bodies **A**	Granular eosinophilic "ground glass" appearance due to accumulation of surface antigen within infected hepatocytes; cytotoxic T cells mediate damage	Lymphoid aggregates with focal areas of macrovesicular steatosis	Similar to HBV	Patchy necrosis
NOTES	Absent (no) carrier state	Carrier state common	Carrier state very common	Defective virus, Depends on HBV HBsAg coat for entry into hepatocytes	Enteric, Epidemic (eg, in parts of Asia, Africa, Middle East), no carrier state

Extrahepatic manifestations of hepatitis B and C

	Hepatitis B	Hepatitis C
HEMATOLOGIC	Aplastic anemia	Essential mixed cryoglobulinemia, ↑ risk B-cell NHL, ITP, autoimmune hemolytic anemia
RENAL	Membranous GN > membranoproliferative GN	Membranoproliferative GN > membranous GN
VASCULAR	Polyarteritis nodosa	Leukocytoclastic vasculitis
DERMATOLOGIC		Sporadic porphyria cutanea tarda, lichen planus
ENDOCRINE		↑ risk of diabetes mellitus, autoimmune hypothyroidism

Hepatitis serologic markers

Anti-HAV (IgM)	IgM antibody to HAV; best test to detect acute hepatitis A.
Anti-HAV (IgG)	IgG antibody indicates prior HAV infection and/or prior vaccination; protects against reinfection.
HBsAg	Antigen found on surface of HBV; indicates hepatitis B infection.
Anti-HBs	Antibody to HBsAg; indicates immunity to hepatitis B due to vaccination or recovery from infection.
HBcAg	Antigen associated with core of HBV.
Anti-HBc	Antibody to HBcAg; IgM = acute/recent infection; IgG = prior exposure or chronic infection. IgM anti-HBc may be the sole ⊕ marker of infection during window period.
HBeAg	Secreted by infected hepatocyte into circulation. Not part of mature HBV virion. Indicates active viral replication and therefore high transmissibility and poorer prognosis.
Anti-HBe	Antibody to HBeAg; indicates low transmissibility.

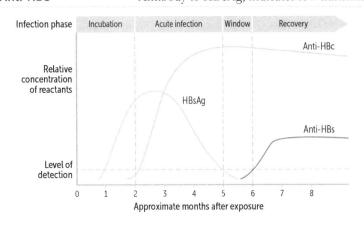

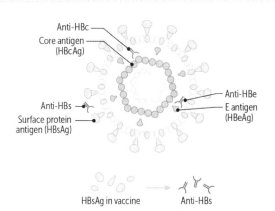

	HBsAg	Anti-HBs	Anti-HBc	HBeAg	Anti-HBe
Incubation	+				
Acute infection	+		+ (IgM)	+	
Window			+ (IgM)		+
Recovery		+	+ (IgM)		+
Chronic infection (high infectivity)	+		+ (IgG)	+	
Chronic infection (low infectivity)	+		+ (IgG)		+
Immunized		+			

HIV

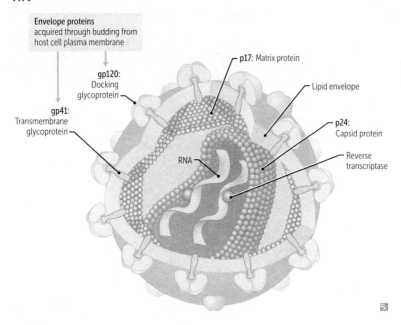

Envelope proteins acquired through budding from host cell plasma membrane

gp120: Docking glycoprotein

gp41: Transmembrane glycoprotein

p17: Matrix protein

Lipid envelope

p24: Capsid protein

Reverse transcriptase

RNA

Diploid genome (2 molecules of RNA).

The 3 structural genes (protein coded for):
- *Env* (gp120 and gp41)—formed from cleavage of gp160 to form envelope glycoproteins.
  - gp120—attachment to host CD4+ T cell.
  - gp41 (forty-one)—fusion and entry.
- *gag* (p24 and p17)—capsid and matrix proteins, respectively.
- *pol*—**R**everse transcriptase, **I**ntegrase, **P**rotease; **RIP** "**Pol**" (Paul)

Reverse transcriptase synthesizes dsDNA from genomic RNA; dsDNA integrates into host genome.

Virus binds CD4 as well as a coreceptor, either CCR5 on macrophages (early infection) or CXCR4 on T cells (late infection).

Homozygous CCR5 mutation = immunity.

Heterozygous CCR5 mutation = slower course.

HIV diagnosis

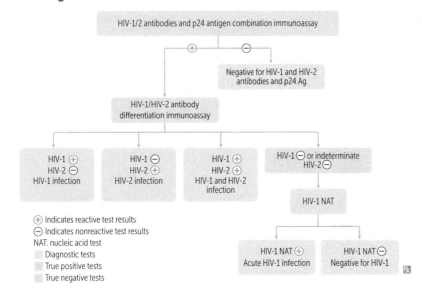

HIV-1/2 antibodies and p24 antigen combination immunoassay

⊕ / ⊖

Negative for HIV-1 and HIV-2 antibodies and p24 Ag

HIV-1/HIV-2 antibody differentiation immunoassay

HIV-1 ⊕ / HIV-2 ⊖ HIV-1 infection

HIV-1 ⊖ / HIV-2 ⊕ HIV-2 infection

HIV-1 ⊕ / HIV-2 ⊕ HIV-1 and HIV-2 infection

HIV-1 ⊖ or indeterminate HIV-2 ⊖

HIV-1 NAT

HIV-1 NAT ⊕ Acute HIV-1 infection

HIV-1 NAT ⊖ Negative for HIV-1

⊕ Indicates reactive test results
⊖ Indicates nonreactive test results
NAT: nucleic acid test
  Diagnostic tests
  True positive tests
  True negative tests

HIV-1/2 Ag/Ab immunoassays detect viral p24 antigen capsid protein and IgG and/or IgM to HIV-1/2.
- Use for diagnosis. Very high sensitivity/specificity, but may miss early HIV disease if tested within first 2 weeks of infection.
- A positive screening test is followed by a confirmatory HIV-1/2 differentiation immunoassay.

HIV RNA tests detect elevated HIV RNA and can be qualitative or quantitative.
- NAAT is qualitative, and is a sensitive method to detect HIV viremia in antibody-negative patients.
- Viral load tests (RT-PCR) are quantitative and determine amount of viral RNA in the plasma. Use to monitor response to treatment and transmissibility.

Western blot tests are no longer recommended by the CDC for confirmatory testing.

HIV-1/2 Ag/Ab testing is not recommended in babies with suspected HIV due to maternally transferred antibody. Use HIV viral load instead.

AIDS diagnosis: ≤ 200 CD4+ cells/mm^3 (normal: 500–1500 cells/mm^3) or HIV ⊕ with AIDS-defining condition (eg, *Pneumocystis pneumonia*).

Common diseases of HIV-positive adults
↓ CD4+ cell count → reactivation of past infections (eg, TB, HSV, shingles), dissemination of bacterial infections and fungal infections (eg, coccidioidomycosis), and non-Hodgkin lymphomas.

PATHOGEN	PRESENTATION	FINDINGS
CD4+ cell count < 500/mm³		
Candida albicans	Oral thrush	Scrapable white plaque, pseudohyphae on microscopy
EBV	Oral hairy leukoplakia	Unscrapable white plaque on lateral tongue
HHV-8	Kaposi sarcoma, localized cutaneous disease	Perivascular spindle cells invading and forming vascular tumors on histology
HPV	Squamous cell carcinoma at site(s) of sexual contact (most commonly anus, cervix, oropharynx)	
Mycobacterium tuberculosis	Increased risk of reactivation of latent TB infection	
CD4+ cell count < 200/mm³		
Histoplasma capsulatum	Fever, weight loss, fatigue, cough, dyspnea, nausea, vomiting, diarrhea	Oval yeast cells within macrophages
HIV	Dementia, HIV-associated nephropathy	Cerebral atrophy on neuroimaging
JC virus (reactivation)	Progressive multifocal leukoencephalopathy	Nonenhancing areas of demyelination on MRI
HHV-8	Kaposi sarcoma, disseminated disease (pulmonary, GI, lymphatic)	
Pneumocystis jirovecii	*Pneumocystis* pneumonia	"Ground-glass" opacities on chest imaging
CD4+ cell count < 100/mm³		
Bartonella spp	Bacillary angiomatosis	Multiple red to purple papules or nodules Biopsy with neutrophilic inflammation
Candida albicans	Esophagitis	White plaques on endoscopy; yeast and pseudohyphae on biopsy
CMV	Colitis, Retinitis, Esophagitis, Encephalitis, Pneumonitis (**CREEP**)	Linear ulcers on endoscopy, cotton-wool spots on fundoscopy Biopsy reveals cells with intranuclear (owl eye) inclusion bodies
Cryptococcus neoformans	Meningitis	Encapsulated yeast on India ink stain or capsular antigen ⊕
Cryptosporidium spp	Chronic, watery diarrhea	Acid-fast oocysts in stool
EBV	B-cell lymphoma (eg, non-Hodgkin lymphoma, CNS lymphoma)	CNS lymphoma—ring enhancing, may be solitary (vs *Toxoplasma*)
Mycobacterium avium–intracellulare, Mycobacterium avium complex	Nonspecific systemic symptoms (fever, night sweats, weight loss, diarrhea) or superficial lymphadenitis	Most common if CD4+ cell count < 50/mm³
Toxoplasma gondii	Brain abscesses	Multiple ring-enhancing lesions on MRI

Prions

Prion diseases are caused by the conversion of a normal (predominantly α-helical) protein termed prion protein (PrP^c) to a β-pleated form (PrP^{sc}), which is transmissible via CNS-related tissue (iatrogenic CJD) or food contaminated by BSE-infected animal products (variant CJD). PrP^{sc} resists protease degradation and facilitates the conversion of still more PrP^c to PrP^{sc}. Resistant to standard sterilizing procedures, including standard autoclaving. Accumulation of PrP^{sc} results in spongiform encephalopathy and dementia, ataxia, startle myoclonus, and death.

Creutzfeldt-Jakob disease—rapidly progressive dementia, typically sporadic (some familial forms).

Bovine spongiform encephalopathy—also called "mad cow disease."

Kuru—acquired prion disease noted in tribal populations practicing human cannibalism.

▶ MICROBIOLOGY—SYSTEMS

Normal microbiota: dominant

Neonates delivered by C-section have microbiota enriched in skin commensals.

LOCATION	MICROORGANISM
Skin	S epidermidis
Nose	S epidermidis; colonized by S aureus
Oropharynx	Viridans group streptococci
Dental plaque	S mutans
Colon	B fragilis > E coli
Vagina	Lactobacillus; colonized by E coli and group B strep

Bugs causing food-borne illness

S aureus and B cereus food poisoning starts quickly and ends quickly (exotoxin-mediated).

MICROORGANISM	SOURCE OF INFECTION
B cereus	Reheated rice. "Food poisoning from reheated rice? **Be serious!**" (**B cereus**)
C botulinum	Improperly canned foods (toxins), raw honey (spores)
C perfringens	Reheated meat
E coli O157:H7	Undercooked meat
L monocytogenes	Deli meats, soft cheeses
Salmonella	Poultry, meat, and eggs
S aureus	Meats, mayonnaise, custard; preformed toxin
V parahaemolyticus and V vulnificus[a]	Raw/undercooked seafood

[a]V vulnificus predominantly causes wound infections from contact with contaminated water or shellfish.

Bugs causing diarrhea

Bloody diarrhea

Campylobacter	Comma- or S-shaped organisms; growth at 42°C
E histolytica	Protozoan; amebic dysentery; liver abscess
Enterohemorrhagic *E coli*	O157:H7; can cause HUS; makes Shiga toxin
Enteroinvasive *E coli*	Invades colonic mucosa
Salmonella (non-typhoidal)	Lactose ⊖; flagellar motility; has animal reservoir, especially poultry and eggs
Shigella	Lactose ⊖; very low ID_{50}; produces Shiga toxin; human reservoir only; bacillary dysentery
Y enterocolitica	Day care outbreaks; pseudoappendicitis

Watery diarrhea

C difficile	Pseudomembranous colitis; associated with antibiotics and PPIs; occasionally bloody diarrhea
C perfringens	Also causes gas gangrene
Enterotoxigenic *E coli*	Travelers' diarrhea; produces heat-labile (LT) and heat-stable (ST) toxins
Protozoa	*Giardia, Cryptosporidium*
V cholerae	Comma-shaped organisms; rice-water diarrhea; often from infected seafood
Viruses	Norovirus (most common cause in developed countries), rotavirus (↓ incidence in developed countries due to vaccination), enteric adenovirus

Common causes of pneumonia

NEONATES (< 4 WK)	CHILDREN (4 WK–18 YR)	ADULTS (18–40 YR)	ADULTS (40–65 YR)	ADULTS (65 YR +)
Group B streptococci *E coli*	Viruses (**R**SV) *Mycoplasma* *C trachomatis* (infants–3 yr) *C pneumoniae* (school-aged children) *S pneumoniae* **R**unts **M**ay **C**ough **C**hunky **S**putum	*Mycoplasma* *C pneumoniae* *S pneumoniae* Viruses (eg, influenza)	*S pneumoniae* *H influenzae* Anaerobes Viruses *Mycoplasma*	*S pneumoniae* Influenza virus Anaerobes *H influenzae* Gram ⊖ rods

Special groups

Alcohol overuse	*Klebsiella*, anaerobes usually due to aspiration (eg, *Peptostreptococcus, Fusobacterium, Prevotella, Bacteroides*)
Injection drug use	*S pneumoniae, S aureus*
Aspiration	Anaerobes
Atypical	*Mycoplasma, Chlamydophila, Legionella*, viruses (RSV, CMV, influenza, adenovirus)
Cystic fibrosis	*Pseudomonas, S aureus, S pneumoniae, Burkholderia cepacia*
Immunocompromised	*S aureus*, enteric gram ⊖ rods, fungi, viruses, *P jirovecii* (with HIV)
Healthcare-associated	*S aureus, Pseudomonas*, other enteric gram ⊖ rods
Postviral	*S pneumoniae, S aureus, H influenzae*
COPD	*S pneumoniae, H influenzae, M catarrhalis, Pseudomonas*

Common causes of meningitis

NEWBORN (0–6 MO)	CHILDREN (6 MO–6 YR)	6–60 YR	60 YR +
Group B *Streptococcus*	*S pneumoniae*	*S pneumoniae*	*S pneumoniae*
E coli	*N meningitidis*	*N meningitidis*	*N meningitidis*
Listeria	*H influenzae* type b	Enteroviruses	*H influenzae* type b
	Group B *Streptococcus*	HSV	Group B *Streptococcus*
	Enteroviruses		*Listeria*

Give ceftriaxone and vancomycin empirically (add ampicillin if *Listeria* is suspected; add acyclovir if viral encephalitis is suspected).

Viral causes of meningitis: enteroviruses (especially coxsackievirus), HSV-2 (HSV-1 = encephalitis), HIV, West Nile virus (also causes encephalitis), VZV.

In HIV: *Cryptococcus* spp.

Note: Incidence of Group B streptococcal meningitis in neonates has ↓ greatly due to screening and antibiotic prophylaxis in pregnancy. Incidence of *H influenzae* meningitis has ↓ greatly due to conjugate *H influenzae* vaccinations. Today, cases are usually seen in unimmunized children.

Cerebrospinal fluid findings in meningitis

	OPENING PRESSURE	CELL TYPE	PROTEIN	GLUCOSE
Bacterial	↑	↑ PMNs	↑	↓
Fungal/TB	↑	↑ lymphocytes	↑	↓
Viral	Normal/↑	↑ lymphocytes	Normal/↑	Normal

Infections causing brain abscess	Most commonly viridans streptococci and *Staphylococcus aureus*. If dental infection or extraction precedes abscess, oral anaerobes commonly involved. Multiple abscesses are usually from bacteremia; single lesions from contiguous sites: otitis media and mastoiditis → temporal lobe and cerebellum; sinusitis or dental infection → frontal lobe. *Toxoplasma* reactivation in AIDS.

Osteomyelitis

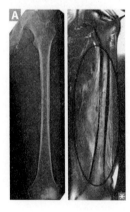

RISK FACTOR	ASSOCIATED INFECTION
Assume if no other information is available	*S aureus* (most common overall)
Sexually active	*Neisseria gonorrhoeae* (rare), septic arthritis more common
Sickle cell disease	*Salmonella*, *S aureus*
Prosthetic joint replacement	*S aureus*, *S epidermidis*
Vertebral involvement	*S aureus*, *M tuberculosis* (Pott disease)
Cat and dog bites	*Pasteurella multocida*
Injection drug use	*S aureus*; also *Pseudomonas*, *Candida*

Elevated ESR and CRP sensitive but not specific.

Radiographs are insensitive early but can be useful in chronic osteomyelitis (**A**, left). MRI is best for detecting acute infection and detailing anatomic involvement (**A**, right). Biopsy or aspiration with culture necessary to identify organism.

Red rashes of childhood

AGENT	ASSOCIATED SYNDROME/DISEASE	CLINICAL PRESENTATION
Coxsackievirus type A	Hand-foot-mouth disease	Oval-shaped vesicles on palms and soles **A**; vesicles and ulcers in oral mucosa (herpangina)
Human herpesvirus 6	Roseola (exanthem subitum)	Asymptomatic rose-colored macules appear on body after several days of high fever; can present with febrile seizures; usually affects infants
Measles virus	Measles (rubeola)	Confluent rash beginning at head and moving down **B**; preceded by cough, coryza, conjunctivitis, and blue-white (Koplik) spots on buccal mucosa
Parvovirus B19	Erythema infectiosum (fifth disease)	"Slapped cheek" rash on face **C**
Rubella virus	Rubella	Pink macules and papules begin at head and move down, remain discrete → fine desquamating truncal rash; postauricular lymphadenopathy
Streptococcus pyogenes	Scarlet fever	Sore throat, Circumoral pallor, group **A** strep, **R**ash (sandpaperlike **D**, from neck to trunk and extremities), **L**ymphadenopathy, **E**rythrogenic toxin, strawberry **T**ongue (**SCARLET**)
Varicella-zoster virus	Chickenpox	Vesicular rash begins on trunk **E**, spreads to face and extremities with lesions of different stages

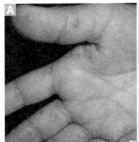
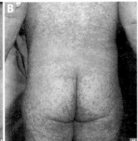
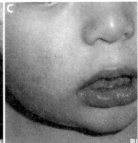
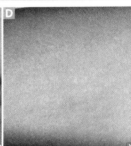
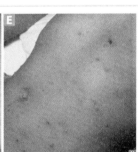

Urinary tract infections	Cystitis presents with dysuria, frequency, urgency, suprapubic pain, and WBCs (but not WBC casts) in urine. Primarily caused by ascension of microbes from urethra to bladder. Ascension to kidney results in pyelonephritis, which presents with fever, chills, flank pain, costovertebral angle tenderness, hematuria, and WBC casts.
	Ten times more common in females (shorter urethras colonized by fecal microbiota).
	Risk factors: obstruction (eg, kidney stones, enlarged prostate), kidney surgery, catheterization, congenital GU malformation (eg, vesicoureteral reflux), diabetes, pregnancy.

SPECIES	FEATURES	COMMENTS
Escherichia coli	Leading cause of UTI. Colonies show strong pink lactose-fermentation on MacConkey agar.	Diagnostic markers:
Staphylococcus saprophyticus	2nd leading cause of UTI, particularly in young, sexually active females.	⊕ Leukocyte esterase = evidence of WBC activity. ⊕ Nitrite test = reduction of urinary nitrates by gram ⊖ bacterial species (eg, *E coli*).
Klebsiella pneumoniae	3rd leading cause of UTI. Large mucoid capsule and viscous colonies.	
Serratia marcescens	Some strains produce a red pigment; often healthcare-associated and drug resistant.	
Enterococcus	Often healthcare-associated and drug resistant.	
Proteus mirabilis	Motility causes "swarming" on agar; associated with struvite stones. Produces urease.	
Pseudomonas aeruginosa	Blue-green pigment and fruity odor; usually healthcare-associated and drug resistant.	

Common vaginal infections

	Bacterial vaginosis	***Trichomonas* vaginitis**	***Candida* vulvovaginitis**
SIGNS AND SYMPTOMS	No inflammation Thin, white discharge 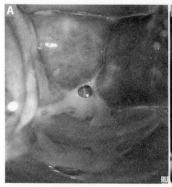 A with fishy odor	Inflammation B ("strawberry cervix") Frothy, yellow-green, foul-smelling discharge	Inflammation Thick, white, "cottage cheese" discharge D
LAB FINDINGS	Clue cells (bacteria-coated epithelial cells) pH > 4.5 ⊕ KOH whiff test	Motile pear-shaped trichomonads C pH > 4.5	Pseudohyphae pH normal (4.0–4.5)
TREATMENT	Metronidazole or clindamycin	Metronidazole Treat sexual partner(s)	Azoles

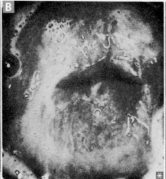
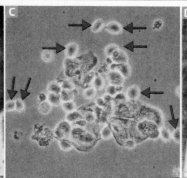
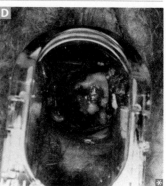

Sexually transmitted infections

DISEASE	CLINICAL FEATURES	PATHOGEN
AIDS	Opportunistic infections, Kaposi sarcoma, lymphoma	HIV
Chancroid	Painful genital ulcer(s) with exudate, inguinal adenopathy 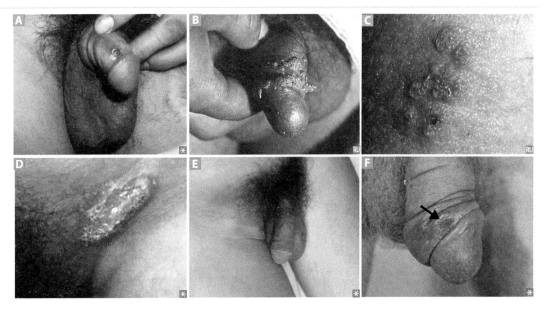	*Haemophilus ducreyi* (it's so painful, you "**do cry**")
Chlamydia	Urethritis, cervicitis, epididymitis, conjunctivitis, reactive arthritis, PID	*Chlamydia trachomatis* (D–K)
Condylomata acuminata	Genital warts B, koilocytes	HPV-6 and -11
Herpes genitalis	Painful penile, vulvar, or cervical vesicles and ulcers C with bilateral tender inguinal lymphadenopathy; can cause systemic symptoms such as fever, headache, myalgia	HSV-2, less commonly HSV-1
Gonorrhea	Urethritis, cervicitis, PID, prostatitis, epididymitis, arthritis, creamy purulent discharge	*Neisseria gonorrhoeae*
Granuloma inguinale (Donovanosis)	Painless, beefy red ulcer that bleeds readily on contact D Uncommon in US	*Klebsiella (Calymmatobacterium) granulomatis*; cytoplasmic Donovan bodies (bipolar staining) seen on microscopy
Hepatitis B	Jaundice	HBV
Lymphogranuloma venereum	Infection of lymphatics; painless genital ulcers, painful lymphadenopathy (ie, buboes E)	*C trachomatis* (L1–L3)
Primary syphilis	Painless chancre F, regional lymphadenopathy	*Treponema pallidum*
Secondary syphilis	Fever, diffuse lymphadenopathy, generalized rash, condylomata lata	
Tertiary syphilis	Gummas, tabes dorsalis, general paresis, aortitis, Argyll Robertson pupil	
Trichomoniasis	Vaginitis, strawberry cervix, motile in wet prep	*Trichomonas vaginalis*

TORCH infections

Microbes that may pass from mother to fetus. Transmission is transplacental in most cases, or via vaginal delivery (especially HSV-2). Nonspecific signs common to many **ToRCHHeS** infections include hepatosplenomegaly, jaundice, thrombocytopenia, and growth restriction.

Other important infectious agents include *Streptococcus agalactiae* (group B streptococci), *E coli*, and *Listeria monocytogenes*—all causes of meningitis in neonates. Parvovirus B19 causes hydrops fetalis.

AGENT	MATERNAL ACQUISITION	MATERNAL MANIFESTATIONS	NEONATAL MANIFESTATIONS
Toxoplasma gondii	Cat feces or ingestion of undercooked meat	Usually asymptomatic; lymphadenopathy (rarely)	Classic triad: chorioretinitis, hydrocephalus, and intracranial calcifications, +/– "blueberry muffin" rash 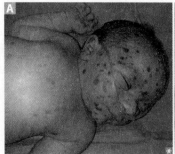
Rubella	Respiratory droplets	Rash, lymphadenopathy, polyarthritis, polyarthralgia	Classic triad: abnormalities of **eye** (cataracts 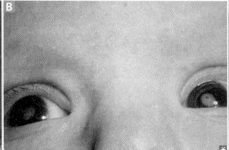) and **ear** (deafness) and congenital **heart** disease (PDA); +/– "blueberry muffin" rash. "**I** (eye) ♥ ruby (**rubella**) earrings"
Cytomegalovirus	Sexual contact, organ transplants	Usually asymptomatic; mononucleosis-like illness	Hearing loss, seizures, petechial rash, "blueberry muffin" rash, chorioretinitis, periventricular calcifications 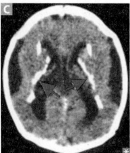 **CMV** = **C**horioretinitis, **M**icrocephaly, peri**V**entricular calcifications
HIV	Sexual contact, needlestick	Variable presentation depending on CD4+ cell count	Recurrent infections, chronic diarrhea
Herpes simplex virus-2	Skin or mucous membrane contact	Usually asymptomatic; herpetic (vesicular) lesions	Meningoencephalitis, herpetic (vesicular) lesions
Syphilis	Sexual contact	Chancre (1°) and disseminated rash (2°) are the two stages likely to result in fetal infection	Often results in stillbirth, hydrops fetalis; if child survives, presents with facial abnormalities (eg, notched teeth, saddle nose, rhinitis, short maxilla), saber shins, CN VIII deafness

Pelvic inflammatory disease

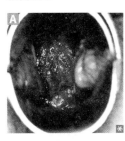

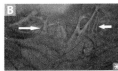

Ascending infection causing inflammation of the female gynecologic tract. PID may include salpingitis, endometritis, hydrosalpinx, and tubo-ovarian abscess.

Signs include cervical motion tenderness, adnexal tenderness, purulent cervical discharge A.

Top bugs—*Chlamydia trachomatis* (subacute, often undiagnosed), *Neisseria gonorrhoeae* (acute).

C trachomatis—most common bacterial STI in the United States.

Salpingitis is a risk factor for ectopic pregnancy, infertility, chronic pelvic pain, and adhesions. Can lead to perihepatitis (**Fitz-Hugh–Curtis syndrome**)—infection and inflammation of liver capsule and "violin string" adhesions of peritoneum to liver B.

Healthcare-associated infections

E coli (UTI) and *S aureus* (wound infection) are the two most common causes.

RISK FACTOR	PATHOGEN	UNIQUE SIGNS/SYMPTOMS
Antibiotic use, PPIs	*C difficile*	Watery diarrhea, leukocytosis
Aspiration (2° to altered mental status, old age)	Polymicrobial, gram ⊖ bacteria, often anaerobes	Right lower lobe infiltrate or right upper/middle lobe (patient recumbent); purulent malodorous sputum
Decubitus ulcers, surgical wounds, drains	*S aureus* (including MRSA), gram ⊖ anaerobes (*Bacteroides*, *Prevotella*, *Fusobacterium*)	Erythema, tenderness, induration, drainage from surgical wound sites
Intravascular catheters	*S aureus* (including MRSA), *S epidermidis* (long term)	Erythema, induration, tenderness, drainage from access sites
Mechanical ventilation, endotracheal intubation	Late onset: *P aeruginosa*, *Klebsiella*, *Acinetobacter*, *S aureus*	New infiltrate on CXR, ↑ sputum production; sweet odor (*Pseudomonas*)
Exposure to blood products, shared medical equipment, needlesticks	HBV, HCV	
Urinary catheterization	*Proteus* spp, *E coli*, *Klebsiella* (PEcK)	Dysuria, leukocytosis, flank pain or costovertebral angle tenderness
Water aerosols	*Legionella*	Signs of pneumonia, GI symptoms (diarrhea, nausea, vomiting), neurologic abnormalities

Bugs affecting unvaccinated children

CLINICAL PRESENTATION	FINDINGS/LABS	PATHOGEN
Dermatologic		
Rash	Beginning at head and moving down with postauricular, posterior cervical, and suboccipital lymphadenopathy	Rubella virus
	Beginning at head and moving down; preceded by cough, coryza, conjunctivitis, and Koplik spots	Measles virus
Neurologic		
Meningitis	Microbe colonizes nasopharynx	*H influenzae* type b
	Can also lead to myalgia and paralysis	Poliovirus
Tetanus	Muscle spasms and spastic paralysis (eg, lockjaw, opisthotonus)	*C tetani*
Respiratory		
Epiglottitis	Fever with dysphagia, drooling, inspiratory stridor, and difficulty breathing due to edema	*H influenzae* type b (also capable of causing epiglottitis in fully immunized children)
Pertussis	Low-grade fevers, coryza → whooping cough, posttussive vomiting → gradual recovery	*Bordetella pertussis*
Pharyngitis	Grayish pseudomembranes (may obstruct airways)	*Corynebacterium diphtheriae*

▶ MICROBIOLOGY—ANTIMICROBIALS

Antimicrobial therapy

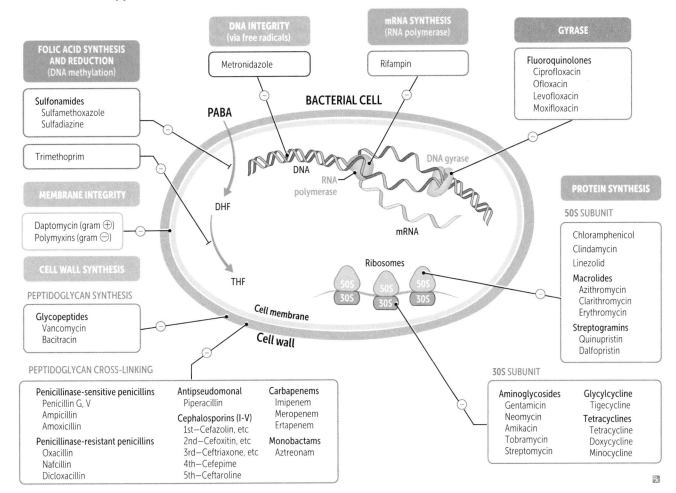

Penicillin G, V	Penicillin G (IV and IM form), penicillin V (oral). Prototype β-lactam antibiotics.
MECHANISM	D-Ala-D-Ala structural analog. Bind penicillin-binding proteins (transpeptidases). Block transpeptidase cross-linking of peptidoglycan in cell wall. Activate autolytic enzymes.
CLINICAL USE	Mostly used for gram ⊕ organisms (*S pneumoniae, S pyogenes, Actinomyces*). Also used for gram ⊖ cocci (mainly *N meningitidis*) and spirochetes (mainly *T pallidum*). Bactericidal for gram ⊕ cocci, gram ⊕ rods, gram ⊖ cocci, and spirochetes. β-lactamase sensitive.
ADVERSE EFFECTS	Hypersensitivity reactions, direct Coombs ⊕ hemolytic anemia, drug-induced interstitial nephritis.
RESISTANCE	β-lactamase cleaves the β-lactam ring. Mutations in PBPs.

Penicillinase-sensitive penicillins	Amoxicillin, ampicillin; aminopenicillins.	
MECHANISM	Same as penicillin. Wider spectrum; penicillinase sensitive. Also combine with clavulanic acid to protect against destruction by β-lactamase.	**Aminopenicillins** are **amped-up** penicillin. Amoxicillin has greater oral bioavailability than ampicillin.
CLINICAL USE	Extended-spectrum penicillin—*H influenzae*, *H pylori*, *E coli*, Enterococci, *Listeria monocytogenes*, *Proteus mirabilis*, *Salmonella*, *Shigella*.	Coverage: ampicillin/amoxicillin **HHEELPSS** kill enterococci.
ADVERSE EFFECTS	Hypersensitivity reactions, rash, pseudomembranous colitis.	
MECHANISM OF RESISTANCE	Penicillinase (a type of β-lactamase) cleaves β-lactam ring.	

Penicillinase-resistant penicillins	Dicloxacillin, nafcillin, oxacillin.	
MECHANISM	Same as penicillin. Narrow spectrum; penicillinase resistant because bulky R group blocks access of β-lactamase to β-lactam ring.	
CLINICAL USE	*S aureus* (except MRSA).	"Use **naf** (nafcillin) for **staph**."
ADVERSE EFFECTS	Hypersensitivity reactions, interstitial nephritis.	
MECHANISM OF RESISTANCE	MRSA has altered penicillin-binding protein target site.	

Piperacillin	Antipseudomonal penicillin.
MECHANISM	Same as penicillin. Extended spectrum. Penicillinase sensitive; use with β-lactamase inhibitors.
CLINICAL USE	*Pseudomonas* spp., gram ⊖ rods, anaerobes.
ADVERSE EFFECTS	Hypersensitivity reactions.

Cephalosporins

MECHANISM	β-lactam drugs that inhibit cell wall synthesis but are less susceptible to penicillinases. Bactericidal.	Organisms typically not covered by 1st–4th generation cephalosporins are LAME: *Listeria*, Atypicals (*Chlamydia*, *Mycoplasma*), MRSA, and Enterococci.
CLINICAL USE	1st generation (cefazolin, cephalexin)—gram ⊕ cocci, *Proteus mirabilis*, *E coli*, *Klebsiella pneumoniae*. Cefazolin used prior to surgery to prevent *S aureus* wound infections.	1st generation—⊕ PEcK.
	2nd generation (cefaclor, cefoxitin, cefuroxime, cefotetan)—gram ⊕ cocci, *H influenzae*, *Enterobacter aerogenes*, *Neisseria* spp., *Serratia marcescens*, *Proteus mirabilis*, *E coli*, *Klebsiella pneumoniae*.	2nd graders wear fake fox fur to tea parties. 2nd generation—⊕ HENS PEcK.
	3rd generation (ceftriaxone, cefpodoxime, ceftazidime, cefixime)—serious gram ⊖ infections resistant to other β-lactams.	Can cross blood-brain barrier. Ceftriaxone—meningitis, gonorrhea, disseminated Lyme disease. Ceftazidime for pseudomonaz.
	4th generation (cefepime)—gram ⊖ organisms, with ↑ activity against *Pseudomonas* and gram ⊕ organisms.	
	5th generation (ceftaroline)—broad gram ⊕ and gram ⊖ organism coverage; unlike 1st–4th generation cephalosporins, ceftaroline covers MRSA, and *Enterococcus faecalis*—does not cover *Pseudomonas*.	
ADVERSE EFFECTS	Hypersensitivity reactions, autoimmune hemolytic anemia, disulfiram-like reaction, vitamin K deficiency. Low rate of cross-reactivity even in penicillin-allergic patients. ↑ nephrotoxicity of aminoglycosides.	
MECHANISM OF RESISTANCE	Inactivated by cephalosporinases (a type of β-lactamase). Structural change in penicillin-binding proteins (transpeptidases).	

β-lactamase inhibitors	Include Clavulanic acid, Avibactam, Sulbactam, Tazobactam. Often added to penicillin antibiotics to protect the antibiotic from destruction by β-lactamase.	CAST (eg, amoxicillin-clavulanate, ceftazidime-avibactam, ampicillin-sulbactam, piperacillin-tazobactam).

Carbapenems

Imipenem, meropenem, ertapenem.

MECHANISM	Imipenem is a broad-spectrum, β-lactamase–resistant carbapenem. Binds penicillin-binding proteins → inhibition of cell wall synthesis → cell death. Always administered with cilastatin (inhibitor of renal dehydropeptidase I) to ↓ inactivation of drug in renal tubules.	With imipenem, "the kill is **lastin'** with ci**lastatin**." Unlike other carbapenems, ertapenem is not active against *Pseudomonas*.
CLINICAL USE	Gram ⊕ cocci, gram ⊖ rods, and anaerobes. Wide spectrum and significant adverse effects limit use to life-threatening infections or after other drugs have failed. Meropenem has a ↓ risk of seizures and is stable to dehydropeptidase I.	
ADVERSE EFFECTS	GI distress, rash, and CNS toxicity (seizures) at high plasma levels.	
MECHANISM OF RESISTANCE	Inactivated by carbapenemases produced by, eg, *K pneumoniae*, *E coli*, *Klebsiella aerogenes*.	

Aztreonam

MECHANISM	Less susceptible to β-lactamases. Prevents peptidoglycan cross-linking by binding to penicillin-binding protein 3. Synergistic with aminoglycosides. No cross-allergenicity with penicillins.
CLINICAL USE	Gram ⊖ rods only—no activity against gram ⊕ rods or anaerobes. For penicillin-allergic patients and those with renal insufficiency who cannot tolerate aminoglycosides.
ADVERSE EFFECTS	Usually nontoxic; occasional GI upset.

Vancomycin

MECHANISM	Inhibits cell wall peptidoglycan formation by binding D-Ala-D-Ala portion of cell wall precursors. Bactericidal against most bacteria (bacteriostatic against *C difficile*). Not susceptible to β-lactamases.
CLINICAL USE	Gram ⊕ bugs only—for serious, multidrug-resistant organisms, including MRSA, *S epidermidis*, sensitive *Enterococcus* species, and *C difficile* (oral route).
ADVERSE EFFECTS	Well tolerated in general but **not** trouble free: **n**ephrotoxicity, **o**totoxicity, **t**hrombophlebitis, diffuse **f**lushing (vancomycin infusion reaction —idiopathic reaction largely preventable by pretreatment with antihistamines and slower infusion rate), DRESS syndrome.
MECHANISM OF RESISTANCE	Occurs in bacteria (eg, *Enterococcus*) via amino acid modification of D-Ala-D-Ala to **D-Ala**-D-**Lac**. "If you **Lac**k a **D-Ala** (dollar), you can't ride the **van** (**van**comycin)."

Protein synthesis inhibitors	Specifically target smaller bacterial ribosome (70S, made of 30S and 50S subunits), leaving human ribosome (80S) unaffected. All are bacteriostatic, except aminoglycosides (bactericidal) and linezolid (variable).	
30S inhibitors	Aminoglycosides Tetracyclines	"Buy **at 30, ccel** (sell) **at 50.**"
50S inhibitors	Chloramphenicol, Clindamycin Erythromycin (macrolides) Linezolid	

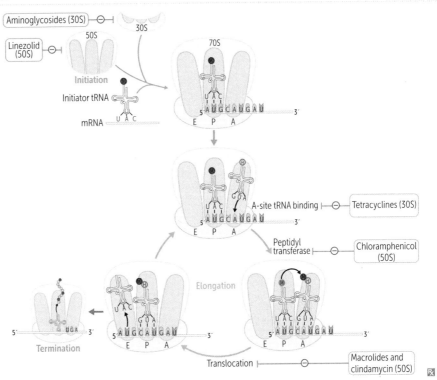

Aminoglycosides	Gentamicin, Neomycin, Amikacin, Tobramycin, Streptomycin. "**Mean**" (aminoglycoside) **GNATS cannot** kill anaerobes.
MECHANISM	Bactericidal; irreversible inhibition of initiation complex through binding of the 30S subunit. Can cause misreading of mRNA. Also block translocation. Require O_2 for uptake; therefore ineffective against anaerobes.
CLINICAL USE	Severe gram ⊖ rod infections. Synergistic with β-lactam antibiotics. Neomycin for bowel surgery.
ADVERSE EFFECTS	Nephrotoxicity, neuromuscular blockade (absolute contraindication with myasthenia gravis), ototoxicity (especially with loop diuretics), teratogenicity.
MECHANISM OF RESISTANCE	Bacterial transferase enzymes inactivate the drug by acetylation, phosphorylation, or adenylation.

Tetracyclines	Tetracycline, doxycycline, minocycline.
MECHANISM	Bacteriostatic; bind to 30S and prevent attachment of aminoacyl-tRNA. Limited CNS penetration. Doxycycline is fecally eliminated and can be used in patients with renal failure. Do not take tetracyclines with milk (Ca^{2+}), antacids (eg, Ca^{2+} or Mg^{2+}), or iron-containing preparations because divalent cations inhibit drugs' absorption in the gut.
CLINICAL USE	*Borrelia burgdorferi*, *M pneumoniae*. Drugs' ability to accumulate intracellularly makes them very effective against *Rickettsia* and *Chlamydia*. Also used to treat acne. Doxycycline effective against community-acquired MRSA.
ADVERSE EFFECTS	GI distress, discoloration of teeth and inhibition of bone growth in children, photosensitivity. "**Terato**cyclines" are **teratogenic**; generally avoided in pregnancy and in children (except doxycycline).
MECHANISM OF RESISTANCE	↓ uptake or ↑ efflux out of bacterial cells by plasmid-encoded transport pumps.

Tigecycline	
MECHANISM	Tetracycline derivative. Binds to 30S, inhibiting protein synthesis. Generally bacteriostatic.
CLINICAL USE	Broad-spectrum anaerobic, gram ⊖, and gram ⊕ coverage. Multidrug-resistant organisms (eg, MRSA, VRE).
ADVERSE EFFECTS	Nausea, vomiting.

Chloramphenicol	
MECHANISM	Blocks peptidyltransferase at 50S ribosomal subunit. Bacteriostatic.
CLINICAL USE	Meningitis (*Haemophilus influenzae*, *Neisseria meningitidis*, *Streptococcus pneumoniae*) and rickettsial diseases (eg, Rocky Mountain spotted fever [*Rickettsia rickettsii*]). Limited use due to toxicity but often still used in developing countries because of low cost.
ADVERSE EFFECTS	Anemia (dose dependent), aplastic anemia (dose independent), gray baby syndrome (in premature infants because they lack liver UDP-glucuronosyltransferase).
MECHANISM OF RESISTANCE	Plasmid-encoded acetyltransferase inactivates the drug.

Clindamycin	
MECHANISM	Blocks peptide transfer (translocation) at 50S ribosomal subunit. Bacteriostatic.
CLINICAL USE	Anaerobic infections (eg, *Bacteroides* spp., *C perfringens*) in aspiration pneumonia, lung abscesses, and oral infections. Also effective against invasive group A streptococcal infection. Treats anaerobic infections above the diaphragm vs metronidazole (anaerobic infections below diaphragm).
ADVERSE EFFECTS	Pseudomembranous colitis (*C difficile* overgrowth), fever, diarrhea.

Linezolid

MECHANISM	Inhibits protein synthesis by binding to the 23S rRNA of the 50S ribosomal subunit and preventing formation of the initiation complex.
CLINICAL USE	Gram ⊕ species including MRSA and VRE.
ADVERSE EFFECTS	Myelosuppression (especially thrombocytopenia), peripheral neuropathy, serotonin syndrome (due to partial MAO inhibition).
MECHANISM OF RESISTANCE	Point mutation of ribosomal RNA.

Macrolides

	Azithromycin, clarithromycin, erythromycin.
MECHANISM	Inhibit protein synthesis by blocking translocation ("macroslides"); bind to the 50S ribosomal subunit. Bacteriostatic.
CLINICAL USE	Atypical pneumonias (*Mycoplasma*, *Chlamydia*, *Legionella*), STIs (*Chlamydia*), gram ⊕ cocci (streptococcal infections in patients allergic to penicillin), and *B pertussis*.
ADVERSE EFFECTS	MACRO: Gastrointestinal Motility issues, Arrhythmia caused by prolonged QT interval, acute Cholestatic hepatitis, Rash, eOsinophilia. Increases serum concentration of theophylline, oral anticoagulants. Clarithromycin and erythromycin inhibit cytochrome P-450.
MECHANISM OF RESISTANCE	Methylation of 23S rRNA-binding site prevents binding of drug.

Polymyxins

	Colistin (polymyxin E), polymyxin B.
MECHANISM	Cation polypeptides that bind to phospholipids on cell membrane of gram ⊖ bacteria. Disrupt cell membrane integrity → leakage of cellular components → cell death.
CLINICAL USE	Salvage therapy for multidrug-resistant gram ⊖ bacteria (eg, *P aeruginosa*, *E coli*, *K pneumoniae*). Polymyxin B is a component of a triple antibiotic ointment used for superficial skin infections.
ADVERSE EFFECTS	Nephrotoxicity, neurotoxicity (eg, slurred speech, weakness, paresthesias), respiratory failure.

Sulfonamides	Sulfamethoxazole (SMX), sulfisoxazole, sulfadiazine.
MECHANISM	Inhibit dihydropteroate synthase, thus inhibiting folate synthesis. Bacteriostatic (bactericidal when combined with trimethoprim).
CLINICAL USE	Gram ⊕, gram ⊖, *Nocardia*. TMP-SMX for simple UTI.
ADVERSE EFFECTS	Stevens-Johnson syndrome, **u**rticaria, **l**iver damage, **f**olate deficiency, **o**ptic neuritis, **n**ephrotoxicity, **a**granulocytosis, hemolysis if G6PD deficient, kernicterus in infants.
MECHANISM OF RESISTANCE	Altered enzyme (bacterial dihydropteroate synthase), ↓ uptake, or ↑ PABA synthesis.

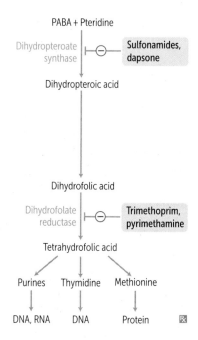

Dapsone	
MECHANISM	Similar to sulfonamides, but structurally distinct agent.
CLINICAL USE	Leprosy (lepromatous and tuberculoid), *Pneumocystis jirovecii* prophylaxis, or treatment when used in combination with TMP.
ADVERSE EFFECTS	Hemolysis if G6PD deficient, methemoglobinemia, agranulocytosis.

Trimethoprim	
MECHANISM	Inhibits bacterial dihydrofolate reductase. Bacteriostatic.
CLINICAL USE	Used in combination with sulfonamides (trimethoprim-sulfamethoxazole [TMP-SMX]), causing sequential block of folate synthesis. Combination used for UTIs, *Shigella*, *Salmonella*, *Pneumocystis jirovecii* pneumonia treatment and prophylaxis, toxoplasmosis prophylaxis.
ADVERSE EFFECTS	Hyperkalemia (at high doses; similar mechanism as potassium-sparing diuretics), megaloblastic anemia, leukopenia, granulocytopenia, which may be avoided with coadministration of leucovorin (folinic acid). **TMP T**reats **M**arrow **P**oorly.

Fluoroquinolones	Ciprofloxacin, ofloxacin; respiratory fluoroquinolones: levofloxacin, moxifloxacin.	
MECHANISM	Inhibit prokaryotic enzymes topoisomerase II (DNA gyrase) and topoisomerase IV. Bactericidal. Concurrent ingestion of divalent cations (eg, dairy, antacids) markedly decreases oral absorption.	
CLINICAL USE	Gram ⊖ rods of urinary and GI tracts (including *Pseudomonas*), some gram ⊕ organisms, otitis externa, community-acquired pneumonia.	
ADVERSE EFFECTS	GI upset, superinfections, skin rashes, headache, dizziness. Less commonly, can cause leg cramps and myalgias. Contraindicated during pregnancy or breastfeeding and in children < 18 years old due to possible damage to cartilage. Some may prolong QT interval.	May cause tendonitis or tendon rupture in people > 60 years old and in patients taking prednisone. Ciprofloxacin inhibits cytochrome P-450. Fluoroquino**lones** hurt attachments to your **bones**.
MECHANISM OF RESISTANCE	Chromosome-encoded mutation in DNA gyrase, plasmid-mediated resistance, efflux pumps.	

Daptomycin		
MECHANISM	Lipopeptide that disrupts cell membranes of gram ⊕ cocci by creating transmembrane channels.	
CLINICAL USE	*S aureus* skin infections (especially MRSA), bacteremia, infective endocarditis, VRE.	Not used for pneumonia (avidly binds to and is inactivated by surfactant). "Dapto-**myo-skin**" is used for **skin** infections but can cause **myopathy**.
ADVERSE EFFECTS	Myopathy, rhabdomyolysis.	

Metronidazole		
MECHANISM	Forms toxic free radical metabolites in the bacterial cell that damage DNA. Bactericidal, antiprotozoal.	
CLINICAL USE	Treats *Giardia*, *Entamoeba*, *Trichomonas*, *Gardnerella vaginalis*, Anaerobes (*Bacteroides*, *C difficile*). Can be used in place of amoxicillin in *H pylori* "triple therapy" in case of penicillin allergy.	**GET GAP** on the **Metro** with **metro**nidazole! Treats anaerobic infection **below** the diaphragm vs clindamycin (anaerobic infections **above** diaphragm).
ADVERSE EFFECTS	Disulfiram-like reaction (severe flushing, tachycardia, hypotension) with alcohol; headache, metallic taste.	

Antituberculous drugs

DRUG	MECHANISM	ADVERSE EFFECTS	NOTES
Rifamycins Rifampin, rifabutin, rifapentine	Inhibit DNA-dependent RNA polymerase → ↓ mRNA synthesis Rifamycin resistance arises due to mutations in gene encoding RNA polymerase	Minor hepatotoxicity, drug interactions (CYP450 induction), red-orange discoloration of body fluids (nonhazardous adverse effect)	Rifabutin favored over rifampin in patients with HIV infection due to less CYP450 induction Monotherapy rapidly leads to resistance
Isoniazid	Inhibits mycolic acid synthesis → ↓ cell wall synthesis Bacterial catalase-peroxidase (encoded by *kat*G) is needed to convert INH to active form INH resistance arises due to mutations in *kat*G	Vitamin B_6 deficiency (peripheral neuropathy, sideroblastic anemia), hepatotoxicity, drug interactions (CYP450 inhibition), drug-induced lupus INH overdose can lead to seizures (often refractory to benzodiazepines)	Administer with pyridoxine (vitamin B_6) **INH** **I**njures **N**eurons and **H**epatocytes (↑ risk of hepatotoxicity with ↑ age and alcohol overuse) Different INH half-lives in fast vs slow acetylators
Pyrazinamide	Mechanism uncertain	Hepatotoxicity, hyperuricemia	Works best at acidic pH (eg, in host phagolysosomes)
Ethambutol	Inhibits arabinosyltransferase → ↓ arabinogalactan synthesis → ↓ cell wall synthesis	**Optic** neuropathy (red-green color blindness or ↓ visual acuity, typically reversible)	Pronounce "**eye**thambutol"

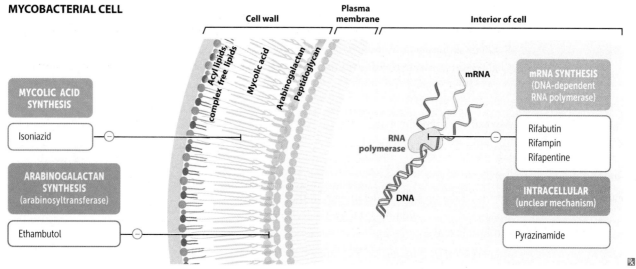

Antimycobacterial therapy

BACTERIUM	PROPHYLAXIS	TREATMENT
M tuberculosis	Rifamycin-based regimen for 3–4 months	**R**ifampin, **I**soniazid, **P**yrazinamide, **E**thambutol (**RIPE** for treatment)
M avium–intracellulare	Azithromycin, rifabutin	Azithromycin or clarithromycin + ethambutol Can add rifabutin or ciprofloxacin
M leprae	N/A	Long-term treatment with dapsone and rifampin for tuberculoid form Add clofazimine for lepromatous form

Antimicrobial prophylaxis

CLINICAL SCENARIO	MEDICATION
Exposure to meningococcal infection	Ceftriaxone, ciprofloxacin, or rifampin
High risk for infective endocarditis and undergoing surgical or dental procedures	Amoxicillin
History of recurrent UTIs	TMP-SMX
Malaria prophylaxis for travelers	Atovaquone-proguanil, mefloquine, doxycycline, primaquine, or chloroquine (for areas with sensitive species)
Pregnant patients carrying group B strep	Intrapartum penicillin G or ampicillin
Prevention of gonococcal conjunctivitis in newborn	Erythromycin ointment on eyes
Prevention of postsurgical infection due to *S aureus*	Cefazolin; vancomycin if ⊕ for MRSA
Prophylaxis of strep pharyngitis in child with prior rheumatic fever	Benzathine penicillin G or oral penicillin V

Prophylaxis in HIV infection/AIDS

CELL COUNT	PROPHYLAXIS	INFECTION
CD4+ < 200 cells/mm^3	TMP-SMX	*Pneumocystis* pneumonia
CD4+ < 100 cells/mm^3	TMP-SMX	*Pneumocystis* pneumonia and toxoplasmosis

Antifungal therapy

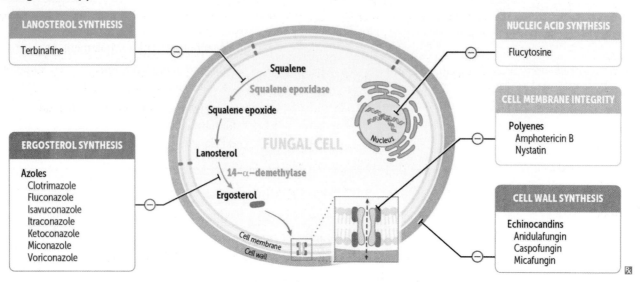

Amphotericin B

MECHANISM	Binds ergosterol (unique to fungi); forms membrane pores that allow leakage of electrolytes.	Amphotericin "**tears**" holes in the fungal membrane by forming pores.
CLINICAL USE	Serious, systemic mycoses. *Cryptococcus* (amphotericin B +/– flucytosine for cryptococcal meningitis), *Blastomyces*, *Coccidioides*, *Histoplasma*, *Candida*, *Mucor*. Intrathecally for coccidioidal meningitis.	Supplement K^+ and Mg^{2+} because of altered renal tubule permeability.
ADVERSE EFFECTS	Fever/chills ("shake and bake"), hypotension, nephrotoxicity, arrhythmias, anemia, IV phlebitis ("**amphoterrible**").	Hydration ↓ nephrotoxicity. Liposomal amphotericin ↓ toxicity.

Nystatin

MECHANISM	Same as amphotericin B. Topical use only as too toxic for systemic use.
CLINICAL USE	"Swish and swallow" for oral candidiasis (thrush); topical for diaper rash or vaginal candidiasis.

Flucytosine

MECHANISM	Inhibits DNA and RNA biosynthesis by conversion to 5-fluorouracil by cytosine deaminase.
CLINICAL USE	Systemic fungal infections (especially meningitis caused by *Cryptococcus*) in combination with amphotericin B.
ADVERSE EFFECTS	Myelosuppression.

Azoles

Clotrimazole, fluconazole, isavuconazole, itraconazole, ketoconazole, miconazole, voriconazole.

MECHANISM	Inhibit fungal sterol (ergosterol) synthesis by inhibiting the cytochrome P-450 enzyme that converts lanosterol to ergosterol.
CLINICAL USE	Local and less serious systemic mycoses. Fluconazole for chronic suppression of cryptococcal meningitis in people living with HIV and candidal infections of all types. Itraconazole may be used for *Blastomyces*, *Coccidioides*, *Histoplasma*, *Sporothrix schenckii*. Clotrimazole and miconazole for topical fungal infections. Voriconazole for *Aspergillus* and some *Candida*. Isavuconazole for serious *Aspergillus* and *Mucor* infections.
ADVERSE EFFECTS	Testosterone synthesis inhibition (gynecomastia, especially with ketoconazole), liver dysfunction (inhibits cytochrome P-450), QT interval prolongation.

Terbinafine

MECHANISM	Inhibits the fungal enzyme squalene epoxidase.
CLINICAL USE	Dermatophytoses (especially onychomycosis—fungal infection of finger or toe nails).
ADVERSE EFFECTS	GI upset, headaches, hepatotoxicity, taste disturbance.

Echinocandins

Anidulafungin, caspofungin, micafungin.

MECHANISM	Inhibit cell wall synthesis by inhibiting synthesis of β-glucan.
CLINICAL USE	Invasive aspergillosis, *Candida*.
ADVERSE EFFECTS	GI upset, flushing (by histamine release).

Griseofulvin

MECHANISM	Interferes with microtubule function; disrupts mitosis. Deposits in keratin-containing tissues (eg, nails).
CLINICAL USE	Oral treatment of superficial infections; inhibits growth of dermatophytes (tinea, ringworm).
ADVERSE EFFECTS	Teratogenic, carcinogenic, confusion, headaches, disulfiram-like reaction, ↑ cytochrome P-450 and warfarin metabolism.

Antiprotozoal therapy

Pyrimethamine-sulfadiazine (toxoplasmosis), suramin and melarsoprol (*Trypanosoma brucei*), nifurtimox (*T cruzi*), sodium stibogluconate (leishmaniasis).

Anti-mite/louse therapy

Permethrin, malathion (acetylcholinesterase inhibitor), topical or oral ivermectin. Used to treat scabies (*Sarcoptes scabiei*) and lice (*Pediculus* and *Pthirus*).

Chloroquine

MECHANISM	Blocks detoxification of heme into hemozoin. Heme accumulates and is toxic to plasmodia.
CLINICAL USE	Treatment of plasmodial species other than *P falciparum* (due to drug resistance from membrane pump that ↓ intracellular concentration of drug).
ADVERSE EFFECTS	Retinopathy (dependent on cumulative dose); pruritus (especially in dark-skinned individuals).

Antihelminthic therapy	Pyrantel pamoate, ivermectin, mebendazole (treats "**bend**y worms" by disrupting microtubules and cellular motility), praziquantel ($\uparrow$ Ca^{2+} permeability, $\uparrow$ vacuolization), diethylcarbamazine.

Oseltamivir, zanamivir

MECHANISM	Inhibit influenza neuraminidase → $\downarrow$ release of progeny virus.
CLINICAL USE	Treatment and prevention of influenza A and B. Beginning therapy within 48 hours of symptom onset may shorten duration of illness.

Baloxavir

MECHANISM	Inhibits the "cap snatching" (transfer of the 5′ cap from cell mRNA onto viral mRNA) endonuclease activity of the influenza virus RNA polymerase → $\downarrow$ viral replication.
CLINICAL USE	Treatment within 48 hours of symptom onset shortens duration of illness.

Remdesivir

MECHANISM	Prodrug of an ATP analog. The active metabolite inhibits viral RNA-dependent RNA polymerase and evades proofreading by viral exoribonuclease (ExoN) → $\downarrow$ viral RNA production.
CLINICAL USE	Recently approved for treatment of COVID-19 requiring hospitalization.

Acyclovir, famciclovir, valacyclovir

MECHANISM	Guanosine analogs. Monophosphorylated by HSV/VZV thymidine kinase and not phosphorylated in uninfected cells → few adverse effects. Triphosphate formed by cellular enzymes. Preferentially inhibit viral DNA polymerase by chain termination.
CLINICAL USE	No activity against CMV because CMV lacks the thymidine kinase necessary to activate guanosine analogs. Used for HSV-induced mucocutaneous and genital lesions as well as for encephalitis. Prophylaxis in patients who are immunocompromised. Also used as prophylaxis for immunocompetent patients with severe or recurrent infection. No effect on latent forms of HSV and VZV. Valacyclovir, a prodrug of acyclovir, has better oral bioavailability. For herpes zoster, use famciclovir.
ADVERSE EFFECTS	Obstructive crystalline nephropathy and acute kidney injury if not adequately hydrated.
MECHANISM OF RESISTANCE	Mutated viral thymidine kinase.

Ganciclovir

MECHANISM	Guanosine analog. 5′-monophosphate formed by a CMV viral kinase. Triphosphate formed by cellular kinases. Preferentially inhibits viral DNA polymerase.
CLINICAL USE	CMV, especially in patients who are immunocompromised. Valganciclovir, a prodrug of ganciclovir, has better oral bioavailability.
ADVERSE EFFECTS	Myelosuppression (leukopenia, neutropenia, thrombocytopenia), renal toxicity. More toxic to host enzymes than acyclovir.
MECHANISM OF RESISTANCE	Mutated viral kinase.

Foscarnet

MECHANISM	Viral DNA/RNA polymerase inhibitor and HIV reverse transcriptase inhibitor. Binds to pyrophosphate-binding site of enzyme. Does not require any kinase activation. Foscarnet = pyrofosphate analog.
CLINICAL USE	CMV retinitis in immunocompromised patients when ganciclovir fails; acyclovir-resistant HSV.
ADVERSE EFFECTS	Nephrotoxicity, multiple electrolyte abnormalities can lead to seizures.
MECHANISM OF RESISTANCE	Mutated DNA polymerase.

Cidofovir

MECHANISM	Preferentially inhibits viral DNA polymerase. Does not require phosphorylation by viral kinase.
CLINICAL USE	CMV retinitis in immunocompromised patients. Long half-life.
ADVERSE EFFECTS	Nephrotoxicity (coadminister **cid**ofovir with proben**ecid** and IV saline to ↓ toxicity).
MECHANISM OF RESISTANCE	Mutations in the viral DNA polymerase gene.

HIV therapy

Antiretroviral therapy (ART): often initiated at the time of HIV diagnosis.

Strongest indication for use with patients presenting with AIDS-defining illness, low CD4+ cell counts (< 500 cells/mm^3), or high viral load. Regimen consists of 3 drugs to prevent resistance: 2 NRTIs and preferably an integrase inhibitor.

Most ARTs are active against both HIV-1 and HIV-2 (exceptions: NNRTIs and enfuvirtide not effective against HIV-2).

Tenofovir + emtricitabine can be administered as pre-exposure prophylaxis.

DRUG	MECHANISM	ADVERSE EFFECTS
NRTIs		
Abacavir (ABC) Emtricitabine (FTC) Lamivudine (3TC) Tenofovir (TDF) Zidovudine (ZDV, formerly AZT)	Competitively inhibit nucleotide binding to reverse transcriptase and terminate the DNA chain (lack a 3′ OH group). Tenofovir is a nucleoTide; the others are nucleosides. All need to be phosphorylated to be active. ZDV can be used for general prophylaxis and during pregnancy to ↓ risk of fetal transmission. Have **you dined** (**vudine**) with my **nuclear** (**nucleosides**) family?	Myelosuppression (can be reversed with granulocyte colony-stimulating factor [G-CSF] and erythropoietin), nephrotoxicity. Abacavir contraindicated if patient has HLA-B*5701 mutation due to ↑ risk of hypersensitivity.
NNRTIs		
Doravirine Efavirenz Rilpivirine	Bind to reverse transcriptase at site different from NRTIs. Do not require phosphorylation to be active or compete with nucleotides.	Rash and hepatotoxicity are common to all NNRTIs. Vivid dreams and CNS symptoms are common with efavirenz.
Integrase strand transfer inhibitors		
Bictegravir Dolutegravir	Also called integrase inhibitors. Inhibit HIV genome integration into host cell chromosome by reversibly inhibiting HIV integrase.	↑ creatine kinase, weight gain.

HIV therapy (continued)

DRUG	MECHANISM	ADVERSE EFFECTS
Protease inhibitors		
Atazanavir Darunavir Lopinavir Ritonavir	Prevents maturation of new virions. Maturation depends on HIV-1 protease (*pol* gene), which cleaves the polypeptide products of HIV mRNA into their functional parts. All protease inhibitors require boosting with either ritonavir or cobicistat. **Navir** (never) **tease a protease.**	Hyperglycemia, GI intolerance (nausea, diarrhea). Rifampin (potent CYP/UGT inducer) ↓ protease inhibitor concentrations; use rifabutin instead. Ritonavir (cytochrome P-450 inhibitor) is only used as a boosting agent.
Entry inhibitors		
Enfuvirtide	Binds gp41, inhibiting viral entry. En**fu**virtide inhibits **fu**sion.	Skin reaction at injection sites.
Maraviroc	Binds CCR-5 on surface of T cells/monocytes, inhibiting interaction with gp120. Maravi**roc** inhibits **doc**king.	

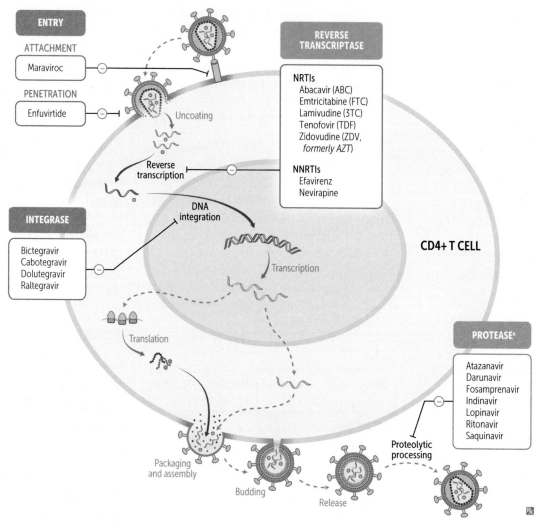

^aAll protease inhibitors require boosting with either ritonavir (protease inhibitor only used as a boosting agent) or cobicistat (cytochrome P450 inhibitor).

Hepatitis C therapy

Chronic HCV infection treated with multidrug therapy that targets specific steps within HCV replication cycle (HCV-encoded nonstructural proteins). Examples of drugs are provided.

DRUG	MECHANISM	TOXICITY
NS5A inhibitors		
Elbasvir Ledipasvir Pibrentasvir Velpatasvir	Inhibits NS5A, a viral phosphoprotein that plays a key role in RNA replication Exact mechanism unknown	Headache, diarrhea
NS5B inhibitors		
Sofosbuvir	Inhibits NS5B, an RNA-dependent RNA polymerase acting as a chain terminator Prevents viral RNA replication	Fatigue, headache
NS3/4A inhibitors		
Glecaprevir Grazoprevir	Inhibits NS3/4A, a viral protease, preventing viral replication	Headache, fatigue
Alternative drugs		
Ribavirin	Inhibits synthesis of guanine nucleotides by competitively inhibiting IMP dehydrogenase	Hemolytic anemia, severe teratogen

Disinfection and sterilization

Goals include the reduction of pathogenic organism counts to safe levels (disinfection) and the inactivation of all microbes including spores (sterilization).

Autoclave[a]	Pressurized steam at $> 120°C$. May not reliably inactivate prions.
Alcohols	Denature proteins and disrupt cell membranes.
Chlorhexidine	Disrupts cell membranes and coagulates intracellular components.
Chlorine[a]	Oxidizes and denatures proteins.
Ethylene oxide[a]	Alkylating agent.
Hydrogen peroxide[a]	Free radical oxidation.
Iodine and iodophors	Halogenation of DNA, RNA, and proteins. May be sporicidal.
Quaternary amines	Impair permeability of cell membranes.

[a]Sporicidal.

Antimicrobials to avoid in pregnancy

ANTIMICROBIAL	ADVERSE EFFECTS
Sulfonamides	Kernicterus
Aminoglycosides	Ototoxicity
Fluoroquinolones	Cartilage damage
Clarithromycin	Embryotoxic
Tetracyclines	Discolored teeth, inhibition of bone growth
Ribavirin	Teratogenic
Griseofulvin	Teratogenic
Chloramphenicol	Gray baby syndrome

Safe **c**hildren **t**ake **r**eally **g**ood **c**are.

▶ NOTES

Pathology

"Digressions, objections, delight in mockery, carefree mistrust are signs of health; everything unconditional belongs in pathology."

—Friedrich Nietzsche

"You cannot separate passion from pathology any more than you can separate a person's spirit from his body."

—Richard Selzer

"My business is not prognosis, but diagnosis. I am not engaged in therapeutics, but in pathology."

—H.L. Mencken

The fundamental principles of pathology are key to understanding diseases in all organ systems. Major topics such as inflammation and neoplasia appear frequently in questions across different organ systems, and such topics are definitely high yield. For example, the concepts of cell injury and inflammation are key to understanding the inflammatory response that follows myocardial infarction, a very common subject of board questions. Similarly, a familiarity with the early cellular changes that culminate in the development of neoplasias—for example, esophageal or colon cancer—is critical. Make sure you recognize the major tumor-associated genes and are comfortable with key cancer concepts such as tumor staging and metastasis. Finally, take some time to learn about the major systemic changes that come with aging, and how these physiologic alterations differ from disease states.

▶ PATHOLOGY—CELLULAR INJURY

Cellular adaptations	Reversible changes that can be physiologic (eg, uterine enlargement during pregnancy) or pathologic (eg, myocardial hypertrophy 2° to systemic HTN). If stress is excessive or persistent, adaptations can progress to cell injury (eg, significant LV hypertrophy → myocardial injury → HF).
Hypertrophy	↑ structural proteins and organelles → ↑ in size of cells. Example: cardiac hypertrophy.
Hyperplasia	Controlled proliferation of stem cells and differentiated cells → ↑ in number of cells (eg, benign prostatic hyperplasia). Excessive stimulation → pathologic hyperplasia (eg, endometrial hyperplasia), which may progress to dysplasia and cancer.
Atrophy	↓ in tissue mass due to ↓ in size (↑ cytoskeleton degradation via ubiquitin-proteasome pathway and autophagy [programmed digestion of damaged/misfolded intracellular proteins]; ↓ protein synthesis) and/or number of cells (apoptosis). Causes include disuse, denervation, loss of blood supply, loss of hormonal stimulation, poor nutrition.
Metaplasia	Reprogramming of stem cells → replacement of one cell type by another that can adapt to a new stressor. Usually due to exposure to an irritant, such as gastric acid (→ esophageal epithelium replaced by intestinal epithelium, called Barrett esophagus) or tobacco smoke (→ respiratory ciliated columnar epithelium replaced by stratified squamous epithelium). May progress to dysplasia → malignant transformation with persistent insult (eg, Barrett esophagus → esophageal adenocarcinoma). Metaplasia of connective tissue can also occur (eg, myositis ossificans, the formation of bone within muscle after trauma).
Dysplasia	Disordered, precancerous epithelial cell growth; not considered a true adaptive response. Characterized by loss of uniformity of cell size and shape (pleomorphism); loss of tissue orientation; nuclear changes (eg, ↑ nuclear:cytoplasmic ratio and clumped chromatin). Mild and moderate dysplasias (ie, do not involve entire thickness of epithelium) may regress with alleviation of inciting cause. Severe dysplasia often becomes irreversible and progresses to carcinoma in situ. Usually preceded by persistent metaplasia or pathologic hyperplasia.

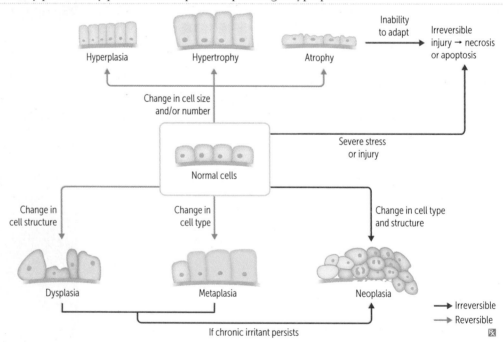

Cell injury

Reversible cell injury	▪ ↓ ATP → ↓ activity of Ca^{2+} and Na$^+$/K$^+$-ATPase pumps → cellular swelling (cytosol, mitochondria, endoplasmic reticulum/Golgi), which is the earliest morphologic manifestation
	▪ Ribosomal/polysomal detachment → ↓ protein synthesis
	▪ Plasma membrane changes (eg, blebbing)
	▪ Nuclear changes (eg, chromatin clumping)
	▪ Rapid loss of function (eg, myocardial cells are noncontractile after 1–2 minutes of ischemia)
	▪ Myelin figures (aggregation of peroxidized lipids)
Irreversible cell injury	▪ Breakdown of plasma membrane → cytosolic enzymes (eg, troponin) leak outside of cell, influx of Ca^{2+} → activation of degradative enzymes
	▪ Mitochondrial damage/dysfunction → loss of electron transport chain → ↓ ATP
	▪ Rupture of lysosomes → autolysis
	▪ Nuclear degradation: pyknosis (nuclear condensation) → karyorrhexis (nuclear fragmentation caused by endonuclease-mediated cleavage) → karyolysis (nuclear dissolution)
	▪ Amorphous densities/inclusions in mitochondria

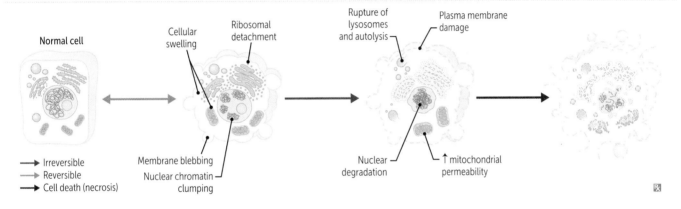

Normal cell

Cellular swelling

Ribosomal detachment

Rupture of lysosomes and autolysis

Plasma membrane damage

Membrane blebbing

Nuclear chromatin clumping

Nuclear degradation

↑ mitochondrial permeability

→ Irreversible
→ Reversible
→ Cell death (necrosis)

Apoptosis	ATP-dependent programmed cell death. Intrinsic, extrinsic, and perforin/granzyme B pathways → activate caspases (cytosolic proteases) → cellular breakdown including cell shrinkage, chromatin condensation, membrane blebbing, and formation of apoptotic bodies, which are then phagocytosed. Characterized by deeply eosinophilic cytoplasm and basophilic nucleus, pyknosis, and karyorrhexis. Cell membrane typically remains intact without significant inflammation (unlike necrosis). DNA laddering (fragments in multiples of 180 bp) is a sensitive indicator of apoptosis.
Intrinsic (mitochondrial) pathway	Involved in tissue remodeling in embryogenesis. Occurs when a regulating factor is withdrawn from a proliferating cell population (eg, ↓ IL-2 after a completed immunologic reaction → apoptosis of proliferating effector cells). Also occurs after exposure to injurious stimuli (eg, radiation, toxins, hypoxia). Regulated by Bcl-2 family of proteins. **Ba**x and **Ba**k are proapoptotic (**Bad** for survival), while **Bcl**-2 and **Bcl**-xL are antiapoptotic (**Be clever, live**). BAX and BAK form pores in the mitochondrial membrane → release of cytochrome C from inner mitochondrial membrane into the cytoplasm → activation of caspases. Bcl-2 keeps the mitochondrial membrane impermeable, thereby preventing cytochrome C release. Bcl-2 overexpression (eg, follicular lymphoma t[14;18]) → ↓ caspase activation → tumorigenesis.
Extrinsic (death receptor) pathway	Ligand receptor interactions: FasL binding to Fas (CD95) or TNF-α binding to its receptor. Fas-FasL interaction is necessary in thymic medullary negative selection. Autoimmune lymphoproliferative syndrome—caused by defective Fas-FasL interaction → failure of clonal deletion → ↑ numbers of self-reacting lymphocytes. Presents with lymphadenopathy, hepatosplenomegaly, autoimmune cytopenias.
Perforin/granzyme B pathway	Release of granules containing perforin and granzyme B by immune cells (cytotoxic T-cell and natural killer cell) → perforin forms a pore for granzyme B to enter the target cell.

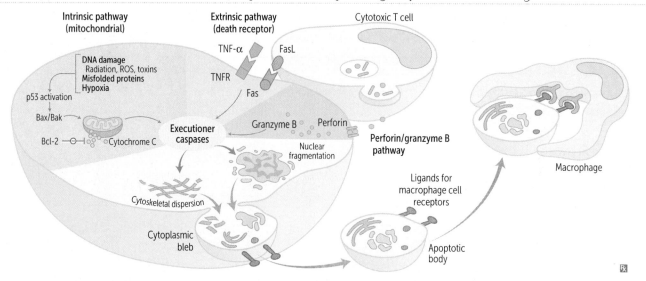

Necrosis	Exogenous injury → plasma membrane damage → intracellular components leak → cell undergoes enzymatic degradation and protein denaturation → local inflammatory reaction (unlike apoptosis).		
TYPE	SEEN IN	DUE TO	HISTOLOGY
Coagulative	Ischemia/infarcts in most tissues (except brain)	Ischemia or infarction; injury denatures enzymes → proteolysis blocked	Preserved cellular architecture (cell outlines seen), but nuclei disappear; ↑ cytoplasmic binding of eosin stain (→ ↑ eosinophilia; red/pink color) A
Liquefactive	Bacterial abscesses, CNS infarcts	Neutrophils release lysosomal enzymes that digest the tissue	Early: cellular debris and macrophages Late: cystic spaces and cavitation (CNS) B Neutrophils and cell debris seen with bacterial infection
Caseous	TB, systemic fungi (eg, *Histoplasma capsulatum*), *Nocardia*	Macrophages wall off the infecting microorganism → granular debris	Fragmented cells and debris surrounded by lymphocytes and macrophages (granuloma) Cheeselike gross appearance C
Fat	Enzymatic: acute pancreatitis (saponification of peripancreatic fat) Nonenzymatic: traumatic (eg, injury to breast tissue)	Damaged pancreatic cells release lipase, which breaks down triglycerides; liberated fatty acids bind calcium → saponification (chalky-white appearance)	Outlines of dead fat cells without peripheral nuclei; saponification of fat (combined with Ca^{2+}) appears dark blue on H&E stain D
Fibrinoid	Immune vascular reactions (eg, polyarteritis nodosa) Nonimmune vascular reactions (eg, hypertensive emergency, preeclampsia)	Immune complex deposition (type III hypersensitivity reaction) and/or plasma protein (eg, fibrin) leakage from damaged vessel	Vessel walls contain eosinophilic layer of proteinaceous material E
Gangrenous	Distal extremity and GI tract, after chronic ischemia	Dry: ischemia F	Coagulative
		Wet: superinfection	Liquefactive superimposed on coagulative

Ischemia

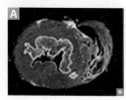

Inadequate blood supply to meet demand. Mechanisms include ↓ arterial perfusion (eg, atherosclerosis), ↓ venous drainage (eg, testicular torsion, Budd-Chiari syndrome), shock. Regions most vulnerable to hypoxia/ischemia and subsequent infarction:

ORGAN	SUSCEPTIBLE REGION
Brain	ACA/MCA/PCA boundary areas[a,b]
Heart	Subendocardium of LV (yellow lines in A outline a subendocardial infarction)
Kidney	Straight segment of proximal tubule (medulla) Thick ascending limb (medulla)
Liver	Area around central vein (zone III)
Colon	Splenic flexure (Griffith point),[a] rectosigmoid junction (Sudeck point)[a]

[a]Watershed areas (border zones) receive blood supply from most distal branches of 2 arteries with limited collateral vascularity. These areas are susceptible to ischemia from hypoperfusion.
[b]Neurons most vulnerable to hypoxic-ischemic insults include Purkinje cells of the cerebellum and pyramidal cells of the hippocampus and neocortex (layers 3, 5, 6).

Types of infarcts

Red infarct

Occurs in venous occlusion and tissues with multiple blood supplies (eg, liver, lung A, intestine, testes), and with reperfusion (eg, after angioplasty). **R**eperfusion injury is due to damage by free radicals.

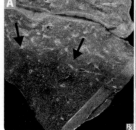
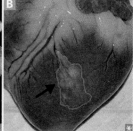

Pale infarct

Occurs in solid organs with a single (end-arterial) blood supply (eg, heart B, kidney).

Free radical injury

Free radicals damage cells via membrane lipid peroxidation, protein modification, DNA breakage. Initiated via radiation exposure (eg, cancer therapy), metabolism of drugs (phase I), redox reactions, nitric oxide (eg, inflammation), transition metals (eg, iron, copper; form free radicals via Fenton reaction), WBC (eg, neutrophils, macrophages) oxidative burst.

Free radicals can be eliminated by scavenging enzymes (eg, catalase, superoxide dismutase, glutathione peroxidase), spontaneous decay, antioxidants (eg, vitamins A, C, E), and certain metal carrier proteins (eg, transferrin, ceruloplasmin).

Examples:
- Oxygen toxicity: retinopathy of prematurity (abnormal vascularization), bronchopulmonary dysplasia, reperfusion injury after thrombolytic therapy
- Drug/chemical toxicity: acetaminophen overdose (hepatotoxicity), carbon tetrachloride (converted by cytochrome P-450 into CCl_3 free radical → fatty liver [cell injury → ↓ apolipoprotein synthesis → fatty change], centrilobular necrosis)
- Metal storage diseases: hemochromatosis (iron) and Wilson disease (copper)

Ionizing radiation toxicity	Ionizing radiation causes DNA (eg, double strand breaks) and cellular damage both directly and indirectly through the production of free radicals. Complications usually arise when patient is exposed to significant doses (eg, radiotherapy, nuclear reactor accidents): <ul><li>Localized inflammation and fibrosis</li><li>Neoplasia (eg, leukemia, thyroid cancer)</li></ul>Acute radiation syndrome—develops after sudden whole-body exposure to high doses of ionizing radiation → nausea, vomiting, diarrhea, hair loss, erythema, cytopenias, headache, altered mental status.	Stem cells of rapidly regenerating tissues (eg, skin, bone marrow, GI tract, gonads) are the most susceptible to radiation injury. Radiotherapy damages cancer cells more than healthy cells because cancer cells have dysfunctional DNA repair mechanisms in addition to high replicative rates.

Types of calcification — Calcium deposits appear deeply basophilic (arrow in A) on H&E stain.

	Dystrophic calcification	Metastatic calcification
Ca^{2+} DEPOSITION	In abnormal (diseased) tissues	In normal tissues
EXTENT	Tends to be localized (eg, calcific aortic stenosis)	Widespread (ie, diffuse, metastatic)
ASSOCIATED CONDITIONS 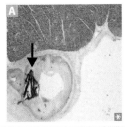	TB (lung and pericardium) and other granulomatous infections, liquefactive necrosis of chronic abscesses, fat necrosis, infarcts, thrombi, schistosomiasis, congenital CMV, toxoplasmosis, rubella, psammoma bodies, CREST syndrome, atherosclerotic plaques can become calcified	Predominantly in interstitial tissues of kidney, lung, and gastric mucosa (these tissues lose acid quickly; ↑ pH favors Ca^{2+} deposition) Nephrocalcinosis of collecting ducts may lead to nephrogenic diabetes insipidus and renal failure
ETIOLOGY	2° to injury or necrosis	2° to hyperphosphatemia (eg, chronic kidney disease) or hypercalcemia (eg, 1° hyperparathyroidism, sarcoidosis, hypervitaminosis D)

Psammoma bodies 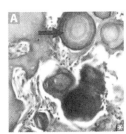	Concentrically laminated calcified spherules A. Usually seen in certain types of tumors: <ul><li>Papillary carcinoma of thyroid gland and kidney</li><li>Somatostatinoma</li><li>Meningioma</li><li>Mesothelioma</li><li>Ovarian serous papillary cystadenocarcinoma</li><li>Milk (prolactinoma)</li></ul>Histology: **B**asophilic staining of Ca^{2+} deposits within tissue.	**PS**o**MM**O**M**a Bodies.

Amyloidosis

Extracellular deposition of protein in abnormal fibrillar form (β-pleated sheet configuration) → cell injury and apoptosis. Manifestations vary depending on involved organ and include:
- Renal—nephrotic syndrome.
- Cardiac—restrictive cardiomyopathy.
- GI—hepatosplenomegaly.
- Neurologic—peripheral neuropathy.
- Musculoskeletal—muscle enlargement (eg, macroglossia), carpal tunnel syndrome.
- Skin—waxy thickening, easy bruising.

Amyloid deposits are visualized by Congo red stain (red/orange on nonpolarized light **A**, apple-green birefringence on polarized light **B**), and H&E stain (amorphous pink).

COMMON TYPES	FIBRIL PROTEIN	NOTES
Systemic		
Primary amyloidosis	AL (from Ig Light chains)	Seen in plasma cell dyscrasias (eg, multiple myeloma)
Secondary amyloidosis	AA (serum Amyloid A)	Seen in chronic inflammatory conditions, (eg, rheumatoid arthritis, IBD, familial Mediterranean fever, protracted infection)
Transthyretin amyloidosis	Transthyretin	Sporadic (wild-type *TTR*)—slowly progressive, associated with aging; mainly affects the heart. Hereditary (mutated *TTR*)—familial amyloid polyneuropathy and/or cardiomyopathy
Dialysis-related amyloidosis	β_2-microglobulin	Seen in patients with ESRD on long-term dialysis
Localized		
Alzheimer disease	β-amyloid protein	Cleaved from amyloid precursor protein
Isolated atrial amyloidosis	ANP	Common, associated with aging; ↑ risk for atrial fibrillation
Type 2 diabetes mellitus	Islet amyloid polypeptide	Caused by deposition of amylin in pancreatic islets
Medullary thyroid cancer	Calcitonin	Secreted from tumor cells

▶ PATHOLOGY—INFLAMMATION

Inflammation	Response to eliminate initial cause of cell injury, to remove necrotic cells resulting from the original insult, and to initiate tissue repair. Divided into acute and chronic. The inflammatory response itself can be harmful to the host if the reaction is excessive (eg, septic shock), prolonged (eg, persistent infections such as TB), or inappropriate (eg, autoimmune diseases such as SLE).

SIGN	MECHANISM
Cardinal signs	
Rubor and calor	Redness and warmth. Vasodilation (relaxation of arteriolar smooth muscle) → ↑ blood flow. Mediated by histamine, prostaglandins, bradykinin, NO.
Tumor	Swelling. Endothelial contraction/disruption (eg, from tissue damage) → ↑ vascular permeability → leakage of protein-rich fluid from postcapillary venules into interstitial space (exudate) → ↑ interstitial oncotic pressure. Endothelial cell contraction is mediated by leukotrienes (C_4, D_4, E_4), histamine, serotonin, bradykinin.
Dolor	Pain. Sensitization of sensory nerve endings. Mediated by bradykinin, PGE_2, histamine.
Functio laesa	Loss of function. Inflammation impairs function (eg, inability to make fist due to hand cellulitis).
Systemic manifestations (acute-phase reaction)	
Fever	Pyrogens (eg, LPS) induce macrophages to release IL-1 and TNF → ↑ COX activity in perivascular cells of anterior hypothalamus → ↑ PGE_2 → ↑ temperature set point.
Leukocytosis	↑ WBC count; type of predominant cell depends on inciting agent or injury (eg, bacteria → ↑ neutrophils).
↑ plasma acute-phase reactants	Serum concentrations significantly change in response to acute and chronic inflammation. Produced by liver. Notably induced by IL-6.

Acute phase reactants

POSITIVE (UPREGULATED)	
C-reactive protein	Opsonin; fixes complement and facilitates phagocytosis. Measured clinically as a nonspecific sign of ongoing inflammation.
Ferritin	Binds and sequesters iron to inhibit microbial iron scavenging.
Fibrinogen	Coagulation factor; promotes endothelial repair; correlates with ESR.
Haptoglobin	Binds extracellular hemoglobin, protects against oxidative stress.
Hepcidin	↓ iron absorption (by degrading ferroportin) and ↓ iron release (from macrophages) → anemia of chronic disease.
Procalcitonin	Increases in bacterial infections.
Serum amyloid A	Prolonged elevation can lead to secondary amyloidosis.
NEGATIVE (DOWNREGULATED)	
Albumin	Reduction conserves amino acids for positive reactants.
Transferrin	Internalized by macrophages to sequester iron.
Transthyretin	Also called prealbumin. Reduction conserves amino acids for positive reactants.

Erythrocyte sedimentation rate	RBCs normally remain separated via ⊖ charges. Products of inflammation (eg, fibrinogen) coat RBCs → ↓ ⊖ charge → ↑ RBC aggregation. Denser RBC aggregates fall at a faster rate within a pipette tube → ↑ ESR. Often co-tested with CRP (more specific marker of inflammation).

↑ ESR	↓ ESR[a]
Most anemias	Sickle cell anemia (altered shape)
Infections	Polycythemia (↑ RBCs "dilute" aggregation
Inflammation (eg, giant cell [temporal] arteritis, polymyalgia rheumatica)	factors)
	HF
Cancer (eg, metastases, multiple myeloma)	Microcytosis
Renal disease (end-stage or nephrotic syndrome)	Hypofibrinogenemia
Pregnancy	

[a]Lower than expected.

Acute inflammation	Transient and early response to injury or infection. Characterized by neutrophils in tissue 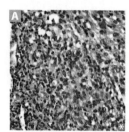, often with associated edema. Rapid onset (seconds to minutes) and short duration (minutes to days). Represents a reaction of the innate immune system (ie, less specific response than chronic inflammation).

STIMULI	Infections, trauma, necrosis, foreign bodies.	
MEDIATORS	Toll-like receptors, arachidonic acid metabolites, neutrophils, eosinophils, antibodies (pre-existing), mast cells, basophils, complement, Hageman factor (factor XII).	Inflammasome—Cytoplasmic protein complex that recognizes products of dead cells, microbial products, and crystals (eg, uric acid crystals) → activation of IL-1 and inflammatory response.
COMPONENTS	■ Vascular: vasodilation (→ ↑ blood flow and stasis) and ↑ endothelial permeability (contraction of endothelial cells opens interendothelial junctions)	To bring cells and proteins to site of injury or infection.
	■ Cellular: extravasation of leukocytes (mainly neutrophils) from postcapillary venules → accumulation of leukocytes in focus of injury → leukocyte activation	Leukocyte extravasation has 4 steps: margination and rolling, adhesion, transmigration, and migration (chemoattraction).
OUTCOMES	■ Resolution and healing (IL-10, TGF-β) ■ Persistent acute inflammation (IL-8) ■ Abscess (acute inflammation walled off by fibrosis) ■ Chronic inflammation (antigen presentation by macrophages and other APCs → activation of CD4+ Th cells) ■ Scarring	Macrophages predominate in the late stages of acute inflammation (peak 2–3 days after onset) and influence outcome by secreting cytokines.

Leukocyte extravasation

Extravasation predominantly occurs at postcapillary venules.

STEP	VASCULATURE/STROMA	LEUKOCYTE
❶ Margination and rolling— defective in leukocyte adhesion deficiency type 2 (↓ Sialyl Lewis^X)	E-selectin (upregulated by TNF and IL-1)	Sialyl Lewis^X
	P-selectin (translocated to endothelial surface via exocytosis from Weibel-Palade bodies)	Sialyl Lewis^X
	GlyCAM-1, CD34	L-selectin
❷ Tight binding (adhesion)— defective in leukocyte adhesion deficiency type 1 (↓ CD18 integrin subunit)	ICAM-1 (CD54)	CD11/18 integrins (LFA-1, Mac-1)
	VCAM-1 (CD106)	VLA-4 integrin
❸ DiaPEdesis (transmigration)— WBC travels between endothelial cells and exits blood vessel	PECAM-1 (CD31)	PECAM-1 (CD31)
❹ Migration—WBC travels through interstitium to site of injury or infection guided by chemotactic signals	Chemotactic factors: C5a, IL-8, LTB$_4$, 5-HETE, kallikrein, platelet-activating factor, N-formylmethionyl peptides	Various

Chronic inflammation	Prolonged inflammation characterized by mononuclear infiltration (macrophages, lymphocytes, plasma cells), which leads to simultaneous tissue destruction and repair (including angiogenesis and fibrosis). May be preceded by acute inflammation.
STIMULI	Persistent infections (eg, TB, *T pallidum*, certain fungi and viruses) → type IV hypersensitivity, autoimmune diseases, prolonged exposure to toxic agents (eg, silica) and foreign material.
MEDIATORS	Macrophages are the dominant cells. Interaction of macrophages and T cells → chronic inflammation. ▪ Th1 cells secrete IFN-γ → macrophage classical activation (proinflammatory) ▪ Th2 cells secrete IL-4 and IL-13 → macrophage alternative activation (repair and anti-inflammatory)
OUTCOMES	Scarring, amyloidosis, and neoplastic transformation (eg, chronic HCV infection → chronic inflammation → hepatocellular carcinoma; *Helicobacter pylori* infection → chronic gastritis → gastric adenocarcinoma).

Wound healing

Tissue mediators	MEDIATOR	ROLE
	FGF	Stimulates angiogenesis
	TGF-β	Angiogenesis, fibrosis
	VEGF	Stimulates angiogenesis
	PDGF	Secreted by activated platelets and macrophages Induces vascular remodeling and smooth muscle cell migration Stimulates fibroblast growth for collagen synthesis
	Metalloproteinases	Tissue remodeling
	EGF	Stimulates cell growth via tyrosine kinases (eg, EGFR/*ErbB1*)

PHASE OF WOUND HEALING	EFFECTOR CELLS	CHARACTERISTICS
Inflammatory (up to 3 days after wound)	Platelets, neutrophils, macrophages	Clot formation, ↑ vessel permeability and neutrophil migration into tissue; macrophages clear debris 2 days later
Proliferative (day 3–weeks after wound)	Fibroblasts, myofibroblasts, endothelial cells, keratinocytes, macrophages	Deposition of granulation tissue and type III collagen, angiogenesis, epithelial cell proliferation, dissolution of clot, and wound contraction (mediated by myofibroblasts) Delayed second phase of wound healing in vitamin C and copper deficiency
Remodeling (1 week–6+ months after wound)	Fibroblasts	Type III collagen replaced by type I collagen, ↑ tensile strength of tissue Collagenases (require zinc to function) break down type III collagen Zinc deficiency → delayed wound healing

| **Granulomatous inflammation** | A pattern of chronic inflammation. Can be induced by persistent T-cell response to certain infections (eg, TB), immune-mediated diseases, and foreign bodies. Granulomas "wall off" a resistant stimulus without completely eradicating or degrading it → persistent inflammation → fibrosis, organ damage. |

| HISTOLOGY | 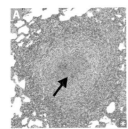 | Focus of epithelioid cells (activated macrophages with abundant pink cytoplasm) surrounded by lymphocytes and multinucleated giant cells (formed by fusion of several activated macrophages). Two types:
Caseating: associated with central necrosis A. Seen with infectious etiologies (eg, TB, fungal).
Noncaseating: no central necrosis. Seen with noninfectious etiologies (eg, sarcoidosis, Crohn disease). |

| MECHANISM | ❶ APCs present antigens to CD4+ Th cells and secrete IL-12 → CD4+ Th cells differentiate into Th1 cells
❷ Th1 secretes IFN-γ → macrophage activation
❸ Macrophages ↑ cytokine secretion (eg, TNF) → formation of epithelioid macrophages and giant cells
Anti-TNF therapy can cause sequestering granulomas to break down → disseminated disease. Always test for latent TB before starting anti-TNF therapy.
Associated with hypercalcemia due to ↑ 1α-hydroxylase activity in activated macrophages, resulting in ↑ vitamin D activity. |

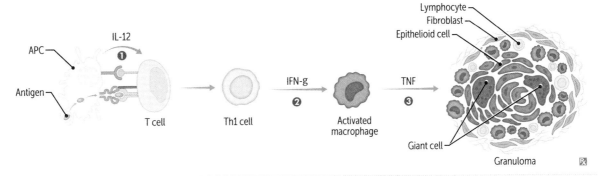

ETIOLOGIES	Infectious	Noninfectious
	Bacterial: *Mycobacteria* (tuberculosis, leprosy), *Bartonella henselae* (cat scratch disease; stellate necrotizing granulomas), *Listeria monocytogenes* (granulomatosis infantiseptica), *Treponema pallidum* (3° syphilis) Fungal: endemic mycoses (eg, histoplasmosis) Parasitic: schistosomiasis Catalase ⊕ organisms in chronic granulomatous disease	Immune-mediated: sarcoidosis, Crohn disease, 1° biliary cholangitis, subacute (de Quervain/ granulomatous) thyroiditis Vasculitis: granulomatosis with polyangiitis, eosinophilic granulomatosis with polyangiitis, giant cell (temporal) arteritis, Takayasu arteritis Foreign bodies: berylliosis, talcosis, hypersensitivity pneumonitis

Scar formation   Occurs when repair cannot be accomplished by cell regeneration alone. Nonregenerated cells (2° to severe acute or chronic injury) are replaced by connective tissue. 70–80% of tensile strength regained at 3 months; little tensile strength regained thereafter. Excess TGF-β is associated with aberrant scarring, such as hypertrophic and keloid scars.

	Hypertrophic scar A	Keloid scar B
COLLAGEN SYNTHESIS	↑ (type III collagen)	↑↑↑ (types I and III collagen)
COLLAGEN ORGANIZATION	Parallel	Disorganized
EXTENT OF SCAR	Confined to borders of original wound	Extends beyond borders of original wound with "clawlike" projections typically on earlobes, face, upper extremities
RECURRENCE	Infrequent	Frequent
PREDISPOSITION	None	↑ incidence in people with darker skin

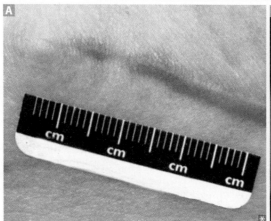
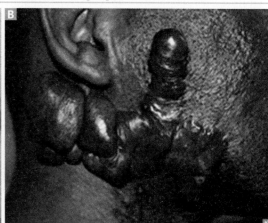

▸ PATHOLOGY—NEOPLASIA

Neoplasia and neoplastic progression	Uncontrolled, often monoclonal proliferation of cells. Can be benign or malignant. Any neoplastic growth has two components: parenchyma (neoplastic cells) and supporting stroma (non-neoplastic; eg, blood vessels, connective tissue).

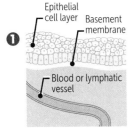 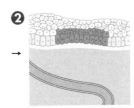 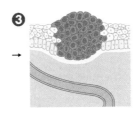 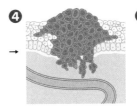 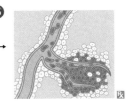

Normal cells	❶ Normal cells with basal → apical polarity. See cervical example, which shows normal cells and spectrum of dysplasia, as discussed below.
Dysplasia	❷ Loss of uniformity in cell size and shape (pleomorphism); loss of tissue orientation; nuclear changes (eg, ↑ nuclear:cytoplasmic ratio); often reversible.
Carcinoma in situ/ preinvasive	❸ Irreversible severe dysplasia that involves the entire thickness of epithelium but does not penetrate the intact basement membrane.
Invasive carcinoma	❹ Cells have invaded basement membrane using collagenases and hydrolases (metalloproteinases). Cell-cell contacts lost by inactivation of E-cadherin.
Metastasis	❺ Spread to distant organ(s) via lymphatics or blood.

Tumor nomenclature

Carcinoma implies epithelial origin, whereas **sarcoma** denotes mesenchymal origin. Both terms generally imply malignancy.

Benign tumors are usually well-differentiated and well-demarcated, with low mitotic activity, no metastases, and no necrosis.

Malignant tumors (cancers) may show poor differentiation, erratic growth, local invasion, metastasis, and ↓ apoptosis.

Terms for non-neoplastic malformations include hamartoma (disorganized overgrowth of tissues in their native location, eg, Peutz-Jeghers polyps) and choristoma (normal tissue in a foreign location, eg, gastric tissue located in distal ileum in Meckel diverticulum).

CELL TYPE	BENIGN	MALIGNANT
Epithelium	Adenoma, papilloma	Adenocarcinoma, papillary carcinoma
Mesenchyme		
Blood cells		Leukemia, lymphoma
Blood vessels	Hemangioma	Angiosarcoma
Smooth muscle	Leiomyoma	Leiomyosarcoma
Striated muscle	Rhabdomyoma	Rhabdomyosarcoma
Connective tissue	Fibroma	Fibrosarcoma
Bone	Osteoma	Osteosarcoma
Fat	Lipoma	Liposarcoma
Melanocyte	Nevus/mole	Melanoma

Tumor grade vs stage

Grade

Degree of cell differentiation (tissue of origin resemblance) and mitotic activity on histology.

Ranges from low-grade (well differentiated) to high-grade (poorly differentiated or undifferentiated [anaplastic]).

Higher grade often correlates with higher aggressiveness.

Low grade　　High grade

Stage

Degree of invasion and spread from initial site. Depth of invasion correlates to risk of metastasis. Based on clinical (c) or pathologic (p) findings.

TNM staging system (importance: M > N > T):
- Primary tumor size/invasion.
- Regional lymph node metastasis.
- Distant metastasis.

Stage generally has more prognostic value than grade (eg, a high-stage yet low-grade tumor is usually worse than a low-stage yet high-grade tumor). Stage (spread) determines survival.

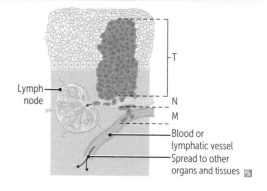

Lymph node — T
N
M
Blood or lymphatic vessel
Spread to other organs and tissues

Hallmarks of cancer	Cancer is caused by (mostly acquired) DNA mutations that affect fundamental cellular processes (eg, growth, DNA repair, survival).
HALLMARK	MECHANISM
Growth signal self-sufficiency	Mutations in genes encoding: ▪ Proto-oncogenes → ↑ growth factors → autocrine loop (eg, ↑ PDGF in brain tumors) ▪ Growth factor receptors → constitutive signaling (eg, HER2 in breast cancer) ▪ Signaling molecules (eg, RAS) ▪ Transcription factors (eg, MYC) ▪ Cell cycle regulators (eg, cyclins, CDKs)
Anti-growth signal insensitivity	▪ Mutations in tumor suppressor genes (eg, Rb) ▪ Loss of E-cadherin function → loss of contact inhibition (eg, NF2 mutations)
Evasion of apoptosis	Mutations in genes that regulate apoptosis (eg, TP53, BCL2 → follicular B cell lymphoma).
Limitless replicative potential	Reactivation of telomerase → maintenance and lengthening of telomeres → prevention of chromosome shortening and cell aging.
Sustained angiogenesis	↑ pro-angiogenic factors (eg, VEGF) or ↓ inhibitory factors. Factors may be produced by tumor or stromal cells. Vessels can sprout from existing capillaries (neoangiogenesis) or endothelial cells are recruited from bone marrow (vasculogenesis). Vessels may be leaky and/or dilated.
Warburg effect	Shift of glucose metabolism away from mitochondrial oxidative phosphorylation toward glycolysis, even in the presence of oxygen. Aerobic glycolysis provides rapidly dividing cancer cells with the carbon needed for synthesis of cellular structures, leading to ↑ lactic acid.
Immune evasion in cancer	Normally, immune cells can recognize and attack tumor cells. For successful tumorigenesis, tumor cells must evade the immune system. Multiple escape mechanisms exist: ▪ ↓ MHC class I expression by tumor cells → cytotoxic T cells are unable to recognize tumor cells. ▪ Tumor cells secrete immunosuppressive factors (eg, TGF-β) and recruit regulatory T cells to down regulate immune response. ▪ Tumor cells up regulate immune checkpoint molecules, which inhibit immune response.
Tissue invasion	Loss of E-cadherin function → loosening of intercellular junctions → metalloproteinases degrade basement membrane and ECM → cells attach to ECM proteins (eg, laminin, fibronectin) → cells migrate through degraded ECM ("locomotion") → vascular dissemination.
Metastasis	Tumor cells or emboli spread via lymphatics or blood → adhesion to endothelium → extravasation and homing. Site of metastasis can be predicted by site of 1° tumor, as the target organ is often the first-encountered capillary bed. Some cancers show organ tropism (eg, lung cancers commonly metastasize to adrenals).

Immune checkpoint interactions

Signals that modulate T-cell activation and function → ↓ immune response against tumor cells. Targeted by several cancer immunotherapies. Examples:

- Interaction between PD-1 (on T cells) and PD-L1/2 (on tumor cells or immune cells in tumor microenvironment) → T-cell dysfunction (exhaustion). Inhibited by antibodies against PD-1 (eg, cemiplimab, nivolumab, pembrolizumab) or PD-L1 (eg, atezolizumab, durvalumab, avelumab).
- CTLA-4 on T cells outcompetes CD28 for B7 on APCs → loss of T-cell costimulatory signal. Inhibited by antibodies against CTLA-4 (eg, ipilimumab).

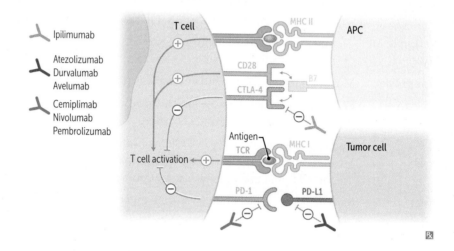

Cancer epidemiology

Skin cancer (basal > squamous >> melanoma) is the most common cancer (not included below).

	MALES	FEMALES	CHILDREN (AGE 0–14)	NOTES
Cancer incidence	1. Prostate 2. Lung 3. Colon/rectum	1. Breast 2. Lung 3. Colon/rectum	1. Leukemia 2. CNS 3. Neuroblastoma	Lung cancer incidence has ↓ in males, but has not changed significantly in females.
Cancer mortality	1. Lung 2. Prostate 3. Colon/rectum	1. Lung 2. Breast 3. Colon/rectum	1. Leukemia 2. CNS 3. Neuroblastoma	Cancer is the 2nd leading cause of death in the United States (heart disease is 1st).

Common metastases	\multicolumn{2}{l}{Most Carcinomas spread via Lymphatics; most Sarcomas spread Hematogenously (CLaSH). However, four carcinomas route hematogenously: follicular thyroid carcinoma, choriocarcinoma, renal cell carcinoma, and hepatocellular carcinoma. Metastasis to bone, liver, lung, and brain is more common than 1° malignancy in these organs. Metastases often appear as multiple lesions (vs 1° tumors which generally appear as solitary lesions).}

SITE OF METASTASIS	1° TUMOR	NOTES
Bone	Prostate, breast >> lung > kidney, colon	Predilection for axial skeleton **A** Bone metastasis can be: ▪ Blastic (eg, prostate, small cell lung cancer) ▪ Mixed (eg, breast) ▪ Lytic (eg, kidney, colon, non-small cell lung cancer)
Liver	Colon > breast >> pancreas, lung, prostate	Scattered throughout liver parenchyma **B**
Lung	Colon, breast >> kidney, prostate	Typically involve both lungs
Brain	Lung > breast >> melanoma > colon, prostate	Usually seen at gray/white matter junction

Oncogenes	Gain of function mutation converts proto-oncogene (normal gene) to oncogene → ↑ cancer risk. Requires damage to only **one** allele of a proto-oncogene.	
GENE	GENE PRODUCT	ASSOCIATED NEOPLASM
ALK	Receptor tyrosine kinase	Lung adenocarcinoma
EGFR (ERBB1)	Receptor tyrosine kinase	Lung adenocarcinoma
HER2 (ERBB2)	Receptor tyrosine kinase	Breast and gastric carcinomas
RET	REceptor Tyrosine kinase	MEN2A and 2B, medullary and papillary thyroid carcinoma, pheochromocytoma
BCR-ABL	Non-receptor tyrosine kinase	CML, ALL
JAK2	Non-receptor tyrosine kinase	Myeloproliferative neoplasms
BRAF	Serine/threonine kinase	Melanoma, non-Hodgkin lymphoma, colorectal carcinoma, papillary thyroid carcinoma, hairy cell leukemia
c-KIT	CytoKIne receptor (CD117)	Gastrointestinal stromal tumor (GIST), mastocytosis
MYCC (c-myc)	Transcription factor	Burkitt lymphoma
MYCN (N-myc)	Transcription factor	Neuroblastoma
KRAS	RAS GTPase	Pancreatic, colorectal, lung, endometrial cancers
BCL-2	Antiapoptotic molecule (inhibits apoptosis)	Follicular and diffuse large B-Cell Lymphomas

Tumor suppressor genes	Loss of function → ↑ cancer risk; both (**two**) alleles of a tumor suppressor gene must be lost for expression of disease (the Knudson 2-hit hypothesis).	
GENE	GENE PRODUCT	ASSOCIATED CONDITION
APC	Negative regulator of β-catenin/WNT pathway	Colorectal cancer (associated with FAP)
BRCA1/BRCA2	BRCA1/BRCA2 proteins	BReast, ovarian, prostate, pancreatic CAncers
CDKN2A	p16, blocks G_1 → S phase	Many cancers (eg, melanoma, lung, pancreatic)
DCC	DCC—Deleted in Colorectal Cancer	Colorectal cancer
SMAD4 (DPC4)	DPC—Deleted in Pancreatic Cancer	Pancreatic cancer, colorectal cancer
MEN1	MENin	Multiple Endocrine Neoplasia type 1
NF1	Neurofibromin (Ras GTPase activating protein)	NeuroFibromatosis type 1
NF2	Merlin (schwannomin) protein	NeuroFibromatosis type 2
PTEN	Negative regulator of PI3k/AKT pathway	Prostate, breasT, and ENdometrial cancers
RB1	Inhibits E2F; blocks G_1 → S phase	Retinoblastoma, osteosarcoma (Bone cancer)
TP53	p53, activates p21, blocks G_1 → S phase	Most cancers, Li-Fraumeni (SBLA) syndrome (multiple malignancies at early age; Sarcoma, Breast/Brain, Lung/Leukemia, Adrenal gland)
TSC1	Hamartin protein	Tuberous sclerosis complex
TSC2	Tuberin ("2berin")	Tuberous sclerosis complex
VHL	Inhibits hypoxia-inducible factor 1α	von Hippel-Lindau disease
WT1	Urogenital development transcription factor	Wilms Tumor (nephroblastoma)

Carcinogens

TOXIN	EXPOSURE	ORGAN	IMPACT
Aflatoxins (*Aspergillus*)	Stored grains and nuts	Liver	Hepatocellular carcinoma
Alkylating agents	Oncologic chemotherapy	Blood	Leukemia/lymphoma
Aromatic amines (eg, benzidine, 2-naphthylamine)	Textile industry (dyes), tobacco smoke (2-naphthylamine)	Bladder	Transitional cell carcinoma
Arsenic	Herbicides (vineyard workers), metal smelting, wood preservation	Liver Lung Skin	Hepatic angiosarcoma Lung cancer Squamous cell carcinoma
Asbestos	Old roofing material, shipyard workers	Lung	Bronchogenic carcinoma > mesothelioma
Tobacco smoke		Bladder Cervix Esophagus Kidney Larynx Lung Oropharynx Pancreas	Transitional cell carcinoma Squamous cell carcinoma Squamous cell carcinoma/ adenocarcinoma Renal cell carcinoma Squamous cell carcinoma Squamous cell and small cell carcinoma Squamous cell carcinoma Pancreatic adenocarcinoma
Ethanol		Esophagus Liver Breast	Squamous cell carcinoma Hepatocellular carcinoma Breast cancer
Ionizing radiation		Blood Thyroid	Leukemia Papillary thyroid carcinoma
Nickel, chromium, beryllium, silica	Occupational exposure	Lung	Lung cancer
Nitrosamines	Smoked foods	Stomach	Gastric cancer (intestinal type)
Radon	Byproduct of uranium decay, accumulates in basements	Lung	Lung cancer (2nd leading cause after tobacco smoke)
Vinyl chloride	Used to make PVC pipes	Liver	Hepatic angiosarcoma

Oncogenic microbes

MICROBE	ASSOCIATED CANCER
EBV	Burkitt lymphoma, Hodgkin lymphoma, nasopharyngeal carcinoma, 1° CNS lymphoma (in immunocompromised patients)
HBV, HCV	Hepatocellular carcinoma
HHV-8	Kaposi ("Ka∞si") sarcoma
HPV (usually types 16, 18)	Cervical and penile/anal carcinoma, head and neck cancer
H pylori	Gastric adenocarcinoma and MALT lymphoma
HTLV-1	Adult T-cell Leukemia/Lymphoma
Liver fluke (Clonorchis sinensis)	Cholangiocarcinoma
Schistosoma haematobium	Squamous cell bladder cancer

Serum tumor markers

Tumor markers should not be used as the 1° tool for cancer diagnosis or screening. They may be used to monitor tumor recurrence and response to therapy, but definitive diagnosis is made via biopsy. Some can be associated with non-neoplastic conditions.

MARKER	IMPORTANT ASSOCIATIONS	NOTES
Alkaline phosphatase	Metastases to bone or liver, Paget disease of bone, seminoma (PLAP).	Exclude hepatic origin by checking LFTs and GGT levels.
α-fetoprotein	Hepatocellular carcinoma, endodermal sinus (yolk sac) tumor, mixed germ cell tumor, ataxia-telangiectasia, neural tube defects.	Normally made by fetus. Transiently elevated in pregnancy. High levels associated with neural tube and abdominal wall defects, low levels associated with Down syndrome.
hCG	Hydatidiform moles and Choriocarcinomas (Gestational trophoblastic disease), testicular cancer, mixed germ cell tumor.	Produced by syncytiotrophoblasts of the placenta.
CA 15-3/CA 27-29	Breast cancer.	
CA 19-9	Pancreatic adenocarcinoma.	
CA 125	Epithelial ovarian cancer.	
Calcitonin	Medullary thyroid carcinoma (alone and in MEN2A, MEN2B).	Calci2nin.
CEA	Colorectal and pancreatic cancers. Minor associations: gastric, breast, and medullary thyroid carcinomas.	CarcinoEmbryonic Antigen. Very nonspecific.
Chromogranin	Neuroendocrine tumors.	
LDH	Testicular germ cell tumors, ovarian dysgerminoma, other cancers.	Can be used as an indicator of tumor burden.
Neuron-specific enolase	Neuroendocrine tumors (eg, small cell lung cancer, carcinoid tumor, neuroblastoma).	
PSA	Prostate cancer.	Prostate-Specific Antigen. Also elevated in BPH and prostatitis. Questionable risk/benefit for screening. Marker for recurrence after treatment.

Liquid biopsy

Noninvasive diagnostic test in body fluid (eg, blood, urine) using circulating tumor DNA (ctDNA), RNA (ctRNA), or circulating tumor cells (CTCs) for cancer profiling (eg, *EGFR* in lung cancer), treatment monitoring, and post-treatment surveillance (eg, colorectal cancer). Aids in early metastatic detection and personalized therapy.

Important immunohistochemical stains

Determine primary site of origin for metastatic tumors and characterize tumors that are difficult to classify. Can have prognostic and predictive value.

STAIN	TARGET	TUMORS IDENTIFIED
Chromogranin and synaptophysin	Neuroendocrine cells	Small cell carcinoma of the lung, carcinoid tumor, neuroblastoma
Cytokeratin	Epithelial cells	Epithelial tumors (eg, squamous cell carcinoma)
Desmin	Muscle	Muscle tumors (eg, rhabdomyosarcoma)
GFAP	NeuroGlia (eg, astrocytes, Schwann cells, oligodendrocytes)	Astrocytoma, Glioblastoma
Neurofilament	Neurons	Neuronal tumors (eg, neuroblastoma)
PSA	Prostatic epithelium	Prostate cancer
PECAM-1/CD-31	Endothelial cells	Vascular tumors (eg, angiosarcoma)
S-100	Neural crest cells	Melanoma, schwannoma, Langerhans cell histiocytosis
TRAP	Tartrate-resistant acid phosphatase	Hairy cell leukemia
Vimentin	Mesenchymal tissue (eg, fibroblasts, endothelial cells, macrophages)	Mesenchymal tumors (eg, sarcoma), but also many other tumors (eg, endometrial carcinoma, renal cell carcinoma, meningioma)

P-glycoprotein

ATP-dependent efflux pump also called multidrug resistance protein 1 (MDR1). Expressed in some cancer cells to pump out toxins, including chemotherapeutic agents (one mechanism of ↓ responsiveness or resistance to chemotherapy over time).

Paraneoplastic syndromes

MANIFESTATION	DESCRIPTION/MECHANISM	MOST COMMONLY ASSOCIATED TUMOR(S)
Musculoskeletal and cutaneous		
Dermatomyositis	Progressive proximal muscle weakness, Gottron papules, heliotrope rash	Adenocarcinomas, especially ovarian
Acanthosis nigricans	Hyperpigmented velvety plaques in axilla and neck	Gastric adenocarcinoma and other visceral malignancies
Sign of Leser-Trélat	Sudden onset of multiple seborrheic keratoses	GI adenocarcinomas and other visceral malignancies
Hypertrophic osteoarthropathy	Abnormal proliferation of skin and bone at distal extremities → clubbing, arthralgia, joint effusions, periostosis of tubular bones	Adenocarcinoma of the lung
Endocrine		
Hypercalcemia	PTHrP	SCa^{2+}mous cell carcinomas of lung, head, and neck; renal, bladder, breast, and ovarian carcinomas
	↑ $1,25\text{-}(OH)_2$ vitamin D_3 (calcitriol)	Lymphoma
Cushing syndrome	↑ ACTH	Small cell lung cancer
Hyponatremia (SIADH)	↑ ADH	
Hematologic		
Polycythemia	↑ Erythropoietin Paraneoplastic rise to High hematocrit levels	Pheochromocytoma, renal cell carcinoma, HCC, hemangioblastoma, leiomyoma
Pure red cell aplasia	Anemia with low reticulocytes	Thymoma
Good syndrome	Hypogammaglobulinemia	
Trousseau syndrome	Migratory superficial thrombophlebitis	Adenocarcinomas, especially pancreatic
Nonbacterial thrombotic endocarditis	Deposition of sterile platelet thrombi on heart valves	
Neuromuscular		
Anti-NMDA receptor encephalitis	Psychiatric disturbance, memory deficits, seizures, dyskinesias, autonomic instability, language dysfunction	Ovarian teratoma
Opsoclonus-myoclonus ataxia syndrome	"Dancing eyes, dancing feet"	Neuroblastoma (children), small cell lung cancer (adults)
Paraneoplastic cerebellar degeneration	Antibodies against antigens in Purkinje cells	Small cell lung cancer (anti-Hu), gynecologic and breast cancers (anti-Yo), and Hodgkin lymphoma (anti-Tr)
Paraneoplastic encephalomyelitis	Antibodies against Hu antigens in neurons	Small cell lung cancer
Lambert-Eaton myasthenic syndrome	Antibodies against presynaptic (P/Q-type) Ca^{2+} channels at NMJ	
Myasthenia gravis	Antibodies against postsynaptic ACh receptors at NMJ	Thymoma

▶ PATHOLOGY—AGING

Normal aging	Time-dependent progressive decline in organ function resulting in ↑ susceptibility to disease. Associated with genetic (eg, telomere shortening), epigenetic (eg, DNA methylation), and metabolic (eg, mitochondrial dysfunction) alterations.
Cardiovascular	↓ arterial compliance (↑ stiffness), ↑ aortic diameter, ↓ left ventricular cavity size and sigmoid-shaped interventricular septum (due to myocardial hypertrophy), ↑ left atrial cavity size, aortic and mitral valve calcification, ↓ maximum heart rate.
Gastrointestinal	↓ LES tone, ↓ gastric mucosal protection, ↓ colonic motility.
Hematopoietic	↓ bone marrow mass, ↑ bone marrow fat; less vigorous response to stressors (eg, blood loss).
Immune	Predominant effect on adaptive immunity: ↓ naïve B cells and T cells, preserved memory B cells and T cells. Immunosenescence impairs response to new antigens (eg, pathogens, vaccines).
Musculoskeletal	↓ skeletal muscle mass (sarcopenia), ↓ bone mass (osteopenia), joint cartilage thinning.
Nervous	↓ brain volume (neuronal loss), ↓ cerebral blood flow; function is preserved despite mild cognitive decline.
Special senses	Impaired accommodation (presbyopia), ↓ hearing (presbycusis), ↓ smell and taste.
Skin	Atrophy with flattening of dermal-epidermal junction; ↓ dermal collagen and ↓ elastin (wrinkles, senile purpura), ↓ sweat glands (heat stroke), ↓ sebaceous glands (xerosis cutis). ▪ Intrinsic aging (chronological aging)—↓ biosynthetic capacity of dermal fibroblasts. ▪ Extrinsic aging (photoaging)—degradation of dermal collagen and elastin from sun exposure (UVA); degradation products accumulate in dermis (solar elastosis).
Renal	↓ GFR (↓ nephrons), ↓ RBF, ↓ hormonal function. Voiding dysfunction (eg, urinary incontinence).
Reproductive	Males—testicular atrophy (↓ spermatogenesis), prostate enlargement, slower erection/ejaculation, longer refractory period. Less pronounced ↓ in libido as compared to females. Females—vulvovaginal atrophy; vaginal shortening, thinning, dryness, ↑ pH. Due to ↓ estrogen from exhaustion of ovarian follicles (menopause).
Respiratory	↑ lung compliance (↓ elastic recoil), ↓ chest wall compliance (↑ stiffness), ↓ respiratory muscle strength; ↓ FEV_1, ↓ FVC, ↑ RV (TLC is unchanged); ↑ A-a gradient, ↑ V/Q mismatch. Ventilatory response to hypoxia/hypercapnia is blunted. Less vigorous cough, slower mucociliary clearance.

Lipofuscin 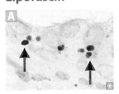	A yellow-brown, "wear and tear" pigment A associated with normal aging. Composed of polymers of lipids and phospholipids complexed with protein. May be derived through lipid peroxidation of polyunsaturated lipids of subcellular membranes. Autopsy of older adult will reveal deposits in heart, colon, liver, kidney, eye, and other organs.

Pharmacology

"Cure sometimes, treat often, and comfort always."
> —Hippocrates

"One pill makes you larger, and one pill makes you small."
> —Jefferson Airplane, *White Rabbit*

"For the chemistry that works on one patient may not work for the next, because even medicine has its own conditions."
> —Suzy Kassem

"I wondher why ye can always read a doctor's bill an' ye niver can read his purscription."
> —Finley Peter Dunne

"Love is the drug I'm thinking of."
> —The Bryan Ferry Orchestra

Preparation for pharmacology questions is not as straightforward as in years past. One major recent change is that the USMLE Step 1 has moved away from testing pharmacotherapeutics. That means you will generally not be required to identify medications indicated for a specific condition. You still need to know mechanisms and important adverse effects of key drugs and their major variants. Obscure derivatives are low-yield. Learn their classic and distinguishing toxicities as well as major drug-drug interactions.

Reviewing associated biochemistry, physiology, and microbiology concepts can be useful while studying pharmacology. The exam has a strong emphasis on ANS, CNS, antimicrobial, and cardiovascular agents as well as on NSAIDs, which are covered throughout the text. Specific drug dosages or trade names are generally not testable. The exam may use graphs to test various pharmacology content, so make sure you are comfortable interpreting them.

▶ **PHARMACOLOGY—PHARMACOKINETICS AND PHARMACODYNAMICS**

Enzyme kinetics

| Michaelis-Menten kinetics | K_m is the substrate concentration needed for an enzyme to reach a rate of $1/2 \, V_{max}$ and is inversely related to the affinity of the enzyme for its substrate.
V_{max} is directly proportional to the enzyme concentration.
Most enzymatic reactions follow a hyperbolic curve (ie, Michaelis-Menten kinetics); however, enzymatic reactions that exhibit a sigmoidal curve usually indicate positive cooperativity in substrate binding (eg, aspartate transcarbamoylase). | [S] = concentration of substrate; V = velocity.
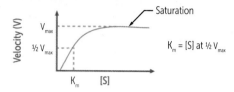
Effects of enzyme inhibition
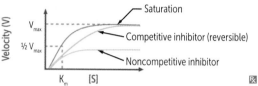 |

| Lineweaver-Burk plot | The closer to 0 on the Y-axis, the higher the V_{max}.
The closer to 0 on the X-axis, the higher the K_m.
The higher the K_m, the lower the affinity.

Reversible competitive inhibitors cross each other, whereas noncompetitive inhibitors do not.

Kompetitive inhibitors increase K_m. | 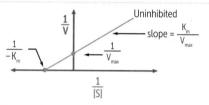
Effects of enzyme inhibition
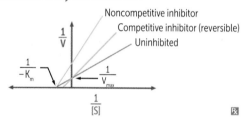 |

	Competitive inhibitors, reversible	Competitive inhibitors, irreversible	Noncompetitive inhibitors
Resemble substrate	Yes	Yes	No
Overcome by ↑ [S]	Yes	No	No
Bind active site	Yes	Yes	No
Effect on V_{max}	Unchanged	↓	↓
Effect on K_m	↑	Unchanged	Unchanged
Pharmacodynamics	↓ potency	↓ efficacy	↓ efficacy

Pharmacokinetics

Bioavailability (F)	Fraction of administered drug reaching systemic circulation. For an IV dose, F = 100%. Orally: F typically < 100% due to incomplete absorption and first-pass metabolism. Can be calculated from the area under the curve in a plot of plasma concentration over time.

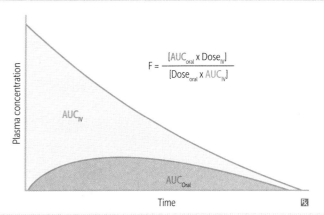

$$F = \frac{[AUC_{oral} \times Dose_{IV}]}{[Dose_{oral} \times AUC_{IV}]}$$

Volume of distribution (V$_d$)	Theoretical value that relates drug amount to plasma concentration. Liver and kidney disease increase V$_d$ (↓ protein binding, ↑ V$_d$). Drugs may be distributed in more than one compartment. Hemodialysis is most effective for drugs with a low V$_d$.

$$V_d = \frac{\text{amount of drug in the body}}{\text{plasma drug concentration}}$$

V$_d$	COMPARTMENT	DRUG TYPES
Low	Intravascular	Large/charged molecules; plasma protein bound
Medium	ECF	Small hydrophilic molecules
High	All tissues including fat	Small lipophilic molecules, especially if bound to tissue protein

Clearance (CL)	The volume of plasma cleared of drug per unit time. Clearance may be impaired with defects in cardiac, hepatic, or renal function.

$$CL = \frac{\text{rate of elimination of drug}}{\text{plasma drug concentration}} = V_d \times K_e \text{ (elimination constant)}$$

Half-life (t$_{1/2}$)	The time required to eliminate 1/2 of the drug from the body. Steady state is a dynamic equilibrium in which drug concentration stays constant (ie, rate of drug elimination = rate of drug administration). In first-order kinetics, a drug infused at a constant rate takes 4–5 half-lives to reach steady state. It takes 3.3 half-lives to reach 90% of the steady-state level.

$$t_{1/2} = \frac{0.7 \times V_d}{CL} \text{ in first-order elimination}$$

# of half-lives	1	2	3	4
% remaining	50%	25%	12.5%	6.25%

Dosage calculations	$$\text{Loading dose} = \frac{C_p \times V_d}{F}$$ $$\text{Maintenance dose} = \frac{C_p \times CL \times \tau}{F}$$ C_p = target plasma concentration τ = dosage interval (time between doses); does not apply for continuous infusions

In renal or liver disease, maintenance dose ↓ and loading dose is usually unchanged.
Time to steady state depends primarily on t$_{1/2}$ and is independent of dose and dosing frequency.

Drug metabolism

Drugs can be metabolized by either or both phase I and phase II reactions. These reactions serve to bioactivate or deactivate substances, and do not have to take place sequentially (eg, phase I can follow phase II, or take place as a single reaction).

Geriatric patients lose phase I first. Patients who are slow acetylators have ↑ adverse effects from certain drugs because of ↓ rate of metabolism (eg, isoniazid).

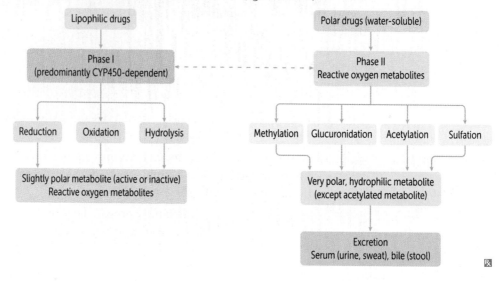

Elimination of drugs

Zero-order elimination	Rate of elimination is constant regardless of C_p (ie, constant **amount** of drug eliminated per unit time). C_p ↓ linearly with time. Examples of drugs—**P**henytoin, **E**thanol, and **A**spirin (at high or toxic concentrations).	Capacity-limited elimination. A **PEA** is round, shaped like the "0" in zero-order.
First-order elimination	Rate of first-order elimination is directly proportional to the drug concentration (ie, constant **fraction** of drug eliminated per unit time). C_p ↓ exponentially with time. Applies to most drugs.	Flow-dependent elimination.

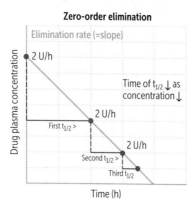

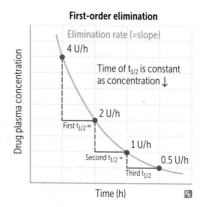

Urine pH and drug elimination	Ionized species are trapped in urine and cleared quickly. Neutral forms can be reabsorbed.
Weak acids	Examples: phenobarbital, methotrexate, aspirin (salicylates). Treat overdose with sodium bicarbonate to alkalinize urine. $$RCOOH \;\rightleftharpoons\; RCOO^- + H^+$$ (lipid soluble) (trapped)
Weak bases	Examples: tricyclic antidepressants (TCAs), amphetamines. Trapped in acidic environments. For severe alkalosis, treat with ammonium chloride to acidify urine. $$RNH_3^+ \;\rightleftharpoons\; RNH_2 + H^+$$ (trapped) (lipid soluble) TCA toxicity is initially treated with sodium bicarbonate to overcome the sodium channel-blocking activity of TCAs. This treats cardiac toxicity, but does not accelerate drug elimination.
pKa	pH at which drugs (weak acid or base) are 50% ionized and 50% nonionized. The pKa represents the strength of the weak acid or base.

Efficacy vs potency

Efficacy

Maximal effect a drug can produce (intrinsic activity). Represented by the y-value (E_{max}). ↑ y-value = ↑ E_{max} = ↑ efficacy. Unrelated to potency (ie, efficacious drugs can have high or low potency). Partial agonists have less efficacy than full agonists.

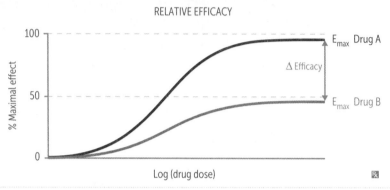

Potency

Amount of drug needed for a given effect. Represented by the x-value (EC_{50}). Left shifting = ↓ EC_{50} = ↑ potency = ↓ drug needed. Unrelated to efficacy (ie, potent drugs can have high or low efficacy).

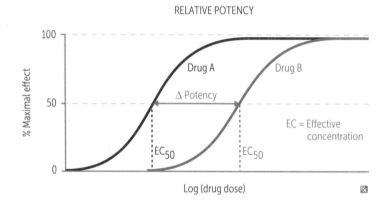

Receptor binding

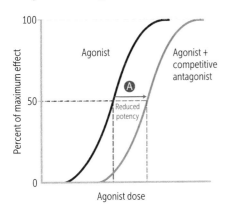

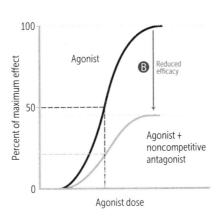

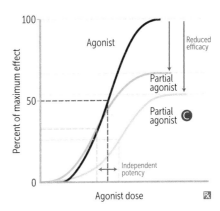

AGONIST WITH	POTENCY	EFFICACY	REMARKS	EXAMPLE
A Competitive antagonist	↓	No change	**Can** be overcome by ↑ agonist concentration	Diazepam (agonist) + flumazenil (competitive antagonist) on $GABA_A$ receptor.
B Noncompetitive antagonist	No change	↓	**Cannot** be overcome by ↑ agonist concentration	Norepinephrine (agonist) + phenoxybenzamine (noncompetitive antagonist) on α-receptors.
C Partial agonist (alone)	Independent	↓	Acts at same site as full agonist	Morphine (full agonist) vs buprenorphine (partial agonist) at opioid μ-receptors.
Inverse agonist (alone)	Independent	Independent	Binds to a constitutively active receptor, thereby reducing its activity; has the opposite effect of an agonist	H_1 antihistamines (eg, diphenhydramine)

Therapeutic index

Measurement of drug safety.

$$\frac{TD_{50}}{ED_{50}} = \frac{\text{median toxic dose}}{\text{median effective dose}}$$

Therapeutic window—range of drug concentrations that can safely and effectively treat disease.

TITE: Therapeutic Index = TD_{50} / ED_{50}.
Safer drugs have higher TI values. Drugs with lower TI values frequently require monitoring (eg, warfarin, theophylline, digoxin, antiepileptic drugs, lithium; Warning! These drugs are lethal!).
LD_{50} (lethal median dose) often replaces TD_{50} in animal studies.

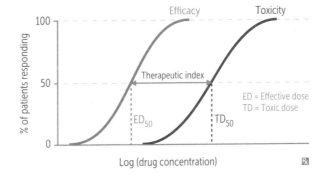

Drug effect modifications

TERM	DEFINITION	EXAMPLE
Additive	Effect of substances A and B together is equal to the sum of their individual effects	Aspirin and acetaminophen "2 + 2 = 4"
Permissive	Presence of substance A is required for the full effects of substance B	Cortisol on catecholamine responsiveness
Synergistic	Effect of substances A and B together is greater than the sum of their individual effects	Clopidogrel with aspirin "2 + 2 > 4"
Potentiation	Similar to synergism, but drug B (with no therapeutic action alone) enhances the therapeutic action of drug A	Carbidopa only blocks enzyme to prevent peripheral conversion of levodopa "2 + 0 > 2"
Antagonistic	Effect of substances A and B together is less than the sum of their individual effects	Morphine with naloxone "2 + 2 < 4"
Tachyphylactic	Acute decrease in response to a drug after initial/repeated administration	Repeat use of intranasal decongestant (eg, oxymetazoline) → ↓ therapeutic response (with rebound congestion)

▶ PHARMACOLOGY—AUTONOMIC DRUGS

Autonomic receptors

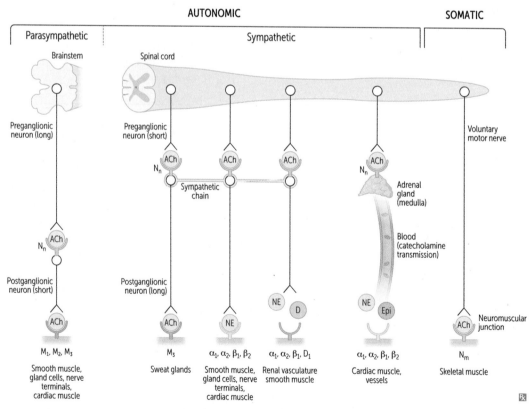

Pelvic splanchnic nerves and CNs III, VII, IX and X are part of the parasympathetic nervous system. Adrenal medulla is directly innervated by preganglionic sympathetic fibers.

Sweat glands are part of the **sympathetic** pathway but are innervated by **chol**inergic fibers (**sympathetic** nervous system results in a "**chold**" sweat).

Acetylcholine receptors	Nicotinic ACh receptors are ligand-gated channels allowing efflux of K^+ and influx of Na^+ and in some cases Ca^{2+}. Two subtypes: N_N (found in autonomic ganglia, adrenal medulla) and N_M (found in neuromuscular junction of skeletal muscle). Muscarinic ACh receptors are G-protein–coupled receptors that usually act through 2nd messengers. 5 subtypes: M_{1-5} found in heart, smooth muscle, brain, exocrine glands, and on sweat glands (cholinergic sympathetic).

Pain transmission

Nociceptive pain	Pain signals transmitted to the CNS in response to mechanical, thermal, or chemical stimuli. Transient receptor potential vanilloid ligand receptors cause Ca^{2+} influx–induced Na^+ channel activation. Signals transmitted by $A\delta$ fibers (sharp, acute pain) or C fibers (dull, throbbing, chronic pain). Processes involved in pain transmission: ■ Transduction—blocked by local anesthetics, α_2-agonists, gabapentinoids, NSAIDs, acetaminophen, glucocorticoids ■ Transmission—blocked by local anesthetics, α_2-agonists, opioids ■ Modulation—blocked by TCAs, SSRIs, SNRIs, gabapentinoids ■ Perception—blocked by α_2-agonists, opioids, TCAs, SSRIs, SNRIs
Neuropathic pain	Caused by neuronal dysfunction of the CNS or PNS. Transmitted via upregulation and persistent activation of voltage-gated Na^+ channels. Example: diabetic peripheral neuropathy.

Micturition control

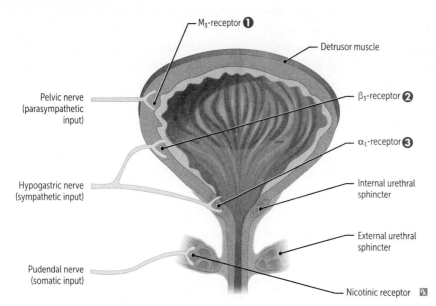

Micturition center in pons regulates involuntary bladder function via coordination of sympathetic and parasympathetic nervous systems.
⊕ sympathetic → ↑ urinary retention.
⊕ parasympathetic → ↑ urine voiding.
Some autonomic drugs act on smooth muscle receptors to treat bladder dysfunction.
Baby one more time.

DRUGS	MECHANISM	APPLICATIONS
❶ **Muscarinic agonists** (eg, bethanechol)	⊕ M_3 receptor → contraction of detrusor smooth muscle → ↑ bladder emptying	Urinary retention
❶ **Muscarinic antagonists** (eg, oxybutynin)	⊖ M_3 receptor → relaxation of detrusor smooth muscle → ↓ detrusor overactivity	Urgency incontinence
❷ **Sympathomimetics** (eg, mirabegron)	⊕ β_3 receptor → relaxation of detrusor smooth muscle → ↑ bladder capacity	Urgency incontinence
❸ **α_1-antagonists** (eg, tamsulosin)	⊖ α_1-receptor → relaxation of smooth muscle (bladder neck, prostate) → ↓ urinary obstruction	BPH

Tissue distribution of adrenergic receptors

RECEPTOR	TISSUE	EFFECT(S)
α_1	Vascular smooth muscle	Vasoconstriction
	Visceral smooth muscle	Smooth muscle contraction
α_2	Pancreas	Inhibition of insulin secretion
	Presynaptic terminals	Inhibition of neurotransmitter release
	Salivary glands	Inhibition of salivary secretion
β_1	Heart	↑ heart rate, contractility
	Kidney	↑ renin secretion
β_2	Bronchioles	Bronchodilation
	Cardiac muscle	↑ heart rate, contractility
	Liver	Glycogenolysis, glucose release
	Arterial smooth muscle	Vasodilation
	Pancreas	Stimulation of insulin secretion
β_3	Adipose	↑ lipolysis

G-protein–linked second messengers

RECEPTOR	G-PROTEIN CLASS	MAJOR FUNCTIONS
Adrenergic		
α_1	q	↑ vascular smooth muscle contraction, ↑ pupillary dilator muscle contraction (mydriasis), ↑ intestinal and bladder sphincter muscle contraction
α_2	i	↓ sympathetic (adrenergic) outflow, ↓ insulin release, ↓ lipolysis, ↑ platelet aggregation, ↓ aqueous humor production
β_1	s	↑ heart rate, ↑ contractility (**one** heart), ↑ renin release, ↑ lipolysis
β_2	s	Vasodilation, bronchodilation (**two** lungs), ↑ lipolysis, ↑ insulin release, ↑ glycogenolysis, ↓ uterine tone (tocolysis), ↑ aqueous humor production, ↑ cellular K^+ uptake
β_3	s	↑ lipolysis, ↑ thermogenesis in skeletal muscle, ↑ bladder relaxation
Cholinergic		
M_1	q	Mediates higher cognitive functions, stimulates enteric nervous system, ↑ exocrine gland secretions
M_2	i	↓ heart rate, AV node conduction velocity, and atrial contractility
M_3	q	↑ exocrine gland secretions, gut peristalsis, bladder contraction, bronchoconstriction, vasodilation, ↑ pupillary sphincter muscle contraction (miosis), ciliary muscle contraction (accommodation)
Dopamine		
D_1	s	Relaxes renal vascular smooth muscle, activates direct pathway of striatum
D_2	i	Modulates transmitter release, especially in brain, inhibits indirect pathway of striatum
Histamine		
H_1	q	↑ bronchoconstriction, airway mucus production, ↑ vascular permeability/vasodilation, pruritus
H_2	s	↑ gastric acid secretion
Vasopressin		
V_1	q	↑ vascular smooth muscle contraction
V_2	s	↑ H_2O permeability and reabsorption via upregulating aquaporin-2 in collecting twobules (tubules) of kidney, ↑ release of vWF

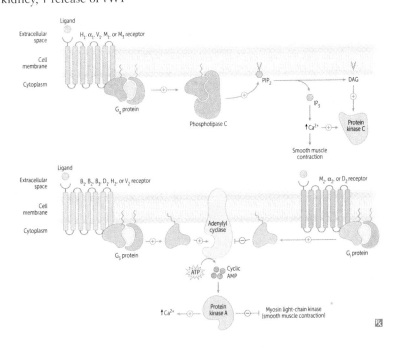

Autonomic drugs   Release of norepinephrine from a sympathetic nerve ending is modulated by NE itself, acting on presynaptic α_2-autoreceptors → negative feedback.

Amphetamines use the NE transporter (NET) to enter the presynaptic terminal, where they utilize the vesicular monoamine transporter (VMAT) to enter neurosecretory vesicles. This displaces NE from the vesicles. Once NE reaches a concentration threshold within the presynaptic terminal, the action of NET is reversed, and NE is expelled into the synaptic cleft, contributing to the characteristics and effects of ↑ NE observed in patients taking amphetamines.

CHOLINERGIC

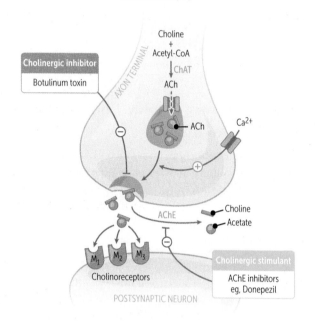

NORADRENERGIC

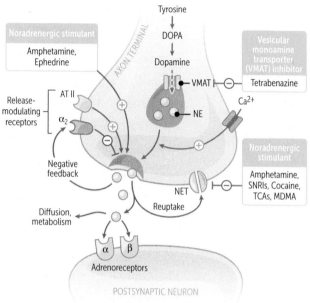

DOPAMINERGIC

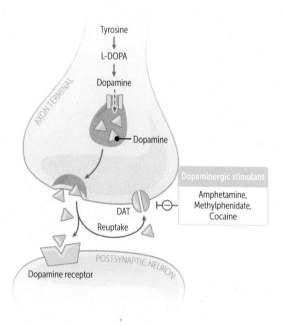

SEROTONERGIC

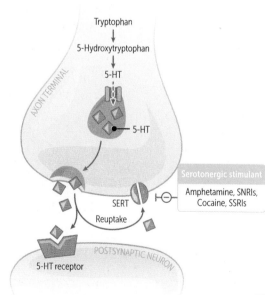

Cholinomimetic agents

Watch for exacerbation of COPD, asthma, and peptic ulcers in susceptible patients.

DRUG	ACTION	APPLICATIONS
Direct agonists		
Bethanechol	Activates **bladder** smooth muscle; resistant to AChE. Acts on muscarinic receptors; no nicotinic activity. "**Bethan**y, call me to activate your **bladder**."	Urinary retention.
Carbachol	Carbon copy of acetyl**chol**ine (but resistant to AChE).	Constricts pupil. Used for intraoperative miosis induction.
Methacholine	Stimulates muscarinic receptors in airway when inhaled.	Challenge test for diagnosis of asthma.
Pilocarpine	Contracts ciliary muscle of eye (open-angle glaucoma), pupillary sphincter (closed-angle glaucoma); resistant to AChE, can cross blood-brain barrier. "You cry, drool, and sweat on your 'pilow.'"	Potent stimulator of sweat, tears, and saliva Open-angle and closed-angle glaucoma, xerostomia (Sjögren syndrome).
Indirect agonists (anticholinesterases)		
Donepezil, rivastigmine, galantamine	↑ ACh.	1st line for Alzheimer disease (**Dona Riva** forgot the **gala**).
Neostigmine	↑ ACh. Neo = **no** blood-brain barrier penetration due to positive charge.	Postoperative and neurogenic ileus and urinary retention, myasthenia gravis, reversal of neuromuscular junction blockade (postoperative).
Pyridostigmine	↑ ACh; ↑ muscle strength. Does not penetrate CNS. Pyridostigmine gets **rid** of myasthenia gravis.	Myasthenia gravis (long acting). Used with glycopyrrolate or hyoscyamine to control pyridostigmine adverse effects.
Physostigmine	↑ ACh. **Ph**reely (freely) crosses blood-brain barrier as not charged → CNS.	Antidote for anticholinergic toxicity; physostigmine "**ph**yxes" atropine overdose.

Anticholinesterase poisoning

Often due to organophosphates (eg, fenthion, parathion, malathion) that irreversibly inhibit AChE. Organophosphates commonly used as insecticides; poisoning usually seen in farmers.

Muscarinic effects	**D**iarrhea, **U**rination, **M**iosis, **B**ronchospasm, **B**radycardia, **E**mesis, **L**acrimation, **S**weating, **S**alivation.	**DUMBBELSS**. Reversed by atropine, a competitive inhibitor. Atropine can cross BBB to relieve CNS symptoms.
Nicotinic effects	Neuromuscular blockade (mechanism similar to succinylcholine).	Reversed by pralidoxime, regenerates AChE via dephosphorylation if given early. Must be coadministered with atropine to prevent transient worsening of symptoms. Pralidoxime does not readily cross BBB.
CNS effects	Respiratory depression, lethargy, seizures, coma.	

Muscarinic antagonists

DRUGS	ORGAN SYSTEMS	APPLICATIONS
Atropine, homatropine, tropicamide	Eye	Produce mydriasis and cycloplegia
Benztropine, trihexyphenidyl	CNS	Parkinson disease ("**park my Benz**") Acute dystonia
Glycopyrrolate	GI, respiratory	Parenteral: preoperative use to reduce airway secretions Oral: reduces drooling, peptic ulcer
Hyoscyamine, dicyclomine	GI	Antispasmodics for irritable bowel syndrome
Ipratropium, tiotropium	Respiratory	COPD, asthma Duration: tiotropium > ipratropium
Solifenacin, Oxybutynin, Flavoxate, Tolterodine	Genitourinary	Reduce bladder spasms and urge urinary incontinence (overactive bladder) Make bladder **SOFT**
Scopolamine	CNS	Motion sickness

Atropine

Muscarinic antagonist. Used to treat bradycardia and for ophthalmic applications.

ORGAN SYSTEM	ACTION	NOTES
Eye	↑ pupil dilation, cycloplegia	Blocks muscarinic effects (**DUMBBELSS**) of anticholinesterases, but not the nicotinic effects
Airway	Bronchodilation, ↓ secretions	
Heart	↑ heart rate	
Stomach	↓ acid secretion	
Gut	↓ motility	
Bladder	↓ urgency in cystitis	
ADVERSE EFFECTS	↑ body **temperature** (due to ↓ sweating); ↑ **HR**; dry mouth; **dry, flushed skin**; cycloplegia; constipation; **disorientation** Can cause acute angle-closure glaucoma in older adults (due to mydriasis), **urinary retention** in men with prostatic hyperplasia, and hyperthermia in infants	Adverse effects: **Hot** as a hare **Fast** as a fiddle **Dry** as a bone **Red** as a beet **Blind** as a bat **Mad** as a hatter **Full** as a flask Jimson weed (*Datura*) → gardener's pupil (mydriasis)

Sympathomimetics

DRUG	SITE	HEMODYNAMIC CHANGES	APPLICATIONS
Direct sympathomimetics			
Albuterol, salmeterol, terbutaline	$\beta_2 > \beta_1$	↑ HR (little effect)	Albuterol for acute asthma/COPD. Salmeterol for serial (long-term) asthma/COPD. Terbutaline for acute bronchospasm in asthma and tocolysis.
Dobutamine	$\beta_1 > \beta_2, \alpha$	–/↓ BP, ↑ HR, ↑ CO	Cardiac stress testing, acute decompensated heart failure (HF) with cardiogenic shock (inotrope)
Dopamine	$D_1 = D_2 > \beta > \alpha$	↑ BP (high dose), ↑ HR, ↑ CO	Unstable bradycardia, shock; inotropic and chronotropic effects at lower doses via β effects; vasoconstriction at high doses via α effects.
Epinephrine	$\beta > \alpha$	↑ BP (high dose), ↑ HR, ↑ CO	Anaphylaxis, asthma, shock, open-angle glaucoma; α effects predominate at high doses. Stronger effect at β_2-receptor than norepinephrine.
Fenoldopam	D_1	↓ BP (vasodilation), ↑ HR, ↑ CO	Postoperative hypertension, hypertensive crisis. Vasodilator (coronary, peripheral, renal, and splanchnic). Promotes natriuresis. Can cause hypotension, tachycardia, flushing, headache.
Isoproterenol	$\beta_1 = \beta_2$	↓ BP (vasodilation), ↑ HR, ↑ CO	Electrophysiologic evaluation of tachyarrhythmias. Can worsen ischemia. Has negligible α effect.
Midodrine	α_1	↑ BP (vasoconstriction), ↓ HR, –/↓ CO	Autonomic insufficiency and postural hypotension. May exacerbate supine hypertension.
Mirabegron	β_3		Urinary urgency or incontinence or overactive bladder. Think "mirab3gron."
Norepinephrine	$\alpha_1 > \alpha_2 > \beta_1$	↑ BP, –/↓ HR (may have minor reflexive change in response to ↑ BP due to α_1 agonism outweighing direct β_1 chronotropic effect), –/↑ CO	Hypotension, septic shock.
Phenylephrine	$\alpha_1 > \alpha_2$	↑ BP (vasoconstriction), ↓ HR, –/↓ CO	Hypotension (vasoconstrictor), ocular procedures (mydriatic), rhinitis (decongestant), ischemic priapism.
Indirect sympathomimetics			
Amphetamine	Indirect general agonist, reuptake inhibitor, also releases stored catecholamines.		Narcolepsy, obesity, ADHD.
Cocaine	Indirect general agonist, reuptake inhibitor. Causes vasoconstriction and local anesthesia. Caution when giving β-blockers if cocaine intoxication is suspected (unopposed α_1 activation → ↑↑↑ BP, coronary vasospasm).		Causes mydriasis in eyes with intact sympathetic innervation → used to confirm Horner syndrome.
Ephedrine	Indirect general agonist, releases stored catecholamines.		Nasal decongestion (pseudoephedrine), urinary incontinence, hypotension.

Physiologic effects of sympathomimetics

NE ↑ systolic and diastolic pressures as a result of α_1-mediated vasoconstriction → ↑ mean arterial pressure → ↑ reflex bradycardia. However, isoproterenol (rarely used) has little α effect but causes β_2-mediated vasodilation, resulting in ↓ mean arterial pressure and ↑ heart rate through β_1 and reflex activity.

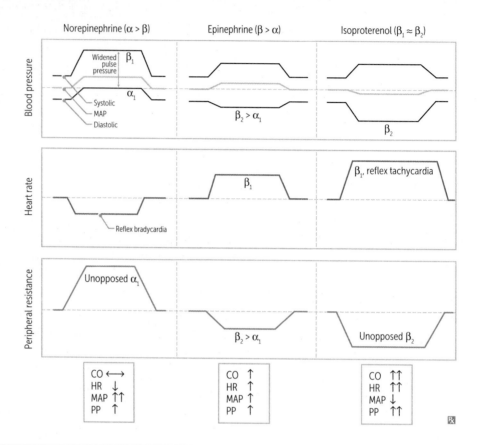

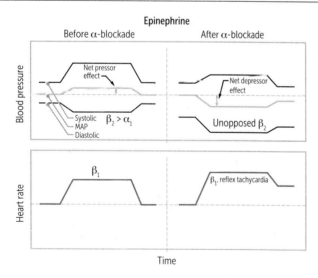

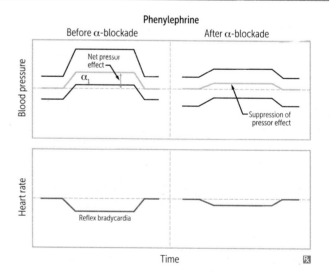

Epinephrine response exhibits reversal of mean arterial pressure from a net increase (the α response) to a net decrease (the β_2 response).

Phenylephrine response is suppressed but not reversed because it is a "pure" α-agonist (lacks β-agonist properties).

Sympatholytics (α₂-agonists)

DRUG	APPLICATIONS	ADVERSE EFFECTS
Clonidine, guanfacine	Hypertensive urgency (limited situations), ADHD, Tourette syndrome, symptom control in opioid withdrawal	CNS depression, bradycardia, hypotension, respiratory depression, miosis, rebound hypertension with abrupt cessation
α-methyldopa	Hypertension in pregnancy	Direct Coombs ⊕ hemolysis, drug-induced lupus, hyperprolactinemia
Tizanidine	Relief of spasticity	Hypotension, weakness, xerostomia

α-blockers

DRUG	APPLICATIONS	ADVERSE EFFECTS
Nonselective		
Phenoxybenzamine	Irreversible. Pheochromocytoma (used preoperatively) to prevent catecholamine (hypertensive) crisis.	Orthostatic hypotension, reflex tachycardia.
Phentolamine	Reversible. Given to patients on MAO inhibitors who eat tyramine-containing foods and for severe cocaine-induced hypertension (2nd line). Also used to treat norepinephrine extravasation.	
α₁ selective (-osin ending)		
Prazosin, terazosin, doxazosin, tamsulosin	Urinary symptoms of BPH; PTSD (prazosin); hypertension (except tamsulosin).	1st-dose orthostatic hypotension, dizziness, headache.
α₂ selective		
Mirtazapine	Depression.	Sedation, ↑ serum cholesterol, ↑ appetite.

β-blockers

Atenolol, betaxolol, bisoprolol, carvedilol, esmolol, labetalol, metoprolol, nadolol, nebivolol, propranolol, timolol.

APPLICATION	ACTIONS	NOTES/EXAMPLES
Angina pectoris	↓ heart rate and contractility → ↓ O_2 consumption	
Glaucoma	↓ production of aqueous humor	Timolol
Heart failure	Blockade of neurohormonal stress → prevention of deleterious cardiac remodeling → ↓ mortality	Bisoprolol, carvedilol, metoprolol (β-blockers curb mortality)
Hypertension	↓ cardiac output, ↓ renin secretion (due to $β_1$-receptor blockade on JG cells)	
Hyperthyroidism/ thyroid storm	Symptom control (↓ heart rate, ↓ tremor)	Propranolol
Hypertrophic cardiomyopathy	↓ heart rate → ↑ filling time, relieving obstruction	
Migraine	↓ nitric oxide production	Effective for prevention
Myocardial infarction	↓ O_2 demand (short-term), ↓ mortality (long-term)	
Supraventricular tachycardia (eg, atrial fibrillation)	↓ AV conduction velocity (class II antiarrhythmic)	Metoprolol, esmolol
Variceal bleeding	↓ hepatic venous pressure gradient and portal hypertension (prophylactic use)	Nadolol, propranolol, carvedilol for **no** portal circulation
ADVERSE EFFECTS	Erectile dysfunction, cardiovascular (bradycardia, AV block, HF), CNS (seizures, sleep alterations), dyslipidemia (metoprolol), masked hypoglycemia, asthma/COPD exacerbations	Use of β-blockers for acute cocaine-associated chest pain remains controversial due to unsubstantiated concern for unopposed α-adrenergic stimulation
SELECTIVITY	$β_1$-selective antagonists ($β_1 > β_2$)—**a**tenolol, **b**etaxolol, **b**isoprolol, **e**smolol, **m**etoprolol	Selective antagonists mostly go from **A** to **M** ($β_1$ with 1st half of alphabet)
	Nonselective antagonists ($β_1 = β_2$)—**n**adolol, **p**ropranolol, **t**imolol	**NonZ**elective antagonists mostly go from **N** to **Z** ($β_2$ with 2nd half of alphabet)
	Nonselective α- and β-antagonists—carve**dilol**, labet**alol**	Nonselective α- and β-antagonists have **modified suffixes** (instead of "-olol")
	Nebivolol combines cardiac-selective $β_1$-adrenergic blockade with stimulation of $β_3$-receptors (activate NO synthase in the vasculature and ↓ SVR)	Nebiv**O**lol increases **NO**

Phosphodiesterase inhibitors	Phosphodiesterase (PDE) inhibitors inhibit PDE, which catalyzes the hydrolysis of cAMP and/or cGMP, and thereby increase cAMP and/or cGMP. These inhibitors have varying specificity for PDE isoforms and thus have different clinical uses.

TYPE OF INHIBITOR	MECHANISM OF ACTION	CLINICAL USES	ADVERSE EFFECTS
Nonspecific PDE inhibitor Theophylline	↓ cAMP hydrolysis → ↑ cAMP → bronchial smooth muscle relaxation → bronchodilation	COPD/asthma (rarely used)	Cardiotoxicity (eg, tachycardia, arrhythmia), neurotoxicity (eg, seizures, headache), abdominal pain
PDE-5 inhibitors Sildenafil, vardenafil, tadalafil, avanafil	↓ hydrolysis of cGMP → ↑ cGMP → ↑ smooth muscle relaxation by enhancing NO activity → pulmonary vasodilation and ↑ blood flow in corpus cavernosum fills the penis	Erectile dysfunction Pulmonary hypertension Benign prostatic hyperplasia (**tadalafil** only)	Facial flushing, headache, dyspepsia, hypotension in patients taking nitrates; "hot and sweaty," then headache, heartburn, hypotension Sildenafil only: cyanopia (blue-tinted vision) via inhibition of PDE-6 (six) in retina
PDE-4 inhibitor Roflumilast	↑ cAMP in neutrophils, granulocytes, and bronchial epithelium	Severe COPD	Abdominal pain, weight loss, depression, anxiety, insomnia
PDE-3 inhibitor Milrinone	In cardiomyocytes: ↑ cAMP → ↑ Ca^{2+} influx → ↑ ionotropy and chronotropy In vascular smooth muscle: ↑ cAMP → MLCK inhibition → vasodilation → ↓ preload and afterload	Acute decompensated HF with cardiogenic shock (inotrope)	Tachycardia, ventricular arrhythmias, hypotension
"Platelet inhibitors" Cilostazol[a] Dipyridamole[b]	In platelets: ↑ cAMP → inhibition of platelet aggregation	Intermittent claudication Stroke or TIA prevention (with aspirin) Cardiac stress testing (dipyridamole only, due to coronary vasodilation) Prevention of coronary stent restenosis	Nausea, headache, facial flushing, hypotension, abdominal pain

[a]Cilostazol is a PDE-3 inhibitor, but due to its indications is categorized as a platelet inhibitor together with dipyridamole.
[b]Dipyridamole is a nonspecific PDE inhibitor, leading to inhibition of platelet aggregation. It also prevents adenosine reuptake by platelets → ↑ extracellular adenosine → ↑ vasodilation.

▶ PHARMACOLOGY—TOXICITIES AND ADVERSE EFFECTS

Ingested seafood toxins

Toxin actions include histamine release, total block of Na^+ channels, or opening of Na^+ channels to cause depolarization.

TOXIN	SOURCE	ACTION	SYMPTOMS	TREATMENT
Histamine (scombroid poisoning)	Spoiled dark-meat fish such as tuna, mahi-mahi, mackerel, and bonito	Bacterial histidine decarboxylase converts histidine to histamine Frequently misdiagnosed as fish allergy	Mimics anaphylaxis: oral burning sensation, facial flushing, erythema, urticaria, itching; may progress to bronchospasm, angioedema, hypotension	Antihistamines Albuterol +/– epinephrine
Tetrodotoxin	Pufferfish	Binds fast voltage-gated Na^+ channels in nerve tissue, preventing depolarization	Nausea, diarrhea, paresthesias, weakness, dizziness, loss of reflexes	Supportive
Ciguatoxin	Reef fish such as barracuda, snapper, and moray eel	Opens Na^+ channels, causing depolarization	Nausea, vomiting, diarrhea; perioral numbness; reversal of hot and cold sensations; bradycardia, heart block, hypotension	Supportive

Age-related changes in pharmacokinetics

Aging alters the passage of drugs through the body and standard doses can result in ↑ plasma concentrations. Older patients often require reduced doses to prevent toxicity.
- Absorption—mostly unaffected.
- Distribution—↓ total body water (↓ V_d of hydrophilic drugs → ↑ concentration), ↑ total body fat (↑ V_d of lipophilic drugs → ↑ half-life).
- Metabolism—↓ hepatic mass and blood flow → ↓ first-pass metabolism, ↓ hepatic clearance. Phase I of drug metabolism is decreased; phase II is relatively preserved.
- Excretion—↓ renal mass and blood flow (↓ GFR) → ↓ renal clearance.

Specific toxicity treatments

TOXIN	TREATMENT
Acetaminophen	N-acetylcysteine (replenishes glutathione)
AChE inhibitors, organophosphates	Atropine > pralidoxime
Antimuscarinic, anticholinergic agents	Physostigmine (crosses BBB), control hyperthermia
Arsenic	Dimercaprol, succimer
Benzodiazepines	Flumazenil
β-blockers	Atropine, glucagon, saline
Carbon monoxide	100% O_2, hyperbaric O_2
Copper	"Penny"cillamine (penicillamine), trientine (3 copper pennies)
Cyanide	Hydroxocobalamin, nitrites + sodium thiosulfate
Dabigatran	Idarucizumab
Digoxin	Digoxin-specific antibody fragments
Direct factor **Xa** inhibitors (eg, apixaban)	Andexanet alfa
Heparin	Protamine sulfate
Iron (**Fe**)	Deferoxamine, deferasirox, deferiprone
Lead	Penicillamine, calcium disodium EDTA, Dimercaprol, Succimer, (correct lead poisoning in **PEDS** patients)
Mercury	Dimercaprol, succimer
Methanol, ethylene glycol (antifreeze)	Fomepizole > ethanol, dialysis
Methemoglobin	Methylene blue, vitamin C (reducing agent)
Methotrexate	Leucovorin
Opioids	Naloxone
Salicylates	$NaHCO_3$ (alkalinizes urine), dialysis
TCAs	$NaHCO_3$ (stabilizes cardiac cell membrane)
Warfarin	Vitamin K (delayed effect), PCC (prothrombin complex concentrate)/FFP (immediate effect)

Drug reactions—cardiovascular

DRUG REACTION	CAUSAL AGENTS
Coronary vasospasm	Cocaine, Amphetamines, Sumatriptan, Ergot alkaloids (**CASE**)
Cutaneous flushing	Vancomycin, Adenosine, Niacin, Ca^{2+} channel blockers, Echinocandins, Nitrates (flushed from **VANCEN** [dancing]) Vancomycin infusion reaction (formerly called red man syndrome)—histamine release → widespread pruritic erythema. Infusion rate–dependent. Manage with slower infusion rate, diphenhydramine.
Dilated cardiomyopathy	Alcohol, anthracycline (eg, doxorubicin, daunorubicin; prevent with dexrazoxane), trastuzumab
Peripheral edema	Dihydropyridine Ca^{2+} channel blockers (eg, amlodipine)
Torsades de pointes	Associated with agents that prolong QT interval: Methadone, antiArrhythmics (class IA, III), antiBiotics (eg, macrolides, fluoroquinolones), anti"C"ychotics (eg, ziprasidone), antiDepressants (eg, TCAs), antiEmetics (eg, ondansetron), antiFungals (eg, fluconazole) (**Memorize your ABCDEF**)

Drug reactions—endocrine/reproductive

DRUG REACTION	CAUSAL AGENTS	NOTES
Adrenocortical insufficiency	HPA suppression secondary to chronic exogenous glucocorticoid use	Abrupt withdrawal of exogenous glucocorticoids leads to adrenal crisis
Diabetes insipidus	Lithium, demeclocycline	
Gynecomastia	Ketoconazole, cimetidine, spironolactone, GnRH analogs/antagonists, androgen receptor inhibitors, 5α-reductase inhibitors	
Hot flashes	SERMs (eg, tamoxifen, clomiphene, raloxifene)	
Hyperglycemia	Tacrolimus, protease inhibitors, niacin, HCTZ, glucocorticoids	The people need High glucose
Hyperprolactinemia	Typical antipsychotics (eg, haloperidol), atypical antipsychotics (eg, risperidone), metoclopramide, methyldopa, verapamil	Presents with hypogonadism (eg, infertility, amenorrhea, erectile dysfunction) and galactorrhea
Hyperthyroidism	Amiodarone, iodine, lithium	
Hypothyroidism	Amiodarone, lithium	I am lethargic
SIADH	Carbamazepine, Cyclophosphamide, SSRIs	Can't Concentrate Serum Sodium

Drug reactions—gastrointestinal

DRUG REACTION	CAUSAL AGENTS	NOTES
Acute cholestatic hepatitis, jaundice	Macrolides (eg, erythromycin)	
Constipation	Antimuscarinics (eg, atropine), antipsychotics, opioids, non-dihydropyridine CCBs, ranolazine, amiodarone, aluminum hydroxide, loperamide, 5HT3 receptor antagonist (ondansetron), vincristine	
Diarrhea	Acamprosate, antidiabetic agents (acarbose, metformin, pramlintide), colchicine, cholinesterase inhibitors, lipid-lowering agents (eg, ezetimibe, orlistat), macrolides (eg, erythromycin), SSRIs, chemotherapy (eg, irinotecan)	
Focal to massive hepatic necrosis	*Amanita phalloides* (death cap mushroom), valproate, acetaminophen	
Hepatitis	Rifampin, isoniazid, pyrazinamide, statins, fibrates	
Pancreatitis	Diuretics (eg, furosemide, HCTZ), glucocorticoids, alcohol, valproate, azathioprine	Drugs generate a violent abdominal distress
Medication-induced esophagitis	Potassium chloride, NSAIDs, bisphosphonates, ferrous sulfate, tetracyclines Pills Not beneficial for food tube	Usually occurs at anatomic sites of esophageal narrowing (eg, near level of aortic arch); caustic effect minimized with upright posture and adequate water ingestion
Pseudomembranous colitis	Ampicillin, cephalosporins, clindamycin, fluoroquinolones, PPIs	Antibiotics predispose to superinfection by resistant *C difficile*

Drug reactions—hematologic

DRUG REACTION	CAUSAL AGENTS	NOTES
Agranulocytosis	Dapsone, clozapine, carbamazepine, propylthiouracil, methimazole, ganciclovir, colchicine	Drugs can cause pretty major granulocytes collapse
Aplastic anemia	Carbamazepine, methimazole, NSAIDs, benzene, chloramphenicol, propylthiouracil	Can't make New blood cells properly
Direct Coombs ⊕ hemolytic anemia	Penicillin, cephalosporins, methyldopa	Pooh classically munches on honey Coombs
Drug Reaction with Eosinophilia and Systemic Symptoms	Phenytoin, carbamazepine, minocycline, sulfa drugs, allopurinol, vancomycin	T cell-mediated hypersensitivity reaction. Also known as drug-induced hypersensitivity syndrome (DIHS) DRESSes partially cover my skin and viscera
Hemolysis in G6PD deficiency	Sulfonamides, dapsone, primaquine, aspirin, nitrofurantoin	
Megaloblastic anemia	Hydroxyurea, Phenytoin, Methotrexate, Sulfa drugs	You're having a mega blast with PMS
Thrombocytopenia	Heparin, quinidine, ganciclovir, vancomycin, linezolid	
Thrombotic complications	Combined oral contraceptives, hormone replacement therapy, SERMs Testosterone supplements, epoetin alfa	Estrogen-mediated ↑ blood viscosity and platelet accumulation

Drug reactions—musculoskeletal/skin/connective tissue

DRUG REACTION	CAUSAL AGENTS	NOTES
Drug-induced lupus	Hydralazine, procainamide, quinidine	
Fat redistribution	Protease inhibitors, glucocorticoids	Fat protects glutes
Gingival hyperplasia	Cyclosporine, Ca^{2+} channel blockers, phenytoin	Can Cause puffy gums
Hyperuricemia (gout)	Pyrazinamide, thiazides, furosemide, niacin, cyclosporine	Painful tophi and feet need care
Malignant hyperthermia	Inhaled anesthetics (eg, isoflurane)	Individuals with ryanodine receptor mutation; antidote is dantrolene
Myopathy	Statins, fibrates, niacin, colchicine, daptomycin, hydroxychloroquine, interferon-α, penicillamine, glucocorticoids	
Osteoporosis	Glucocorticoids, depot medroxyprogesterone acetate, GnRH agonists, aromatase inhibitors, anticonvulsants, heparin, PPIs	
Photosensitivity	Sulfonamides, amiodarone, tetracyclines, fluoroquinolones	Sat for photo
Rash (Stevens-Johnson syndrome)	Anti-epileptic drugs (especially lamotrigine), allopurinol, sulfa drugs, penicillin	Steven Johnson has epileptic allergy to sulfa drugs and penicillin
Teeth discoloration	Tetracyclines	Teethracyclines
Tendon/cartilage damage	Fluoroquinolones	

Drug reactions—neurologic

DRUG REACTION	CAUSAL AGENTS	NOTES
Cinchonism	Quinidine, quinine	Can present with tinnitus, hearing/vision loss, psychosis, and cognitive impairment
Parkinson-like syndrome	Antipsychotics, metoclopramide	Cogwheel rigidity of arm
Peripheral neuropathy	Platinum agents (eg, **cis**platin), isoniazid, vincristine, paclitaxel, phenytoin	**Cis, it's** very painful peripherally
Idiopathic intracranial hypertension	Corticosteroids, danazol, vitamin A, growth hormones, tetracyclines	**C**rime and **d**ebt **A**lways **g**row **h**ead **t**ension
Seizures	Isoniazid, bupropion, imipenem/cilastatin, tramadol	With **seizures, I bit** my tongue
Tardive dyskinesia	Antipsychotics, metoclopramide	
Visual disturbances	Topiramate (blurred vision/diplopia, haloes), hydroxychloroquine (↓ visual acuity, visual field defects), digoxin (yellow-tinged vision), isoniazid (optic neuritis), ivabradine (luminous phenomena), PDE-5 inhibitors (blue-tinged vision), ethambutol (color vision changes)	**T**hese **h**orrible **d**rugs **i**irritate **P**recious **e**yes

Drug reactions—renal/genitourinary

DRUG REACTION	CAUSAL AGENTS	NOTES
Fanconi syndrome	Cisplatin, ifosfamide, expired tetracyclines, tenofovir	
Hemorrhagic cystitis	Cyclophosphamide, ifosfamide	Prevent by coadministering with mesna
Interstitial nephritis	Diuretics (**P**ee), NSAIDs (**P**ain-free), **P**enicillins and cephalosporins, **P**PIs, rifam**P**in, sulfa drugs	Remember the 5 P's
Nephrotoxicity	Cisplatin, aminoglycosides, amphotericin, vancomycin	

Drug reactions—respiratory

DRUG REACTION	CAUSAL AGENTS	NOTES
Dry cough	ACE inhibitors	
Pulmonary fibrosis	**M**ethotrexate, **n**itrofurantoin, **c**armustine, **b**leomycin, **b**usulfan, **a**miodarone	**M**y **n**ose **c**annot **b**reathe **b**ad **a**ir

Drug reactions—multiorgan

DRUG REACTION	CAUSAL AGENTS	NOTES
Antimuscarinic	Atropine, TCAs, H$_1$-blockers, antipsychotics	
Disulfiram-like reaction	1st-generation sulfonylureas, procarbazine, certain cephalosporins, griseofulvin, metronidazole	**S**orry **p**als, **c**an't **g**o **m**ingle

Drugs affecting pupil size	↑ pupil size (mydriasis)	↓ pupil size (miosis)
	Anticholinergics (eg, atropine, TCAs, tropicamide, scopolamine, antihistamines)	Sympatholytics (eg, α₂-agonists)
	Indirect sympathomimetics (eg, amphetamines, cocaine, LSD), meperidine	Opioids (except meperidine)
	Direct sympathomimetics	Parasympathomimetics (eg, pilocarpine), organophosphates

Anticholinergics (eg, atropine, TCAs, tropicamide, scopolamine, antihistamines)
Indirect sympathomimetics (eg, amphetamines, cocaine, LSD), meperidine
Direct sympathomimetics

Sympatholytics (eg, α_2-agonists)
Opioids (except meperidine)
Parasympathomimetics (eg, pilocarpine), organophosphates

Radial muscle contraction
(α_1 receptor mediated)

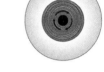

Sphincter muscle contraction
(M_3 receptor mediated)

Cytochrome P-450 interactions (selected)

Inducers (+)	Substrates	Inhibitors (−)
St. John's wort	Theophylline	Sodium valproate
Phenytoin	OCPs	Isoniazid
Phenobarbital	Anti-epileptics	Cimetidine
Modafinil	Warfarin	Ketoconazole
Nevirapine		Fluconazole
Rifampin		Acute alcohol overuse
Griseofulvin		Chloramphenicol
Carbamazepine		Erythromycin/clarithromycin
Chronic alcohol overuse		Sulfonamides
		Ciprofloxacin
		Omeprazole
		Amiodarone
		Ritonavir
		Grapefruit juice
St. John's funny funny (phen-phen) mom never refuses greasy carbs and chronic alcohol	The OCPs are anti-war	**SICK FACES** come when I am really drinking grapefruit juice

---

Sulfa drugs

Sulfonamide antibiotics, Sulfasalazine, Probenecid, Furosemide, Acetazolamide, Celecoxib, Thiazides, Sulfonylureas.
Patients with sulfa allergies may develop fever, urinary tract infection, Stevens-Johnson syndrome, hemolytic anemia, thrombocytopenia, agranulocytosis, acute interstitial nephritis, and urticaria (hives), and photosensitivity.

Scary Sulfa Pharm **FACTS**

▶ PHARMACOLOGY—MISCELLANEOUS

Drug names

ENDING	CATEGORY	EXAMPLE
Antimicrobial		
-asvir	NS5A inhibitor	Ledipasvir
-bendazole	Antiparasitic/antihelminthic	Mebendazole
-buvir	NS5B inhibitor	Sofosbuvir
-cillin	Transpeptidase inhibitor	Ampicillin
-conazole	Ergosterol synthesis inhibitor	Ketoconazole
-cycline	Protein synthesis inhibitor	Tetracycline
-floxacin	Fluoroquinolone	Ciprofloxacin
-mivir	Neuraminidase inhibitor	Oseltamivir
-navir	Protease inhibitor	Ritonavir
-ovir	Viral DNA polymerase inhibitor	Acyclovir
-previr	NS3/4A inhibitor	Grazoprevir
-tegravir	Integrase inhibitor	Dolutegravir
-thromycin	Macrolide	Azithromycin
Antineoplastic		
-case	Recombinant uricase	Rasburicase
-mustine	Nitrosourea	Carmustine
-platin	Platinum compound	Cisplatin
-poside	Topoisomerase II inhibitor	Etoposide
-rubicin	Anthracycline	Doxorubicin
-taxel	Taxane	Paclitaxel
-tecan	Topoisomerase I inhibitor	Irinotecan
CNS		
-flurane	Inhaled anesthetic	Sevoflurane
-apine, -idone	Atypical antipsychotic	Quetiapine, risperidone
-azine	Typical antipsychotic	Thioridazine
-barbital	Barbiturate	Phenobarbital
-benazine	VMAT inhibitor	Tetrabenazine
-caine	Local anesthetic	Lidocaine
-capone	COMT inhibitor	Entacapone
-curium, -curonium	Nondepolarizing neuromuscular blocker	Atracurium, pancuronium
-giline	MAO-B inhibitor	Selegiline
-ipramine, -triptyline	TCA	Imipramine, amitriptyline
-triptan	5-HT$_{1B/1D}$ agonist	Sumatriptan
-zepam, -zolam	Benzodiazepine	Diazepam, alprazolam

Drug names (*continued*)

ENDING	CATEGORY	EXAMPLE
Autonomic		
-chol	Cholinergic agonist	Bethanechol
-olol	β-blocker	Propranolol
-stigmine	AChE inhibitor	Neostigmine
-terol	β_2-agonist	Albuterol
-zosin	α_1-blocker	Prazosin
Cardiovascular		
-afil	PDE-5 inhibitor	Sildenafil
-dipine	Dihydropyridine Ca^{2+} channel blocker	Amlodipine
-parin	Low-molecular-weight heparin	Enoxaparin
-plase	Thrombolytic	Alteplase
-pril	ACE inhibitor	Captopril
-sartan	Angiotensin-II receptor blocker	Losartan
-xaban	Direct factor Xa inhibitor	Apixaban
Metabolic		
-gliflozin	SGLT-2 inhibitor	Dapagliflozin
-glinide	Meglitinide	Repaglinide
-gliptin	DPP-4 inhibitor	Sitagliptin
-glitazone	PPAR-γ activator	Pioglitazone
-glutide	GLP-1 analog	Liraglutide
-statin	HMG-CoA reductase inhibitor	Atorvastatin
Other		
-caftor	CFTR modulator	Lumacaftor
-dronate	Bisphosphonate	Alendronate
-lukast	CysLT1 receptor blocker	Montelukast
-lutamide	Androgen receptor inhibitor	Flutamide
-pitant	NK_1 blocker	Aprepitant
-prazole	Proton pump inhibitor	Omeprazole
-prost	Prostaglandin analog	Latanoprost
-sentan	Endothelin receptor antagonist	Bosentan
-setron	$5\text{-}HT_3$ blocker	Ondansetron
-steride	5α-reductase inhibitor	Finasteride
-tadine	H_1-antagonist	Loratadine
-tidine	H_2-antagonist	Cimetidine
-trozole	Aromatase inhibitor	Anastrozole
-vaptan	ADH antagonist	Tolvaptan

Biologic agents

ENDING	CATEGORY	EXAMPLE
Monoclonal antibodies (-mab)—target overexpressed cell surface receptors		
-ximab	**Chi**meric human-mouse monoclonal antibody	Rituximab
-zumab	**Hu**manized monoclonal antibody	Bevacizumab
-umab	**Hu**man monoclonal antibody	Denosumab
Small molecule inhibitors (-ib)—target intracellular molecules		
-ciclib	**Cycl**in-dependent kinase inhibitor	Palbociclib
-coxib	**COX**-2 inhibitor	Celecoxib
-parib	Poly(**ADP-ri**bose) polymerase inhibitor	Olaparib
-rafenib	**BRAF** inhibitor	Vemurafenib
-tinib	**T**yrosine **kin**ase inhibitor	Imatinib
-zomib	Protea**som**e inhibitor	Bortezomib
Interleukin receptor modulators (-kin)—agonists and antagonists of interleukin receptors		
-leukin	Inter**leuk**in-2 agonist/analog	Aldesleukin
-kinra	Interleukin **r**eceptor antagonist	Anakinra

Public Health Sciences

"Medicine is a science of uncertainty and an art of probability."
—Sir William Osler

"People will forget what you said, people will forget what you did, but people will never forget how you made them feel."
—Maya Angelou

"On a long enough timeline, the survival rate for everyone drops to zero."
—Chuck Palahniuk, *Fight Club*

A heterogenous mix of epidemiology, biostatistics, ethics, law, healthcare delivery, patient safety, quality improvement, and more falls under the heading of public health sciences. Biostatistics and epidemiology are the foundations of evidence-based medicine and are very high yield. Make sure you can quickly apply biostatistical equations such as sensitivity, specificity, and predictive values in a problem-solving format. Also, know how to set up your own 2 × 2 tables, and look out for questions that switch the rows and columns. Quality improvement and patient safety topics were introduced a few years ago on the exam and represent trends in health system science. Medical ethics questions often require application of principles. Typically, you are presented with a patient scenario and then asked how you would respond. In this edition, we provide further details on communication skills and patient care given their growing emphasis on the exam. Effective communication is essential to the physician-patient partnership. Physicians must seek opportunities to connect with patients, understand their perspectives, express empathy, and form shared decisions and realistic goals.

▶ PUBLIC HEALTH SCIENCES—EPIDEMIOLOGY AND BIOSTATISTICS

Observational studies

STUDY TYPE	DESIGN	MEASURES/EXAMPLE
Case series	Describes several individual patients with the same diagnosis, treatment, or outcome.	Description of clinical findings and symptoms. Has no comparison group, thus cannot show risk factor association with disease.
Cross-sectional study	Frequency of disease and frequency of risk-related factors are assessed in the present. Asks, "What is happening?"	Disease prevalence. Can show risk factor association with disease, but does not establish causality.
Case-control study	Retrospectively compares a group of people with disease to a group without disease. Looks to see if odds of prior exposure or risk factor differ by disease state. Asks, "What happened?"	Odds ratio (**OR**). **Control** the case in the **OR**. Patients with COPD had higher odds of a smoking history than those without COPD.
Cohort study	Compares a group with a given exposure or risk factor to a group without such exposure. Looks to see if exposure or risk factor is associated with later development of disease. Can be prospective or retrospective, but risk factor has to be present prior to disease development.	Disease incidence. Relative risk (RR). People who smoke had a higher risk of developing COPD than people who do not. Cohort = relative risk.
Twin concordance study	Compares the frequency with which both monozygotic twins vs both dizygotic twins develop the same disease.	Measures heritability and influence of environmental factors ("nature vs nurture").
Adoption study	Compares behavioral traits/genetics in siblings raised by biological vs adoptive parents.	Measures heritability and influence of environmental factors.
Ecological study	Compares frequency of disease and frequency of risk-related factors across populations. Measures population data not necessarily applicable to individuals (ecological fallacy).	Used to monitor population health. COPD prevalence was higher in more polluted cities.

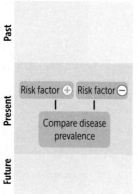
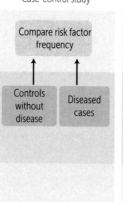
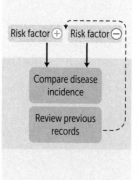
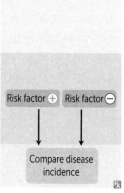

Clinical therapeutic trial	Experimental study involving humans. Compares therapeutic benefits of ≥ 2 interventions (eg, treatment vs placebo, treatment vs treatment). Study quality improves when clinical trial is randomized, controlled, and double-blinded (ie, neither subject nor researcher knows whether the subject is in the treatment or control group). Triple-blind refers to additional blinding of the researchers analyzing the data.

Crossover clinical trial—compares the effect of a series of ≥ 2 treatments on a subject. Order in which subjects receive treatments is randomized. Washout period occurs between treatments. Allows subjects to serve as their own controls.

Intention-to-treat analysis—all subjects are analyzed according to their original, randomly assigned treatment. No one is excluded, ie, once randomized, always analyzed. Attempts to avoid bias from attrition, crossover, and nonrandom noncompliance, but may dilute the true effects of intervention.

As-treated analysis—all subjects are analyzed according to the treatment they actually received. ↑ risk of bias.

Per-protocol analysis—subjects who fail to complete treatment as originally, randomly assigned are excluded. ↑ risk of bias.

Clinical trials occur after preclinical studies and consist of five phases ("Can **I SWIM**?").

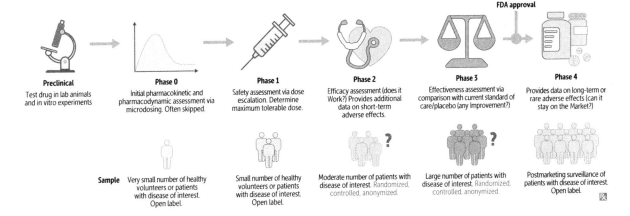

Preclinical
Test drug in lab animals and in vitro experiments

Phase 0
Initial pharmacokinetic and pharmacodynamic assessment via microdosing. Often skipped.

Phase 1
Safety assessment via dose escalation. Determine maximum tolerable dose.

Phase 2
Efficacy assessment (does it Work?) Provides additional data on short-term adverse effects.

Phase 3
Effectiveness assessment via comparison with current standard of care/placebo (any Improvement?)

FDA approval

Phase 4
Provides data on long-term or rare adverse effects (can it stay on the Market?)

Sample
Very small number of healthy volunteers or patients with disease of interest. Open label.

Small number of healthy volunteers or patients with disease of interest. Open label.

Moderate number of patients with disease of interest. Randomized, controlled, anonymized.

Large number of patients with disease of interest. Randomized, controlled, anonymized.

Postmarketing surveillance of patients with disease of interest. Open label.

Off-label drug use	Use of a drug to treat a disease in a form, population group, or dosage that is not specifically approved by the FDA. Reasons for off-label use include treatment of an illness with no approved pharmacologic treatment or exploring alternative treatments after failure of approved options. Example: use of tricyclic antidepressants for treating neuropathic/chronic pain.

Bradford Hill criteria	A group of principles that provide limited support (ie, necessary but not sufficient criteria) for establishing evidence of a causal relationship between presumed cause and effect.
Strength	Association does not necessarily imply causation, but the stronger the association, the more evidence for causation.
Consistency	Repeated observations of the findings in multiple distinct samples.
Specificity	The more specific the presumed cause is to the effect, the stronger the evidence for causation.
Temporality	The presumed cause precedes the effect by an expected amount of time.
Biological gradient	Greater effect observed with greater exposure to the presumed cause (dose-response relationship).
Plausibility	A conceivable mechanism exists by which the cause may lead to the effect.
Coherence	The presumed cause and effect do not conflict with existing scientific consensus.
Experiment	Empirical evidence supporting the presumed cause and effect (eg, animal studies, in vitro studies).
Analogy	The presumed cause and effect are comparable to a similar, established cause and effect.

Quantifying risk　　Definitions and formulas are based on the classic 2×2 or contingency table.

	Disease or outcome $\oplus$	Disease or outcome $\ominus$
Exposure or intervention $\oplus$	a	b
Exposure or intervention $\ominus$	c	d

TERM	DEFINITION	EXAMPLE	FORMULA
Odds ratio	Typically used in case-control studies. Represents the odds of exposure among cases (a/c) vs odds of exposure among controls (b/d). $OR = 1 \rightarrow$ odds of exposure are equal in cases and controls. $OR > 1 \rightarrow$ odds of exposure are greater in cases. $OR < 1 \rightarrow$ odds of exposure are greater in controls.	If in a **case-control** study, 20/30 patients with lung cancer and 5/25 healthy individuals report smoking, the **OR** is 8; so the patients with lung cancer are 8 times more likely to have a history of smoking. You take a **case** to the **OR**.	$OR = \dfrac{a/c}{b/d} = \dfrac{ad}{bc}$ <table><tr><td>a 20</td><td>b 5</td></tr><tr><td>c 10</td><td>d 20</td></tr></table>
Relative risk	Typically used in cohort studies. Risk of developing disease in the exposed group divided by risk in the unexposed group. $RR = 1 \rightarrow$ no association between exposure and disease. $RR > 1 \rightarrow$ exposure associated with ↑ disease occurrence. $RR < 1 \rightarrow$ exposure associated with ↓ disease occurrence.	If 5/10 people exposed to radiation are diagnosed with cancer, and 1/10 people not exposed to radiation are diagnosed with cancer, the RR is 5; so people exposed to radiation have a 5 times greater risk of developing cancer. For rare diseases (low prevalence), OR approximates RR.	$RR = \dfrac{a/(a+b)}{c/(c+d)}$ <table><tr><td>a 5</td><td>b 5</td></tr><tr><td>c 1</td><td>d 9</td></tr></table>
Relative risk reduction	The proportion of risk reduction attributable to the intervention/treatment (ART) as compared to a control (ARC).	If 2% of patients who receive a flu shot develop the flu, while 8% of unvaccinated patients develop the flu, then RR = 2/8 = 0.25, and RRR = 0.75.	$RRR = 1 - RR$ $RRR = \dfrac{(ARC - ART)}{ARC}$
Attributable risk	The difference in risk between exposed and unexposed groups.	If risk of lung cancer in people who smoke is 21% and risk in people who don't smoke is 1%, then the attributable risk is 20%.	$AR = \dfrac{a}{a+b} - \dfrac{c}{c+d}$ $AR\% = \dfrac{RR-1}{RR} \times 100$
Absolute risk reduction	The difference in risk (not the proportion) attributable to the intervention as compared to a control.	If 8% of people who receive a placebo vaccine develop the flu vs 2% of people who receive a flu vaccine, then ARR = 8%–2% = 6% = 0.06.	$ARR = \dfrac{c}{c+d} - \dfrac{a}{a+b}$
Number needed to treat	Number of patients who need to be treated for 1 patient to benefit. Lower number = better treatment.		$NNT = 1/ARR$
Number needed to harm	Number of patients who need to be exposed to a risk factor for 1 patient to be harmed. Higher number = safer exposure.		$NNH = 1/AR$
Case fatality rate	Percentage of deaths occurring among those with disease.	If 4 patients die among 10 cases of meningitis, case fatality rate is 40%.	$CFR\% = \dfrac{deaths}{cases} \times 100$

Quantifying risk (continued)

TERM	DEFINITION	EXAMPLE	FORMULA
Mortality rate	Number of deaths (in general or due to specific cause) within a population over a defined period.	If 80 people in a town of 10,000 die over 2 years, mortality rate is 4 per 1000 per year.	Deaths/1000 people per year.
Attack rate	Proportion of exposed people who become ill.	If 80 people in a town are exposed and 60 people become ill, attack rate is 75%.	$\dfrac{\text{People who become ill}}{\text{Total people exposed}}$

Demographic transition	As a country proceeds to higher levels of development, birth and mortality rates decline to varying degrees, changing the age composition of the population.		
Population pyramid	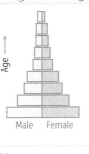	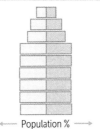	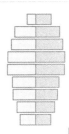
Birth rate	↑↑	↓	↓↓
Mortality rate	↑	↓	↓
Life expectancy	Short	Long	Long
Population	Growing	Stable	Declining

Likelihood ratio	$$LR^+ = \frac{\text{probability of positive result in patient with disorder}}{\text{probability of positive result in patient without disorder}} = \frac{\text{sensitivity}}{1-\text{specificity}} = \frac{\text{TP rate}}{\text{FP rate}}$$ $$LR^- = \frac{\text{probability of negative result in patient with disorder}}{\text{probability of negative result in patient without disorder}} = \frac{1-\text{sensitivity}}{\text{specificity}} = \frac{\text{FN rate}}{\text{TN rate}}$$ $LR^+ > 10$ indicates a highly specific test, while $LR^- < 0.1$ indicates a highly sensitive test. Pretest odds × LR = posttest odds. Posttest probability = posttest odds / (posttest odds + 1).

Kaplan-Meier curve	Used to estimate probability of survival over time. Graphic representation shows the survival probabilities (y-axis) vs length of time (x-axis). Useful for displaying "time-to-event" data. Outcomes examined may include any event, but frequently include mortality. Survival probability = 1 – (event probability). P value for the survival difference can be calculated using log rank test or Cox regression.	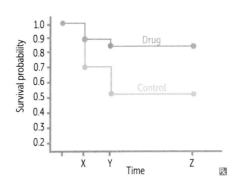

| **Evaluation of diagnostic tests** | Sensitivity and specificity are fixed properties of a test. PPV and NPV vary depending on disease prevalence in population being tested. Test efficiency = $(TP + TN)/(TP + FN + FP + TN)$ | 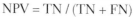 |

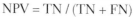

Sensitivity (true-positive rate)	Proportion of all people with disease who test positive, or the ability of a test to correctly identify those with the disease. Value approaching 100% is desirable for **ruling out** disease and indicates a **low false-negative rate**.	$= TP / (TP + FN)$ $= 1 - FN$ rate **SN-N-OUT** = highly **SeN**sitive test, when Negative, rules **OUT** disease High sensitivity test used for screening
Specificity (true-negative rate)	Proportion of all people without disease who test negative, or the ability of a test to correctly identify those without the disease. Value approaching 100% is desirable for **ruling in** disease and indicates a **low false-positive rate**.	$= TN / (TN + FP)$ $= 1 - FP$ rate **SP-P-IN** = highly **SP**ecific test, when Positive, rules **IN** disease High specificity test used for confirmation after a positive screening test
Positive predictive value	Probability that a person who has a positive test result actually has the disease.	PPV = $TP / (TP + FP)$ PPV varies directly with pretest probability (baseline risk, such as prevalence of disease): high pretest probability → high PPV
Negative predictive value	Probability that a person with a negative test result actually does not have the disease.	NPV = $TN / (TN + FN)$ NPV varies inversely with prevalence or pretest probability

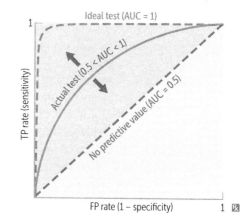

Possible cutoff values for ⊕ vs ⊖ test result
A = 100% sensitivity cutoff value
B = practical compromise between specificity and sensitivity
C = 100% specificity cutoff value

| Lowering the cutoff value:
B → A (↑ FP ↓ FN) | ↑ Sensitivity ↑ NPV
↓ Specificity ↓ PPV |
| Raising the cutoff value:
B → C (↑ FN ↓ FP) | ↑ Specificity ↑ PPV
↓ Sensitivity ↓ NPV |

Note: In diseases where diagnosis is based on lower values (eg, anemia), the TP and TN are switched in the graph, ie, ↓ sensitivity and ↓ NPV, and vice-versa.

| **Receiver operating characteristic curve** | ROC curve demonstrates how well a diagnostic test can distinguish between 2 groups (eg, disease vs healthy). Plots the true-positive rate (sensitivity) against the false-positive rate (1 − specificity). The better performing test will have a higher area under the curve (AUC), with the curve closer to the upper left corner. | |

Precision vs accuracy

Precision (reliability)	The consistency and reproducibility of a test. The absence of random variation in a test.	Random error ↓ precision in a test. ↑ precision → ↓ standard deviation. ↑ precision → ↑ statistical power (1 − β).
Accuracy (validity)	The closeness of test results to the true values. The absence of systematic error or bias in a test.	Systematic error ↓ accuracy in a test.

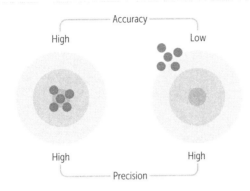

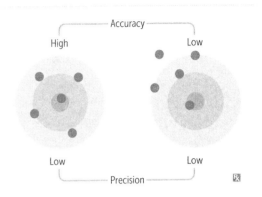

Incidence vs prevalence

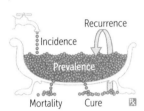

$$\text{Incidence} = \frac{\text{\# of new cases}}{\text{\# of people at risk}} \quad \text{(per unit of time)}$$

$$\text{Prevalence} = \frac{\text{\# of existing cases}}{\text{Total \# of people in a population}} \quad \begin{array}{c}\text{(at a point in}\\ \text{time)}\end{array}$$

$$\frac{\text{Prevalence}}{1 - \text{prevalence}} = \text{Incidence rate} \times \begin{array}{c}\text{average duration}\\ \text{of disease}\end{array}$$

Prevalence = incidence × duration of the disease.
Prevalence > incidence for chronic diseases, due to large # of existing cases (eg, diabetes).

Incidence looks at new cases (incidents).

Prevalence looks at all current cases.

Prevalence ~ pretest probability.
↑ prevalence → ↑ PPV and ↓ NPV.
Prevalence ≈ incidence for short duration disease (eg, common cold).

SITUATION	INCIDENCE	PREVALENCE
↑ survival time	—	↑
↑ mortality rate	—	↓
Faster recovery time	—	↓
Extensive vaccine administration	↓	↓
↓ risk factors	↓	↓
↑ diagnostic sensitivity	↑	↑
New effective treatment started	—	↓
↓ contact between infected and noninfected patients with airborne infectious disease	↓	↓

Bias and study errors

TYPE	DEFINITION	EXAMPLES	STRATEGIES TO REDUCE BIAS
Recruiting participants			
Selection bias	Nonrandom sampling or treatment allocation of subjects such that study population is not representative of target population Most commonly a sampling bias Convenience sampling—patients are enrolled on basis of ease of contact	Berkson bias—cases and/or controls selected from hospitals (**bedside bias**) are less healthy and have different exposures Attrition bias—participants lost to follow up have a different prognosis than those who complete the study	Randomization (creates groups with similar distributions of known and unknown variables) Ensure the choice of the right comparison/reference group
Performing study			
Recall bias	Awareness of disorder alters recall by subjects; common in retrospective studies	Patients with disease recall exposure after learning of similar cases	Decrease time from exposure to follow-up; use medical records as sources
Measurement bias	Information is gathered in a systemically distorted manner	Using a faulty automatic sphygmomanometer Hawthorne effect—participants change behavior upon awareness of being **observed** (**Haw**thorne **watches** you like a **hawk**).	Use objective, standardized, and previously tested methods of data collection that are planned ahead of time Use placebo group
Procedure bias	Subjects in different groups are not treated the same	Patients in treatment group spend more time in highly specialized hospital units	Blinding (masking) and use of placebo reduce influence of participants and researchers on procedures and interpretation of outcomes as neither are aware of group assignments
Observer-expectancy bias	Researcher's belief in the efficacy of a treatment changes the outcome of that treatment (also called Pygmalion effect)	An observer expecting treatment group to show signs of recovery is more likely to document positive outcomes	
Interpreting results			
Lead-time bias	Early detection interpreted as ↑ survival, but the disease course has not changed	Breast cancer diagnosed early by mammography may appear to exaggerate survival time because patients are known to have the cancer for longer	Measure "back-end" survival (adjust survival according to the severity of disease at the time of diagnosis); a caveat of adjusting for severity is the potential masking of causality
Length-time bias	Screening test detects diseases with long latency period, while those with shorter latency period become symptomatic earlier	A slowly progressive cancer is more likely detected by a screening test than a rapidly progressive cancer	A randomized controlled trial assigning subjects to the screening program or to no screening

Confounding vs effect modification

TYPE	DEFINITION	EXAMPLES	STRATEGIES TO REDUCE BIAS
Confounding	Factor related to **both exposure and outcome** (not on a causal pathway) distorts the effect on the outcome No association after stratification	Coffee appears to be linked to lung cancer, but smoking is the true cause, as coffee drinkers tend to smoke more	Crossover studies (subject serves as self-control) Matching (patients with similar characteristics in both treatment and control groups) Analytic techniques (eg, regression analysis when confounding variables are known and were measured)
Effect modification	Exposure leads to different outcomes in subgroups stratified by factor True association exists	A study among women using OCPs showed significant risk of DVT, but when these data were stratified by smoking habits, there was a very strong association between OCP use and DVT among smokers, but there was no such association in people who do not smoke	Stratified analysis (eg, after testing for interaction between OCP and smoking, analyze risk among smokers and nonsmokers)

Confounding

Crude analysis

Drinking coffee ⟶ Lung cancer

Stratified analysis

Smokers Drinking coffee ⟶ Lung cancer

Nonsmokers Drinking coffee ⤍ Lung cancer

Note: Association disappeared after stratification.

Effect modification

Crude analysis

OCP use ⟶ DVT

Stratified analysis

Smokers OCP use ⟶ DVT

Nonsmokers OCP use ⤍ DVT

Note: Association was strong in one subgroup with weak/no association in the other subgroup.

⟶ Strong association

⟶ Significant association

⤍ Weak/no association

Statistical distribution

Measures of central tendency	Mean = (sum of values)/(total number of values).	Most affected by outliers (extreme values).
	Median = middle value of a list of data sorted from least to greatest.	If there is an even number of values, the median will be the average of the middle two values.
	Mode = most common value.	Least affected by outliers.
Measures of dispersion	Standard deviation = how much variability exists in a set of values, around the mean of these values. Standard error = an estimate of how much variability exists in a (theoretical) set of sample means around the true population mean.	σ = SD; n = sample size. Variance = $(SD)^2$. SE = $\sigma/\sqrt{n}$. SE ↓ as n ↑.
Normal distribution	Gaussian, also called bell-shaped. Mean = median = mode. For normal distribution, mean is the best measure of central tendency. For skewed data, median is a better measure of central tendency than mean.	

Nonnormal distributions

Bimodal distribution	Suggests two different populations (eg, metabolic polymorphism such as fast vs slow acetylators; age at onset of Hodgkin lymphoma; suicide rate by age).	
Positive skew	Typically, mean > median > mode. Asymmetry with longer tail on right; mean falls closer to tail.	
Negative skew	Typically, mean < median < mode. Asymmetry with longer tail on left; mean falls closer to tail.	

Statistical hypothesis testing

Null hypothesis	Also called H_0. Hypothesis with no difference or association (eg, there is **zero** association between disease and risk factor in the population).
Alternative hypothesis	Also called H_1. Hypothesis with at least **one** difference or relationship (eg, there is some association between disease and risk factor in the population).
P **value**	Probability of obtaining test results at least as extreme as those observed in the sample, assuming that H_0 is correct. Commonly accepted as 0.05 (< 5% of such repeated tests would show results that extreme just by chance alone).

Outcomes of statistical hypothesis testing

Correct result	Stating that there is an effect or difference when one exists (H_0 rejected in favor of H_1). Stating that there is no effect or difference when none exists (H_0 not rejected).	

	Reality	
	H_1	H_0
Study rejects H_0	Power $(1 - \beta)$	α Type I error
Study does not reject H_0	β Type II error	

Blue shading = correct result.

Testing errors

Type I error (α)	Stating that there is an effect or difference when none exists (H_0 incorrectly rejected in favor of H_1). α is the probability of making a type I error (usually 0.05 is chosen). If $P < \alpha$, then assuming H_0 is true, the probability of obtaining the test results would be less than the probability of making a type I error. H_0 is therefore rejected as false. Statistical significance $\neq$ clinical significance.	Also called false-positive error. 1st time boy cries wolf, the town believes there is a wolf, but there is not (false positive). You can never "prove" H_1, but you can reject the H_0 as being very unlikely.
Type II error (β)	Stating that there is not an effect or difference when one exists (H_0 is not rejected when it is in fact false). β is the probability of making a type II error. β is related to statistical power $(1 - \beta)$, which is the probability of rejecting H_0 when it is false. ↑ power and ↓ β by: <ul><li>↑ sample size</li><li>↑ expected effect size</li><li>↑ precision of measurement</li><li>↑ α level (↑ statistical significance level).</li></ul>	Also called false-negative error. 2nd time boy cries wolf, the town believes there is no wolf, but there is one. If you ↑ sample size, you ↑ power. There is **power in numbers**. Generally, when type I error increases, type II error decreases.

Statistical vs clinical significance	Statistical significance—defined by the likelihood of study results being due to chance. If there is a high statistical significance, then there is a low probability that the results are due to chance. Clinical significance—measure of effect on treatment outcomes. An intervention with high clinical significance is likely to have a large impact on patient outcomes/measures. Some studies have a very high statistical significance, but the proposed intervention may have limited clinical impact/significance, eg, a study might show a statistical significance of lowered blood sugar levels by 1 mg/dL correlated with better outcomes, but this may not be clinically as important.

Confidence interval	Range of values within which the true mean of the population is expected to fall, with a specified probability. $CI = 1 - \alpha$. The 95% CI (corresponding to $\alpha = 0.05$) is often used. As sample size increases, CI narrows. CI for sample mean $= \bar{x} \pm Z(SE)$ For the 95% CI, $Z = 1.96$. For the 99% CI, $Z = 2.58$.	H_0 is rejected (and results are significant) when: • 95% CI for mean difference excludes 0 • 95% CI OR or RR excludes 1 • CIs between two groups do not overlap H_0 is not rejected (and results are not significant) when: • 95% CI for mean difference includes 0 • 95% CI OR or RR includes 1 • CIs between two groups do overlap

Meta-analysis	A method of statistical analysis that pools summary data (eg, means, RRs) from multiple studies for a more precise estimate of the size of an effect. Also estimates heterogeneity of effect sizes between studies. Improves power, strength of evidence, and generalizability (external validity) of study findings. Limited by quality of individual studies and bias in study selection.

Common statistical tests

t-test	Checks differences between **means** of 2 groups.	Tea is **meant** for 2. Example: comparing the mean blood pressure between men and women.
ANOVA	Checks differences between means of 3 or more groups.	3 words: **AN**alysis **O**f **VA**riance. Example: comparing the mean blood pressure between members of 3 different ethnic groups.
Chi-square (χ^2)	Checks differences between 2 or more percentages or proportions of **categorical** outcomes (not mean values).	Pronounce **chi-tegorical**. Example: comparing the proportion of members of 3 age groups who have essential hypertension.
Fisher's exact test	Checks differences between 2 percentages or proportions of categorical, nominal outcomes. Use instead of chi-square test with small samples.	Example: comparing the percentage of 20 men and 20 women with hypertension.

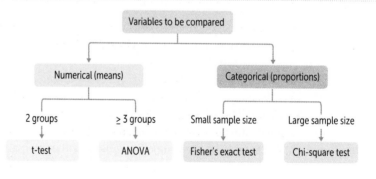

Pearson correlation coefficient	A measure of the linear correlation between two variables. r is always between -1 and $+1$. The closer the absolute value of r is to 1, the stronger the linear correlation between the 2 variables. Variance is how much the measured values differ from the average value in a data set. Positive r value → positive correlation (as one variable ↑, the other variable ↑). Negative r value → negative correlation (as one variable ↑, the other variable ↓). Coefficient of determination = r^2 (proportion of variance in one variable that can be explained by variance in the other variable). Correlation does not necessarily imply causation.

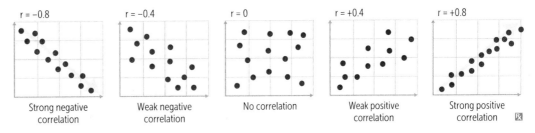

▸ PUBLIC HEALTH SCIENCES—ETHICS

Core ethical principles

Autonomy	Obligation to respect patients as individuals (truth-telling, confidentiality), to create conditions necessary for autonomous choice (informed consent), and to honor their preference in accepting or not accepting medical care.
Beneficence	"Do good." Physicians have a special ethical (fiduciary) duty to act in the patient's best interest. May conflict with autonomy (an informed patient has the right to decide) or what is best for society (eg, mandatory TB treatment). Traditionally, patient interest supersedes. Principle of double effect—facilitating comfort is prioritized over potential side effects (eg, respiratory depression with opioid use) for patients receiving end-of-life care.
Nonmaleficence	"Do no harm." Must be balanced against beneficence; if the benefits outweigh the risks, a patient may make an informed decision to proceed (most surgeries and medications fall into this category).
Justice	To treat persons fairly and equitably. This does not always imply equally (eg, triage).

Decision-making capacity	Physician must determine whether the patient is psychologically and legally capable of making a particular healthcare decision. Note that decisions made with capacity cannot be revoked simply if the patient later loses capacity. Intellectual disabilities and mental illnesses are not exclusion criteria unless the patient's condition presently impairs their ability to make healthcare decisions. Capacity is determined by a physician for a specific healthcare-related decision (eg, to refuse medical care). Competency is determined by a judge and usually refers to more global categories of decision-making (eg, legally unable to make any healthcare-related decision).	Four major components of decision-making: ▪ Understanding (what do you know about your condition/proposed procedure/ treatment?) ▪ Appreciation (what does your condition mean to you? why do you think your doctor is recommending this course of treatment?) ▪ Reasoning (how are you weighing your options?) ▪ Expressing a choice (what would you like to do?)

Informed consent	A process (not just a document/signature) that requires:
	  ▪ Disclosure: discussion of pertinent information, including risks/benefits (using medical interpreter, if needed)
	  ▪ Understanding: ability to comprehend
	  ▪ Capacity: ability to reason and make one's own decisions (distinct from competence, a legal determination)
	  ▪ Voluntariness: freedom from coercion and manipulation
	Patients must have a comprehensive understanding of their diagnosis and the risks/benefits of proposed treatment and alternative options, including no treatment.
	Patients must be informed of their right to revoke written consent at any time, even orally.
		Exceptions to informed consent (**WIPE** it away):
		  ▪ **W**aiver—patient explicitly relinquishes the right of informed consent
		  ▪ Legally **I**ncompetent—patient lacks decision-making capacity (obtain consent from legal surrogate)
		  ▪ Therapeutic **P**rivilege—withholding information when disclosure would severely harm the patient or undermine informed decision-making capacity
		  ▪ **E**mergency situation—implied consent may apply

Consent for minors	A minor is generally any person < 18 years old. Parental consent laws in relation to healthcare vary by state. In general, parental consent should be obtained, but exceptions exist for emergency treatment (eg, blood transfusions) or if minor is legally emancipated (eg, married, self-supporting, or in the military).	Situations in which parental consent is usually not required:
		  ▪ **Sex** (contraception, STIs, prenatal care—usually not abortion)
		  ▪ **Drugs** (substance use disorder treatment)
		  ▪ **Rock and roll** (emergency/trauma)
		Physicians should always encourage healthy minor-guardian communication.
		Physician should seek a minor's assent (agreement of someone unable to legally consent) even if their consent is not required.

Advance directives	Instructions given by a patient in anticipation of the need for a medical decision. Details vary per state law.	
Oral advance directive	Incapacitated patient's prior oral statements commonly used as guide. Problems arise from variance in interpretation. If patient was informed, directive was specific, patient made a choice, and decision was repeated over time to multiple people, then the oral directive is more valid.	
Written advance directive	Delineates specific healthcare interventions that patient anticipates accepting or rejecting during treatment for a critical or life-threatening illness. A living will is an example.	
Medical power of attorney	Patient designates an agent to make medical decisions in the event that the patient loses decision-making capacity. Patient may also specify decisions in clinical situations. Can be revoked by patient if decision-making capacity is intact. More flexible than a living will.	
Do not resuscitate order	DNR order prohibits cardiopulmonary resuscitation (CPR). Patient may still consider other life-sustaining measures (eg, intubation, feeding tube, chemotherapy).	

Ventilator-assisted life support	Ideally, discussions with patients occur before ventilator support is necessary. However, information about patient preferences may be absent at the time patients require this intervention to survive. Medical decision-making frequently relies on surrogate decision-makers (patient identified or legally appointed) when discussing the continuation or withdrawal of ventilatory support, focusing on both the prognosis of the condition and the believed wishes of the patient. If surrogates indicate patient would not have wanted to receive life support with ventilation → withhold or withdraw life support regardless of what the surrogate prefers. If the decision is made to withhold or withdraw life support, involve palliative care, chaplain services, and the primary care physician in medical discussions with the family and provide emotional support.
Surrogate decision-maker	If a patient loses decision-making capacity and has not prepared an advance directive, individuals (surrogates) who know the patient must determine what the patient would have done. Priority of surrogates: **spouse** → adult **children** → **parents** → adult **siblings** → other **relatives** (the **spouse chips** in).
Confidentiality	Confidentiality respects patient privacy and autonomy. If the patient is incapacitated or the situation is emergent, disclosing information to family and friends should be guided by professional judgment of patient's best interest. The patient may voluntarily waive the right to confidentiality (eg, insurance company request). General principles for exceptions to confidentiality: ▪ Potential physical harm to self or others is serious and imminent ▪ Alternative means to warn or protect those at risk is not possible ▪ Steps can be taken to prevent harm Examples of exceptions to patient confidentiality (many are state specific) include the following ("The physician's good judgment **SAVED** the day"): ▪ Patients with active **S**uicidal/homicidal ideation ▪ **A**buse (children, older adults, and/or prisoners) ▪ Duty to protect—state-specific laws that sometimes allow physician to inform or somehow protect potential **V**ictim from harm ▪ Patients with **E**pilepsy and other impaired automobile drivers ▪ Reportable **D**iseases (eg, STIs, hepatitis, food poisoning); physicians may have a duty to warn public officials, who will then notify people at risk. Dangerous communicable diseases, such as TB or Ebola, may require involuntary treatment.
Accepting gifts from patients	A complex subject without definitive regulations. Some argue that the patient-physician relationship is strengthened through accepting a gift from a patient, while others argue that negative consequences outweigh the benefits of accepting any gift. In practice, patients often present items such as cards, baked goods, and inexpensive gifts to physicians. The physician's decision to accept or decline is based on an individual assessment of whether or not the risk of harm outweighs the potential benefit. ▪ Physicians should not accept gifts that are inappropriately large or valuable. ▪ Gifts should not be accepted if the physician identifies that the gift could detrimentally affect patient care. ▪ Gifts that may cause emotional or financial stress for the patient should not be accepted. If a gift violates any of the guidelines above, the best practice is to thank the patient for offering a kind gift, but politely indicate that it must be declined. During this conversation it should be emphasized that the incident does not influence the physician-patient relationship in any way.

▶ PUBLIC HEALTH SCIENCES—COMMUNICATION SKILLS

Patient-centered interviewing techniques

Introduction	Introduce yourself and ask the patient their name and how they would like to be addressed. Address the patient by the name and pronouns given. Avoid making gender assumptions. Sit at eye level, near the patient, while facing them directly.
Agenda setting	Identify concerns and set goals by developing joint agenda between the physician and the patient.
Reflection	Actively listen and synthesize information offered by the patient, particularly with respect to primary concern(s).
Validation	Legitimize or affirm the patient's perspectives.
Recapitulation	Summarize what the patient has said so far to ensure correct interpretation.
Facilitation	Encourage the patient to speak freely without guiding responses or leading questions. Allow the patient to ask questions throughout the encounter.

Establishing rapport — PEARLS

Partnership	Work together with patient to identify primary concerns and develop preferred solutions.
Empathy	Acknowledge the emotions displayed and demonstrate understanding of why the patient is feeling that way.
Apology	Take personal responsibility when appropriate.
Respect	Commend the patient for coming in to discuss a problem, pushing through challenging circumstances, keeping a positive attitude, or other constructive behaviors.
Legitimization	Assure patient that emotional responses are understandable or common.
Support	Reassure patient that you will work together through difficult times and offer appropriate resources.

Delivering bad news — SPIKES

Setting	Offer in advance for the patient to bring support. Eliminate distractions, ensure privacy, and sit down with the patient to talk.
Perception	Determine the patient's understanding and expectations of the situation.
Invitation	Obtain the patient's permission to disclose the news and what level of detail is desired.
Knowledge	Share the information in small pieces without medical jargon, allowing time to process. Assess the patient's understanding.
Emotions	Acknowledge the patient's emotions, and provide opportunity to express them. Listen and offer empathetic responses.
Strategy	If the patient feels ready, discuss treatment options and goals of care. Offer an agenda for the next appointment. Giving control to the patient may be empowering. Ask how they feel a problem might be solved and what they would like to do about the plan of action.

Gender- and sexuality-inclusive history taking	Avoid making assumptions about sexual orientation, gender identity, gender expression, and behavior (eg, a patient who identifies as heterosexual may engage in same-sex sexual activity).
	Use gender-neutral terms when referring to the patient or the patient's family (eg, "partner" rather than "husband" or "wife") upon first meeting the patient until the patient instructs otherwise or uses specific pronouns. A patient's assigned sex at birth and gender identity may differ. Do not bring up gender or sexuality if it is not relevant to the visit (eg, a gender-nonconforming patient seeking care for a hand laceration).
	Consider stating what pronouns you use when you introduce yourself (eg, "I'm Dr. Smith, and I use she/her pronouns") and asking patients how they would like to be addressed. Also consider ways of being inclusive (eg, ensuring correct name and pronouns are in the electronic medical record).
	Reassure them about the confidentiality of their visits and be sensitive to the fact that patients may not be open about their sexual orientation or gender identity to others in their life.
	Remember: trust is built over time, and listening to and learning from patients about how they would like to approach the topics discussed above is key.
Cultural formulation interview	Identify the problem through the patient's perspective. Ask the patient to describe the problem in their own words, or how the patient would describe the problem to their family and friends.
	Identify cultural perceptions of factors leading to a problem. Ask the patient to explain why they think they are experiencing their problem.
	Identify how the patient's background influences their problem. Ask the patient about what makes their problem better or worse. Investigate roles of family, community, and spirituality.
	Identify how culture may impact current and future interventions. Ask the patient if they have any concerns or suggestions about the current plan of treatment. If they do not want to follow medical advice, investigate if there is a way to combine their plans with the standard medical regimen.
	Identify possible barriers to care based on culture. Ask the patient if there is anything that would prevent them from seeking care in a standard medical institution. Probe for explanations and what may increase the chance of maintaining a good patient-physician relationship.
Motivational interviewing	Counseling technique to facilitate behavior modification by helping patients resolve ambivalence about change. Useful for many conditions (eg, nicotine dependence, obesity). Helpful when patient has some desire to change, but it does not require that the patient be committed to making the change. May involve asking patients to examine how their behavior interferes with their life or why they might want to change it. Assess barriers (eg, food access, untreated trauma) that may make behavior change difficult.
	Assessing a patient's readiness for change is also important for guiding physician-suggested goals. These goals should be **S**pecific, **M**easurable, **A**chievable, **R**elevant, and **T**ime bound (**SMART**).
Trauma-informed care	Patients with history of psychological trauma should receive thorough behavioral health screenings. Regularly assess mood, substance use, social supports, and suicide risk.
	Focus assessments on trauma-related symptoms that interfere with social and occupational function. Always be empathetic. Do not ask invasive questions requiring the patient to describe trauma in detail. Ask permission prior to discussion.
	Before the physical exam, reassure patients that they may signal to end it immediately if they experience too much physical or emotional discomfort. Offer the presence of additional staff for support. Psychological counseling may be indicated. Follow-up counseling is offered (or advised) as appropriate. Remember **4 R's**: **R**ealize, **R**ecognize, **R**espond, **R**esist retraumatization.

Challenging patient and ethical scenarios

The most appropriate response is usually one that is patient-centered, open-ended, and empathetic; acknowledges the obstacles in care; and validates emotions. It often honors one or more of the principles of autonomy, beneficence, nonmaleficence, and justice. Appropriate responses are respectful of patients and other members of the healthcare team. Consider the patient's point of view.

SITUATION	APPROPRIATE RESPONSE
Patient does not follow the medical plan.	Determine whether there are financial, logistical, or other obstacles preventing the patient's adherence. Do not coerce the patient into adhering or refer the patient to another physician. Schedule regular follow-up visits to track patient progress.
Patient desires an unnecessary procedure.	Attempt to understand why the patient wants the procedure and address underlying concerns. Do not refuse to see the patient or refer to another physician. Avoid performing unnecessary procedures.
Patient has difficulty taking medications.	Determine what factors are involved in the patient's difficulties. If comprehension or memory are issues, use techniques such as providing written instructions, using the teach-back method, or simplifying treatment regimens.
Family members ask for information about patient's prognosis.	Avoid discussing issues with relatives without the patient's permission.
A patient's family member asks you not to disclose the results of a test if the prognosis is poor because the patient will be "unable to handle it."	Explore why the family member believes this would be detrimental, including possible cultural factors. Explain that if the patient would like to know information concerning care, it will not be withheld. However, if you believe the patient might seriously harm self or others if informed, you may invoke therapeutic privilege and withhold the information.
A 17-year-old is pregnant and requests an abortion.	Many states require parental notification or consent for minors for an abortion. Unless there are specific medical risks associated with pregnancy, a physician should not sway the patient's decision for, or against, an elective abortion (regardless of patient's age or fetal condition). Discuss options for terminating the pregnancy and refer to abortion care, if needed.
A 15-year-old is pregnant and wants to raise the child. The patient's parents want you to tell the patient to give the child up for adoption.	The patient retains the right to make decisions regarding the child, even if the patient's parents disagree. Provide information to the teenager about the practical aspects of caring for a baby. Discuss options for terminating the pregnancy, if requested. Encourage discussion between the patient and parents to reach the best decision.
A terminally ill patient requests physician-assisted dying.	The overwhelming majority of states prohibit most forms of physician-assisted dying. Physicians may, however, prescribe medically appropriate analgesics even if they potentially shorten the patient's life.
Patient is suicidal.	Assess the seriousness of the threat. If patient is actively suicidal with a plan, suggest remaining in the hospital voluntarily; patient may be hospitalized involuntarily if needed.
Patient states that you are attractive and asks if you would go on a date.	Use a chaperone if necessary. Romantic relationships with patients are never appropriate. Set firm professional boundaries with direct communication. Transition care to another physician if necessary.
A woman who had a mastectomy says she now feels "ugly."	Find out why the patient feels this way. Do not offer falsely reassuring statements (eg, "You still look good").
Patient is angry about the long time spent in the waiting room.	Acknowledge the patient's anger, but do not take a patient's anger personally. Thank the patient for being patient and apologize for any inconvenience. Stay away from efforts to explain the delay.
Patient is upset with treatment received from another physician.	Suggest that the patient speak directly to that physician regarding the concern. If the problem is with a member of the office staff, reassure the patient you will speak to that person.

Challenging patient and ethical scenarios *(continued)*

SITUATION	APPROPRIATE RESPONSE
An invasive test is performed on the wrong patient.	Regardless of the outcome, a physician is ethically obligated to inform a patient that a mistake has been made.
A patient requires a treatment not covered by insurance.	Discuss all treatment options with patients, even if some are not covered by their insurance companies. Inform patient of financial assistance programs.
A 7-year-old boy loses a sister to cancer and now feels responsible.	At ages 5–7, children begin to understand that death is permanent, all life functions end completely at death, and everything that is alive eventually dies. Provide a direct, concrete description of his sister's death. Avoid clichés and euphemisms. Reassure the boy that he is not responsible. Identify and normalize fears and feelings. Encourage play and healthy coping behaviors (eg, remembering her in his own way).
Patient is victim of intimate partner violence.	Ask if patient is safe and help devise an emergency plan if there isn't one. Ask patient direct, open-ended questions about exam findings and summarize patient's answers back to them. Ask if patient has any questions. Do not necessarily pressure patient to leave a partner or disclose the incident to the authorities (unless required by state law).
Patient wants to try alternative or holistic medicine.	Explore any underlying reasons with the patient in a supportive, nonjudgmental manner. Advise the patient of known benefits and risks of treatment, including adverse effects, contraindications, and medication interactions. Consider referral to an appropriate complementary or alternative medicine provider.
Physician colleague presents to work impaired.	This presents a potential risk to patient safety. You have an ethical and usually a legal obligation to report impaired colleagues so they can cease patient care and receive appropriate assistance in a timely manner. Seek guidance in reporting as procedures and applicable law vary by institution and state.
Patient's family insists on maintaining life support after brain death has occurred, citing patient's movements when touched.	Gently explain to family that there is no chance of recovery, and that brain death is equivalent to death. Movement is due to spinal arc reflex and is not voluntary. Bring case to appropriate ethics board regarding futility of care and withdrawal of life support.
A pharmaceutical company offers you a sponsorship in exchange for advertising its new drug.	Reject this offer. Generally, decline gifts and sponsorships to avoid any conflict of interest. The AMA Code of Ethics does make exceptions for gifts directly benefitting patients; special funding for medical education of students, residents, fellows; grants whose recipients are chosen by independent institutional criteria; and funds that are distributed without attribution to sponsors.
Patient requests a nonemergent procedure that is against your personal or religious beliefs.	Provide accurate and unbiased information so patients can make an informed decision. In a neutral, nonjudgmental manner, explain to the patient that you do not perform the procedure but offer to refer to another physician.
Mother and 15-year-old daughter are unresponsive and bleeding heavily, but father refuses transfusion because they are Jehovah's Witnesses.	Transfuse daughter, but do not transfuse mother. Emergent care can be refused by the healthcare proxy for an adult, particularly when patient preferences are known or reasonably inferred, but not for a minor based solely on faith.
A dependent patient presents with injuries inconsistent with caretaker's story.	Document detailed history and physical. If possible and appropriate, interview the patient alone. Provide any necessary medical care. If suspicion remains, contact the appropriate agencies or authorities (eg, child or adult protective services) for an evaluation. Inform the caretaker of your obligation to report. Physicians are required by law to report any reasonable suspicion of abuse, neglect, or endangerment.
A pediatrician recommends standard vaccinations for a patient, but the child's parent refuses.	Address any concerns the parent has. Explain the risks and benefits of vaccinations and why they are recommended. Do not administer routine vaccinations without the parent's consent.

Communicating with patients with disabilities	Patients may identify with person-first (ie, "a person with a disability") or identity-first (ie, "a disabled person") language. Ask patients what terms they use.
	Under most circumstances, talk directly to the patient. Do not assume that nonverbal patients do not understand. Accompanying caregivers can add information to any discussion as needed.
	Ask if assistance is desired rather than assuming the patient cannot do something alone. Most people, including people with disabilities, value their independence.
	For patients with speech difficulties, provide extra time for the interview. If their speech is difficult to understand, consider asking them to write down a few words or ask them to rephrase their sentence. Repeat what they said to ensure you understood it correctly.
	For patients with a cognitive impairment, use concrete, specific language. Ask simple, direct questions. Eliminate background noise and distractions. Do not assume the patient can read. Adjust to how the patient understands best (eg, use hand gestures or ask them to demonstrate a task).
	Ask patients who are deaf or hard of hearing their preferred mode of communication. Use light touch or waving to get their attention. For patients who prefer to speak and lipread, eliminate background noise, face the patient, and do not change your mode of speaking. Consider using an interpreter when necessary.
	As with other parts of a medical history, do not bring up a disability if it is not relevant to a visit (eg, a patient in a wheelchair with an ear infection). Do not skip relevant parts of the physical exam even if the disability makes the exam challenging.
Use of interpreters	Visits with a patient who speaks little English should utilize a professionally trained medical interpreter unless the physician is conversationally fluent in the patient's preferred language. If an interpreter is unavailable in person, interpretation services may be provided by telephone or video call. If the patient prefers to utilize a family member, this should be recorded in the chart.
	Do not assume that a patient is a poor English speaker because of name, skin tone, or accent. Ask the patient what language is preferred.
	The physician should make eye contact with the patient and speak to them directly, without use of third-person statements such as "tell him."
	Allow extra time for the interview, and ask one question at a time.
	For in-person spoken language interpretation, the interpreter should ideally be next to or slightly behind the patient. For sign language interpretation, the interpreter should be next to or slightly behind the physician.
	In cases of emergency, facilitate communication by any tools available (eg, friends, family, sketches, interpreter apps) even though they do not comprise standard procedure otherwise.

▶ PUBLIC HEALTH SCIENCES—HEALTHCARE DELIVERY

Disease prevention

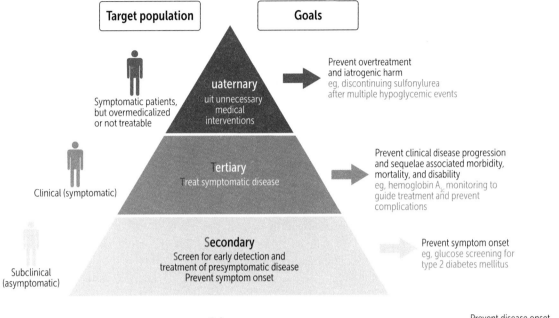

Target population		Goals
Symptomatic patients, but overmedicalized or not treatable	**uaternary** uit unnecessary medical interventions	Prevent overtreatment and iatrogenic harm eg, discontinuing sulfonylurea after multiple hypoglycemic events
Clinical (symptomatic)	**Tertiary** Treat symptomatic disease	Prevent clinical disease progression and sequelae associated morbidity, mortality, and disability eg, hemoglobin A$_{1c}$ monitoring to guide treatment and prevent complications
Subclinical (asymptomatic)	**Secondary** Screen for early detection and treatment of presymptomatic disease Prevent symptom onset	Prevent symptom onset eg, glucose screening for type 2 diabetes mellitus
Susceptible/general population	**Primary** Prevent disease onset by reducing risks or increasing immunity	Prevent disease onset eg, healthy diet and exercise to prevent diabetes

Major medical insurance plans

Exclusive provider organization (EPO)	Requires in-network care; out-of-network coverage available for emergencies.
Health maintenance organization (HMO)	Lower premiums, limited to in-network providers, requires primary care referral for specialists, lower out-of-pocket cost.
Point of service (PoS)	Combination of HMO and PPO, allows out-of-network care at higher cost, and requires primary care referrals.
Preferred provider organization (PPO)	Flexibility with in-network and out-of-network care, higher cost for out-of-network services, no referral requirement.
Accountable care organization (ACO)	Group of providers who voluntarily coordinate care for Medicare patients.
High deductible health plan (HDHP)	Low premiums, high out-of-pocket cost, compatible with health savings account (HSA).

Healthcare payment models

Bundled payment	Healthcare organization receives a set amount per service, regardless of ultimate cost, to be divided among all providers and facilities involved.
Capitation	Physicians receive a set amount per patient assigned to them per period of time, regardless of how much the patient uses the healthcare system. Used by some HMOs.
Discounted fee-for-service	Insurer and/or patient pays for each individual service at a discounted rate predetermined by providers and payers (eg, PPOs).
Fee-for-service	Insurer and/or patient pays for each individual service.
Global payment	Insurer and/or patient pays for all expenses associated with a single incident of care with a single payment. Most commonly used during elective surgeries, as it covers the cost of surgery as well as the necessary pre- and postoperative visits.

Medicare and Medicaid	Medicare and Medicaid—federal social healthcare programs that originated from amendments to the Social Security Act. Medicare is available to patients ≥ 65 years old, < 65 with certain disabilities, and those with end-stage renal disease. Medicaid is joint federal and state health assistance for people with limited income and/or resources.	MedicarE is for Elderly. MedicaiD is for Disadvantaged. The 4 parts of Medicare: ▪ Part **A**: hospital **A**dmissions, including hospice, skilled nursing ▪ Part **B**: **B**asic medical bills (eg, physician fees, diagnostic testing) ▪ Part **C**: (parts A + B = **C**ombo) delivered by approved private companies ▪ Part **D**: prescription **D**rugs

Palliative care	Medical care aiming to provide comfort, relieve suffering, and improve quality of life in patients with complex or life-threatening illness regardless of their diagnosis or prognosis. Often concurrent with curative or life-prolonging treatment. Delivered by interdisciplinary team (eg, physicians, nurses, social workers) in hospitals, outpatient clinics, or at home. Hospice care (end-of-life care)—form of palliative care for patients with prognosis ≤ 6 months when curative or life-prolonging treatment is no longer wanted or beneficial.

Types of medical errors	May involve patient identification, diagnosis, monitoring, healthcare-associated infection, medications, procedures, devices, documentation, handoffs. Medical errors should be disclosed to patients, independent of immediate outcome (harmful or not).	
Active error	Occurs at level of frontline operator (eg, wrong IV pump dose programmed).	Immediate impact.
Latent error	Occurs in processes indirect from operator but impacts patient care (eg, different types of IV pumps used within same hospital).	Accident waiting to happen.
Never event	Adverse event that is identifiable, serious, and usually preventable (eg, scalpel retained in a surgical patient's abdomen).	Major error that should never occur. Sentinel event—a never event that leads to death, permanent harm, or severe temporary harm.
Near miss	Unplanned event that does not result in harm but has the potential to do so (eg, pharmacist recognizes a medication interaction and cancels the order).	Narrow prevention of harm that exposes dangers.

Medical error analysis

	DESIGN	METHODS
Root cause analysis	Retrospective approach. Applied after failure event to prevent recurrence.	Uses records and participant interviews (eg, 5 whys approach, fishbone/cause-and-effect diagrams, process maps) to identify all the underlying problems (eg, process, people, environment, equipment, materials, management) that led to an error.
Failure mode and effects analysis	Forward-looking approach. Applied before process implementation to prevent failure occurrence.	Uses inductive reasoning to identify all the ways a process might fail and prioritizes them by their probability of occurrence and impact on patients.

Causes of medical errors

Burnout	Prolonged, excessive stress leading to emotional exhaustion, depersonalization, leading to reduced professional efficacy.
Fatigue	Sleep/rest deprivation resulting in cognitive impairment and decreased attention to detail.

▶ NOTES

SECTION III

High-Yield Organ Systems

"Symptoms, then, are in reality nothing but the cry from suffering organs."
—Jean-Martin Charcot

"Man is an intelligence in servitude to his organs."
—Aldous Huxley

"When every part of the machine is correctly adjusted and in perfect harmony, health will hold dominion over the human organism by laws as natural and immutable as the laws of gravity."
—Andrew T. Still

▶ APPROACHING THE ORGAN SYSTEMS

In this section, we have divided the High-Yield Facts into the major **Organ Systems**. Within each Organ System are several subsections, including **Embryology, Anatomy, Physiology, Pathology,** and **Pharmacology.** As you progress through each Organ System, refer back to information in the previous subsections to organize these basic science subsections into a "vertically integrated" framework for learning. Below is some general advice for studying the organ systems by these subsections.

Embryology

Relevant embryology is included in each organ system subsection. Embryology tends to correspond well with the relevant anatomy, especially with regard to congenital malformations.

Anatomy

Several topics fall under this heading, including gross anatomy, histology, and neuroanatomy. Do not memorize all the small details; however, do not ignore anatomy altogether. Review what you have already learned and what you wish you had learned. Many questions require two or more steps. The first step is to identify a structure on anatomic cross section, electron micrograph, or photomicrograph. The second step may require an understanding of the clinical significance of the structure.

While studying, emphasize clinically relevant material. For example, be familiar with gross anatomy and radiologic anatomy related to specific diseases (eg, Pancoast tumor, Horner syndrome), traumatic injuries (eg, fractures, sensory and motor nerve deficits), procedures (eg, lumbar puncture), and common surgeries (eg, cholecystectomy). There are also many questions on the exam involving x-rays, CT scans, and neuro MRI scans. Many students suggest browsing through a general radiology atlas, pathology atlas, and histology atlas. Focus on learning basic anatomy at key levels in the body (eg, sagittal brain MRI; axial CT of the midthorax, abdomen, and pelvis). Basic neuroanatomy (especially pathways, blood supply, and functional anatomy), associated neuropathology, and neurophysiology have good yield. Please note that many of the photographic images in this book are for illustrative purposes and are not necessarily reflective of Step 1 emphasis.

Physiology

The portion of the examination dealing with physiology is broad and concept oriented and thus does not lend itself as well to fact-based review. Graphs and diagrams are often the best study aids, especially given the increasing number of questions requiring their interpretation. Learn to apply basic physiologic relationships in a variety of ways (eg, the Fick equation, clearance equations). You are seldom asked to perform complex calculations, though simple calculations and key relationships are important to grasp. Hormones are the focus of many questions; learn where, why, and how they are synthesized and released, their regulatory mechanisms and sites of action.

A large portion of the physiology tested on the USMLE Step 1 is clinically relevant and involves understanding physiologic changes associated with pathologic processes (eg, changes in pulmonary function with COPD). Thus, it is worthwhile to review the physiologic changes that are found with common pathologies of the major organ systems (eg, heart, lungs, kidneys, GI tract) and endocrine glands.

Pathology

Questions dealing with this discipline are difficult to prepare for because of the sheer volume of material involved. Review the underlying physiology, basic principles, and hallmark characteristics of the key diseases. Given the clinical orientation of Step 1, it is no longer sufficient to know only the "buzzword" associations of certain diseases (eg, café-au-lait macules and neurofibromatosis); you must also recognize the clinical descriptions of these high-yield physical exam findings.

Given the clinical slant of the USMLE Step 1, it is also important to review the classic presenting signs and symptoms of diseases as well as their associated laboratory findings. Delve into the signs, symptoms, and pathophysiology of major diseases that have a high prevalence in the United States (eg, alcohol use disorder, diabetes, hypertension, heart failure, ischemic heart disease, infectious disease). Be prepared to think one step beyond the simple diagnosis to treatment or complications.

The examination includes a number of color photomicrographs and photographs of gross specimens that are presented in the setting of a brief clinical history. However, read the question and the choices carefully before looking at the illustration, because the history will help you identify the pathologic process. Flip through an illustrated pathology textbook, color atlases, and appropriate Web sites in order to look at the pictures in the days before the exam. Pay attention to potential clues such as age, sex, ethnicity, occupation, recent activities and exposures, and specialized lab tests.

Pharmacology

Preparation for questions on pharmacology is straightforward. Learning all the key drugs and their characteristics (eg, mechanisms, clinical use, and important adverse effects) is high yield. Focus on understanding the prototype drugs in each class. Avoid memorizing obscure derivatives. Learn the "classic" and distinguishing toxicities of the major drugs. Do not bother with drug dosages or brand names. Reviewing associated biochemistry, physiology, and microbiology can be useful while studying pharmacology. There is a strong emphasis on ANS, CNS, antimicrobial, and cardiovascular agents as well as NSAIDs. Much of the material is clinically relevant. Newer drugs on the market are also fair game.

Cardiovascular

"As for me, except for an occasional heart attack, I feel as young as I ever did."

—Robert Benchley

"Hearts will never be practical until they are made unbreakable."

—The Wizard of Oz

"As the arteries grow hard, the heart grows soft."

—H. L. Mencken

"Nobody has ever measured, not even poets, how much the heart can hold."

—Zelda Fitzgerald

"The art of medicine has its roots in the heart."

—Paracelsus

"It is not the size of the man but the size of his heart that matters."

—Evander Holyfield

The cardiovascular system is one of the highest yield areas for the boards and, for some students, may be the most challenging. Focusing on understanding the mechanisms instead of memorizing the details can make a big difference. Pathophysiology of atherosclerosis and heart failure, mechanism of action of drugs (particularly, their interplay with cardiac physiology) and their adverse effects, ECGs of heart blocks, the cardiac cycle, and the Starling curve are some of the more high-yield topics. Differentiating between systolic and diastolic dysfunction is also very important. Heart murmurs and maneuvers that affect these murmurs have also been high yield and may be asked in a multimedia format.

▶ CARDIOVASCULAR—EMBRYOLOGY

Heart morphogenesis	First functional organ in vertebrate embryos; beats spontaneously by week 4 of development.	
Cardiac looping	Primary heart tube loops to establish left-right polarity; begins in week 4 of development.	Defect in left-right dynein (involved in left-right asymmetry) can lead to dextrocardia, as seen in Kartagener syndrome.

Septation of the chambers

Atria

❶ Septum primum grows toward endocardial cushions, narrowing ostium primum.

❷ Ostium secundum forms in septum primum due to cell death (ostium primum regresses).

❸ Septum secundum develops on the right side of septum primum, as ostium secundum maintains right-to-left shunt.

❹ Septum secundum expands and covers most of ostium secundum. The residual foramen is the foramen ovale.

❺ Remaining portion of septum primum forms the one-way valve of the foramen ovale.

6. Septum primum closes against septum secundum, sealing the foramen ovale soon after birth because of ↑ LA pressure and ↓ RA pressure.

7. Septum secundum and septum primum fuse during infancy/early childhood, forming the atrial septum.

Patent foramen ovale—failure of septum primum and septum secundum to fuse after birth; seen in 25% of population. Most are asymptomatic and remain undetected. Can lead to paradoxical emboli (venous thromboemboli entering the systemic arterial circulation through right-to-left shunt) as can occur in atrial septal defect (ASD).

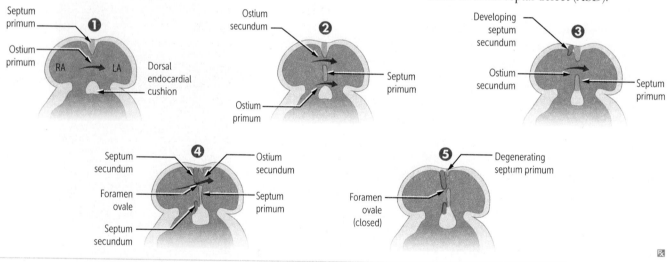

Heart morphogenesis (continued)

Ventricles	❶ Muscular interventricular septum forms. Opening is called interventricular foramen. ❷ Aorticopulmonary septum rotates and fuses with muscular ventricular septum to form membranous interventricular septum, closing interventricular foramen. ❸ Growth of endocardial cushions separates atria from ventricles and contributes to both atrial septation and membranous portion of the interventricular septum.	Ventricular septal defect—most common congenital cardiac anomaly, usually occurs in membranous septum. Atrioventricular septal defect (AVSD)—also known as endocardial cushion or AV canal defect. Acyanotic congenital heart defect with single common AV valve plus either ASD alone (partial AVSD) or both ASD and VSD (complete AVSD). Associated with Down syndrome, maternal diabetes, and obesity.

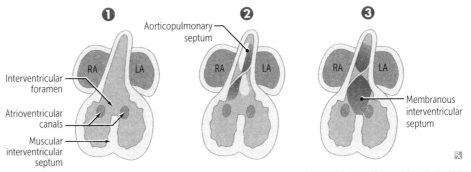

Outflow tract formation	Neural crest cell migrations → truncal and bulbar ridges that spiral and fuse to form aorticopulmonary septum → ascending aorta and pulmonary trunk.	Conotruncal abnormalities associated with failure of neural crest cells to migrate: ▪ Transposition of great arteries (TGA). ▪ Tetralogy of Fallot. ▪ Persistent truncus arteriosus.
Valve development	Aortic/pulmonary: derived from endocardial cushions of outflow tract. Mitral/tricuspid: derived from fused endocardial cushions of the AV canal.	Valvular anomalies may be stenotic, regurgitant, atretic (eg, tricuspid atresia), or displaced (eg, Ebstein anomaly).

Heart embryology

EMBRYONIC STRUCTURE	GIVES RISE TO
Right common cardinal vein and right anterior cardinal vein	Superior vena cava (SVC)
Posterior cardinal, subcardinal, and supracardinal veins	Inferior vena cava (IVC)
Right horn of sinus venosus	Smooth part of right atrium (sinus venarum)
Left horn of sinus venosus	Coronary sinus
Primitive pulmonary vein	Smooth part of left atrium
Primitive atrium	Trabeculated part of left and right atria
Endocardial cushion	Atrial septum, membranous interventricular septum; AV and semilunar valves
Primitive ventricle	Trabeculated part of left and right ventricles
Bulbus cordis	Smooth parts (outflow tract) of left and right ventricles
Truncus arteriosus	Ascending aorta and pulmonary trunk

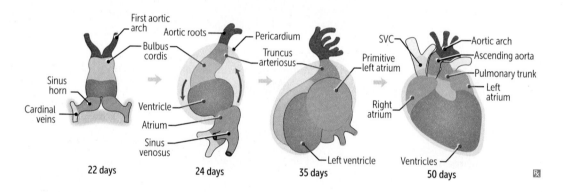

Fetal-postnatal derivatives

FETAL STRUCTURE	POSTNATAL DERIVATIVE	NOTES
Ductus arteriosus	Ligamentum arteriosum	Near the left recurrent laryngeal nerve
Ductus venosus	Ligamentum venosum	
Foramen ovale	Fossa ovalis	
Allantois → urachus	Median umbilical ligament	Urachus is part of allantois between bladder and umbilicus
Umbilical arteries	Medial umbilical ligaments	
Umbilical vein	Ligamentum teres hepatis (round ligament)	Contained in falciform ligament

Fetal circulation

3 important shunts:
1. Umbilical vein → **ductus venosus** → IVC (bypassing hepatic circulation).
2. Most of the highly oxygenated blood from IVC → **foramen ovale** → LA.
3. Deoxygenated blood from SVC → RA → RV → main pulmonary artery → **ductus arteriosus** → descending aorta; shunt is due to ↑ fetal pulmonary artery resistance.

At birth, infant takes a breath → ↓ resistance in pulmonary vasculature → ↑ LA pressure vs RA pressure → foramen ovale closes (now called fossa ovalis); ↑ in O₂ (from respiration) and ↓ in prostaglandins (from placental separation) → closure of ductus arteriosus.

NSAIDs (eg, indomethacin, ibuprofen) or acetaminophen help close the patent ductus arteriosus (PDA) → ligamentum arteriosum (remnant of ductus arteriosus). "**Endo**methacin" **ends** the PDA.

Prostaglandins **E₁** and **E₂** k**EE**p PDA open.

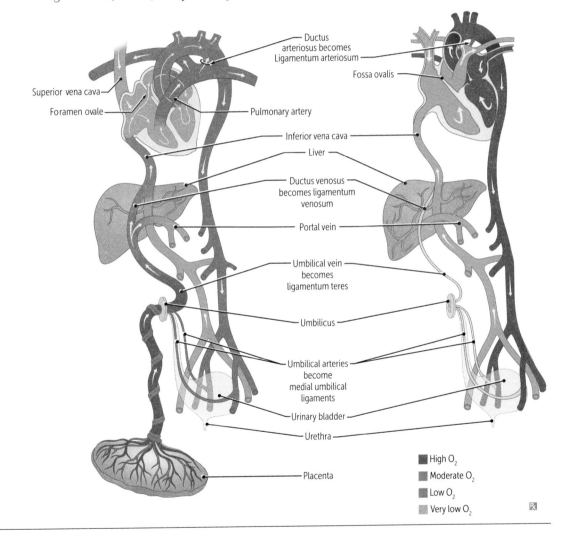

Ductus arteriosus becomes Ligamentum arteriosum
Fossa ovalis
Superior vena cava
Foramen ovale
Pulmonary artery
Inferior vena cava
Liver
Ductus venosus becomes ligamentum venosum
Portal vein
Umbilical vein becomes ligamentum teres
Umbilicus
Umbilical arteries become medial umbilical ligaments
Urinary bladder
Urethra
Placenta

High O₂
Moderate O₂
Low O₂
Very low O₂

▸ CARDIOVASCULAR—ANATOMY

Heart anatomy

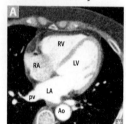

LA is the most posterior part of the heart 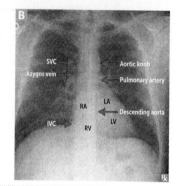; LA enlargement (eg, in mitral stenosis) can lead to:
- Compression of esophagus → dysphagia
- Compression of left recurrent laryngeal nerve (branch of vagus nerve → hoarseness (**Ortner syndrome**)

RV is the most anterior part of the heart and most commonly injured in trauma. LV is about 2/3 and RV is about 1/3 of the inferior (diaphragmatic) cardiac surface **B**.

Pericardium

Consists of 3 layers (from outer to inner):
- Fibrous pericardium
- Parietal pericardium
- Epicardium (visceral pericardium)

Pericardial space lies between parietal pericardium and epicardium.

Pericardium innervated by phrenic nerve.

Pericarditis can cause referred pain to the neck, arms, or one or both shoulders (often left).

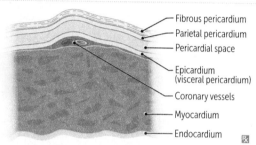

Coronary blood supply

LAD and its branches supply anterior 2/3 of interventricular septum, anterolateral papillary muscle, and anterior surface of LV. Most commonly occluded.

Posterior descending artery (PDA) supplies posterior 1/3 of interventricular septum, posterior 2/3 of ventricular walls, posteromedial papillary muscle, and SA and AV nodes (as determined by dominance). Infarct may cause nodal dysfunction (bradycardia or heart block).

Right (acute) marginal artery supplies RV.

Dominance:
- Right-dominant circulation (most common) = PDA arises from RCA
- Left-dominant circulation = PDA arises from LCX (~5%–10% of patients)
- Codominant circulation = PDA arises from both LCX and RCA (~10%–20% of patients)

Coronary blood flow to LV and interventricular septum peaks in early diastole.

Coronary sinus runs in the left AV groove and drains into the RA.

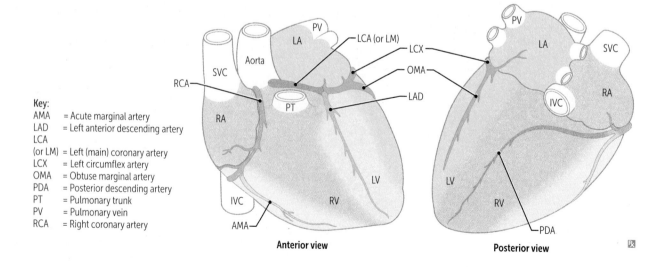

Key:
AMA = Acute marginal artery
LAD = Left anterior descending artery
LCA
(or LM) = Left (main) coronary artery
LCX = Left circumflex artery
OMA = Obtuse marginal artery
PDA = Posterior descending artery
PT = Pulmonary trunk
PV = Pulmonary vein
RCA = Right coronary artery

Anterior view   **Posterior view**

▶ CARDIOVASCULAR—PHYSIOLOGY

Cardiac output variables

Stroke volume	Stroke Volume affected by Contractility, Afterload, and Preload.
	↑ SV with:
	  ▪ ↑ Contractility (eg, anxiety, exercise)
	  ▪ ↑ Preload (eg, early pregnancy)
	  ▪ ↓ Afterload
		SV CAP.
		Stroke work (SW) is work done by ventricle to eject SV.
		SW $\propto$ SV $\times$ MAP
		A failing heart has ↓ SV (systolic and/or diastolic dysfunction).

Contractility	Contractility (and SV) ↑ with:
	  ▪ Catecholamine stimulation via β_1 receptor:
	    ▪ Activated protein kinase A
	      → phospholamban phosphorylation
	      → active Ca^{2+} ATPase → ↑ Ca^{2+} storage in sarcoplasmic reticulum
	    ▪ Activated protein kinase A → Ca^{2+} channel phosphorylation → ↑ Ca^{2+} entry → ↑ Ca^{2+}-induced Ca^{2+} release
	  ▪ ↑ intracellular Ca^{2+}
	  ▪ Digoxin (blocks Na^+/K^+ pump → ↑ intracellular Na^+ → ↓ Na^+/Ca^{2+} exchanger activity → ↑ intracellular Ca^{2+})
		Contractility (and SV) ↓ with:
		  ▪ β_1-blockade (↓ cAMP)
		  ▪ Heart failure (HF) with systolic dysfunction
		  ▪ Acidosis
		  ▪ Hypoxia/hypercapnia (↓ P_{O_2}/↑ P_{CO_2})
		  ▪ Nondihydropyridine Ca^{2+} channel blockers

Preload	Preload approximated by ventricular end-diastolic volume (EDV); depends on venous tone and circulating blood volume, both of which affect venous return.	Venous vasodilators (eg, nitroglycerin) ↓ preload.

Cardiac oxygen demand	Myocardial O_2 demand is ↑ by:
	  ▪ ↑ contractility
	  ▪ ↑ afterload (proportional to arterial pressure)
	  ▪ ↑ heart rate
	  ▪ ↑ diameter of ventricle (↑ wall tension)
	Coronary sinus contains most deoxygenated blood in body.
		Wall tension follows Laplace's law:
		Wall tension = pressure $\times$ radius
		Wall stress = $\dfrac{\text{pressure} \times \text{radius}}{2 \times \text{wall thickness}}$

Afterload	Afterload approximated by MAP. ↑ pressure → ↑ wall tension per Laplace's law → ↑ afterload. LV compensates for ↑ afterload by thickening (hypertrophy) in order to ↓ wall stress.	Arterial vasodilators (eg, hydralazine) ↓ afterload. ACE inhibitors and ARBs ↓ both preload and afterload. Chronic hypertension (↑ MAP) → LV hypertrophy.

Cardiac output equations

	EQUATION	NOTES
Stroke volume	$SV = EDV - ESV$	ESV = end-systolic volume.
Ejection fraction	$EF = \dfrac{SV}{EDV} = \dfrac{EDV - ESV}{EDV}$	EF is an index of ventricular contractility (↓ in systolic HF; usually normal in diastolic HF). Normal EF is 50%–70%.
Cardiac output	$CO = \dot{Q} = SV \times HR$ Fick principle: $CO = \dfrac{\text{rate of } O_2 \text{ consumption}}{(\text{arterial } O_2 \text{ content} - \text{venous } O_2 \text{ content})}$	In early stages of exercise, CO maintained by ↑ HR and ↑ SV. In later stages, CO maintained by ↑ HR only (SV plateaus). Diastole is shortened with ↑↑ HR (eg, ventricular tachycardia) → ↓ diastolic filling time → ↓ SV → ↓ CO.
Pulse pressure	PP = systolic blood pressure (SBP) – diastolic blood pressure (DBP)	PP directly proportional to SV and inversely proportional to arterial compliance. ↑ PP in aortic regurgitation, aortic stiffening (isolated systolic hypertension in older adults), obstructive sleep apnea (↑ sympathetic tone), high-output state (eg, anemia, hyperthyroidism), exercise (transient). ↓ PP in aortic stenosis, cardiogenic shock, cardiac tamponade, advanced HF.
Mean arterial pressure	MAP = CO × total peripheral resistance (TPR)	MAP (at resting HR) = 2/3 DBP + 1/3 SBP = DBP + 1/3 PP.

Starling curves

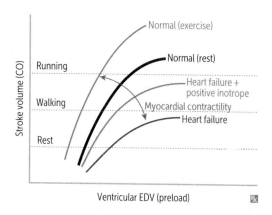

Force of contraction is proportional to end-diastolic length of cardiac muscle fiber (preload).

↑ contractility with catecholamines, positive inotropes (eg, dobutamine, milrinone, digoxin).

↓ contractility with loss of functional myocardium (eg, MI), β-blockers (acutely), nondihydropyridine Ca^{2+} channel blockers, HF.

Resistance, pressure, flow

Volumetric flow rate $(\dot{Q})$ = flow velocity (v) × cross-sectional area (A)

Resistance (R)

$$= \frac{\text{driving pressure } (\Delta P)}{\dot{Q}} = \frac{8\eta \text{ (viscosity)} \times \text{length}}{\pi r^4}$$

Total resistance of vessels in series:

$$R_T = R_1 + R_2 + R_3 \ldots$$

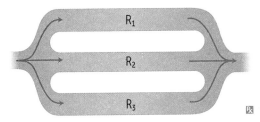

Total resistance of vessels in parallel:

$$\frac{1}{R_T} = \frac{1}{R_1} + \frac{1}{R_2} + \frac{1}{R_3} \ldots$$

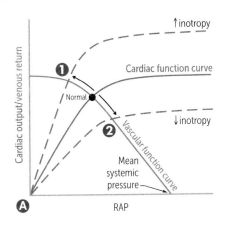

$\Delta P = \dot{Q} \times R$ is analogous to Ohm's Law for electrical circuits $(V = I \times R)$.

$\dot{Q} \propto r^4$

$R \propto 1/r^4$

Capillaries have highest total cross-sectional area and lowest flow velocity.

Pressure gradient drives flow from high pressure to low pressure.

Arterioles account for most of TPR. Veins provide most of blood storage capacity.

Viscosity depends mostly on hematocrit.

Viscosity ↑ in hyperproteinemic states (eg, multiple myeloma), polycythemia.

Viscosity ↓ in anemia.

Cardiac and vascular function curves

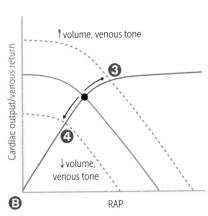
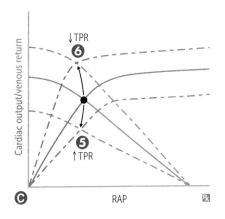

Intersection of curves = operating point of heart (ie, venous return and CO are equal, as circulatory system is a closed system).

GRAPH	EFFECT	EXAMPLES
Ⓐ Inotropy	Changes in contractility → altered SV → altered CO/venous return (VR) and RA pressure (RAP)	❶ Catecholamines, dobutamine, digoxin, exercise ⊕ ❷ HF with reduced EF, narcotic overdose, sympathetic inhibition ⊖
Ⓑ Venous return	Changes in circulating volume → altered RAP → altered SV → change in CO	❸ Fluid infusion, sympathetic activity, arteriovenous shunt ⊕ ❹ Acute hemorrhage, spinal anesthesia ⊖
Ⓒ Total peripheral resistance	Changes in TPR → altered CO Change in RAP unpredictable	❺ Vasopressors ⊕ ❻ Exercise, arteriovenous shunt ⊖

Changes often occur in tandem, and may be reinforcing (eg, exercise ↑ inotropy and ↓ TPR to maximize CO) or compensatory (eg, HF ↓ inotropy → fluid retention to ↑ preload to maintain CO).

Pressure-volume loops and cardiac cycle

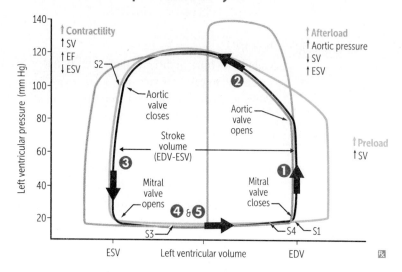

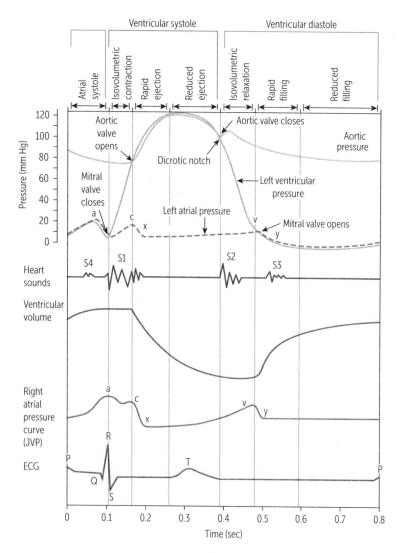

The black loop represents normal cardiac physiology.

Phases—left ventricle:

❶ Isovolumetric contraction—period between mitral valve closing and aortic valve opening; period of highest O_2 consumption

❷ Systolic ejection—period between aortic valve opening and closing

❸ Isovolumetric relaxation—period between aortic valve closing and mitral valve opening

❹ Rapid filling—period just after mitral valve opening

❺ Reduced filling—period just before mitral valve closing

Heart sounds:

S1—mitral and tricuspid valve closure. Loudest at mitral area.

S2—aortic and pulmonary valve closure. Loudest at left upper sternal border.

S3—in early diastole during rapid ventricular filling phase. Best heard at apex with patient in left lateral decubitus position. Associated with ↑ filling pressures (eg, MR, AR, HF, thyrotoxicosis) and more common in dilated ventricles (but can be normal in children, young adults, athletes, and pregnancy). Turbulence caused by blood from LA mixing with ↑ ESV.

S4—in late diastole ("atrial kick"). Turbulence caused by blood entering stiffened LV. Best heard at apex with patient in left lateral decubitus position. High atrial pressure. Associated with ventricular noncompliance (eg, hypertrophy). Considered abnormal if palpable. Common in older adults.

Jugular venous pulse (JVP):

a wave—atrial contraction. Prominent in AV dissociation (cannon a wave) and ↑ RV end-diastolic pressure from any cause. Absent in atrial fibrillation.

c wave—RV contraction (closed tricuspid valve bulging into atrium).

x descent—atrial relaxation and downward displacement of closed tricuspid valve during rapid ventricular ejection phase. Reduced or absent in tricuspid regurgitation and right HF because pressure gradients are reduced.

v wave—↑ RA pressure due to ↑ volume against closed tricuspid valve.

y descent—RA emptying into RV. Prominent in constrictive pericarditis, absent in cardiac tamponade.

Jugular venous pressure tracings

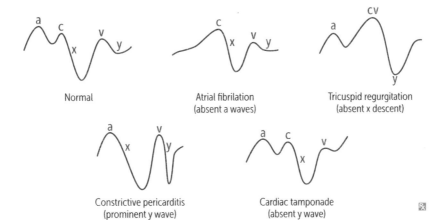

Normal

Atrial fibrilation
(absent a waves)

Tricuspid regurgitation
(absent x descent)

Constrictive pericarditis
(prominent y wave)

Cardiac tamponade
(absent y wave)

Pressure-volume loops and valvular disease

Aortic stenosis

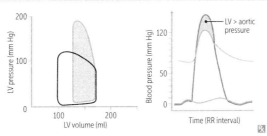

↑ LV pressure

↑ ESV

No change in EDV (if mild)

↓ SV

Ventricular hypertrophy → ↓ ventricular
compliance → ↑ EDP for given EDV

Aortic regurgitation

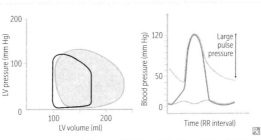

No true isovolumetric phase

↑ EDV

↑ SV

Loss of dicrotic notch

Mitral stenosis

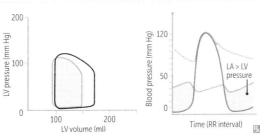

↑ LA pressure

↓ EDV because of impaired ventricular
filling

↓ ESV

↓ SV

Mitral regurgitation

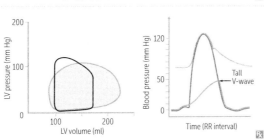

No true isovolumetric phase

↓ ESV due to ↓ resistance and
↑ regurgitation into LA during systole

↑ EDV due to ↑ LA volume/pressure from
regurgitation → ↑ ventricular filling

↑ SV (forward flow into systemic circulation
plus backflow into LA)

Splitting of S2

Physiologic splitting	Inspiration → drop in intrathoracic pressure → ↑ venous return → ↑ RV filling → ↑ RV stroke volume → ↑ RV ejection time → delayed closure of pulmonic valve. ↓ pulmonary impedance (↑ capacity of the pulmonary circulation) also occurs during inspiration, which contributes to delayed closure of pulmonic valve.	Normal delay E = Expiration I = Inspiration
Wide splitting	Seen in conditions that delay RV emptying (eg, pulmonic stenosis, right bundle branch block). Causes delayed pulmonic sound (especially on inspiration). An exaggeration of normal splitting.	Abnormal delay
Fixed splitting	Heard in ASD. ASD → left-to-right shunt → ↑ RA and RV volumes → ↑ flow through pulmonic valve → delayed pulmonic valve closure (independent of respiration).	
Paradoxical splitting	Heard in conditions that delay aortic valve closure (eg, aortic stenosis, left bundle branch block). Normal order of semilunar valve closure is reversed: in paradoxical splitting P2 occurs before A2. On inspiration, P2 closes later and moves closer to A2, "paradoxically" eliminating the split. On expiration, the split can be heard (opposite to physiologic splitting).	

Auscultation of the heart

Where to listen: **APT M**

(A) Aortic area:
Systolic murmur
 Aortic stenosis
 Flow murmur
  (eg, physiologic murmur)
 Aortic valve sclerosis

(T) Tricuspid area:
Holosystolic murmur
 Tricuspid regurgitation
 Ventricular septal defect
Diastolic murmur
 Tricuspid stenosis

Aortic
Pulmonic
Tricuspid
Mitral

Aortic stenosis

Mitral regurgitation

(P) Pulmonic area:
Systolic ejection murmur
 Pulmonic stenosis
 Atrial septal defect
 Flow murmur

(M) Mitral area (apex):
Systolic murmur
 Mitral regurgitation
 Mitral valve prolapse
Diastolic murmur
 Mitral stenosis

Left sternal border:
Systolic murmur
 Hypertrophic
  cardiomyopathy
Diastolic murmur
 Aortic regurgitation
 Pulmonic regurgitation

MANEUVER	CARDIOVASCULAR CHANGES	MURMURS THAT INCREASE WITH MANEUVER	MURMURS THAT DECREASE WITH MANEUVER
Standing, Valsalva (strain phase)	↓ preload (↓ LV volume)	MVP (↓ LV volume) with earlier midsystolic click HCM (↓ LV volume)	Most murmurs (↓ flow through stenotic or regurgitant valve)
Passive leg raise	↑ preload (↑ LV volume)	Most murmurs (↑ flow through stenotic or regurgitant valve)	MVP (↑ LV volume) with later midsystolic click HCM (↑ LV volume)
Squatting	↑ preload, ↑ afterload (↑ LV volume)		
Hand grip	↑↑ afterload → ↑ reverse flow across aortic valve (↑ LV volume)	Most other left-sided murmurs (AR, MR, VSD)	AS (↓ transaortic valve pressure gradient) HCM (↑ LV volume)
Inspiration	↑ venous return to right heart, ↓ venous return to left heart	Most right-sided murmurs (increase with inspiration)	Most left-sided murmurs (increase with expiration)

Heart murmurs

	AUSCULTATION	CLINICAL ASSOCIATIONS	NOTES
Systolic			
Aortic stenosis	Crescendo-decrescendo ejection murmur, loudest at heart base, radiates to carotids Soft S2 +/– ejection click "Pulsus parvus et tardus"—weak pulses with delayed peak	Age-related calcification (> 60 years old) Early-onset calcification of bicuspid aortic valve (~ 50–60 years old)	Can lead to **S**yncope, **A**ngina, **D**yspnea on exertion (**SAD**) LV pressure > aortic pressure during systole
Mitral/tricuspid regurgitation	Holosystolic, high-pitched "blowing" murmur MR: loudest at apex, radiates toward axilla TR: loudest at tricuspid area	MR: often due to ischemic heart disease (post-MI), MVP, LV dilatation, rheumatic fever (RF) TR: often due to RV dilatation; may be 2° to permanent pacemaker placement MR or TR: infective endocarditis	
Mitral valve prolapse	Late crescendo murmur with midsystolic click (MC) that occurs after carotid pulse Best heard over apex Loudest just before S2	Usually benign, but can predispose to infective endocarditis Can be caused by RF, chordae rupture, mitral annular disjunction, or myxomatous degeneration (1° or 2° to connective tissue disease)	MC due to sudden tensing of chordae tendineae as mitral leaflets prolapse into LA (**c**hordae cause **c**rescendo with **c**lick)
Ventricular septal defect	Holosystolic, harsh-sounding murmur Loudest at tricuspid area	Congenital	Larger VSDs have lower intensity murmur than smaller VSDs
Diastolic			
Aortic regurgitation	Early diastolic, decrescendo, high-pitched "blowing" murmur best heard at base (aortic root dilation) or left sternal border (valvular disease)	Causes include **BEAR**: **B**icuspid aortic valve, **E**ndocarditis, **A**ortic root dilation, **R**F Wide pulse pressure, pistol shot femoral pulse, pulsing nail bed	Hyperdynamic pulse and head bobbing when severe and chronic Can progress to left HF
Mitral stenosis	Follows opening snap (OS) Delayed rumbling mid-to-late murmur (↓ interval between S2 and OS correlates with ↑ severity)	Late and highly specific sequelae of RF Chronic MS can result in LA dilation and pulmonary congestion, atrial fibrillation, Ortner syndrome, hemoptysis, right HF	OS due to abrupt halt in leaflet motion in diastole after rapid opening due to fusion at leaflet tips LA >> LV pressure during diastole
Continuous			
Patent ductus arteriosus	Continuous **machine**like murmur, best heard at left infraclavicular area Loudest at S2	Often due to congenital rubella or prematurity	You need a **patent** for that **machine**.

Myocardial action potential

Phase 0 = rapid upstroke and depolarization—fast voltage-gated Na⁺ channels open.

Phase 1 = initial repolarization—inactivation of voltage-gated Na⁺ channels. Transient outward voltage-gated K⁺ channels begin to open.

Phase 2 = plateau ("platwo")—Ca²⁺ influx through voltage-gated Ca²⁺ channels balances K⁺ efflux. Ca²⁺ influx triggers Ca²⁺ release from sarcoplasmic reticulum and myocyte contraction (excitation-contraction coupling).

Phase 3 = rapid repolarization—K⁺ efflux due to opening of voltage-gated slow delayed-rectifier K⁺ channels and closure of voltage-gated Ca²⁺ channels.

Phase 4 = resting potential—high K⁺ permeability through K⁺ channels.

In contrast to skeletal muscle, cardiac muscle has the following characteristics:
- Action potential has a plateau due to Ca²⁺ influx and opposing K⁺ efflux.
- Contraction requires Ca²⁺ influx from ECF to induce Ca²⁺ release from sarcoplasmic reticulum (Ca²⁺-induced Ca²⁺ release).
- Myocytes conduct excitation throughout the heart via gap junctions.

Occurs in all cardiac myocytes except for those in the SA and AV nodes.

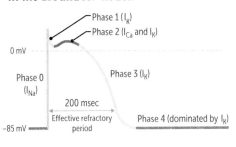

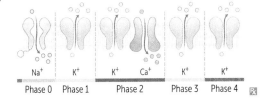

Pacemaker action potential

Key differences from the ventricular action potential include:

Phase 4 = slow spontaneous diastolic depolarization due to I_f ("funny current"). HCN channels are responsible for a slow, mixed Na⁺/K⁺ inward current; different from I_Na in phase 0 of ventricular action potential. Accounts for automaticity of SA and AV nodes. The slope of phase 4 in the SA node determines HR. ACh/adenosine ↓ the rate of diastolic depolarization and ↓ HR, while catecholamines ↑ depolarization and ↑ HR. Sympathetic stimulation ↑ the chance that HCN channels are open and thus ↑ HR.

Phase 0 = upstroke—opening of voltage-gated Ca²⁺ channels. Fast voltage-gated Na⁺ channels are permanently inactivated due to the less negative resting potential of these cells → slow conduction velocity, used by AV node to prolong transmission from atria to ventricles.

Phase 3 = repolarization—inactivation of Ca²⁺ channels and ↑ activation of K⁺ channels → ↑ K⁺ efflux.

Occurs in the SA and AV nodes. Phases 1 and 2 are absent.

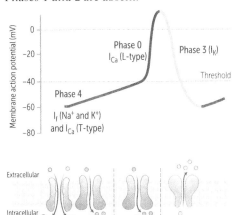

Electrocardiogram

Conduction pathway: SA node → atria → AV node → bundle of His → right bundle branch and left bundle branch (which divides into left anterior and posterior fascicles) → Purkinje fibers → ventricles; left bundle branch divides into left anterior and posterior fascicles.

SA node—located in upper crista terminalis near SVC; typically serves as dominant "pacemaker" for HR, with slow phase of upstroke.

AV node—located in interatrial septum near coronary sinus opening. Blood supply via PDA. 100-msec delay allows time for ventricular filling.

Pacemaker rates: SA > atria > AV > bundle of His/Purkinje/ventricles.

Speed of conduction: **His-Purkinje > Atria > Ventricles > AV** node. **He Parks At Ventura AVenue.**

P wave—atrial depolarization.

PR interval—time from start of atrial depolarization to start of ventricular depolarization (normally 120-200 msec).

QRS complex—ventricular depolarization (normally ≤ 100 msec).

QT interval—ventricular depolarization, contraction, repolarization.

T wave—ventricular repolarization. Inversion may indicate ischemia or recent MI.

J point—junction between end of QRS complex and start of ST segment.

ST segment—isoelectric, ventricles depolarized.

U wave—prominent in hypokalemia (think hyp"U"kalemia), bradycardia.

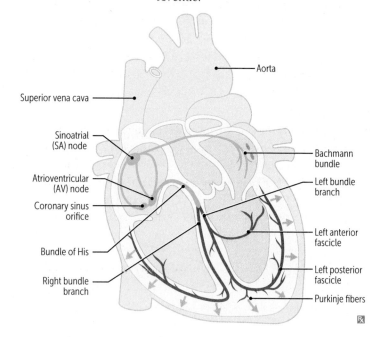

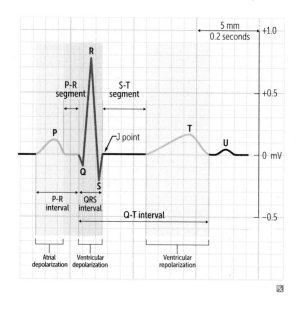

Atrial natriuretic peptide	Released from **atrial myocytes** in response to ↑ blood volume and atrial pressure. Acts via cGMP. Causes vasodilation and ↓ Na^+ reabsorption at the renal collecting tubule. Dilates afferent renal arterioles and constricts efferent arterioles, promoting diuresis and contributing to "aldosterone escape" mechanism.
B-type (brain) natriuretic peptide	Released from **ventricular myocytes** in response to ↑ tension. Similar physiologic action to ANP, with longer half-life. BNP blood test used for diagnosing HF (very good negative predictive value).

Baroreceptors and chemoreceptors

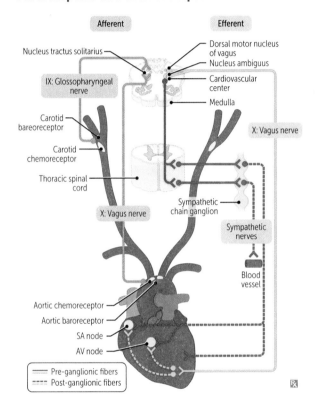

Receptors:
- Aortic arch transmits via vagus nerve to nucleus tractus solitarius of medulla (responds to changes in BP).
- Carotid sinus (dilated region superior to bifurcation of carotid arteries) transmits via glossopharyngeal nerve to nucleus tractus solitarius of medulla (responds to changes in BP).

Chemoreceptors:
- Peripheral—carotid and aortic bodies are stimulated by ↑ P_{CO_2}, ↓ pH of blood, and ↓ P_{O_2} (< 60 mm Hg).
- Central—are stimulated by changes in pH and P_{CO_2} of brain interstitial fluid, which in turn are influenced by arterial CO_2 as H^+ cannot cross the blood-brain barrier. Do not respond to P_{O_2}. Central chemoreceptors become less sensitive with chronically ↑ P_{CO_2} (eg, COPD) → ↑ dependence on peripheral chemoreceptors to detect ↓ O_2 to drive respiration.

Baroreceptors:
- Hypotension—↓ arterial pressure → ↓ stretch → ↓ afferent baroreceptor firing → ↑ efferent sympathetic firing and ↓ efferent parasympathetic stimulation → vasoconstriction, ↑ HR, ↑ contractility, ↑ BP. Important in the response to hypovolemic shock.
- Carotid sinus hypersensitivity—elicited by carotid massage, shaving, tight necktie or shirt collar → ↑ carotid sinus pressure → ↑ afferent baroreceptor firing → ↑ AV node refractory period → ↓ HR → ↓ CO. Also leads to peripheral vasodilation. Can cause presyncope/syncope. Exaggerated in underlying atherosclerosis, prior neck surgery, older age.
- Component of Cushing reflex (triad of hypertension, bradycardia, and respiratory depression)—↑ intracranial pressure constricts arterioles → cerebral ischemia → ↑ pCO_2 and ↓ pH → central reflex sympathetic ↑ in perfusion pressure (hypertension) → ↑ stretch → peripheral reflex baroreceptor–induced bradycardia.

Normal resting cardiac pressures

Pulmonary capillary wedge pressure (PCWP; in mm Hg) is a good approximation of left atrial pressure, except in mitral stenosis when PCWP > LV end diastolic pressure. PCWP is measured with pulmonary artery catheter (Swan-Ganz catheter).

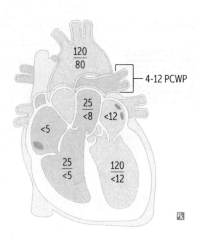

Autoregulation

How blood flow to an organ remains constant over a wide range of perfusion pressures.

ORGAN	FACTORS DETERMINING AUTOREGULATION	
Lungs	Hypoxia causes vasoconstriction	The pulmonary vasculature is unique in that alveolar hypoxia causes vasoconstriction so that only well-ventilated areas are perfused. In other organs, hypoxia causes vasodilation
Heart	Local metabolites (vasodilatory): NO, CO_2, ↓ O_2	
Brain	Local metabolites (vasodilatory): CO_2 (pH)	
Kidneys	Myogenic (stretch-dependent response of afferent arteriole) and tubuloglomerular feedback	
Skeletal muscle	Local metabolites during exercise (vasodilatory): CO_2, H^+, Adenosine, Lactate, K^+ At rest: sympathetic tone in arteries	**CHALK**
Skin	Sympathetic vasoconstriction most important mechanism for temperature control	

Capillary fluid exchange

Starling forces determine fluid movement through capillary walls:

- P_c = capillary hydrostatic pressure—pushes fluid out of capillary
- P_i = interstitial hydrostatic pressure—pushes fluid into capillary
- π_c = plasma oncotic pressure—pulls fluid into capillary
- π_i = interstitial fluid oncotic pressure—pulls fluid out of capillary

J_v = net fluid flow = $K_f [(P_c - P_i) - \sigma(\pi_c - \pi_i)]$

K_f = capillary permeability to fluid

σ = reflection coefficient (measure of capillary impermeability to protein)

Edema—excess fluid outflow into interstitium commonly caused by:

- ↑ capillary hydrostatic pressure (↑ P_c; eg, HF)
- ↑ capillary permeability (↑ K_f; eg, toxins, infections, burns)
- ↑ interstitial fluid oncotic pressure (↑ π_i; eg, lymphatic blockage)
- ↓ plasma proteins (↓ π_c; eg, nephrotic syndrome, liver failure, protein malnutrition)

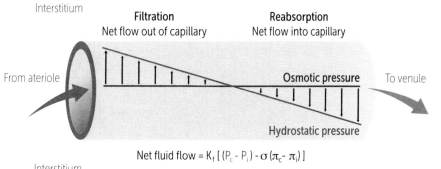

Interstitium

Filtration
Net flow out of capillary

Reabsorption
Net flow into capillary

From ateriole

Osmotic pressure

To venule

Hydrostatic pressure

Net fluid flow = $K_f [(P_c - P_i) - \sigma (\pi_c - \pi_i)]$

Interstitium

▶ CARDIOVASCULAR—PATHOLOGY

Congenital heart diseases

RIGHT-TO-LEFT SHUNTS	Early cyanosis—"blue babies." Often diagnosed prenatally or become evident immediately after birth. Usually require urgent surgical treatment and/or maintenance of a PDA via prostaglandin therapy.	The **5 T's:** 1. Truncus arteriosus (**1** vessel) 2. Transposition (**2** switched vessels) 3. Tricuspid atresia (**3** = **Tri**) 4. Tetralogy of Fallot (**4** = **Tetra**) 5. TAPVR (**5** letters in the name)
Persistent truncus arteriosus	Truncus arteriosus fails to divide into pulmonary trunk and aorta due to failure of aorticopulmonary septum formation; most patients have accompanying VSD.	
D-transposition of great arteries 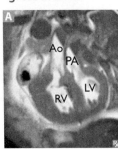	Aorta leaves RV (anterior) and pulmonary trunk leaves LV (posterior) → separation of systemic and pulmonary circulations **A**. Not compatible with life unless a shunt is present to allow mixing of blood (eg, VSD, PDA, or patent foramen ovale). Due to failure of the aorticopulmonary septum to spiral (narrow superior mediastinum causes "egg on a string" appearance on CXR). Without surgical intervention, most infants die within the first few months of life.	
Tricuspid atresia	Absence of tricuspid valve, hypoplastic RV; requires both ASD and VSD/PDA for viability.	ECG shows hypertrophy of RA (tall P-waves) and LV (left axis deviation).
Tetralogy of Fallot 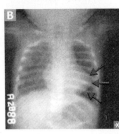	Caused by anterosuperior displacement of the infundibular septum. Most common cause of early childhood cyanosis. ❶ Pulmonary infundibular stenosis (most important determinant for prognosis) ❷ Right ventricular hypertrophy (RVH)—boot-shaped heart on CXR **B** ❸ Overriding aorta—straddles VSD, receives blood from both LV and RV ❹ VSD Pulmonary stenosis forces right-to-left flow across VSD → RVH, "tet spells" (often caused by crying, fever, and exercise due to exacerbation of RV outflow obstruction).	PROVe. Squatting: ↑ SVR, ↓ right-to-left shunt, improves cyanosis. Associated with 22q11 syndromes.
Total anomalous pulmonary venous return	Pulmonary veins drain into right heart circulation (SVC, coronary sinus, etc); associated with ASD and sometimes PDA to allow for right-to-left shunting to maintain CO.	
Ebstein anomaly	Displacement of tricuspid valve leaflets downward into RV, artificially "atrializing" the ventricle. Associated with tricuspid regurgitation, accessory conduction pathways, right-sided HF.	Rare. Can be caused by lithium exposure in utero.

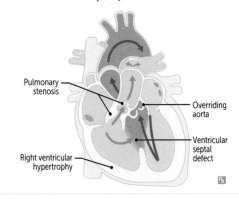

Congenital heart diseases *(continued)*

LEFT-TO-RIGHT SHUNTS	Acyanotic at presentation; cyanosis may occur years later. Frequency: VSD > ASD > PDA.	**Right-to-left** shunts: early cyanosis. **Left-to-right** shunts: "later" cyanosis.
Ventricular septal defect	Asymptomatic at birth, may manifest weeks later or remain asymptomatic throughout life. Most smaller defects self-resolve; larger defects, if left surgically untreated, cause ↑ pulmonary blood flow and LV overload (Eisenmenger syndrome), which may progress to HF.	O_2 saturation ↑ in RV and pulmonary artery.
Atrial septal defect 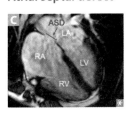	Defect in interatrial septum C; systolic ejection murmur with wide, fixed split S2. Ostium secundum defects most common and usually an isolated finding; ostium primum defects rarer and usually occur with other cardiac anomalies. Symptoms range from none to HF. Distinct from patent foramen ovale, which is due to failed fusion.	O_2 saturation ↑ in RA, RV, and pulmonary artery. May lead to paradoxical emboli (systemic venous emboli use ASD to bypass lungs and become systemic arterial emboli) in the setting of temporary shunt reversal (eg, when lifting weights or in Eisenmenger syndrome). Associated with Down syndrome.
Patent ductus arteriosus 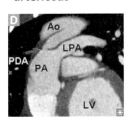	In fetal period, shunt is right to left (normal). In neonatal period, ↓ pulmonary vascular resistance → shunt becomes left to right → progressive RVH and/or LVH and HF. Associated with a continuous, "machinelike" murmur. Patency is maintained by PGE synthesis and low O_2 tension. Uncorrected PDA D can eventually result in late cyanosis in the lower extremities (differential cyanosis).	PDA is normal in utero and normally closes soon after birth. 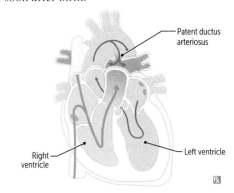
Eisenmenger syndrome	Uncorrected left-to-right shunt (VSD, ASD, PDA) → ↑ pulmonary blood flow → pathologic remodeling of vasculature → pulmonary arterial hypertension. RVH occurs to compensate → shunt becomes right to left when RV > LV pressure (see illustration). Causes late cyanosis, clubbing, and polycythemia. Age of onset varies depending on size and severity of initial left-to-right shunt.	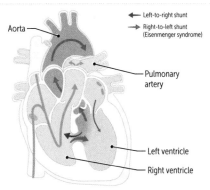 Eisenmenger syndrome from chronic VSD

Coarctation of the aorta 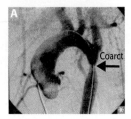	Aortic narrowing 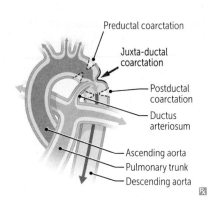 near insertion of ductus arteriosus ("juxtaductal"). Associated with bicuspid aortic valve, other heart defects, and Turner syndrome. Hypertension in upper extremities. Cyanosis, claudication, coolness, and weak, delayed pulses (brachiofemoral delay) in lower extremities. With age, intercostal arteries enlarge due to collateral circulation → rib-notching on x-ray. Complications include HF, ↑ risk of cerebral hemorrhage (berry aneurysms), aortic rupture, and infective endocarditis.

Preductal coarctation
Juxta-ductal coarctation
Postductal coarctation
Ductus arteriosum
Ascending aorta
Pulmonary trunk
Descending aorta

Persistent pulmonary hypertension of the newborn	Persistence of ↑ pulmonary vascular resistance after birth. Associated with abnormal development and postpartum adaptation of pulmonary vasculature. Risk factors include aspiration of meconium-stained amniotic fluid and neonatal pneumonia. Leads to right-to-left shunt through foramen ovale and ductus arteriosus. Preductal O_2 saturation is often > postductal. Newborn presents with signs of respiratory distress (eg, tachypnea) and (often differential) cyanosis. Equal pulses (no delay).

Congenital cardiac defect associations

ASSOCIATION	DEFECT
Prenatal alcohol exposure (fetal alcohol syndrome)	VSD, PDA, ASD, tetralogy of Fallot
Congenital rubella	PDA, pulmonary artery stenosis, septal defects
Down syndrome	AVSD, VSD, ASD
Infant of patient with diabetes during pregnancy	TGA, truncus arteriosus, tricuspid atresia, VSD
Marfan syndrome	MVP, thoracic aortic aneurysm/dissection, AR
Prenatal lithium exposure	Ebstein anomaly
Turner syndrome	Bicuspid aortic valve, aortic coarctation/dissection
Williams syndrome	Supravalvular aortic stenosis
22q11 syndromes	Truncus arteriosus, tetralogy of Fallot

Hypertension

	Persistent systolic BP ≥ 130 mm Hg and/or diastolic BP ≥ 80 mm Hg.
RISK FACTORS	↑ age, obesity, diabetes, physical inactivity, high-sodium diet, excess alcohol intake, tobacco smoking, family history; incidence greatest in Black > White > Asian populations.
FEATURES 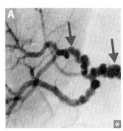	90% of hypertension is 1° (essential) and related to ↑ CO or ↑ TPR. Remaining 10% mostly 2° to renal/renovascular diseases such as fibromuscular dysplasia (characteristic "string of beads" appearance of renal artery A, usually seen in adult females) and atherosclerotic renal artery stenosis, 1° hyperaldosteronism, or obstructive sleep apnea. **Hypertensive urgency**—severe (≥ 180/≥ 120 mm Hg) hypertension without acute end-organ damage. **Hypertensive emergency**—severe hypertension with evidence of acute end-organ damage (eg, encephalopathy, stroke, retinal hemorrhages and exudates, papilledema, MI, HF, aortic dissection, kidney injury, microangiopathic hemolytic anemia, eclampsia). Arterioles may show fibrinoid necrosis.
PREDISPOSES TO	CAD, concentric LVH (mediated by angiotensin II and endothelin), HF, atrial fibrillation; aortic dissection/aneurysm; stroke; CKD (hypertensive nephropathy); retinopathy.

Hyperlipidemia signs

Xanthomas	Plaques or nodules composed of lipid-laden histiocytes in skin A, especially the eyelids (xanthelasma B).
Tendinous xanthoma	Lipid deposit in tendon C, especially Achilles tendon and finger extensors. Associated with familial hypercholesterolemia.
Corneal arcus	Lipid deposit in cornea. Common in older adults (arcus senilis D), but appears earlier in life with hypercholesterolemia.

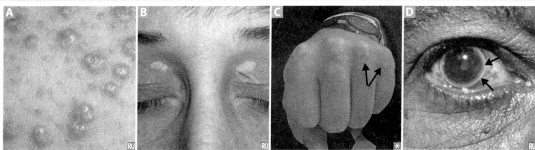

Atherosclerosis	Very common form of arteriosclerosis (hardening of arteries). Disease of elastic arteries and large- and medium-sized muscular arteries; caused by buildup of cholesterol plaques in tunica intima.
LOCATION	Abdominal aorta > coronary artery > popliteal artery > carotid artery > circle of **Willis**. **A copy cat named Willis**.
RISK FACTORS	Modifiable: hypertension, tobacco smoking, dyslipidemia (↑ LDL, ↓ HDL), diabetes. Non-modifiable: age, male sex, postmenopausal status, family history.
SYMPTOMS	Angina, claudication, but can be asymptomatic.
PROGRESSION	Inflammation important in pathogenesis: endothelial cell dysfunction → macrophage and LDL accumulation → foam cell formation → fatty streaks → smooth muscle cell migration (involves PDGF and FGF), proliferation, and extracellular matrix deposition → fibrous plaque → complex atheromas A → calcification (calcium content correlates with risk of complications).
COMPLICATIONS	Ischemia, infarction, aneurysm formation, peripheral vascular disease, thrombosis, embolism, renovascular hypertension, coarctation of the aorta, subclavian steal syndrome.

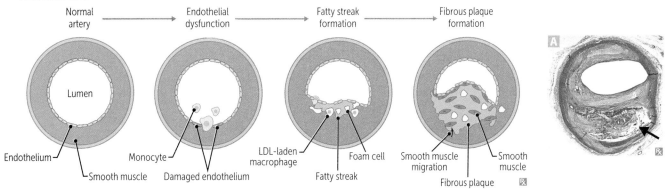

Cholesterol emboli syndrome

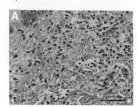

Microembolization of cholesterol displaced from atherosclerotic plaques **A** in large arteries (usually the aorta). Results in end-organ damage due to small artery emboli and an inflammatory response (eg, livedo reticularis, digital ischemia [blue toe syndrome], acute renal failure, cerebrovascular accident, gut ischemia). Pulses remain palpable because larger arteries are unaffected. May follow invasive vascular procedures (angiography, angioplasty, endovascular grafting).

Arteriolosclerosis

Common form of arteriosclerosis. Affects small arteries and arterioles. Two types:
- **Hyaline**—vessel wall thickening 2° to plasma protein leak into subendothelium in hypertension or diabetes mellitus **A**.
- **Hyperplastic**—"onion skinning" **B** in severe hypertension with proliferation of smooth muscle cells.

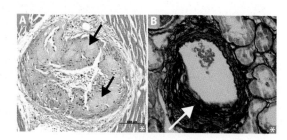

Aortic aneurysm

Localized pathologic dilation of the aorta. May cause abdominal and/or back pain, which is a sign of leaking, dissection, or imminent rupture.

Thoracic aortic aneurysm

Associated with cystic medial degeneration. Risk factors include hypertension, bicuspid aortic valve, connective tissue disease (eg, Marfan syndrome). Also associated with 3° syphilis (obliterative endarteritis of the vasa vasorum). Aortic root dilatation may lead to aortic valve regurgitation.

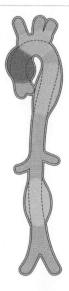

Abdominal aortic aneurysm

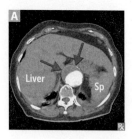

Associated with transmural (all 3 layers) inflammation and extracellular matrix degradation. Risk factors include tobacco smoking (strongest risk factor), ↑ age, male sex, family history. May present as palpable pulsatile abdominal mass (arrows in **A** point to outer dilated aortic wall). Rupture may present as triad of pulsatile abdominal mass, acute abdominal/back pain, and resistant hypotension. Most often infrarenal (distribution of vasa vasorum is reduced).

- Ascending thoracic aorta
- Aortic arch
- Descending thoracic aorta
- Abdominal aorta

Traumatic aortic rupture	Due to trauma and/or deceleration injury (MVA or significant fall), most commonly at aortic isthmus (proximal descending aorta just distal to origin of left subclavian artery). X-ray may reveal widened mediastinum.

Aortic dissection

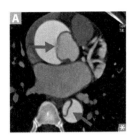

Longitudinal intimal tear forming a false lumen. Associated with hypertension (strongest risk factor), bicuspid aortic valve, inherited connective tissue disorders (eg, Marfan syndrome). Can present with tearing, sudden-onset chest pain radiating to the back +/– markedly unequal BP in arms. CXR can show mediastinal widening. Can result in organ ischemia, embolic stroke, aortic rupture, death.

Stanford type **A** (proximal): involves **A**scending aorta (red arrow in **A**). May extend to aortic arch or descending aorta (blue arrow in **A**). May result in acute aortic regurgitation or cardiac tamponade. Treatment: surgery.

Stanford type **B** (distal): involves only descending aorta (**B**elow left subclavian artery). Treatment: β-blockers, then vasodilators.

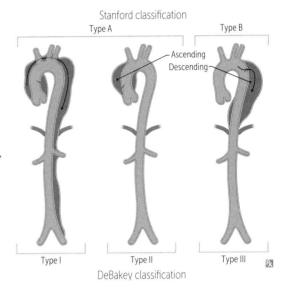

Subclavian steal syndrome

Stenosis of subclavian artery proximal to origin of vertebral artery → hypoperfusion distal to stenosis → reversed blood flow in ipsilateral vertebral artery → reduced cerebral perfusion on exertion of affected arm. Causes arm ischemia, pain, paresthesia, vertebrobasilar insufficiency (dizziness, vertigo), > 15 mm Hg difference in systolic BP between arms. Associated with atherosclerosis (most common cause), Takayasu arteritis, heart surgery.

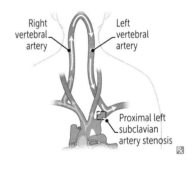

Coronary artery disease

Angina	Chest pain due to ischemic myocardium 2° to coronary artery narrowing or spasm; no necrosis. ▪ Stable—usually 2° to atherosclerosis (≥ 70% occlusion); exertional chest pain in classic distribution resolving with rest or nitroglycerin. ▪ Unstable—thrombosis with incomplete coronary artery occlusion; ↑ in frequency or intensity of exertional chest pain or any chest pain at rest. No cardiac biomarker elevation (vs non–ST-segment elevation MI [NSTEMI]). ▪ Vasospastic (formerly Prinzmetal or variant)—occurs at rest 2° to coronary artery spasm; transient ischemic ST changes on ECG. Tobacco smoking is a major risk factor. Triggers include cocaine, amphetamines, alcohol, triptans. Treat with Ca^{2+} channel blockers, nitrates, and smoking cessation (if applicable).
Myocardial infarction	Most often due to an acute coronary syndrome (ACS): rupture of coronary artery atherosclerotic plaque → acute thrombosis. MI can also occur with prolonged supply-demand mismatch (eg, stable angina → prolonged tachycardia and hypotension from pneumonia → elevated troponin but no acute plaque rupture).

	Stable angina	Unstable angina	NSTEMI	STEMI
PAIN	On exertion	Mild exertion or at rest	At rest	At rest
TROPONIN LEVEL	No elevation	No elevation	Elevated	Elevated
INFARCTION	None	None	Subendocardial	Transmural
ECG CHANGES	Possible ST depression and/or T-wave inversion	Possible ST depression and/or T-wave inversion	ST depression and/or T-wave inversion	ST elevation, pathologic Q waves

Ischemic heart disease manifestations

Coronary steal syndrome	Distal to coronary stenosis, vessels are maximally dilated at baseline to compensate for reduced blood flow. Administration of vasodilators (eg, dipyridamole, adenosine, regadenoson) dilates normal vessels → ↓ hydrostatic pressure in normal coronary arteries → blood is shunted toward well-perfused areas → ↓ flow to myocardium perfused by stenosed vessels ("steal") → ischemia of myocardium downstream to pathologically dilated vessels. Vasodilator stress tests rely on differential in flow to detect potential ischemia. Rarely, they can cause coronary steal and true ischemia. Vasodilation of healthy vessels **steal**s blood from stenosed vessels.
Sudden cardiac death	Unexpected death due to cardiac causes within 1 hour of symptom onset or within 24 hours with no cardiovascular symptoms, most commonly due to lethal ventricular arrhythmia (eg, ventricular fibrillation) impairing blood flow to the brain. Associated with CAD (up to 70% of cases), cardiomyopathy (hypertrophic, dilated), myocarditis, coronary artery anomalies, and hereditary channelopathies (eg, long QT syndrome, Brugada syndrome). Prevent with implantable cardioverter-defibrillator.
Chronic ischemic heart disease	Progressive exertional symptoms and/or development of HF due to chronic ischemic myocardial damage. Myocardial hibernation—LV systolic dysfunction in the setting of chronic ischemia. Potentially reversible with myocardial reperfusion. Seen in stable angina, acute MI, or HF. Contrast with myocardial stunning—transient, reversible LV systolic dysfunction after brief, acute ischemia.

Evolution of myocardial infarction

Commonly occluded coronary arteries: LAD > RCA > circumflex.
Symptoms: diaphoresis, nausea, vomiting, severe retrosternal pain, pain in left arm and/or jaw, shortness of breath, fatigue.

TIME	GROSS	LIGHT MICROSCOPE	COMPLICATIONS
0–24 hours	Occluded artery; Dark mottling; pale with tetrazolium stain	Wavy fibers (0–4 hr), early coagulative necrosis (4–24 hr) **A** → cell content released into blood; edema, hemorrhage. Reperfusion injury → free radicals and ↑ Ca^{2+} influx → hypercontraction of myofibrils (dark eosinophilic stripes)	Ventricular arrhythmia, HF, cardiogenic shock
1–3 days	Hyperemia	Extensive coagulative necrosis. Tissue surrounding infarct shows acute inflammation with neutrophils **B**	Postinfarction fibrinous pericarditis
3–14 days	Hyperemic border; central yellow-brown softening	Macrophages, then granulation tissue at margins **C**	Free wall rupture → tamponade; papillary muscle rupture → mitral regurgitation; interventricular septal rupture due to macrophage-mediated structural degradation → left-to-right shunt. LV pseudoaneurysm (risk of rupture)
2 weeks to several months	Gray-white scar	Contracted scar complete **D**	Postcardiac injury syndrome, HF, arrhythmias, true ventricular aneurysm (risk of mural thrombus)

Diagnosis of myocardial infarction

In the first 6 hours, ECG is the gold standard. Cardiac troponin I rises after 4 hours (peaks at 24 hr) and is ↑ for 7–10 days; more specific than other protein markers.

CK-MB increases after 6–12 hours (peaks at 16–24 hr) and is predominantly found in myocardium but can also be released from skeletal muscle. Useful in diagnosing reinfarction following acute MI because levels return to normal after 48 hours.

ECG changes can include ST elevation (STEMI, transmural infarct), ST depression (NSTEMI, subendocardial infarct), hyperacute (peaked) T waves, T-wave inversion, and pathologic Q waves or poor R wave progression (evolving or old transmural infarct).

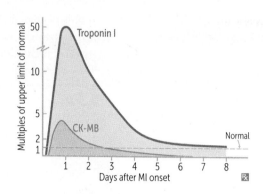

ECG localization of STEMI

INFARCT LOCATION	LEADS WITH ST-SEGMENT ELEVATIONS OR Q WAVES
Anteroseptal (LAD)	V_1–V_2
Anteroapical (distal LAD)	V_3–V_4
Anterolateral (LAD or LCX)	V_5–V_6
Lateral (LCX)	I, aVL
Inferior (RCA)	II, III, aVF
Posterior (PDA)	V_7–V_9, ST depression in V_1–V_3 with tall R waves

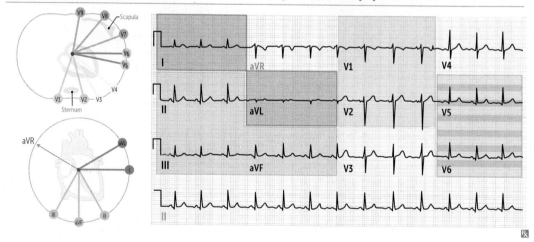

Narrow complex tachycardias

Narrow QRS complex < 120 msec, rapid ventricular activation via normal ventricular conduction system, tachycardia originates within or above AV node (supraventricular arrhythmia).

ARRHYTHMIA	DESCRIPTION	ECG FINDINGS
Atrial fibrillation	Irregularly irregular rate and rhythm with no discrete P waves. Arrhythmogenic activity usually originates from automatic foci near pulmonary vein ostia in left atrium. Common risk factors include hypertension, CAD, advanced age, atrial dilation. May predispose to thromboembolic events due to LA blood stasis, particularly stroke. LA appendage is the most common site of thrombus formation in atrial fibrillation. Management of **A**trial fibrillation involves rate and rhythm control using **B**eta-Blockers, **C**alcium **C**hannel blockers, and **D**igoxin (**ABCD**) and cardioversion.	$RR_1 \neq RR_2 \neq RR_3 \neq RR_4$ Irregular baseline (absent P waves)
Multifocal atrial tachycardia	Irregularly irregular rate and rhythm with at least 3 distinct P wave morphologies, due to multiple ectopic foci in atria. Associated with underlying conditions such as COPD, pneumonia, HF.	
Atrial flutter	Rapid succession of identical, consecutive atrial depolarization waves → "sawtooth" appearance of P waves. Arrhythmogenic activity usually originates from reentry circuit around tricuspid annulus. Treat like atrial fibrillation +/– catheter ablation of region between tricuspid annulus and IVC.	$RR_1 = RR_2 = RR_3$ 4:1 sawtooth pattern
Paroxysmal supraventricular tachycardia	Most often due to a reentrant tract between atrium and ventricle, most commonly in AV node. Commonly presents with sudden-onset palpitations, lightheadedness, diaphoresis. Terminate by slowing AV nodal conduction (vagal maneuvers, adenosine). Definitively treat with catheter ablation.	

Wolff-Parkinson-White syndrome

Most common type of ventricular preexcitation syndrome. Abnormal fast accessory conduction pathway from atria to ventricle (bundle of Kent) bypasses rate-slowing AV node → ventricles partially depolarize earlier → characteristic delta wave with widened QRS complex and shortened PR interval. May result in reentry circuit → supraventricular tachycardia.

Treatment: procainamide, ibutilide. Avoid AV nodal–blocking drugs (eg, adenosine, calcium channel blockers, β-blockers).

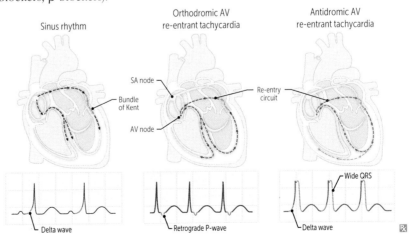

Sinus rhythm — SA node, Bundle of Kent, AV node — Delta wave

Orthodromic AV re-entrant tachycardia — Re-entry circuit — Retrograde P-wave

Antidromic AV re-entrant tachycardia — Wide QRS — Delta wave

Wide complex tachycardias

Wide QRS complex ≥ 120 msec, slow ventricular activation outside normal ventricular conduction system, tachycardia originates below AV node (ventricular arrhythmia).

ARRHYTHMIA	DESCRIPTION	ECG FINDINGS
Ventricular tachycardia	Typically regular rhythm, rate > 100. Most commonly due to structural heart disease (eg, cardiomyopathy, scarring after myocardial infarction). High risk of sudden cardiac death.	
Torsades de pointes	Polymorphic ventricular tachycardia. Shifting sinusoidal waveforms. May progress to ventricular fibrillation. Long QT interval (eg, sinus bradycardia, congenital long QT syndromes) predisposes to torsades de pointes. Caused by drugs, ↓ K^+, ↓ Mg^{2+}, ↓ Ca^{2+}. Torsades de pointes = twisting of the points Treatment: defibrillation for unstable patients, magnesium sulfate for stable patients. Drug-induced long QT (**ABCDEF+NO**): ▪ anti-**A**rrhythmics (Ia and III), **A**rsenic ▪ anti-**B**iotics (macrolides, fluoroquinolones) ▪ anti-**C**ychotics (haloperidol), **C**hloroquine ▪ anti-**D**epressants (TCAs), **D**iuretics (thiazides) ▪ anti-**E**metics (ondansetron) ▪ anti-**F**ungals (Fluconazole) ▪ **N**avir (protease inhibitors) ▪ **O**pioids (methadone)	
Ventricular fibrillation	Disorganized rhythm with no identifiable waves. Treatment: fatal without immediate CPR and defibrillation.	No discernible rhythm

Hereditary channelopathies

Inherited mutations of cardiac ion channels → abnormal myocardial action potential → ↑ risk of ventricular tachyarrhythmias and sudden cardiac death (SCD).

Brugada syndrome	Autosomal dominant; most commonly due to loss of function mutation of Na^+ channels. ↑ prevalence in Asian males. ECG pattern of pseudo-right bundle branch block and ST-segment elevations in leads V_1–V_2. Prevent SCD with ICD.
Congenital long QT syndrome	Most commonly due to loss of function mutation of K^+ channels (affects repolarization). Includes: ▪ Romano-Ward syndrome—autosomal dominant, pure cardiac phenotype (**no** deafness). ▪ Jervell and Lange-Nielsen syndrome—autosomal recessive, **sensori**neural deafness.

Sick sinus syndrome

Age-related degeneration of SA node. ECG can show bradycardia, sinus pauses (delayed P waves), sinus arrests (dropped P waves), junctional escape beats.

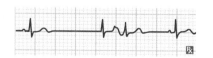

Conduction blocks

ARRHYTHMIA	DESCRIPTION	ECG FINDINGS
First-degree AV block	Prolonged PR interval (>200 msec). Treatment: none required (benign and asymptomatic).	
Second-degree AV block Mobitz type I (Wenckeback)	Progressive lengthening of PR interval until a beat is "dropped" (P wave not followed by QRS complex). Variable RR interval with a pattern (regularly irregular). Treatment: none required (usually asymptomatic)	
Second-degree AV block Mobitz type II	Dropped beats that are not preceded by a change in PR interval. May progress to 3rd-degree block, as it usually indicates a structural abnormality such as ischemia or fibrosis. Treatment: usually a pacemaker.	
Third-degree (complete) AV block	P waves and QRS complexes rhythmically dissociated. Atria and ventricles beat independently of each other. Atrial rate > ventricular rate. May be caused by Lyme disease. Treatment: pacemaker.	
Bundle branch block	Interruption of conduction of normal left or right bundle branches. Affected ventricle depolarizes via slower myocyte-to-myocyte conduction from the unaffected ventricle, which depolarizes via the faster His-Purkinje system. Commonly due to degenerative changes (eg, cardiomyopathy, infiltrative disease).	

Premature beats

ARRHYTHMIA	DESCRIPTION	ECG FINDINGS
Premature atrial contraction	Extra beats arising from ectopic foci in atria instead of the SA node. Often 2° to ↑ adrenergic drive (eg, caffeine consumption). Benign, but may increase risk for atrial fibrillation and flutter. Narrow QRS complex with preceding P wave on ECG.	
Premature ventricular contraction	Ectopic beats arising from ventricle instead of the SA node. Shortened diastolic filling time → ↓ SV compared to a normal beat. Prognosis is largely influenced by underlying heart disease. Wide QRS complex with no preceding P wave on ECG.	

Myocardial infarction complications

COMPLICATION	TIMEFRAME	FINDINGS	NOTES
Cardiac arrhythmia	First few days to several months	Can be supraventricular arrhythmias, ventricular arrhythmias, or conduction blocks.	Due to myocardial death and scarring. Important cause of death before reaching the hospital and within the first 48 hours post-MI.
Peri-infarction pericarditis	1–3 days	Pleuritic chest pain, pericardial friction rub, ECG changes, and/or small pericardial effusion.	Usually self-limited.
Papillary muscle rupture	2–7 days	Can result in acute mitral regurgitation → cardiogenic shock, severe pulmonary edema.	Posteromedial >> anterolateral papillary muscle rupture A, as the posteromedial has single artery blood supply (posterior descending artery) whereas anterolateral has dual (LAD, LCX).
Interventricular septal rupture	3–5 days	Symptoms can range from mild to severe with cardiogenic shock and pulmonary edema.	Macrophage-mediated degradation → VSD → ↑ O_2 saturation and ↑ pressure in RV.
Ventricular pseudoaneurysm	3–14 days	May be asymptomatic. Symptoms may include chest pain, murmur, arrhythmia, syncope, HF, embolus from mural thrombus. Rupture → cardiac tamponade.	Free wall rupture contained by adherent pericardium or scar tissue—does not contain endocardium or myocardium. More likely to rupture than true aneurysm.
Ventricular free wall rupture	5–14 days	Free wall rupture B → cardiac tamponade or internal hemorrhage, often fatal.	LV hypertrophy and previous MI protect against free wall rupture.
True ventricular aneurysm	2 weeks to several months	Symptoms similar to pseudoaneurysm.	Outward bulge with contraction ("dyskinesia"). Associated with fibrosis.
Postcardiac injury syndrome	Weeks to several months	Pericarditis due to autoimmune reaction.	Also called Dressler syndrome. Cardiac antigens released after injury → deposition of immune complexes in pericardium → inflammation.

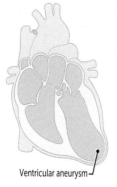

Ventricular aneurysm

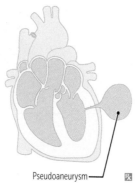

Pseudoaneurysm

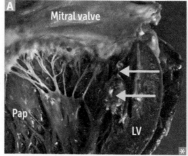

A Mitral valve Pap LV

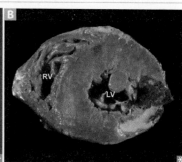

B RV LV

| **Acute coronary syndrome treatments** | Unstable angina/NSTEMI—Anticoagulation (eg, heparin), antiplatelet therapy (eg, aspirin) + ADP receptor inhibitors (eg, clopidogrel), β-blockers, ACE inhibitors, statins. Symptom control with nitroglycerin +/– morphine. |
| | STEMI—In addition to above, reperfusion therapy most important (percutaneous coronary intervention preferred over fibrinolysis). If RV affected (eg, RCA occlusion), support venous return/preload to maintain cardiac output (eg, IV fluids, avoiding nitroglycerin). |

Cardiomyopathies

Dilated cardiomyopathy	Most common cardiomyopathy (90% of cases). Often idiopathic or familial (eg, due to mutation of *TTN* gene encoding the sarcomeric protein titin). Other etiologies include drugs (eg, alcohol, cocaine, doxorubicin), infection (eg, coxsackie B virus, Chagas disease), ischemia (eg, CAD), systemic conditions (eg, hemochromatosis, sarcoidosis, thyrotoxicosis, wet beriberi), peripartum cardiomyopathy. Findings: HF, S3, systolic regurgitant murmur, dilated heart on echocardiogram, balloon appearance of heart on CXR. Treatment: Na^+ restriction, ACE inhibitors/ARBs, β-blockers, sacubitril, diuretics, mineralocorticoid receptor blockers (eg, spironolactone), ICD, heart transplant.	Systolic dysfunction ensues. Displays eccentric hypertrophy 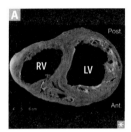 (sarcomeres added in series). Compare to athlete's heart, where LV and RV enlargement facilitates ↑ SV and ↑ CO. Stress cardiomyopathy (also called takotsubo cardiomyopathy, broken heart syndrome)—ventricular apical ballooning likely due to ↑ sympathetic stimulation (eg, stressful situations).
Hypertrophic cardiomyopathy	60–70% of cases are familial, autosomal dominant (most commonly due to mutations in genes encoding sarcomeric proteins, such as myosin binding protein C and β-myosin heavy chain). Causes syncope during exercise and may lead to sudden death (eg, in young athletes) due to ventricular arrhythmia. Findings: S4, systolic murmur. May see mitral regurgitation due to impaired mitral valve closure. Treatment: use of β-blockers or nondihydropyridine Ca^{2+} channel blockers (eg, verapamil) and, in some cases, cessation of high-intensity athletics. ICD if high risk. Avoid drugs that decrease preload (eg, diuretics, vasodilators).	Diastolic dysfunction ensues. Displays ventricular concentric hypertrophy (sarcomeres added in parallel) 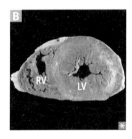, often septal predominance. Myofibrillar disarray and fibrosis. Classified as hypertrophic obstructive cardiomyopathy when LV outflow tract is obstructed. Asymmetric septal hypertrophy and systolic anterior motion of mitral valve → outflow obstruction → dyspnea, possible syncope.
Restrictive/infiltrative cardiomyopathy	Postradiation fibrosis, **L**öffler endocarditis, **E**ndocardial fibroelastosis (thick fibroelastic tissue in endocardium of young children), **A**myloidosis, **S**arcoidosis, **H**emochromatosis (**PLEAS**e **H**elp!).	Diastolic dysfunction ensues. Can have low-voltage ECG despite thick myocardium (especially in amyloidosis). Löffler endocarditis—associated with hypereosinophilic syndrome; histology shows eosinophilic infiltrates in myocardium.

Heart failure

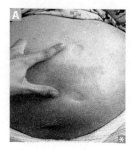

Clinical syndrome of cardiac pump dysfunction → congestion and low perfusion. Symptoms include dyspnea, orthopnea, fatigue; signs include S3 heart sound, rales, jugular venous distention (JVD), pitting edema .

Systolic dysfunction—heart failure with reduced ejection fraction (HFrEF), ↑ EDV; ↓ contractility often 2° to ischemia/MI or dilated cardiomyopathy.

Diastolic dysfunction—heart failure with preserved ejection fraction (HFpEF); ↓ compliance (↑ EDP) often 2° to myocardial hypertrophy.

Right HF most often results from left HF. Cor pulmonale refers to isolated right HF due to pulmonary cause.

ACE inhibitors, ARBs, angiotensin receptor–neprilysin inhibitors, β-blockers (except in acute decompensated HF), and aldosterone receptor antagonists ↓ mortality in HFrEF. Loop and thiazide diuretics are used mainly for symptomatic relief. Hydralazine with nitrate therapy and SGLT2 inhibitors improve both symptoms and mortality in select patients.

Left heart failure	
Orthopnea	Shortness of breath when supine: ↑ venous return from redistribution of blood (immediate gravity effect) exacerbates pulmonary vascular congestion.
Paroxysmal nocturnal dyspnea	Breathless awakening from sleep: ↑ venous return from redistribution of blood, reabsorption of peripheral edema, etc.
Pulmonary edema	↑ pulmonary venous pressure → pulmonary venous distention and transudation of fluid. Presence of hemosiderin-laden macrophages ("HF" cells) in lungs.

Right heart failure	
Congestive hepatomegaly	↑ central venous pressure → ↑ resistance to portal flow. Rarely, leads to "cardiac cirrhosis." Associated with nutmeg liver (mottled appearance) on gross exam.
Jugular venous distention	↑ venous pressure.
Peripheral edema	↑ venous pressure → fluid transudation.

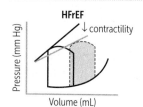

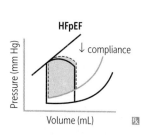

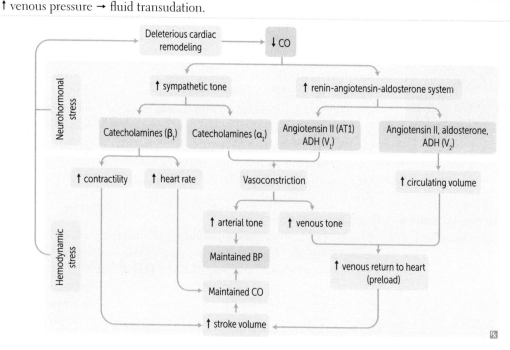

High-output heart failure

Uncommon form of HF characterized by ↑ CO. High-output state is due to ↓ SVR from either vasodilation or arteriovenous shunting. Causes include severe obesity, advanced cirrhosis, severe anemia, hyperthyroidism, wet beriberi, Paget disease of bone.

Presents with symptoms and signs of pulmonary and/or systemic venous congestion.

Shock

Inadequate organ perfusion and delivery of nutrients necessary for normal tissue and cellular function. Initially may be reversible but life threatening if not treated promptly.

TYPE	CAUSED BY	MECHANISM	SKIN	CVP	PCWP	CO	SVR	SVO₂
Hypovolemic shock	Hemorrhage, dehydration, burns	Volume depletion		↓	↓	↓	↑	↓
Cardiogenic shock	MI, HF, valvular dysfunction, arrhythmia	Left heart dysfunction	Cold, clammy	↑	↑	↓	↑	↓
Obstructive shock	PE, tension pneumothorax	Impeded cardiopulmonary blood flow		↑	↓	↓	↑	↓
	Cardiac tamponade			↑	↑	↓	↑	↓
Distributive shock	Sepsis (early), anaphylaxis	Systemic vasodilation	Warm, dry	↓	↓	↑	↓	↑
	CNS injury			↓	↓	↓	↓	normal/↑

↓ = 1° disturbance driving the shock.

Cardiac tamponade

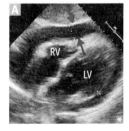

Compression of the heart by fluid (eg, blood, effusions) → ↓ CO. Equilibration of diastolic pressures in all 4 chambers.

Findings: Beck triad (hypotension, distended neck veins, distant heart sounds), ↑ HR, pulsus paradoxus. ECG may show low-voltage QRS and/or electrical alternans (due to "swinging" movement of heart in large effusion). Echocardiogram shows pericardial effusion (arrows in Ⓐ), systolic RA collapse, diastolic RV collapse, and IVC plethora.

Treatment: pericardiocentesis or surgical drainage.

Pulsus paradoxus

↓ in amplitude of systolic BP by > 10 mm Hg during inspiration. ↑ venous return during inspiration → ↑ RV filling → interventricular septum bows toward LV (due to ↓ pericardial compliance) → ↓ LV ejection volume → ↓ systolic BP. Seen in constrictive pericarditis, obstructive pulmonary disease (eg, Croup, OSA, Asthma, COPD), cardiac Tamponade (pea **COAT**).

Syncope

Transient loss of consciousness caused by a period of ↓ cerebral blood flow. Types:
- Reflex (most common)—vasovagal (prodromal symptoms [eg, warmth, pallor, nausea]; episodes are short with rapid recovery), situational (eg, coughing/sneezing, swallowing, defecation, micturition), carotid sinus hypersensitivity (eg, wearing tight collar).
- Orthostatic—hypovolemia, drugs (eg, antihypertensives), autonomic dysfunction. Orthostatic hypotension is defined as a drop in systolic BP ≥ 20 mm Hg and/or diastolic BP ≥ 10 mm Hg within 3 minutes of standing.
- Cardiac—arrhythmias, structural (eg, aortic stenosis, HCM).

Infective endocarditis

Infection of the endocardial surface of the heart, typically involving ≥1 heart valves. Caused by bacteria >> fungi. Forms:
- Acute—classically *S aureus* (high virulence). Large destructive vegetations 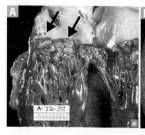 on previously normal valves. Rapid onset.
- Subacute—classically viridans streptococci (low virulence). Smaller vegetations on congenitally abnormal or diseased valves. Sequela of dental procedures. Gradual onset.

Presents with fever (most common), new murmur, vascular and immunologic phenomena.

Vascular phenomena—septic embolism, petechiae, splinter hemorrhages (linear hemorrhagic lesions on nail bed 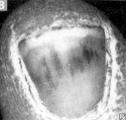), Janeway lesions (painless, flat, erythematous lesions on palms or soles).

Immunologic phenomena—immune complex deposition, glomerulonephritis, **O**sler nodes (painful ["**O**uchy"], raised, violaceous lesions on finger or toe pads 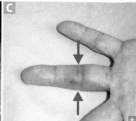), **R**oth spots (**R**etinal hemorrhagic lesions with pale centers 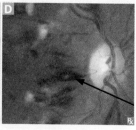).

Mitral valve (most common) > aortic valve. Tricuspid valve involvement is associated with injection **drug** use (don't "**tri**" **drugs**). Common associations:
- Prosthetic valves—*S epidermidis*
- GI/GU procedures—*Enterococcus*
- Colon cancer—*S gallolyticus*
- Gram ⊖—**HACEK** organisms (*Haemophilus, Aggregatibacter* [formerly *Actinobacillus*], *Cardiobacterium, Eikenella, Kingella*)
- Culture ⊖—*Coxiella, Bartonella*
- Injection drug use—*S aureus, Pseudomonas, Candida*

Endothelial injury → formation of vegetations consisting of platelets, fibrin, and microbes on heart valves → valve regurgitation, septic embolism (systemic circulation in left-sided endocarditis, pulmonary in right-sided).

Diagnosis requires multiple blood cultures and echocardiography.

Nonbacterial thrombotic endocarditis

Also called marantic endocarditis. Rare, noninfective. Vegetations typically arise on mitral or aortic valve and consist of sterile, platelet-rich thrombi that dislodge easily. Usually asymptomatic until embolism occurs.

Associated with the hypercoagulable state seen in advanced malignancy (especially pancreatic adenocarcinoma) or SLE (called Libman-Sacks endocarditis in this setting).

Rheumatic fever

A nonsuppurative consequence of pharyngeal infection with group A β-hemolytic streptococci. Late sequelae include rheumatic heart disease, which affects heart valves—**mi**tral > **a**ortic >> **t**ricuspid (high-pressure valves affected most). Early valvular regurgitation, late valvular stenosis.

Associated with Aschoff bodies (granuloma with giant cells), Anitschkow cells (enlarged macrophages with ovoid, wavy, rodlike nucleus), ↑ anti-streptolysin O (ASO) and ↑ anti-DNase B titers.

Immune mediated (type II hypersensitivity); not a direct effect of bacteria. Antibodies to **M** protein cross-react with self antigens, often **m**yosin (**m**olecular **m**imicry).

Treatment/prophylaxis: penicillin.

J♥NES (major criteria):
Joint (migratory polyarthritis)
♥ (pancarditis)
Nodules in skin (subcutaneous)
Erythema marginatum (evanescent rash with ring margin)
Sydenham chorea (involuntary irregular movements of limbs and face)

Syphilitic heart disease

3° syphilis disrupts the vasa vasorum of the aorta with consequent atrophy of vessel wall and dilation of aorta and valve ring.

May see calcification of aortic root, ascending aortic arch, and thoracic aorta. Leads to "tree bark" appearance of aorta.

Can result in aneurysm of ascending aorta or aortic arch, aortic insufficiency.

Acute pericarditis

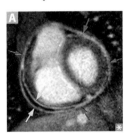

Inflammation of the pericardium (red arrows in Ⓐ). Commonly presents with sharp pain, aggravated by inspiration, and relieved by sitting up and leaning forward. Often complicated by pericardial effusion (between yellow arrows in Ⓐ). Presents with friction rub. ECG changes include widespread/diffuse ST-segment elevation and/or PR depression.

Usually idiopathic, but may be due to viral infections (eg, coxsackievirus B), malignancy (metastasis), cardiac surgery, thoracic radiotherapy (early), MI (eg, postcardiac injury syndrome), autoimmune diseases (eg, SLE, drug-induced lupus, rheumatoid arthritis), renal failure (uremia).

Treatment: NSAIDs, colchicine, glucocorticoids, dialysis (uremia).

Constrictive pericarditis

Chronic inflammation of pericardium → pericardial fibrosis +/− calcification → limited space for expansion → ↓ ventricular filling. Usually idiopathic, but may be due to viral infections, cardiac surgery, thoracic radiotherapy (late). TB is the most common cause in resource-limited countries. ↓ EDV → ↓ CO → ↓ venous return. Presents with dyspnea, peripheral edema, jugular venous distention, Kussmaul sign, pulsus paradoxus, pericardial knock.

Kussmaul sign	Paradoxical ↑ in JVP on inspiration (normally, inspiration → negative intrathoracic pressure → ↑ venous return → ↓ JVP).
	Impaired RV filling → RV cannot accommodate ↑ venous return during inspiration → blood backs up into vena cava → Kussmaul sign. May be seen with constrictive pericarditis, restrictive cardiomyopathy, right HF, massive pulmonary embolism, right atrial or ventricular tumors.

Myocarditis	Inflammation of myocardium. Major cause of SCD in adults < 40 years old.
	Presentation highly variable, can include dyspnea, chest pain, fever, arrhythmias (persistent tachycardia out of proportion to fever is characteristic).
	Multiple causes:
	▪ Viral (eg, adenovirus, coxsackie B, parvovirus B19, HIV, HHV-6, COVID-19); lymphocytic infiltrate with focal necrosis highly indicative of viral myocarditis
	▪ Parasitic (eg, *Trypanosoma cruzi*, *Toxoplasma gondii*)
	▪ Bacterial (eg, *Borrelia burgdorferi*, *Mycoplasma pneumoniae*, *Corynebacterium diphtheriae*)
	▪ Toxins (eg, carbon monoxide, black widow venom)
	▪ RF
	▪ Drugs (eg, doxorubicin, cocaine)
	▪ Autoimmune (eg, Kawasaki disease, sarcoidosis, SLE, polymyositis/dermatomyositis)
	Complications include sudden death, arrhythmias, heart block, dilated cardiomyopathy, HF, mural thrombus with systemic emboli.

Hereditary hemorrhagic telangiectasia 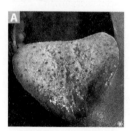	Also called Osler-Weber-Rendu syndrome. Autosomal dominant disorder of blood vessels. Findings: blanching lesions (eg, tongue telangiectasias A) on skin and mucous membranes, recurrent epistaxis, arteriovenous malformations (eg, brain, lung, liver), GI bleeding, hematuria.
	Arteriovenous malformation—abnormal, high-flow connection between artery and vein. ↑ risk of high output cardiac failure. Most common cause of intracranial hemorrhage in children.

Cardiac tumors	Most common cardiac tumor is a metastasis (eg, melanoma).
Myxomas 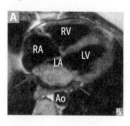	Most common 1° cardiac tumor in **adults** (arrows in A). 90% occur in the atria (mostly left atrium). Myxomas are usually described as a "ball valve" obstruction in the left atrium (associated with multiple syncopal episodes). IL-6 production by tumor → constitutional symptoms (eg, fever, weight loss). May auscultate early diastolic "tumor plop" sound (mimics mitral stenosis). Histology: gelatinous material, myxoma cells immersed in glycosaminoglycans.
	Adults make **6 myx**ed drinks.
Rhabdomyomas	Most frequent 1° cardiac tumor in children (associated with tuberous sclerosis). Histology: hamartomatous growths. More common in the ventricles.

Deep venous thrombosis

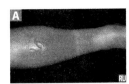

Blood clot within a deep vein → swelling, redness , warmth, pain. Predisposed by Virchow triad (SHE):

- Stasis (eg, post-op, long drive/flight)
- Hypercoagulability (eg, defect in coagulation cascade proteins, such as factor V Leiden; oral contraceptive use; pregnancy)
- Endothelial damage (exposed collagen triggers clotting cascade)

DVT of proximal deep veins of lower extremity (iliac, femoral, popliteal) → embolic source.

D-dimer test may be used clinically to rule out DVT if disease probability is low or moderate (high sensitivity, low specificity). Imaging test of choice is compression ultrasound with Doppler.

Use unfractionated heparin or low-molecular weight heparins (eg, enoxaparin) for prophylaxis and acute management. Use direct anticoagulants (eg, rivaroxaban, apixaban) for treatment and long-term prevention.

▸ CARDIOVASCULAR—PHARMACOLOGY

Hypertension treatment

Primary (essential) hypertension	Thiazide diuretics, ACE inhibitors, angiotensin II receptor blockers (ARBs), Ca^{2+} channel blockers.	
Hypertension with heart failure	ACE inhibitors/ARBs, β-blockers (compensated HF), aldosterone antagonists (mortality benefit), diuretics (improve symptoms and reduce hospitalization)	β-blockers must be used cautiously in decompensated HF and are contraindicated in cardiogenic shock.
Hypertension with diabetes mellitus	ACE inhibitors/ARBs, Ca^{2+} channel blockers, thiazide diuretics, β-blockers.	ACE inhibitors/ARBs are protective against diabetic nephropathy. β-blockers can mask hypoglycemia symptoms.
Hypertension with asthma	ARBs, Ca^{2+} channel blockers, thiazide diuretics, cardioselective β-blockers.	Avoid non-selective β-blockers to prevent β_2-receptor–induced bronchoconstriction. Avoid ACE inhibitors to prevent confusion between drug- or asthma-related cough.
Hypertension with pregnancy	Hydralazine, methyldopa, labetalol, nifedipine.	Hypertensive moms love nifedipine.
Hypertension with gout	ACE inhibitors, Ca^{2+} channel blockers, ARBs (especially losartan).	Avoid loop and thiazide diuretics as these can cause gout flares.
Hypertension with osteoporosis	Thiazides preferred as monotherapy; combine with ACE inhibitors or ARBs if needed.	Thiazides preferred due to increased Ca^{2+} reabsorption.
Hypertension with pheochromocytoma	Phentolamine, phenoxybenzamine (α-blockade first) prior to resection and β-blockade.	Avoid β-blockade first to mitigate unopposed α-mediated hypertensive crisis.

Cardiovascular agents and molecular targets

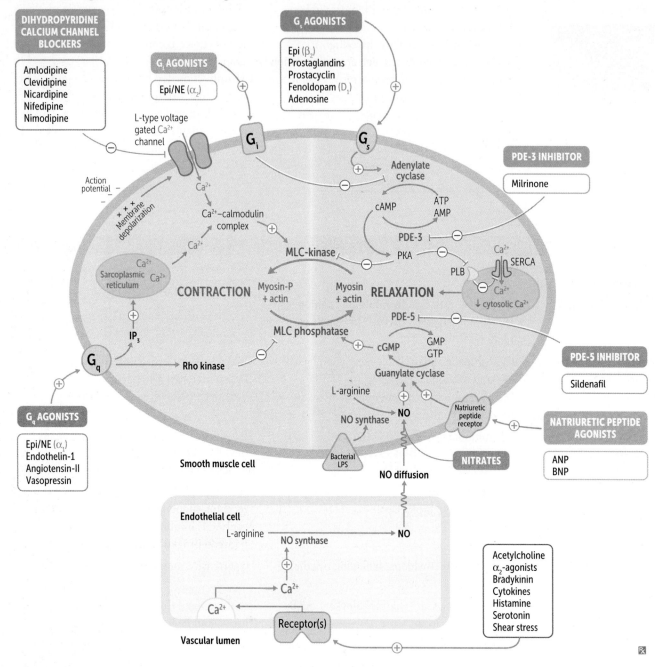

Nitrates	Nitroglycerin, isosorbide dinitrate, isosorbide mononitrate.
MECHANISM	Vasodilate by ↑ NO in vascular smooth muscle → ↑ in cGMP and smooth muscle relaxation. Dilate veins >> arteries. ↓ preload.
CLINICAL USE	Angina, ACS, pulmonary edema.
ADVERSE EFFECTS	Reflex tachycardia (treat with β-blockers), methemoglobinemia, hypotension, flushing, headache, "Monday disease" in industrial nitrate exposure: development of tolerance for the vasodilating action during the work week and loss of tolerance over the weekend → tachycardia, dizziness, headache upon reexposure. Contraindicated in right ventricular infarction, hypertrophic cardiomyopathy, and with concurrent PDE-5 inhibitor use.

Calcium channel blockers	Amlodipine, clevidipine, nicardipine, nifedipine, nimodipine (dihydropyridines, act on vascular smooth muscle); diltiazem, verapamil (nondihydropyridines, act on heart).
MECHANISM	Block voltage-dependent L-type calcium channels of cardiac and smooth muscle → ↓ muscle contractility. Vascular smooth muscle—amlodipine = nifedipine > diltiazem > verapamil. Heart—verapamil > diltiazem > amlodipine = nifedipine.
CLINICAL USE	Dihydropyridines (except nimodipine): hypertension, angina (including vasospastic type), Raynaud phenomenon. **Dihydropyridine mainly dilates arteries.** Nimodipine: subarachnoid hemorrhage (prevents delayed ischemia). Nicardipine, clevidipine: hypertensive urgency or emergency. Nondihydropyridines: hypertension, angina, rate control in atrial fibrillation/flutter, prevention of nodal arrhythmias.
ADVERSE EFFECTS	Gingival hyperplasia. Dihydropyridine: peripheral edema, flushing, dizziness. Nondihydropyridine: cardiac depression, AV block, hyperprolactinemia (verapamil), constipation.

Hydralazine	
MECHANISM	↑ cGMP → smooth muscle relaxation. Hydralazine vasodilates arterioles > veins; afterload reduction.
CLINICAL USE	Severe hypertension (particularly acute), HF (with organic nitrate). Safe to use during pregnancy. Frequently coadministered with a β-blocker to prevent reflex tachycardia.
ADVERSE EFFECTS	Compensatory tachycardia (contraindicated in angina/CAD), fluid retention, headache, angina, drug-induced lupus.

Hypertensive emergency	Treat with labetalol, clevidipine, fenoldopam, nicardipine, nitroprusside.
Nitroprusside	Short acting vasodilator (arteries = veins); ↑ cGMP via direct release of NO. Can cause cyanide toxicity (releases cyanide).
Fenoldopam	Dopamine D_1 receptor agonist—coronary, peripheral, renal, and splanchnic vasodilation. ↓ BP, ↑ natriuresis. Also used postoperatively as an antihypertensive. Can cause hypotension, tachycardia, flushing, headache, nausea.

Antianginal therapy	Goal is reduction of myocardial O_2 consumption (MVO_2) by ↓ 1 or more of the determinants of MVO_2: end-diastolic volume, BP, HR, contractility.

COMPONENT	NITRATES	β-BLOCKERS	NITRATES + β-BLOCKERS
End-diastolic volume	↓	No effect or ↑	No effect or ↓
Blood pressure	↓	↓	↓
Contractility	↑ (reflex response)	↓	Little/no effect
Heart rate	↑ (reflex response)	↓	No effect or ↓
Ejection time	↓	↑	Little/no effect
MVO_2	↓	↓	↓↓

Nondihydropyridine calcium channel blockers (verapamil, diltiazem) are similar to β-blockers in effect.

Ranolazine

MECHANISM	Inhibits the late phase of inward sodium current thereby reducing diastolic wall tension and oxygen consumption. Does not affect heart rate or blood pressure.
CLINICAL USE	Refractory angina.
ADVERSE EFFECTS	Constipation, dizziness, headache, nausea, QT prolongation.

Sacubitril

MECHANISM	A neprilysin inhibitor; prevents degradation of bradykinin, natriuretic peptides, angiotensin II, and substance P → ↑ vasodilation, ↓ ECF volume.
CLINICAL USE	Used in combination with valsartan (an ARB) to treat HFrEF.
ADVERSE EFFECTS	Hypotension, hyperkalemia (due to ARB component of HFrEF therapy), cough, dizziness; contraindicated with ACE inhibitors due to angioedema (both drugs ↑ bradykinin).

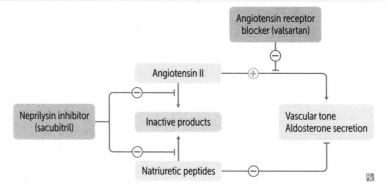

Lipid-lowering agents

DRUG	LDL	HDL	TRIGLYCERIDES	MECHANISM	ADVERSE EFFECTS
Statins Atorvastatin, lovastatin, pravastatin, rosuvastatin, simvastatin	↓↓↓	↑	↓	Inhibit HMG-CoA reductase → ↓ cholesterol synthesis; → ↓ intrahepatic cholesterol → ↑ LDL receptor recycling → ↑ LDL catabolism ↓ in mortality in patients with CAD	Hepatotoxicity (↑ LFTs), myopathy (especially when used with fibrates or niacin)
Bile acid resins Cholestyramine, colesevelam, colestipol	↓↓	↑ slightly	↑ slightly	Disrupt enterohepatic bile acid circulation → compensatory ↑ conversion of cholesterol to bile → ↓ intrahepatic cholesterol → ↑ LDL receptor recycling	GI upset, ↓ absorption of other drugs and fat-soluble vitamins
Ezetimibe	↓↓	↑/—	↓/—	Prevents cholesterol absorption at small intestine brush border	Rare ↑ LFTs, diarrhea

Lipid-lowering agents (continued)

DRUG	LDL	HDL	TRIGLYCERIDES	MECHANISM	ADVERSE EFFECTS
Fibrates Fenofibrate, gemfibrozil	↓	↑	↓↓↓	Activate PPAR-α → upregulate LPL → ↑ TG clearance Activate PPAR-α → induce HDL synthesis	Myopathy (↑ risk with statins), cholesterol gallstones (via inhibition of cholesterol 7α-hydroxylase)
Niacin	↓↓	↑↑	↓	Inhibits lipolysis (hormone-sensitive lipase) in adipose tissue; reduces hepatic VLDL synthesis	Flushed face (prostaglandin mediated; ↓ by NSAIDs or long-term use) Hyperglycemia Hyperuricemia
PCSK9 inhibitors Alirocumab, evolocumab	↓↓↓	↑	↓	Inactivation of LDL-receptor degradation → ↑ removal of LDL from bloodstream	Myalgias, delirium, dementia, other neurocognitive effects
Fish oil and marine omega-3 fatty acids	↑ slightly	↑ slightly	↓ at high doses	Believed to ↓ FFA delivery to liver, ↓ activity of TG-synthesizing enzymes, ↓ VLDL production, and inhibit synthesis of ApoB	Nausea, fishlike taste

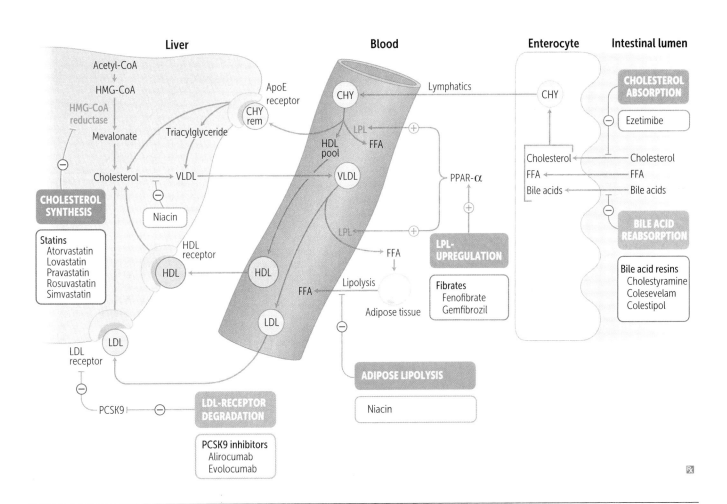

Digoxin

MECHANISM	Direct inhibition of Na⁺/K⁺-ATPase. → indirect inhibition of Na⁺/Ca²⁺ exchanger. ↑ [Ca²⁺]ᵢ → positive inotropy. Stimulates vagus nerve → ↓ HR.

CLINICAL USE	HF (↑ contractility); atrial fibrillation (↓ conduction at AV node and depression of SA node).
ADVERSE EFFECTS	Cholinergic effects (nausea, vomiting, diarrhea), blurry **yellow** vision ("van **Glow**"), arrhythmias, atrial tachycardia with AV block. Can lead to hyperkalemia, which indicates poor prognosis. Factors predisposing to toxicity: renal failure (↓ excretion), hypokalemia (permissive for digoxin binding at K⁺-binding site on Na⁺/K⁺-ATPase), drugs that displace digoxin from tissue-binding sites, and ↓ clearance (eg, verapamil, amiodarone, quinidine).
ANTIDOTE	Slowly normalize K⁺, cardiac pacer, anti-digoxin Fab fragments, Mg²⁺.

Antiarrhythmics—sodium channel blockers (class I)	Slow or block conduction (especially in depolarized cells). ↓ slope of phase 0 depolarization. ↑ action at **faster** HR. State dependent ↑ HR → shorter diastole, Na⁺ channels spend less time in resting state (drugs dissociate during this state) → less time for drug to dissociate from receptor. Effect most pronounced in IC>IA>IB due to relative binding strength. **Fast taxi CAB.**

Class IA	Quinidine, **procainamid**e, **disopyramid**e. "The **queen proclaims Diso's pyramid**."

MECHANISM	Moderate Na⁺ channel blockade. ↑ AP duration, ↑ effective refractory period (ERP) in ventricular action potential, ↑ QT interval, some K⁺ channel blocking effects.
CLINICAL USE	Both atrial and ventricular arrhythmias, especially reentrant and ectopic SVT and VT.
ADVERSE EFFECTS	Cinchonism (headache, tinnitus with quinidine), reversible SLE-like syndrome (procainamide), HF (disopyramide), thrombocytopenia, torsades de pointes due to ↑ QT interval.

Class IB	**L**idocaine, **m**exi**l**etine. "**I'd Buy Liddy's Mexican** tacos."

MECHANISM	Weak Na⁺ channel blockade. ↓ AP duration. Preferentially affect ischemic or depolarized Purkinje and ventricular tissue.
CLINICAL USE	Acute ventricular arrhythmias (especially post-MI), digitalis-induced arrhythmias. **IB** is **B**est post-MI.
ADVERSE EFFECTS	CNS stimulation/depression, cardiovascular depression.

Antiarrhythmics—sodium channel blockers (class I) *(continued)*

Class IC	Flecainide, propafenone. "Can I have fries, please?"
MECHANISM	Strong Na^+ channel blockade. Significantly prolongs ERP in AV node and accessory bypass tracts. No effect on ERP in Purkinje and ventricular tissue. Minimal effect on AP duration.
CLINICAL USE	SVTs, including atrial fibrillation. Only as a last resort in refractory VT.
ADVERSE EFFECTS	Proarrhythmic, especially post-MI (contraindicated). IC is Contraindicated in structural and ischemic heart disease.

0 mV

Slope of phase 0
I_{Na}

℞

Antiarrhythmics—β-blockers (class II)

	Metoprolol, propranolol, esmolol, atenolol, timolol, carvedilol.
MECHANISM	Decrease SA and AV nodal activity by ↓ cAMP, ↓ Ca^{2+} currents. Suppress abnormal pacemakers by ↓ slope of phase 4. AV node particularly sensitive—↑ PR interval. Esmolol very short acting.
CLINICAL USE	SVT, ventricular rate control for atrial fibrillation and atrial flutter, prevent ventricular arrhythmia post-MI.
ADVERSE EFFECTS	Impotence, exacerbation of COPD and asthma, cardiovascular effects (bradycardia, AV block, HF), CNS effects (sedation, sleep alterations). May mask the signs of hypoglycemia. Metoprolol can cause dyslipidemia. Propranolol can exacerbate vasospasm in vasospastic angina. β-blockers (except the nonselective α- and β-antagonists carvedilol and labetalol) cause unopposed α_1-agonism if given alone for pheochromocytoma or for cocaine toxicity (unsubstantiated). Treat β-blocker overdose with Glucagon, Atropine, Saline (**GAS**).

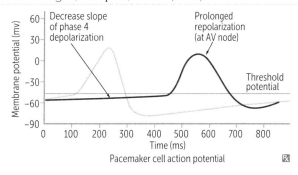

Pacemaker cell action potential

Antiarrhythmics— potassium channel blockers (class III)	Amiodarone, Ibutilide, Dofetilide, Sotalol.	AIDS.
MECHANISM	↑ AP duration, ↑ ERP, ↑ QT interval.	
CLINICAL USE	Atrial fibrillation, atrial flutter; ventricular tachycardia (amiodarone, sotalol).	
ADVERSE EFFECTS	Sotalol—torsades de pointes, excessive β blockade. Ibutilide—torsades de pointes. Amiodarone—pulmonary fibrosis, hepatotoxicity, hypothyroidism or hyperthyroidism (amiodarone is 40% iodine by weight), acts as hapten (corneal deposits, blue/gray skin deposits resulting in photodermatitis), neurologic effects, constipation, cardiovascular effects (bradycardia, heart block, HF).	Remember to check PFTs, LFTs, and TFTs when using amiodarone. Amiodarone is lipophilic and has class I, II, III, and IV effects. 0 mV Markedly prolonged repolarization (I$_K$) −85 mV Cell action potential

Antiarrhythmics— calcium channel blockers (class IV)	Diltiazem, verapamil.	
MECHANISM	Decrease conduction velocity, ↑ ERP, ↑ PR interval.	
CLINICAL USE	Rate control in atrial fibrillation/flutter, prevention of nodal arrhythmias.	Slow rise of action potential Prolonged repolarization (at AV node) Threshold potential
ADVERSE EFFECTS	Constipation, gingival hyperplasia, flushing, edema, cardiovascular effects (HF, AV block, sinus node depression).	

Other antiarrhythmics

Adenosine	↑ K$^+$ out of cells → hyperpolarizing the cell and ↓ I$_{Ca}$, decreasing AV node conduction. Drug of choice in diagnosing/terminating certain forms of SVT. Very short acting (~ 15 sec). Effects blunted by theophylline and caffeine (both are adenosine receptor antagonists). Adverse effects include flushing, hypotension, chest pain, sense of impending doom, bronchospasm.
Magnesium	Effective in torsades de pointes and digoxin toxicity.

Ivabradine

MECHANISM	IVabradine prolongs slow depolarization (phase "IV") by selectively inhibiting "funny" sodium channels (I$_f$).
CLINICAL USE	Chronic HFrEF.
ADVERSE EFFECTS	Luminous phenomena/visual brightness, hypertension, bradycardia.

Endocrine

"If you skew the endocrine system, you lose the pathways to self."
—Hilary Mantel

"Sometimes you need a little crisis to get your adrenaline flowing and help you realize your potential."
—Jeannette Walls, *The Glass Castle*

"Chocolate causes certain endocrine glands to secrete hormones that affect your feelings and behavior by making you happy."
—Elaine Sherman, *Book of Divine Indulgences*

The endocrine system comprises widely distributed organs that work in a highly integrated manner to orchestrate a state of hormonal equilibrium within the body. Generally speaking, endocrine diseases can be classified either as diseases of underproduction or overproduction, or as conditions involving the development of mass lesions—which themselves may be associated with underproduction or overproduction of hormones. Therefore, study the endocrine system first by learning the glands, their hormones, and their regulation, and then by integrating disease manifestations with diagnosis and management. Take time to learn the multisystem connections.

Thyroid development

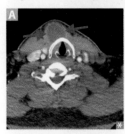

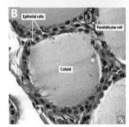

Thyroid diverticulum arises from floor of primitive pharynx and descends into neck. Connected to tongue by thyroglossal duct, which normally disappears but may persist as cysts or the pyramidal lobe of thyroid. Foramen cecum is normal remnant of thyroglossal duct.

Most common ectopic thyroid tissue site is the tongue (lingual thyroid). Removal may result in hypothyroidism if it is the only thyroid tissue present.

Thyroglossal duct cyst **A** presents as an anterior midline neck mass that moves with swallowing or protrusion of the tongue (vs persistent cervical sinus leading to pharyngeal cleft cyst in lateral neck).

Thyroid follicular cells **B** derived from endoderm.

Parafollicular cells arise from 4th pharyngeal pouch.

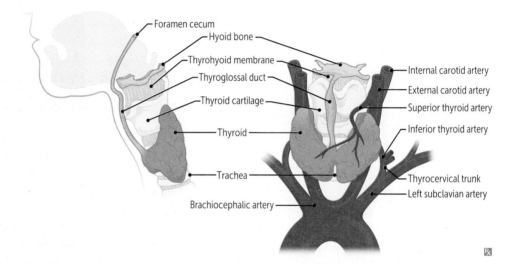

▶ ENDOCRINE—ANATOMY

Pituitary gland

Anterior pituitary (adenohypophysis)	Secretes FSH, LH, ACTH, TSH, prolactin, GH, and β-endorphin. Melanotropin (MSH) secreted from intermediate lobe of pituitary. Derived from oral ectoderm (Rathke pouch). ▪ α subunit—hormone subunit common to TSH, LH, FSH, and hCG. ▪ β subunit—determines hormone specificity.	**Pro**opiomelanocortin (POMC) derivatives—β-endorphin, **A**CTH, and **M**SH. Go **pro** with a **BAM**! **FLAT PeG**: FSH, LH, ACTH, TSH, PRL, GH. **B-FLAT**: Basophils—FSH, LH, ACTH, TSH. **Acid PiG**: Acidophils — PRL, GH.
Posterior pituitary (neurohypophysis)	Stores and releases vasopressin (antidiuretic hormone, or ADH) and oxytocin, both made in the hypothalamus (supraoptic and paraventricular nuclei) and transported to posterior pituitary via neurophysins (carrier proteins). Derived from **neuro**ectoderm.	

Adrenal cortex and medulla

Adrenal cortex (derived from mesoderm) and medulla (derived from neural crest).

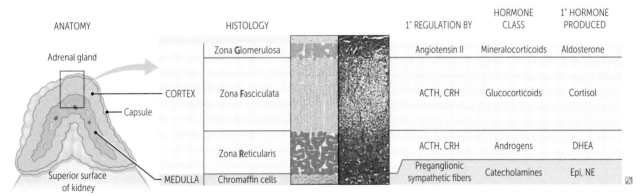

ANATOMY		HISTOLOGY		1° REGULATION BY	HORMONE CLASS	1° HORMONE PRODUCED
		Zona **G**lomerulosa		Angiotensin II	Mineralocorticoids	Aldosterone
CORTEX		Zona **F**asciculata		ACTH, CRH	Glucocorticoids	Cortisol
		Zona **R**eticularis		ACTH, CRH	Androgens	DHEA
MEDULLA		Chromaffin cells		Preganglionic sympathetic fibers	Catecholamines	Epi, NE

GFR corresponds with salt (mineralocorticoids), sugar (glucocorticoids), and sex (androgens).

Endocrine pancreas cell types

Islets of Langerhans are collections of α, β, and δ endocrine cells. Islets arise from pancreatic buds.

α = gluc**α**gon (peripheral)
β = insulin (central)
δ = somatostatin (interspersed)

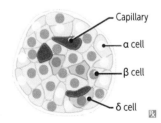

▸ ENDOCRINE—PHYSIOLOGY

Hypothalamic-pituitary hormones

HORMONE	FUNCTION	CLINICAL NOTES
ADH	↑ water permeability of distal convoluted tubule and collecting duct cells in kidney to ↑ water reabsorption	Alcohol consumption → ↓ ADH secretion → polyuria and dehydration
CRH	↑ ACTH, ↑ MSH, ↑ β-endorphin	↓ in chronic glucocorticoid use
Prolactin-inhibiting factor	↓ prolactin, ↓ TSH	Commonly referred to as dopamine Dopamine antagonists (eg, antipsychotics) can cause galactorrhea due to hyperprolactinemia
GHRH	↑ GH	Analog (tesamorelin) used to treat HIV-associated lipodystrophy
GnRH	↑ FSH, ↑ LH	Suppressed by hyperprolactinemia Tonic GnRH analog (eg, leuprolide) suppresses hypothalamic–pituitary–gonadal axis. Pulsatile GnRH leads to puberty, fertility
MSH	↑ melanogenesis by melanocytes	Causes hyperpigmentation in Cushing disease, as MSH and ACTH share the same precursor molecule, POMC
Oxytocin	Causes uterine contractions during labor. Responsible for milk letdown reflex in response to suckling.	Modulates fear, anxiety, social bonding, mood, and depression
Prolactin	↓ GnRH Stimulates lactogenesis.	Pituitary prolactinoma → amenorrhea, osteoporosis, hypogonadism, galactorrhea Breastfeeding → ↑ prolactin → ↓ GnRH → delayed postpartum ovulation (natural contraception)
Somatostatin	↓ GH, ↓ TSH	Also called growth hormone inhibiting hormone (GHIH)
TRH	↑ TSH, ↑ prolactin	↑ TRH (eg, in 1°/2° hypothyroidism) may increase prolactin secretion → galactorrhea

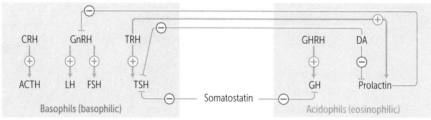

Growth hormone

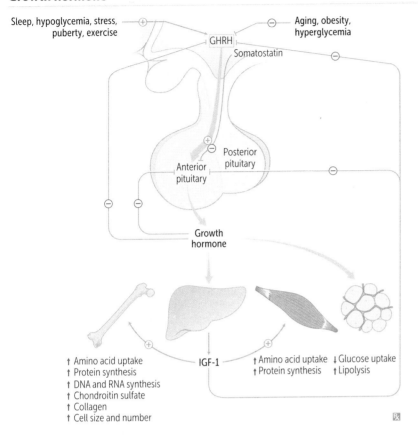

Also called somatotropin. Secreted by anterior pituitary.

Stimulates linear growth and muscle mass through IGF-1 (somatomedin C) secretion by liver. ↑ insulin resistance (diabetogenic).

Released in pulses in response to growth hormone–releasing hormone (GHRH).

Secretion ↑ during (deep) sleep, hypoglycemia, stress, puberty, exercise.

Secretion ↓ with aging, obesity, hyperglycemia, somatostatin, somatomedin (regulatory molecule secreted by liver in response to GH acting on target tissues).

Excess secretion of GH (eg, pituitary adenoma) may cause acromegaly (adults) or gigantism (children). Treatment: somatostatin analogs (eg, octreotide) or surgery.

Antidiuretic hormone	Also called vasopressin.
SOURCE	Synthesized in hypothalamus (supraoptic and paraventricular nuclei), stored and secreted by posterior pituitary.
FUNCTION	Regulates blood pressure (V$_1$-receptors) and serum osmolality (V$_2$-receptors). Primary function is serum osmolality regulation (ADH ↓ serum osmolality, ↑ urine osmolality) via regulation of aquaporin channel insertion in principal cells of renal collecting duct. ADH level is ↓ in central diabetes insipidus (DI), normal or ↑ in nephrogenic DI. Desmopressin (ADH analog) is a treatment for central DI and nocturnal enuresis. **Vasopressin** is a potent **vasopressor** that can be used to increase organ perfusion in septic shock.
REGULATION	Plasma osmolality (1°); hypovolemia.

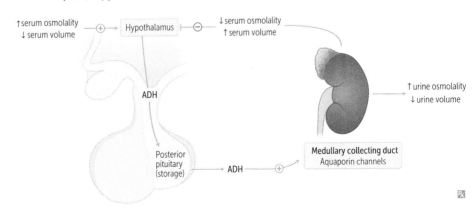

Prolactin

SOURCE	Secreted mainly by anterior pituitary.	Structurally homologous to growth hormone.
FUNCTION	Stimulates milk production in breast; inhibits ovulation in females and spermatogenesis in males by inhibiting GnRH synthesis and release.	Excessive amounts of prolactin associated with galactorrhea, amenorrhea, infertility, osteoporosis (in females); gynecomastia, infertility, decreased libido, impotence (in males).
REGULATION	Prolactin secretion from anterior pituitary is tonically inhibited by dopamine from tuberoinfundibular pathway of hypothalamus. Prolactin in turn inhibits its own secretion by ↑ dopamine synthesis and secretion from hypothalamus. TRH ↑ prolactin secretion (eg, in 1° or 2° hypothyroidism). Dopamine has stronger effect on prolactin regulation than TRH does.	Dopamine agonists (eg, bromocriptine, cabergoline) inhibit prolactin secretion and can be used in treatment of prolactinoma. Dopamine antagonists (eg, most antipsychotics, metoclopramide) and estrogens (eg, OCPs, pregnancy) stimulate prolactin secretion.

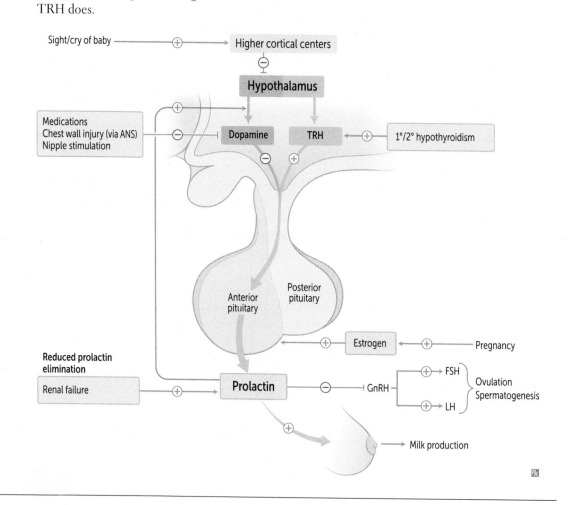

Thyroid hormones	Thyroid produces triiodothyronine (T_3) and thyroxine (T_4), iodine-containing hormones that control the body's metabolic rate.
SOURCE	Follicles of thyroid. 5′-deiodinase converts T_4 (the major thyroid product) to T_3 in peripheral tissue (**5, 4, 3**). Peripheral conversion is inhibited by glucocorticoids, β-blockers, and propylthiouracil (PTU). Reverse T_3 (rT_3) is a metabolically inactive byproduct of the peripheral conversion of T_4 and its production is increased by growth hormone and glucocorticoids. Functions of thyroid peroxidase include oxidation, organification of iodine, and coupling of monoiodotyrosine (MIT) and diiodotyrosine (DIT). Inhibited by PTU and methimazole. DIT + DIT = T_4. DIT + MIT = T_3. Wolff-Chaik**off** effect—protective autoregulation; sudden exposure to excess iodine temporarily turns **off** thyroid peroxidase → ↓ T_3/T_4 production.
FUNCTION	Only free hormone is active. T_3 binds nuclear receptor with greater affinity than T_4. T_3 functions —7 **B**'s: ▪ **B**rain maturation ▪ **B**one growth (synergism with GH and IGF-1) ▪ β-adrenergic effects. ↑ $β_1$ receptors in heart → ↑ CO, HR, SV, contractility; β-blockers alleviate adrenergic symptoms in thyrotoxicosis ▪ **B**asal metabolic rate ↑ (via ↑ Na^+/K^+-ATPase → ↑ O_2 consumption, RR, body temperature) ▪ **B**lood sugar (↑ glycogenolysis, gluconeogenesis) ▪ **B**reak down lipids (↑ lipolysis) ▪ Stimulates surfactant synthesis in **B**abies
REGULATION	TRH → ⊕ TSH release → ⊕ follicular cells. Thyroid-stimulating immunoglobulin (TSI) may ⊕ follicular cells in Graves disease. Negative feedback primarily by free T_3/T_4: ▪ Anterior pituitary → ↓ sensitivity to TRH ▪ Hypothalamus → ↓ TRH secretion Thyroxine-binding globulin (TBG) binds most T_3/T_4 in blood. Bound T_3/T_4 = inactive. ▪ ↑ TBG in pregnancy, OCP use (estrogen → ↑ TBG) → ↑ total T_3/T_4 ▪ ↓ TBG in steroid use, nephrotic syndrome T_3 and T_4 are the only lipophilic hormones with charged amino acids and require specific transporters to diffuse into the cell (facilitated diffusion).

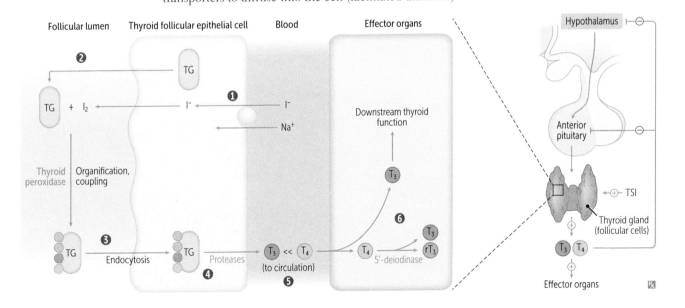

Parathyroid hormone

SOURCE	Chief cells of parathyroid
FUNCTION	↑ free Ca^{2+} in the blood (1° function) ↑ Ca^{2+} and PO_4^{3-} absorption in GI system ↑ Ca^{2+} and PO_4^{3-} from bone resorption ↑ Ca^{2+} reabsorption from DCT ↓ PO_4^{3-} reabsorption in PCT ↑ 1,25-$(OH)_2D_3$ (calcitriol) production by activating 1α-hydroxylase in **PCT** (**tri** to make D_3 in the **PCT**)	PTH ↑ serum Ca^{2+}, ↓ serum PO_4^{3-}, ↑ urine PO_4^{3-}, ↑ urine cAMP ↑ RANK-L (receptor activator of NF-κB ligand) secreted by osteoblasts and osteocytes; binds RANK (receptor) on osteoclasts and their precursors to stimulate osteoclasts and ↑ Ca^{2+} → bone resorption (intermittent PTH release can also stimulate bone formation) **PTH** = **P**hosphate-**T**rashing **H**ormone PTH-related peptide (PTHrP) functions like PTH and is commonly increased in malignancies (eg, squamous cell carcinoma of the lung, renal cell carcinoma)
REGULATION	↓ serum Ca^{2+} → ↑ PTH secretion ↑ serum PO_4^{3-} → ↑ PTH secretion ↓ serum Mg^{2+} → ↑ PTH secretion ↓↓ serum Mg^{2+} → ↓ PTH secretion Common causes of ↓ Mg^{2+} include diarrhea, aminoglycosides, diuretics, alcohol use disorder	Ca^{2+} is the major regulator of PTH release

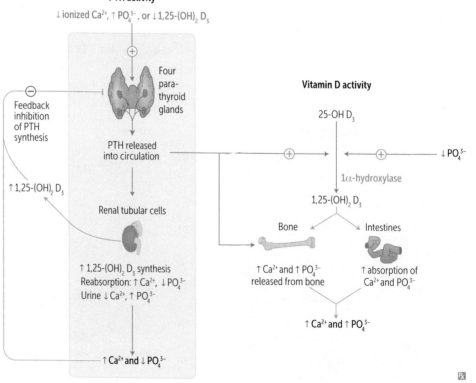

PTH activity

↓ ionized Ca^{2+}, ↑ PO_4^{3-}, or ↓ 1,25-$(OH)_2 D_3$

Four parathyroid glands

Feedback inhibition of PTH synthesis

↑ 1,25-$(OH)_2 D_3$

PTH released into circulation

Renal tubular cells

↑ 1,25-$(OH)_2 D_3$ synthesis
Reabsorption: ↑ Ca^{2+}, ↓ PO_4^{3-}
Urine ↓ Ca^{2+}, ↑ PO_4^{3-}

↑ Ca^{2+} and ↓ PO_4^{3-}

Vitamin D activity

25-OH D_3

↓ PO_4^{3-}

1α-hydroxylase

1,25-$(OH)_2 D_3$

Bone

Intestines

↑ Ca^{2+} and ↑ PO_4^{3-} released from bone

↑ absorption of Ca^{2+} and PO_4^{3-}

↑ Ca^{2+} and ↑ PO_4^{3-}

Calcium homeostasis

Plasma Ca^{2+} exists in three forms:
- Ionized/free (~ 45%, active form)
- Bound to albumin (~ 40%)
- Bound to anions (~ 15%)

Ionized/free Ca^{2+} is 1° regulator of PTH; changes in pH alter PTH secretion, whereas changes in albumin concentration do not

Ca^{2+} competes with H^+ to bind to albumin

↑ pH (less H^+) → albumin binds more Ca^{2+} → ↓ ionized Ca^{2+} (eg, cramps, pain, paresthesias, carpopedal spasm) → ↑ PTH

↓ pH (more H^+) → albumin binds less Ca^{2+} → ↑ ionized Ca^{2+} → ↓ PTH

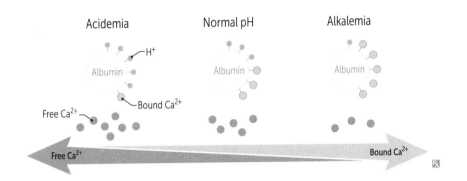

Calcitonin

SOURCE	Parafollicular cells (C cells) of thyroid.
FUNCTION	↓ bone resorption.
REGULATION	↑ serum Ca^{2+} → ↑ calcitonin secretion.

Calcitonin opposes actions of PTH. Not important in normal Ca^{2+} homeostasis

Calcitonin **t**ones down serum Ca^{2+} levels and keeps it in **b**ones

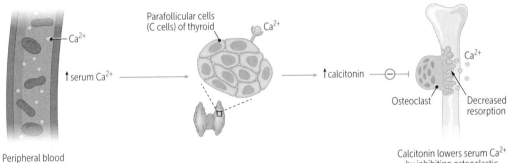

Glucagon

SOURCE	Made by α cells of pancreas.
FUNCTION	Promotes glycogenolysis, gluconeogenesis, lipolysis, ketogenesis. Elevates blood sugar levels to maintain homeostasis when bloodstream glucose levels fall too low (ie, fasting state).
REGULATION	Secreted in response to hypoglycemia. Inhibited by insulin, amylin, somatostatin, hyperglycemia.

Insulin

SYNTHESIS

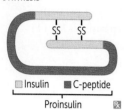

Insulin   ■ C-peptide

Proinsulin   ℞

Preproinsulin (synthesized in RER of pancreatic β cells) → cleavage of "presignal" → proinsulin (stored in secretory granules) → cleavage of proinsulin → exocytosis of insulin and C-peptide equally. Both insulin and C-peptide are ↑ in endogenous insulin secretion (eg, type 2 DM, insulin secretagogues, insulinoma), whereas exogenous insulin lacks C-peptide (helps differentiate factitious hypoglycemia).

Insulin is synthesized in pancreas and cleared by both liver and kidneys.

FUNCTION

Binds insulin receptors (tyrosine kinase activity ❶), inducing glucose uptake (carrier-mediated transport) into insulin-dependent tissue ❷ and gene transcription.

Anabolic effects of insulin:

- ↑ glucose transport in skeletal muscle and adipose tissue
- ↑ glycogen synthesis and storage
- ↑ triglyceride synthesis
- ↑ Na^+ retention (kidneys)
- ↑ protein synthesis (muscles)
- ↑ cellular uptake of K^+ and amino acids
- ↓ glucagon release
- ↓ lipolysis in adipose tissue

Unlike glucose, insulin does not cross placenta. In mothers with diabetes, excess glucose can cross placenta and ↑↑ fetal insulin.

Insulin-dependent glucose transporters:

- GLUT4: adipose tissue, striated muscle (exercise can also ↑ GLUT4 expression)

Insulin-independent transporters:

- GLUT1: RBCs, brain, cornea, placenta
- GLUT2 (bidirectional): β islet cells, liver, kidney, GI tract (think 2-way street)
- GLUT3: brain, placenta
- GLUT5 (fructose): spermatocytes, GI tract
- SGLT1/SGLT2 (Na^+-glucose cotransporters): kidney, small intestine

Brain prefers glucose, but may use ketone bodies during starvation. RBCs utilize only glucose, as they lack mitochondria for aerobic metabolism.

BRICK LIPS (insulin-independent glucose uptake): Brain, RBCs, Intestine, Cornea, Kidney, Liver, Islet (β) cells, Placenta, Spermatocytes.

REGULATION

Glucose is the major regulator of insulin release. ↑ insulin response with oral vs IV glucose due to incretins (eg, glucagonlike peptide 1 [GLP-1], glucose-dependent insulinotropic polypeptide [GIP]), which are released after meals and ↑ β cell sensitivity to glucose. Release ↓ by α_2, ↑ by β_2 stimulation (2 = regulates insulin).

Glucose enters β cells ❸ → ↑ ATP generated from glucose metabolism ❹ closes K^+ channels (target of sulfonylureas) ❺ and depolarizes β cell membrane ❻. Voltage-gated Ca^{2+} channels open → Ca^{2+} influx ❼ and stimulation of insulin exocytosis ❽.

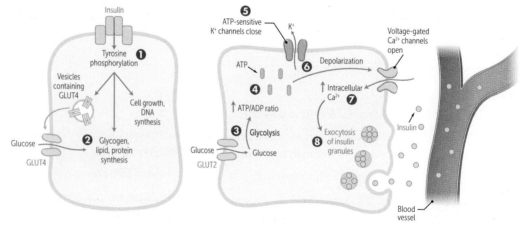

Insulin-dependent glucose uptake   Insulin secretion by pancreatic β cells   ℞

Adrenal steroids and congenital adrenal hyperplasias

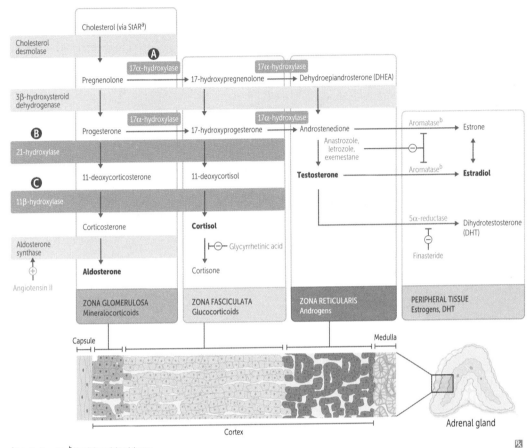

a Rate-limiting step, b Mostly in peripheral tissues.

ENZYME DEFICIENCY	MINERALOCORTICOIDS	[K⁺]	BP	CORTISOL	SEX HORMONES	LABS	PRESENTATION
Ⓐ 17α-hydroxylase[a]	↓ aldosterone ↑ 11-deoxycorti-costerone[b]	↓	↑	↓	↓	↓ androstenedione	XY: atypical genitalia, undescended testes XX: lacks 2° sexual development
Ⓑ 21-hydroxylase[a]	↓		↑	↓	↓	↑	↑ renin activity ↑ 17-hydroxy-progesterone	Most common Presents in infancy (salt wasting) or childhood (precocious puberty) XX: virilization
Ⓒ 11β-hydroxylase[a]	↓ aldosterone ↑ 11-deoxycorti-costerone[b]	↓	↑	↓	↑	↓ renin activity	Presents in infancy (severe hypertension) or childhood (precocious puberty) XX: virilization

[a]All congenital adrenal enzyme deficiencies are autosomal recessive disorders and most are characterized by skin hyperpigmentation (due to ↑ MSH production, which is coproduced and secreted with ACTH) and bilateral adrenal gland enlargement (due to ↑ ACTH stimulation).

[b]Results in ↑ BP.

If deficient enzyme starts with 1, it causes hypertension; if deficient enzyme ends with 1, it causes virilization in females.

Cortisol

SOURCE	Adrenal zona fasciculata.	Bound to corticosteroid-binding globulin.

FUNCTION	↑ Appetite
	↑ Blood pressure:
	  ▪ Upregulates α_1-receptors on arterioles → ↑ sensitivity to norepinephrine and epinephrine (permissive action)
	  ▪ At high concentrations, can bind to mineralocorticoid (aldosterone) receptors
	↑ Insulin resistance (diabetogenic)
	↑ Gluconeogenesis, lipolysis, and proteolysis (↓ glucose utilization)
	↓ Fibroblast activity (poor wound healing, ↓ collagen synthesis, ↑ striae)
	↓ Inflammatory and Immune responses:
	  ▪ Inhibits production of leukotrienes and prostaglandins
	  ▪ Inhibits WBC adhesion → neutrophilia
	  ▪ Blocks histamine release from mast cells
	  ▪ Eosinopenia, lymphopenia
	  ▪ Blocks IL-2 production
	↓ Bone formation (↓ osteoblast activity)
		Cortisol is **A BIG FIB**.
		Exogenous glucocorticoids can cause reactivation of TB and candidiasis (blocks IL-2 production).

REGULATION	CRH (hypothalamus) stimulates ACTH release (pituitary) → cortisol production in adrenal zona fasciculata. Excess cortisol ↓ CRH, ACTH, and cortisol secretion.	Chronic stress may induce prolonged cortisol secretion, cortisol resistance, impaired immunocompetency, and dysregulation of HPA axis.

Appetite regulation

Ghrelin	Stimulates hunger (orexigenic effect) and GH release (via GH secretagog receptor). Produced by stomach. Sleep deprivation, fasting, or Prader-Willi syndrome → ↑ ghrelin production. **Ghrelin** makes you **ghr**ow hun**ghr**y. Acts on lateral area of hypothalamus (hunger center) to ↑ appetite.
Leptin	Satiety hormone. Produced by adipose tissue. Mutation of leptin gene → severe obesity. Obese people have ↑ leptin due to ↑ adipose tissue but are tolerant or resistant to leptin's anorexigenic effect. Sleep deprivation or starvation → ↓ leptin production. **Leptin** keeps you **thin**. Acts on ventromedial area of hypothalamus (satiety center) to ↓ appetite.
Endocannabinoids	Act at cannabinoid receptors in hypothalamus and nucleus accumbens, two key brain areas for the homeostatic and hedonic control of food intake → ↑ appetite. Exogenous cannabinoids cause "the munchies."

Signaling pathways of endocrine hormones

cAMP	FSH, LH, ACTH, TSH, CRH, hCG, ADH (V_2-receptor), MSH, PTH, Calcitonin, Histamine (H_2-receptor), Glucagon, GHRH	FLAT ChAMPs CHuGG
cGMP	BNP, ANP, EDRF (NO)	BAD GraMPa Think vasodilation and diuresis
IP_3	GnRH, Oxytocin, ADH (V_1-receptor), TRH, Histamine (H_1-receptor), Angiotensin II, Gastrin	GOAT HAG
Intracellular receptor	Progesterone, Estrogen, Testosterone, Cortisol, Aldosterone, T_3/T_4, Vitamin D	PET CAT in TV
Receptor tyrosine kinase	IGF-1, FGF, PDGF, EGF, Insulin	MAP kinase pathway Get Found In the MAP
Nonreceptor tyrosine kinase	G-CSF, Erythropoietin, Thrombopoietin Prolactin, Immunomodulators (eg, cytokines IL-2, IL-6, IFN), GH	JAK/STAT pathway Think acidophils and cytokines GET a JAKed PIG

Signaling pathways of steroid hormones

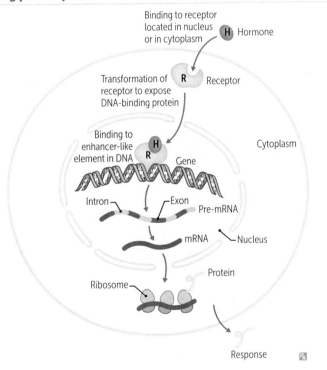

Steroid hormones are lipophilic and therefore must circulate bound to specific binding globulins, which ↑ their solubility.

In males, ↑ sex hormone–binding globulin (SHBG) lowers free testosterone → gynecomastia.

In females, ↓ SHBG raises free testosterone → hirsutism.

↑ estrogen (eg, OCPs, pregnancy) → ↑ SHBG.

▶ ENDOCRINE—PATHOLOGY

Syndrome of inappropriate antidiuretic hormone secretion

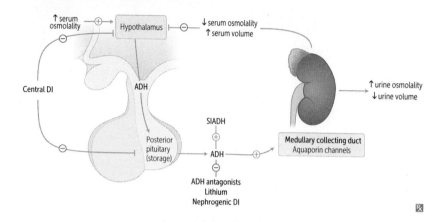

Characterized by excessive free water retention, euvolemic hyponatremia with continued urinary Na^+ excretion, urine osmolality > serum osmolality.

Body responds to water retention with ↓ aldosterone and ↑ ANP and BNP → ↑ urinary Na^+ secretion → normalization of extracellular fluid volume → euvolemic hyponatremia.

Treatment: fluid restriction (first line), salt tablets, IV hypertonic saline, diuretics, ADH antagonists (eg, conivaptan, tolvaptan, demeclocycline).

SIADH causes include (**HEELD**-up water):
- Head trauma/CNS disorders
- Ectopic ADH (eg, small cell lung cancer)
- Exogenous hormones (eg, vasopressin, desmopressin, oxytocin)
- Lung disease
- Drugs (eg, SSRIs, carbamazepine, cyclophosphamide)

Primary polydipsia and diabetes insipidus

Characterized by the production of large amounts of dilute urine +/– thirst. Urine specific gravity < 1.006. Urine osmolality usually < 300 mOsm/kg. Central DI may be transient if damage is below hypothalamic median eminence or in the posterior pituitary (ADH in hypothalamus can still be secreted systemically via portal capillaries in median eminence). Central DI, also known as arginine vasopressin deficiency; nephrogenic DI, also known as arginine vasopressin resistance.

	Primary polydipsia	Central DI	Nephrogenic DI
DEFINITION	Excessive water intake	↓ ADH release	ADH resistance
CAUSES	Psychiatric illnesses, hypothalamic lesions affecting thirst center	Idiopathic, brain injury (trauma, hypoxia, tumor, surgery, infiltrative diseases)	Hereditary (V_2-receptor mutation), drugs (eg, lithium, demeclocycline), hypercalcemia, hypokalemia
SERUM OSMOLALITY	↓	↑	↑
ADH LEVEL	↓ or normal	↓	Normal or ↑
WATER RESTRICTION[a]	Significant ↑ in urine osmolality (> 700 mOsm/kg)	No change or slight ↑ in urine osmolality	No change or slight ↑ in urine osmolality
DESMOPRESSIN ADMINISTRATION[b]	—	Significant ↑ in urine osmolality (> 50%)	Minimal change in urine osmolality
TREATMENT	Water restriction	Desmopressin (DDAVP)	Manage the underlying cause; low-solute diet, HCTZ, amiloride, indomethacin

[a]No water intake for 2–3 hours followed by hourly measurements of urine volume and osmolality as well as plasma Na^+ concentration and osmolality.

[b]Desmopressin (ADH analog) is administered if serum osmolality > 295–300 mOsm/kg, plasma Na^+ ≥ 145 mEq/L, or urine osmolality does not increase despite ↑ plasma osmolality.

Hypopituitarism	Undersecretion of pituitary hormones due to: ▪ Hypothalamic disease (ie, mass lesion, radiation, infiltrative lesions) ▪ Pituitary surgery ▪ Pituitary disorders (eg, mass effect due to nonsecreting pituitary adenoma, craniopharyngioma) ▪ Empty sella ▪ Sheehan syndrome—ischemic infarct of pituitary following severe postpartum hemorrhage; pregnancy-induced pituitary growth → ↑ susceptibility to hypoperfusion. Usually presents with failure to lactate, amenorrhea, cold intolerance (anterior pituitary hormones mainly affected). Treatment: hormone replacement therapy (glucocorticoids, thyroxine, sex steroids, human growth hormone)

Acromegaly	Excess GH in adults. Typically caused by pituitary adenoma.
FINDINGS	Large tongue with deep furrows, frontal bossing, coarsening of facial features with aging A, deep voice, diaphoresis (excessive sweating), hypertrophic arthropathy, impaired glucose tolerance (insulin resistance), HTN, LVH, HFpEF (most common cause of death).
DIAGNOSIS	↑ serum IGF-1 (GH levels unreliable as they fluctuate throughout the day); failure to suppress serum GH following oral glucose tolerance test; pituitary mass seen on brain MRI.
TREATMENT	Pituitary adenoma resection. If not cured, treat with octreotide (somatostatin analog), pegvisomant (GH receptor antagonist), or dopamine agonists (eg, cabergoline).

↑ GH in children → gigantism (↑ linear bone growth due to unfused epiphysis).
Acromegaly in adults, gigantism in j(g)uniors.

Baseline / RU

Hypothyroidism vs hyperthyroidism

	Hypothyroidism	Hyperthyroidism
METABOLIC	Cold intolerance, ↓ sweating, weight gain (↓ basal metabolic rate → ↓ calorigenesis), hyponatremia (↓ free water clearance)	Heat intolerance, ↑ sweating, weight loss (↑ synthesis of Na^+/K^+-ATPase → ↑ basal metabolic rate → ↑ calorigenesis)
SKIN/HAIR	Dry, cool skin (due to ↓ blood flow); coarse, brittle hair; diffuse alopecia; brittle nails; puffy facies and generalized nonpitting edema (myxedema) due to ↑ GAGs in interstitial spaces → ↑ osmotic pressure → water retention	Warm, moist skin (due to vasodilation); fine hair; onycholysis (A); pretibial myxedema in Graves disease B
OCULAR	Periorbital edema C	Ophthalmopathy in Graves disease (including periorbital edema, exophthalmos), lid lag/retraction (↑ sympathetic stimulation of superior tarsal muscle)
GASTROINTESTINAL	Constipation (↓ GI motility), ↓ appetite	Hyperdefecation/diarrhea (↑ GI motility), ↑ appetite
MUSCULOSKELETAL	Hypothyroid myopathy (proximal weakness, ↑ CK), carpal tunnel syndrome, myoedema (small lump rising on the surface of a muscle when struck with a hammer)	Thyrotoxic myopathy (proximal weakness, normal CK), osteoporosis/↑ fracture rate (T_3 stimulates osteoclast differentiation, ↑ bone resorption, and release of calcium; may also affect osteoblasts)
REPRODUCTIVE	Abnormal uterine bleeding, ↓ libido, infertility	Abnormal uterine bleeding, gynecomastia, ↓ libido, infertility
NEUROPSYCHIATRIC	Hypoactivity, lethargy, fatigue, weakness, depressed mood, ↓ reflexes (delayed/slow relaxing)	Hyperactivity, restlessness, anxiety, insomnia, fine tremors (due to ↑ β-adrenergic activity), ↑ reflexes (brisk)
CARDIOVASCULAR	Bradycardia, dyspnea on exertion (↓ cardiac output)	Tachycardia, palpitations, dyspnea, arrhythmias (eg, atrial fibrillation), chest pain and systolic HTN due to ↑ number and sensitivity of β-adrenergic receptors, ↑ expression of cardiac sarcolemmal ATPase and ↓ expression of phospholamban
LABS	↑ TSH (if 1°) ↓ free T_4 Hypercholesterolemia (due to ↓ LDL receptor expression)	↓ TSH (if 1°) ↑ free T_3 and T_4 ↓ LDL, HDL, and total cholesterol

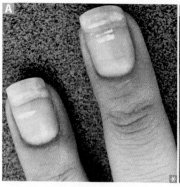
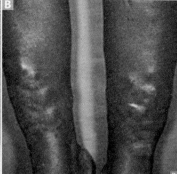
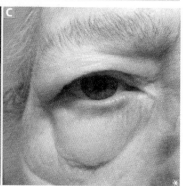

Hypothyroidism

Hashimoto thyroiditis	Also called chronic autoimmune thyroiditis. Most common cause of hypothyroidism in iodine-sufficient regions. Associated with HLA-DR3 (differs by ethnicity), ↑ risk of primary thyroid lymphoma (typically diffuse large B-cell lymphoma). Findings: moderately enlarged, **nontender** thyroid. May be preceded by transient hyperthyroid state ("Hashitoxicosis") due to follicular rupture and thyroid hormone release. Serology: ⊕ antithyroid peroxidase (antimicrosomal) and antithyroglobulin antibodies. Histology: Hürthle cells A, lymphoid aggregates with germinal centers B. Postpartum thyroiditis—mild, self-limited variant of Hashimoto thyroiditis arising < 1 year after delivery. Natural history: hyperthyroidism (within 3 months of birth) → hypothyroidism → recovery/euthyroid state.
Subacute granulomatous thyroiditis	Also called de Quervain thyroiditis. Usually, a self-limited disease. Natural history: transient hyperthyroidism → euthyroid state → hypothyroidism → euthyroid state. Often preceded by viral infection. Findings: ↑ ESR, jaw pain, very **tender** thyroid (de Quervain is associated with **pain**). Histology: granulomatous inflammation C.
Riedel thyroiditis	Also called invasive fibrous thyroiditis. May occur as part of IgG$_4$-related disease spectrum (eg, autoimmune pancreatitis, retroperitoneal fibrosis, noninfectious aortitis). Hypothyroidism occurs in ⅓ of patients. Fibrosis may extend to local structures (eg, trachea, esophagus), mimicking anaplastic carcinoma. Findings: slowly enlarging, hard (rocklike), fixed, **nontender** thyroid. Histology: thyroid replaced by fibrous tissue and inflammatory infiltrate D.
Congenital hypothyroidism	Formerly called cretinism. Most commonly caused by thyroid dysgenesis (abnormal thyroid gland development; eg, agenesis, hypoplasia, ectopy) or dyshormonogenesis (abnormal thyroid hormone synthesis; eg, mutations in thyroid peroxidase) in iodine-sufficient regions. Findings (6 P's): pot-bellied, pale, puffy-faced child E with protruding umbilicus, protuberant tongue F, and poor brain development.
Other causes	Iodine deficiency (most common cause worldwide; typically presents with goiter G), iodine excess (Wolff-Chaikoff effect), drugs (eg, amiodarone, lithium), nonthyroidal illness syndrome (also called euthyroid sick syndrome; ↓ T$_3$ with normal/↓ T$_4$ and TSH in critically ill patients).

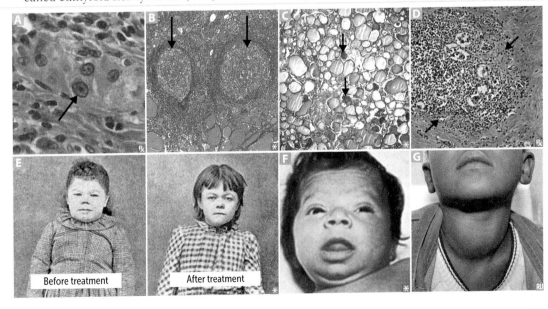

Before treatment After treatment

Hyperthyroidism

Graves disease	Most common cause of hyperthyroidism. Thyroid-stimulating immunoglobulin (IgG, can cause transient neonatal hyperthyroidism; type II hypersensitivity) stimulates TSH receptors on thyroid (hyperthyroidism, diffuse goiter), dermal fibroblasts (pretibial myxedema), and orbital fibroblasts (Graves orbitopathy; treat with glucocorticoids). Activation of T-cells → lymphocytic infiltration of retroorbital space → ↑ cytokines (eg, TNF-α, IFN-γ) → ↑ fibroblast secretion of hydrophilic GAGs → ↑ osmotic muscle swelling, muscle inflammation, and adipocyte count → exophthalmos 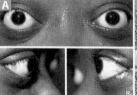. Often presents during stress (eg, pregnancy). Associated with HLA-DR3 and HLA-B8.

Histology: tall, crowded follicular epithelial cells; scalloped colloid 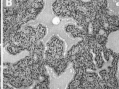 .

Toxic multinodular goiter	Focal patches of hyperfunctioning follicular cells distended with colloid working independently of TSH (due to TSH receptor mutations in 60% of cases). ↑ release of T_3 and T_4. Hot nodules (hyperfunctioning nodules visualized on radioactive iodine scan) are rarely malignant.
Thyroid storm	Uncommon but serious complication that occurs when hyperthyroidism is incompletely treated/untreated and then significantly worsens in the setting of acute stress such as infection, trauma, surgery. Presents with agitation, delirium, fever, diarrhea, coma, and tachyarrhythmia (cause of death). May see ↑ LFTs. Treat with the **4 P's**: β-blockers (eg, propranolol), propylthiouracil, glucocorticoids (eg, prednisolone), potassium iodide (Lugol iodine). Iodide load → ↓ T_4 synthesis → Wolff-Chaikoff effect.
Other causes	Exogenous thyrotoxicosis (excessive intake of thyroid hormone; suspect in patient trying to lose weight), ectopic thyroid production (struma ovarii), contrast-induced thyroiditis (Jod-Basedow phenomenon), drug-induced thyroiditis (amiodarone, lithium).

Causes of goiter	Smooth/diffuse: Graves disease, Hashimoto thyroiditis, iodine deficiency, TSH-secreting pituitary adenoma. Nodular: toxic multinodular goiter, thyroid adenoma, thyroid cancer, thyroid cyst.

Thyroid adenoma 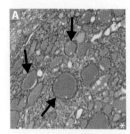	Benign solitary growth of the thyroid. Most are nonfunctional ("cold" on radioactive iodine scan), can rarely cause hyperthyroidism via autonomous thyroid hormone production ("hot" or "toxic"). Most common histology is follicular (arrows in 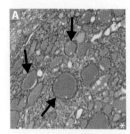); absence of capsular or vascular invasion (unlike follicular carcinoma).

Thyroid cancer	Typically diagnosed with fine needle aspiration; treated with thyroidectomy. Complications of surgery include hypocalcemia (due to removal of parathyroid glands), transection of recurrent laryngeal nerve during ligation of inferior thyroid artery (leads to dysphagia and dysphonia [hoarseness]), and injury to the external branch of the superior laryngeal nerve during ligation of superior thyroid vascular pedicle (may lead to loss of tenor usually noticeable in professional voice users).
Papillary carcinoma	Most common. Empty-appearing nuclei with central clearing ("**Orphan Annie**" eyes) **A**, psam**Moma** bodies, nuclear grooves (**Papi** and **Moma** adopted **Orphan Annie**). ↑ risk with *RET/PTC* rearrangements and *BRAF* mutations, childhood irradiation. Papillary carcinoma: most prevalent, palpable lymph nodes. Good prognosis.
Follicular carcinoma	Good prognosis. Invades tumor capsule and vasculature (unlike follicular adenoma), uniform follicles **B**; hematogenous spread is common. Associated with *RAS* mutation and *PAX8-PPAR-γ* translocations. Fine needle aspiration cytology may not be able to distinguish between follicular adenoma and carcinoma.
Medullary carcinoma	From parafollicular "C cells"; produces calcitonin, sheets of polygonal cells in an amyloid stroma **C** (stains with Congo red). Associated with **MEN 2A** and **2B** (*RET* mutations; **MEN2**llary carcinoma).
Undifferentiated/ anaplastic carcinoma	Older patients; presents with rapidly enlarging neck mass → compressive symptoms (eg, dyspnea, dysphagia, hoarseness); very poor prognosis. Typically composed of pleomorphic cells with frequent mitoses **D**. May arise de novo, but most often arises from dedifferentiation of a preexisting follicular or papillary thyroid carcinoma.

Diagnosing parathyroid disease

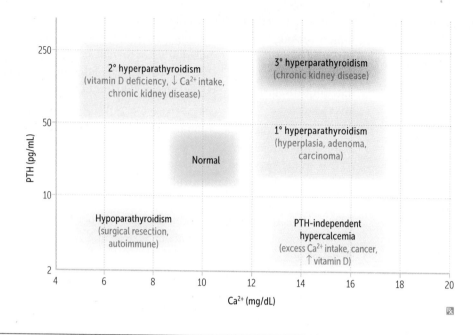

Hypoparathyroidism

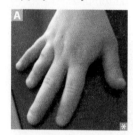

Due to injury to parathyroid glands or their blood supply (usually during thyroid surgery), autoimmune destruction, or DiGeorge syndrome. Findings: tetany, hypocalcemia, hyperphosphatemia.

Chvostek sign—tapping of facial nerve (tap the Cheek) → contraction of facial muscles.
Trousseau sign—occlusion of brachial artery with BP cuff (cuff the Triceps) → carpal spasm.

Pseudohypoparathyroidism type 1A—autosomal dominant, maternally transmitted mutations (imprinted *GNAS* gene). GNAS1-inactivating mutation (coupled to PTH receptor) that encodes the G_s protein α subunit → inactivation of adenylate cyclase when PTH binds to its receptor → end-organ resistance (kidney and bone) to PTH.
Physical findings: Albright hereditary osteodystrophy (shortened 4th/5th digits , short stature, round face, subcutaneous calcifications, developmental delay).
Labs: ↑ PTH, ↓ Ca^{2+}, ↑ PO_4^{3-}.

Pseudopseudohypoparathyroidism—autosomal dominant, paternally transmitted mutations (imprinted *GNAS* gene) but without end-organ resistance to PTH due to normal maternal allele maintaining renal responsiveness to PTH.
Physical findings: same as Albright hereditary osteodystrophy.
Labs: normal PTH, Ca^{2+}, PO_4^{3-}.

Lab values in hypocalcemic disorders

DISORDER	Ca^{2+}	PO_4^{3-}	PTH	ALP	25(OH) VITAMIN D	1,25(OH)₂ VITAMIN D
Vitamin D deficiency	—/↓	—/↓	↑	↑	↓	—/↑
2° hyperpara-thyroidism (CKD)	↓	↑	↑	↑	—	↓
Hypoparathyroidism	↓	↑	↓	—	—	—/↓
Pseudohypo-parathyroidism	↓	↑	↑	↑	—	—/↓

Hyperparathyroidism

Primary hyperparathyroidism 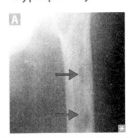	Usually due to parathyroid adenoma or hyperplasia. **Hypercalcemia**, hypercalciuria (renal **stones**), polyuria (**thrones**), hypophosphatemia, ↑ PTH, ↑ ALP, ↑ urinary cAMP. Most often asymptomatic. May present with **bone pain**, weakness, constipation ("**groans**"), abdominal/flank pain (kidney stones, acute pancreatitis), neuropsychiatric disturbances ("**psychiatric overtones**").	**Osteitis fibrosa cystica**—cystic bone spaces filled with brown fibrous tissue 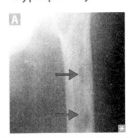 ("brown tumor" consisting of osteoclasts and deposited hemosiderin from hemorrhages; causes bone pain). Due to ↑ PTH, classically associated with 1° (but also seen with 2°) hyperparathyroidism. "Stones, thrones, bones, groans, and psychiatric overtones."
Secondary hyperparathyroidism	2° hyperplasia due to ↓ Ca^{2+} absorption and/or ↑ PO_4^{3-}, most often in chronic kidney disease (causes hypovitaminosis D and hyperphosphatemia → ↓ Ca^{2+}). **Hypocalcemia**, hyperphosphatemia in chronic kidney disease (vs hypophosphatemia with most other causes), ↑ ALP, ↑ PTH.	**Renal osteodystrophy**—renal disease → 2° and 3° hyperparathyroidism → bone lesions.
Tertiary hyperparathyroidism	Refractory (autonomous) hyperparathyroidism resulting from end-stage renal disease. ↑↑ PTH, ↑ Ca^{2+}.	

Familial hypocalciuric hypercalcemia	Autosomal dominant. Defective G-coupled Ca^{2+}-sensing receptors in multiple tissues (eg, parathyroids, kidneys). Higher than normal Ca^{2+} levels required to suppress PTH. Excessive renal Ca^{2+} reabsorption → mild hypercalcemia and hypocalciuria with normal to ↑ PTH levels.

Diabetes mellitus

ACUTE MANIFESTATIONS	Polydipsia, polyuria, polyphagia (**3 P's**), weight loss, DKA (type 1), hyperosmolar hyperglycemic state (type 2).
	Rarely, can be caused by unopposed secretion of GH and epinephrine. Also seen in patients on glucocorticoid therapy (steroid diabetes).
CHRONIC COMPLICATIONS	Nonenzymatic glycation:
	▪ Small vessel disease (hyaline arteriolosclerosis) → retinopathy, neuropathy, nephropathy.
	▪ Large vessel disease (atherosclerosis) → CAD, cerebrovascular disease, peripheral vascular disease. MI is the most common cause of death.
	Osmotic damage (sorbitol accumulation in organs with aldose reductase and ↓ or absent sorbitol dehydrogenase):
	▪ Neuropathy: motor, sensory (glove and stocking distribution), autonomic degeneration (eg, GERD, gastroparesis, diabetic diarrhea).
	▪ Cataracts.

DIAGNOSIS	TEST	DIAGNOSTIC CUTOFF	NOTES
	HbA$_{1c}$	≥ 6.5%	Reflects average blood glucose over prior 3 months (influenced by RBC turnover)
	Fasting plasma glucose	≥ 126 mg/dL	Fasting for > 8 hours
	2-hour oral glucose tolerance test	≥ 200 mg/dL	2 hours after consumption of 75 g of glucose in water
	Random plasma glucose	≥ 200 mg/dL	Presence of hyperglycemic symptoms is required

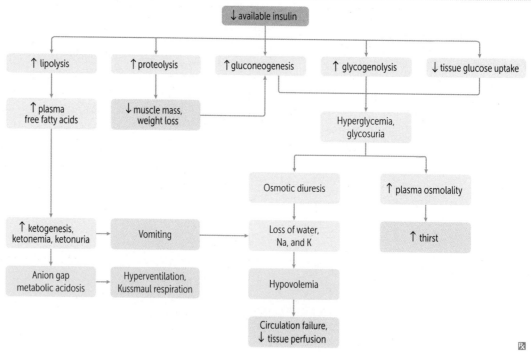

Type 1 vs type 2 diabetes mellitus

	Type 1	Type 2
1° DEFECT	Autoimmune T-cell–mediated destruction of β cells (islet cell cytoplasmic +/– antiglutamic acid decarboxylase +/– insulin autoantibodies often present)	↑ resistance to insulin, progressive pancreatic β-cell failure
INSULIN NECESSARY IN TREATMENT	Always	Sometimes
AGE (EXCEPTIONS COMMON)	< 30 yr	> 40 yr
ASSOCIATION WITH OBESITY	No	Yes
GENETIC PREDISPOSITION	Relatively weak (50% concordance in identical twins), polygenic	Relatively strong (90% concordance in identical twins), polygenic
ASSOCIATION WITH HLA SYSTEM	Yes, HLA-DR4 and -DR3 (4 – 3 = type 1)	No
GLUCOSE INTOLERANCE	Severe	Mild to moderate
INSULIN SENSITIVITY	High	Low
KETOACIDOSIS	Common	Rare
β-CELL NUMBERS IN THE ISLETS	↓	Variable (with amyloid deposits)
SERUM INSULIN LEVEL	↓	↑ initially, but ↓ in advanced disease
CLASSIC SYMPTOMS[a]	Common	Sometimes
HISTOLOGY	Islet leukocytic infiltrate	Islet amyloid polypeptide deposits

[a]Polydipsia, polyuria, polyphagia, weight loss

Hyperglycemic emergencies

	Diabetic ketoacidosis	Hyperosmolar hyperglycemic state
PATHOGENESIS	Insulin noncompliance or ↑ requirements due to ↑ stress (eg, infection) → lipolysis and oxidation of free fatty acids → ↑ ketone bodies (β-hydroxybutyrate > acetoacetate). **Insulin deficient, ketones present.**	Profound hyperglycemia → excessive osmotic diuresis → dehydration and ↑ serum osmolality → HHS. Classically seen in older patients with type 2 DM and limited ability to drink. **Insulin present, ketones deficient.**
SIGNS/SYMPTOMS	**DKA is Deadly: D**elirium/psychosis, **K**ussmaul respirations (rapid, deep breathing), **A**bdominal pain/nausea/vomiting, **D**ehydration. Fruity breath odor due to exhaled acetone.	Thirst, polyuria, lethargy, focal neurologic deficits, seizures.
LABS	Hyperglycemia, ↑ H^+, ↓ HCO_3^- (↑ anion gap metabolic acidosis), ↑ urine and blood ketone levels, leukocytosis. Normal/↑ serum K^+, but depleted intracellular K^+ due to transcellular shift from ↓ insulin and acidosis. Osmotic diuresis → ↑ K^+ loss in urine → total body K^+ depletion.	Hyperglycemia (often > 600 mg/dL), ↑ serum osmolality (> 320 mOsm/kg), normal pH (no acidosis), no ketones. Normal/↑ serum K^+, ↓ intracellular K^+.
COMPLICATIONS	Life-threatening mucormycosis, cerebral edema, cardiac arrhythmias.	Can progress to coma and death if untreated.
TREATMENT	IV fluids, IV insulin, and K^+ (to replete intracellular stores). Glucose may be required to prevent hypoglycemia from insulin therapy.	

Hypoglycemia in diabetes mellitus	Usually occurs in patients treated with insulin or insulin secretagogues (eg, sulfonylureas, meglitinides) in the setting of high-dose treatment, inadequate food intake, and/or exercise.

- Neurogenic (autonomic) symptoms: diaphoresis, tachycardia, tremor, anxiety, hunger. Allow perception of ↓ glucose (hypoglycemia awareness).
- Neuroglycopenic symptoms: altered mental status, seizures, death due to insufficient glucose in CNS. May occur in the absence of preceding neurogenic symptoms in patients with attenuated autonomic response, eg, β-blocker use (ie, hypoglycemia unawareness).

Treatment: simple carbohydrates (eg, glucose tablets, fruit juice), IM glucagon, IV dextrose.

Cushing syndrome

ETIOLOGY	↑ cortisol due to a variety of causes:

- Exogenous glucocorticoids → ↓ ACTH → bilateral adrenal atrophy. Most common cause.
- Primary adrenal adenoma, hyperplasia, or carcinoma → ↓ ACTH → atrophy of uninvolved adrenal gland.
- ACTH-secreting pituitary adenoma (Cushing disease); paraneoplastic ACTH secretion (eg, small cell lung cancer, bronchial carcinoids) → bilateral adrenal hyperplasia. Cushing disease is responsible for the majority of endogenous cases of Cushing syndrome.

FINDINGS	**MOON FACIES:** Metabolic syndrome (hypertension, hyperglycemia, hyperlipidemia), Obesity (truncal weight gain with wasting of extremities, round "moon" facies 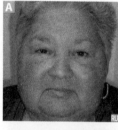, dorsocervical fat pad "buffalo hump"), Osteoporosis, Neuropsychiatric (depression, anxiety, irritability), Facial plethora, Androgen excess (acne, hirsutism), Cataract, Immunosuppression, Ecchymoses (easy bruising), Skin changes (thinning, striae 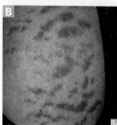, hyperpigmentation).

DIAGNOSIS	Screening tests include: ↑ free cortisol on 24-hr urinalysis, ↑ late night salivary cortisol, and no suppression with overnight low-dose dexamethasone test.

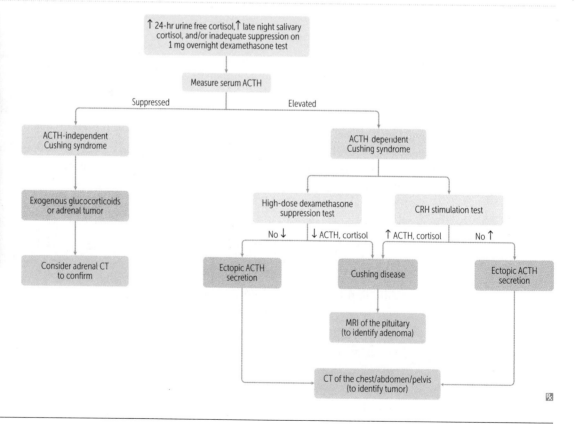

Adrenal insufficiency	Inability of adrenal glands to generate enough glucocorticoids +/– mineralocorticoids for the body's needs. Can be acute or chronic. Symptoms include weakness, fatigue, orthostatic hypotension, muscle aches, weight loss, GI disturbances, sugar and/or salt cravings. Treatment: glucocorticoid +/– mineralocorticoid replacement.
Primary adrenal insufficiency 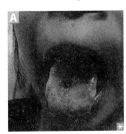	↓ gland function → ↓ cortisol, ↓ aldosterone → hypotension (hyponatremic volume contraction), hyperkalemia, metabolic acidosis, skin/mucosal (pressure areas and buccal mucosa) hyperpigmentation **A**. ↓ cortisol → ↓ negative feedback effect on the pituitary → ↑ production of POMC derivatives (β-endorphin, ACTH, MSH) → ↑ melanin synthesis due to ↑ MSH. Primary pigments the skin/mucosa. Addison disease—chronic 1° adrenal insufficiency; caused by adrenal atrophy or destruction. Most commonly due to autoimmune adrenalitis (high-income countries) or TB (low-income countries).
Secondary and tertiary adrenal insufficiency	↓ pituitary ACTH secretion (secondary) or ↓ hypothalamic CRH secretion (tertiary). No hyperkalemia (aldosterone synthesis preserved due to functioning adrenal gland, intact RAAS), no hyperpigmentation. 2° adrenal insufficiency is due to pituitary pathologies, 3° adrenal insufficiency is most commonly due to abrupt cessation of chronic glucocorticoid therapy (HPA suppression). Tertiary from treatment.
Acute adrenal insufficiency	Also called adrenal (addisonian) crisis; often precipitated by acute stressors that ↑ glucocorticoid requirements (eg, infection) in patients with pre-existing adrenal insufficiency or on glucocorticoid therapy. May present with acute abdominal pain, nausea, vomiting, altered mental status, shock. Waterhouse-Friderichsen syndrome—bilateral adrenal hemorrhage in the setting of sepsis (eg, meningococcemia) → acute 1° adrenal insufficiency.

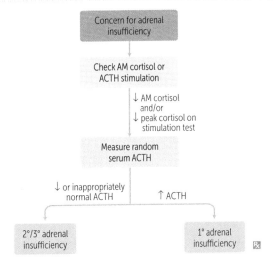

Hyperaldosteronism	Increased secretion of aldosterone from adrenal gland. Clinical features include hypertension, ↓ or normal K⁺, metabolic alkalosis. 1° hyperaldosteronism does not directly cause edema due to aldosterone escape mechanism. However, certain 2° causes of hyperaldosteronism (eg, heart failure) impair the aldosterone escape mechanism, leading to worsening of edema.
Primary hyperaldosteronism	Seen in patients with bilateral adrenal hyperplasia or adrenal adenoma (Conn syndrome). ↑ aldosterone, ↓ renin. Leads to treatment-resistant hypertension.
Secondary hyperaldosteronism	Seen in patients with renovascular hypertension, juxtaglomerular cell tumors (renin-producing), and edema (eg, cirrhosis, heart failure, nephrotic syndrome). ↑ aldosterone, ↑ renin.

Neuroendocrine tumors	Heterogeneous group of neoplasms originating from neuroendocrine cells (which have traits similar to nerve cells and hormone-producing cells).

Most neoplasms occur in the GI system (eg, carcinoid, gastrinoma), pancreas (eg, insulinoma, glucagonoma), and lungs (eg, small cell carcinoma). Also in thyroid (eg, medullary carcinoma) and adrenals (eg, pheochromocytoma).

Neuroendocrine cells (eg, pancreatic β cells, enterochromaffin cells) share a common biologic function through amine precursor uptake decarboxylase (APUD) despite differences in embryologic origin, anatomic site, and secretory products (eg, chromogranin A, neuron-specific enolase [NSE], synaptophysin, serotonin, histamine, calcitonin). Treatment: surgical resection, somatostatin analogs. |

Neuroblastoma 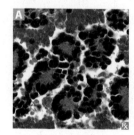	Most common solid extracranial tumor in children (typically < 4 years old). Usually arises in adrenal medulla, but may occur anywhere along the sympathetic chain. Originates from neural crest cells.

Most common presentation is abdominal distension and a firm, irregular mass that can cross the midline (vs Wilms tumor, which is smooth and unilateral). Less likely to develop hypertension than with pheochromocytoma (neuroblastoma is normotensive). Can also present with opsoclonus-myoclonus syndrome ("dancing eyes-dancing feet").

↑ HVA and VMA (catecholamine metabolites) in urine. Homer-Wright rosettes (neuroblasts surrounding a central area of neuropil **A**) characteristic of neuroblastoma and medulloblastoma. Bombesin and NSE ⊕. Associated with amplification of N-*myc* oncogene. |

Pheochromocytoma

ETIOLOGY	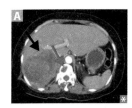 Most common tumor of the adrenal medulla in adults (black arrow in A; red arrow points to bone metastases). Derived from chromaffin cells (arise from neural crest). Rare. May be associated with germline mutations (eg, *NF-1*, *VHL*, *RET* [MEN 2A, 2B]).	Rule of 10's: 10% malignant 10% bilateral 10% extra-adrenal (paraganglioma; eg, bladder wall, organ of Zuckerkandl) 10% calcify 10% kids
SYMPTOMS	Most tumors secrete epinephrine, norepinephrine, and dopamine, which can cause episodic hypertension. May also secrete EPO → polycythemia. Symptoms occur in "spells"—relapse and remit.	Episodic hyperadrenergic symptoms (**5 P's**): Pressure (↑ BP) Pain (headache) Perspiration Palpitations (tachycardia) Pallor
FINDINGS	↑ catecholamines and metanephrines (eg, homovanillic acid, vanillylmandelic acid) in urine and plasma; episodic hyperglycemia may be an uncommon finding.	Chromogranin, synaptophysin and NSE ⊕.
TREATMENT	Irreversible α-antagonists (eg, phenoxybenzamine) followed by β-blockers prior to tumor resection. α-blockade must be achieved before giving β-blockers to avoid a hypertensive crisis. **A** before **B**.	**P**henoxybenzamine for **p**heochromocytoma.

Multiple endocrine neoplasias	All **MEN** syndromes have autosomal **dominant** inheritance. The X-MEN are **dominant** over villains.
SUBTYPE	CHARACTERISTICS
MEN1	Pituitary tumors (prolactin or GH) Pancreatic endocrine tumors—Zollinger-Ellison syndrome, insulinomas, VIPomas, glucagonomas (rare) Parathyroid adenomas Associated with mutation of *MEN1* (tumor suppressor, codes for menin, chromosome 11), angiofibromas, collagenomas, meningiomas
MEN2A	Parathyroid hyperplasia Medullary thyroid carcinoma—neoplasm of parafollicular C cells; secretes calcitonin; prophylactic thyroidectomy required Pheochromocytoma (secretes catecholamines) Associated with mutation in *RET* (protooncogene, codes for receptor tyrosine kinase, chromosome 10)
MEN2B	Medullary thyroid carcinoma Pheochromocytoma Mucosal neuromas A (oral/intestinal ganglioneuromatosis) Associated with marfanoid habitus; mutation in *RET* gene

MEN1 = 3 P's   MEN2A = 2 P's, 1 M   MEN2B = 1 P, 2 M's

Pituitary
Pancreas
Parathyroid
Medullary thyroid carcinoma
Pheochromocytoma
Mucosal neuromas

Pancreatic islet cell tumors

Insulinoma	Tumor of pancreatic β cells → overproduction of insulin → hypoglycemia. May see Whipple triad: low blood glucose, symptoms of hypoglycemia (eg, lethargy, syncope, diplopia), and resolution of symptoms after normalization of plasma glucose levels. Symptomatic patients have ↓ blood glucose and ↑ C-peptide levels (vs exogenous insulin use). ~ 10% of cases associated with MEN1 syndrome. Treatment: surgical resection.
Glucagonoma	Tumor of pancreatic α cells → overproduction of glucagon. Presents with **6 D's**: dermatitis (necrolytic migratory erythema), diabetes (hyperglycemia), DVT, declining weight, depression, diarrhea. Treatment: octreotide, surgical resection.
Somatostatinoma	Tumor of pancreatic δ cells → overproduction of somatostatin → ↓ secretion of secretin, cholecystokinin, glucagon, insulin, gastrin, gastric inhibitory peptide (GIP). May present with diabetes/glucose intolerance, steatorrhea, gallstones, achlorhydria. Treatment: surgical resection; somatostatin analogs (eg, octreotide) for symptom control.

Carcinoid tumors 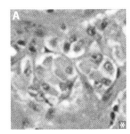	Carcinoid tumors arise from neuroendocrine cells, most commonly in the intestine or lung. Neuroendocrine cells secrete 5-HT, which undergoes hepatic first-pass metabolism and enzymatic breakdown by MAO in the lung. If 5-HT reaches the systemic circulation (eg, after liver metastasis), carcinoid tumor may present with **carcinoid syndrome**—episodic flushing, diarrhea, wheezing, right-sided valvular heart disease (eg, tricuspid regurgitation, pulmonic stenosis), ↑ urinary 5-HIAA. Excess 5-HT production depletes tryptophan stores, leading to niacin deficiency (pellagra). Histology: rosettes **A**, chromogranin A ⊕, synaptophysin ⊕. Diagnosis: ↑ 24-hour urinary excretion of 5-HIAA. Octreotide scintigraphy → tumor localization and staging. Treatment: surgical resection, somatostatin analog (eg, octreotide) or tryptophan hydroxylase inhibitor (eg, telotristat) for symptom control. **Rule of thirds:** 1/3 metastasize 1/3 present with 2nd malignancy 1/3 are multiple

Zollinger-Ellison syndrome	Constellation of symptoms resulting in acid hypersecretion from gastrin-secreting tumor (gastrinomas) in duodenum (most common) or pancreas → single or multiple, recurrent ulcers in the duodenum/jejunum (often refractory to proton pump inhibitors) with resulting malabsorption (acid inactivation of pancreatic enzymes secreted into the small bowel). Presents with abdominal pain, heartburn, diarrhea/steatorrhea, weight loss. Positive secretin stimulation test (↑ gastrin levels after secretin administration, which normally inhibits gastrin release). Chromogranin A ⊕. May be associated with MEN1.

Diabetes mellitus therapy

All patients with diabetes mellitus should receive education on diet, exercise, blood glucose monitoring, and complication management. Treatment differs based on the type of diabetes and glycemic control:

- Type 1 DM—insulin replacement
- Type 2 DM—oral agents (metformin is first line), non-insulin injectables, insulin replacement; weight loss particularly helpful in lowering blood glucose
- Gestational DM—insulin replacement if nutrition therapy and exercise alone fail

Regular (short-acting) insulin is preferred for DKA (via IV), hyperkalemia (with glucose to prevent concomitant hypoglycemia), and stress hyperglycemia.

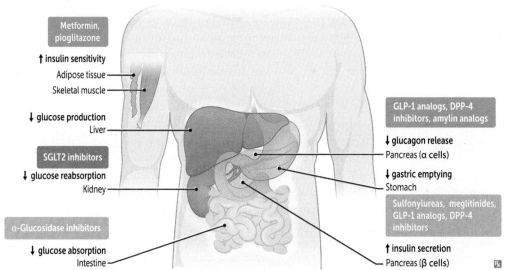

DRUG	MECHANISM	ADVERSE EFFECTS
Insulin preparations		
Rapid acting (no **lag**): lispro, aspart, glulisine Short acting: regular Intermediate acting: NPH Long acting: detemir, glargine Very long acting: degludec	Bind insulin receptor (tyrosine kinase activity). Liver: ↑ glucose storage as glycogen. Muscle: ↑ glycogen, protein synthesis. Fat: ↑ TG storage. Cell membrane: ↑ K⁺ uptake.	Hypoglycemia, lipodystrophy, hypersensitivity reactions (rare), weight gain.

Diabetes mellitus therapy *(continued)*

DRUG	MECHANISM	ADVERSE EFFECTS
Increase insulin sensitivity		
Metformin	Inhibits mitochondrial glycerol-3-phosphate dehydrogenase (mGPD) → inhibition of hepatic gluconeogenesis and the action of glucagon. ↑ glycolysis, peripheral glucose uptake (↑ insulin sensitivity).	GI upset, lactic acidosis (in patients with renal insufficiency, cirrhosis, sepsis, or hypoperfusion), vitamin B_{12} deficiency. Weight loss (often desired).
Pioglitazone	Activate PPAR-γ (a nuclear receptor) → ↑ insulin sensitivity and levels of adiponectin → regulation of glucose metabolism and fatty acid storage.	Weight gain, edema, HF, ↑ risk of fractures. Delayed onset of action (several weeks).
Increase insulin secretion		
Sulfonylureas (1st gen) Chlorpropamide, tolbutamide **Sulfonylureas (2nd gen)** Glipizide, glyburide **Meglitinides** Nateglinide, repaglinide	Close K^+ channels in pancreatic B cell membrane → cell depolarizes → insulin release via ↑ Ca^{2+} influx.	Disulfiram-like reaction with first-generation sulfonylureas only (rarely used). Hypoglycemia (↑ risk in renal insufficiency), weight gain.
Increase glucose-induced insulin secretion		
GLP-1 analogs Exenatide, liraglutide, semaglutide	↓ glucagon release, ↓ gastric emptying, ↑ glucose-dependent insulin release.	Nausea, vomiting, pancreatitis. Weight loss (often desired). ↑ satiety (often desired).
DPP-4 inhibitors Linagliptin, saxagliptin, sitagliptin	Inhibit DPP-4 enzyme that deactivates GLP-1 → ↓ glucagon release, ↓ gastric emptying. ↑ glucose-dependent insulin release.	Respiratory and urinary infections, weight neutral. ↑ satiety (often desired).
Decrease glucose absorption		
Sodium-glucose co-transporter 2 inhibitors Canagliflozin, dapagliflozin, empagliflozin	Block reabsorption of glucose in proximal convoluted tubule (glucosuria). Also cause natriuresis, osmotic diuresis → ↓ blood glucose, ↓ serum Na^+, ↓ ECF volume, ↓ blood pressure.	Glucosuria (UTIs, vulvovaginal candidiasis), dehydration (orthostatic hypotension), weight loss. Glucose **flows in** urine. Use with caution in renal insufficiency (↓ efficacy with ↓ GFR).
α-glucosidase inhibitors Acarbose, miglitol	Inhibit intestinal brush-border α-glucosidases → delayed carbohydrate hydrolysis and glucose absorption → ↓ postprandial hyperglycemia.	GI upset, bloating. Not recommended in renal insufficiency.
Others		
Amylin analogs Pramlintide	↓ glucagon release, ↓ gastric emptying.	Hypoglycemia, nausea. ↑ satiety (often desired).

Thionamides	Propylthiouracil, methimazole.
MECHANISM	Block thyroid peroxidase, inhibiting the oxidation of iodide as well as the organification and coupling of iodine → inhibition of thyroid hormone synthesis. PTU also blocks 5′-deiodinase → ↓ Peripheral conversion of T_4 to T_3.
CLINICAL USE	Hyperthyroidism. **P**TU used in **P**rimary (first) trimester of pregnancy (due to methimazole teratogenicity); methimazole used in second and third trimesters of pregnancy (due to risk of PTU-induced hepatotoxicity). Not used to treat Graves ophthalmopathy (treated with glucocorticoids).
ADVERSE EFFECTS	Skin rash, agranulocytosis (rare), aplastic anemia, hepatotoxicity. PTU use has been associated with ANCA-positive vasculitis. Methimazole is a possible teratogen (can cause aplasia cutis).

Levothyroxine, liothyronine	
MECHANISM	Hormone replacement for T_4 (**levo**thyroxine; **levo** = 4 letters) or T_3 (**lio**thyronine; **lio** = 3 letters). Avoid levothyroxine with antacids, bile acid resins, or ferrous sulfate (↓ absorption).
CLINICAL USE	Hypothyroidism, myxedema. May be misused for weight loss. Distinguish exogenous hyperthyroidism from endogenous hyperthyroidism by using a combination of TSH receptor antibodies, radioactive iodine uptake, and/or measurement of thyroid blood flow on ultrasound.
ADVERSE EFFECTS	Tachycardia, heat intolerance, tremors, arrhythmias.

Hypothalamic/pituitary drugs

DRUG	CLINICAL USE
Conivaptan, tolvaptan	ADH antagonists SIADH (block action of ADH at V_2-receptor)
Demeclocycline	ADH antagonist, a tetracycline SIADH (interferes with ADH signaling)
Desmopressin	ADH analog Central DI, von Willebrand disease, sleep enuresis, hemophilia A
GH	GH deficiency, Turner syndrome
Oxytocin	Induction of labor (stimulates uterine contractions), control uterine hemorrhage
Octreotide	Somatostatin analog Acromegaly, carcinoid syndrome, gastrinoma, glucagonoma, esophageal varices

Fludrocortisone	
MECHANISM	Synthetic analog of aldosterone with glucocorticoid effects. **Fluid**rocortisone retains **fluid**.
CLINICAL USE	Mineralocorticoid replacement in 1° adrenal insufficiency.
ADVERSE EFFECTS	Similar to glucocorticoids; also edema, exacerbation of heart failure, hyperpigmentation.

Cinacalcet

MECHANISM	Sensitizes **calcium**-sensing receptor (CaSR) in parathyroid gland to circulating Ca^{2+} → ↓ PTH. Pronounce "**Sena**calcet."
CLINICAL USE	2° hyperparathyroidism in patients with CKD receiving hemodialysis, hypercalcemia in 1° hyperparathyroidism (if parathyroidectomy fails), or in parathyroid carcinoma.
ADVERSE EFFECTS	Hypocalcemia.

Sevelamer

MECHANISM	Nonabsorbable phosphate binder that prevents phosphate absorption from the GI tract.
CLINICAL USE	Hyperphosphatemia in CKD.
ADVERSE EFFECTS	Hypophosphatemia, GI upset.

Cation exchange resins Patiromer, sodium polystyrene sulfonate, zirconium cyclosilicate.

MECHANISM	Bind K^+ in colon in exchange for other cations (eg, Na^+, Ca^{2+}) → K^+ excreted in feces.
CLINICAL USE	Hyperkalemia.
ADVERSE EFFECTS	Hypokalemia, GI upset.

Gastrointestinal

"A good set of bowels is worth more to a man than any quantity of brains."
—Josh Billings

"Man should strive to have his intestines relaxed all the days of his life."
—Moses Maimonides

"All right, let's not panic. I'll make the money by selling one of my livers. I can get by with one."
—Homer Simpson, *The Simpsons*

"The truth does not change according to our ability to stomach it emotionally."
—Flannery O'Connor

When studying the gastrointestinal system, be sure to understand the normal embryology, anatomy, and physiology and how the system is affected by various pathologies. Study not only disease pathophysiology, but also its specific findings, so that you can differentiate between two similar diseases. For example, what specifically makes ulcerative colitis different from Crohn disease? Also, be comfortable with basic interpretation of abdominal x-rays, CT scans, and endoscopic images.

▶ GASTROINTESTINAL—EMBRYOLOGY

Tongue development

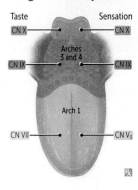

1st pharyngeal arch forms anterior 2/3 of tongue (sensation via CN V_3, taste via CN VII).

3rd and 4th pharyngeal arches form posterior 1/3 of tongue (sensation and taste mainly via CN IX, extreme posterior via CN X).

Motor innervation is via CN XII to hyoglossus (retracts and depresses tongue), **geni**oglossus (**protrudes** tongue), and **sty**loglossus (draws sides of tongue upward to create a trough for swallowing).

Motor innervation is via CN X to palatoglossus (elevates posterior tongue during swallowing).

Taste—CN VII, IX, X (nucleus tractus solitarius [NTS]).

Pain—CN V_3, IX, X.

Motor—CN X, XII.

The **geni**e comes **out** of the lamp in **sty**le.

CN 10 innervates pala**ten**glossus.

Normal gastrointestinal embryology

Foregut—esophagus to duodenum at level of pancreatic duct and common bile duct insertion (ampulla of Vater).

- 4th-6th week of development—stomach rotates 90° clockwise.
- Left vagus becomes anteriorly positioned, and right vagus becomes posteriorly positioned.

Midgut—lower duodenum to proximal 2/3 of transverse colon.

- 6th week of development—physiologic herniation of midgut through the umbilical ring. Yolk sac and midgut are connected via the vitelline (omphalomesenteric) duct.
- 10th week of development—returns to abdominal cavity rotating around superior mesenteric artery (SMA), 270° counterclockwise (~90° before 10th week, remaining ~180° in 10th week when contents retract back into abdominal cavity).

Hindgut—distal 1/3 of transverse colon to anal canal above pectinate line.

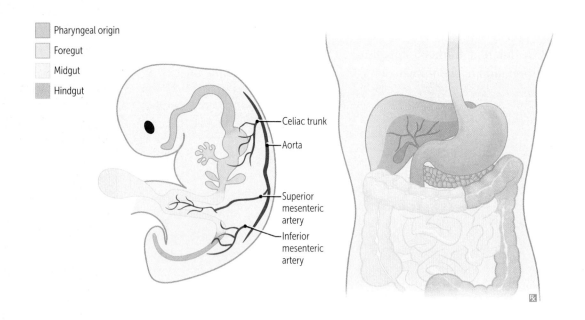

- Pharyngeal origin
- Foregut
- Midgut
- Hindgut

Celiac trunk

Aorta

Superior mesenteric artery

Inferior mesenteric artery

Ventral wall defects	Developmental defects due to failure of rostral fold closure (eg, sternal defects [ectopia cordis]), lateral fold closure (eg, omphalocele, gastroschisis), or caudal fold closure (eg, bladder exstrophy).	
	Gastroschisis	Omphalocele
PRESENTATION	Paraumbilical herniation of abdominal contents through abdominal wall defect	Herniation of abdominal contents through umbilical ring
COVERAGE	Not covered by peritoneum or amnion **A**; right sided/paraumbilical	Covered by peritoneum and amnion **B** (light gray shiny sac); midline, membrane covered
ASSOCIATIONS	Not commonly associated with chromosomal abnormalities; good prognosis	Associated with congenital anomalies (eg, trisomies 13 and 18, Beckwith-Wiedemann syndrome) and other structural abnormalities (eg, cardiac, GU, neural tube)

Congenital umbilical hernia	Delay of umbilical ring to close spontaneously following physiological herniation of midgut → patent umbilical orifice. Covered by skin **C**. Often reducible, but protrudes with ↑ intra-abdominal pressure (eg, crying). May be associated with congenital disorders (eg, Down syndrome, congenital hypothyroidism). Small defects usually close spontaneously.

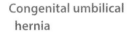
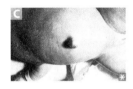

Tracheoesophageal anomalies

Esophageal atresia (EA) with distal tracheoesophageal fistula (TEF) is the most common (85%) and often presents as polyhydramnios in utero (due to inability of fetus to swallow amniotic fluid). Neonates drool, choke, and vomit with first feeding. TEFs allow excess air to enter stomach (visible on CXR as a prominent gastric bubble). Cyanosis is 2° to laryngospasm (to avoid reflux-related aspiration). Clinical test: failure to pass nasogastric tube into stomach. Associated with VATER/VACTERL defects.

In **H**-type, the fistula resembles the letter **H**. In pure EA, CXR shows gasless abdomen.

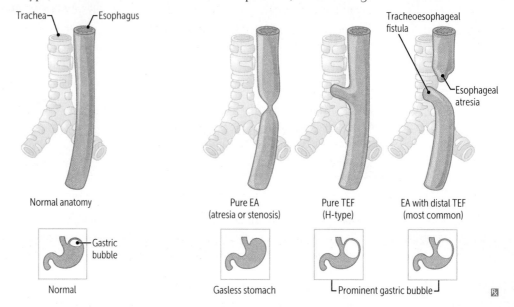

Hypertrophic pyloric stenosis

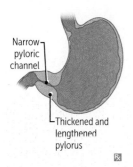

Most common cause of gastric outlet obstruction in infants. Palpable olive-shaped mass (due to hypertrophy and hyperplasia of pyloric sphincter muscle) in epigastric region, visible peristaltic waves, and postprandial nonbilious projectile vomiting at ~ 2–6 weeks old. More common in firstborn males; associated with exposure to macrolides.

Results in hypokalemic hypochloremic metabolic alkalosis (2° to vomiting of gastric acid and subsequent volume contraction).

Ultrasound shows thickened and lengthened pylorus.

Treatment: surgical incision of pyloric muscles (pyloromyotomy).

Intestinal atresia

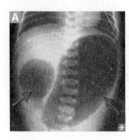

Presents with bilious vomiting and abdominal distension within first 1–2 days of life.

Duodenal atresia—failure to recanalize lumen from solid cord stage. X-ray A shows "double bubble" (dilated stomach, proximal duodenum). Associated with Down syndrome.

Jejunal and ileal atresia—disruption of mesenteric vessels (typically SMA) → ischemic necrosis of fetal intestine → segmental resorption: bowel becomes discontinuous. X-ray may show "triple bubble" (dilated stomach, duodenum, proximal jejunum) and gasless colon. Associated with cystic fibrosis and gastroschisis. May be caused by maternal tobacco smoking or use of vasoconstrictive drugs (eg, cocaine) during pregnancy.

Pancreas and spleen embryology

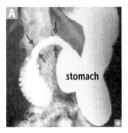

Pancreas—derived from foregut. Ventral pancreatic bud contributes to uncinate process. Both ventral and dorsal buds contribute to pancreatic head and main pancreatic duct.

Annular pancreas—abnormal rotation of ventral pancreatic bud forms a ring of pancreatic tissue → encircles 2nd part of duodenum; may cause duodenal narrowing (arrows in A) and vomiting. Associated with Down syndrome.

Pancreas divisum—ventral and dorsal parts fail to fuse at 7 weeks of development. Common anomaly; mostly asymptomatic, but may cause chronic abdominal pain and/or pancreatitis. Spleen—arises in mesentery of the stomach (dorsal mesogastrium, hence, mesodermal), but has foregut supply (celiac trunk → splenic artery).

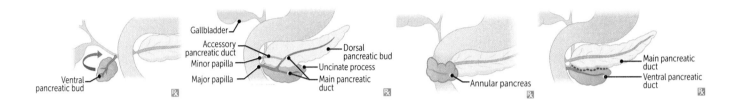

▶ GASTROINTESTINAL—ANATOMY

Retroperitoneal structures

Retroperitoneal structures A are posterior to (and outside of) the peritoneal cavity. Injuries to retroperitoneal structures can cause blood or gas accumulation in retroperitoneal space.

SAD PUCKER:
Suprarenal (adrenal) glands [not shown]
Aorta and IVC
Duodenum (2nd through 4th parts)
Pancreas (except tail)
Ureters [not shown]
Colon (descending and ascending)
Kidneys
Esophagus (thoracic portion) [not shown]
Rectum (partially) [not shown]

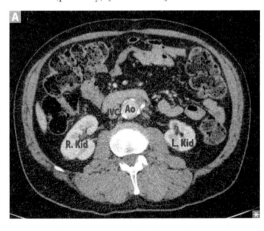

Important gastrointestinal ligaments

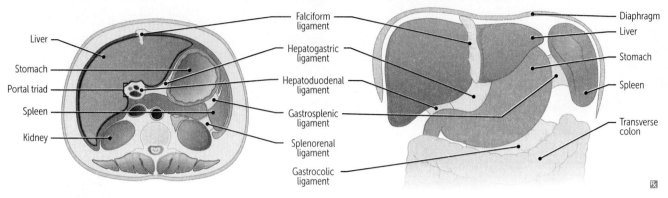

LIGAMENT	CONNECTS	STRUCTURES CONTAINED	NOTES
Falciform ligament	Liver to anterior abdominal wall	Ligamentum teres hepatis (derivative of fetal umbilical vein), patent paraumbilical veins	Derivative of ventral mesentery
Hepatoduodenal ligament	Liver to duodenum	Portal triad: proper hepatic artery, portal vein, common bile duct	Derivative of ventral mesentery Pringle maneuver—ligament is compressed manually or with a vascular clamp in omental foramen to control bleeding from hepatic inflow source (portal vein, hepatic artery) vs outflow (hepatic veins, IVC) Borders the omental foramen, which connects the greater and lesser sacs Part of lesser omentum
Hepatogastric ligament	Liver to lesser curvature of stomach	Gastric vessels	Derivative of ventral mesentery Separates greater and lesser sacs on the right May be cut during surgery to access lesser sac Part of lesser omentum
Gastrocolic ligament	Greater curvature and transverse colon	Gastroepiploic arteries	Derivative of dorsal mesentery Part of greater omentum
Gastrosplenic ligament	Greater curvature and spleen	Short gastrics, left gastroepiploic vessels	Derivative of dorsal mesentery Separates greater and lesser sacs on the left Part of greater omentum
Splenorenal ligament	Spleen to left pararenal space	Splenic artery and vein, tail of pancreas	Derivative of dorsal mesentery

Digestive tract anatomy

Layers of gut wall 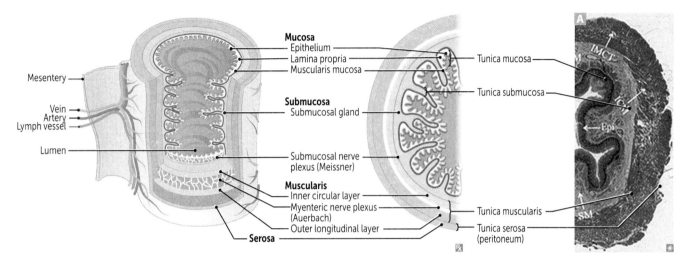 (inside to outside—MSMS):

- Mucosa—epithelium, lamina propria, muscularis mucosa
- Submucosa—includes submucosal nerve plexus (Meissner), secretes fluid; contains vessels
- Muscularis externa—includes myenteric nerve plexus (Auerbach), motility
- Serosa (when intraperitoneal), adventitia (when retroperitoneal)

Ulcers can extend into submucosa, inner or outer muscular layer. Erosions are in mucosa only.

Frequency of basal electric rhythm (slow waves), which originate in the interstitial cells of Cajal: duodenum > ileum > stomach.

Digestive tract histology

Esophagus	Nonkeratinized stratified squamous epithelium. Upper 1/3, striated muscle; middle and lower 2/3 smooth muscle, with some overlap at the transition.
Stomach	Gastric glands **A**. Parietal cells are eosinophilic (pink), chief cells are basophilic.
Duodenum	Villi **B** and microvilli ↑ absorptive surface. Brunner glands (bicarbonate-secreting cells of submucosa), crypts of Lieberkühn (contain stem cells that replace enterocytes/goblet cells and Paneth cells that secrete defensins, lysozyme, and TNF), and plicae circulares (distal duodenum).
Jejunum	Villi, crypts of Lieberkühn, and plicae circulares (taller, more prominent, numerous [vs ileum]) → feathered appearance with oral contrast and ↑ surface area.
Ileum	Villi, Peyer patches (arrow in **C**; lymphoid aggregates in lamina propria, submucosa), plicae circulares (proximal ileum), crypts of Lieberkühn. Largest number of goblet cells in small intestine.
Colon	Crypts of Lieberkühn with abundant goblet cells, but no villi **D**.

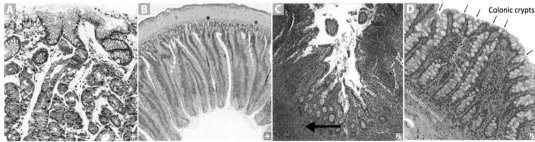

Abdominal aorta and branches

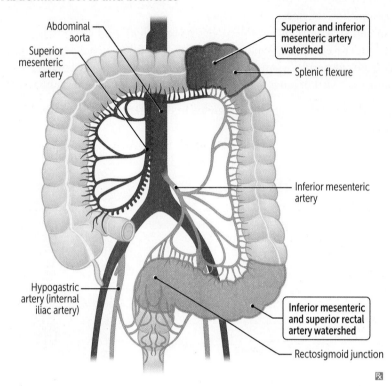

Arteries supplying GI structures are single and branch anteriorly.

Arteries supplying non-GI structures are paired and branch laterally and posteriorly.

Two areas of the colon have dual blood supply from distal arterial branches ("watershed areas") → susceptible in colonic ischemia (hypotensive states, thromboemboli, or atheroemboli):

- Splenic flexure—SMA and IMA
- Rectosigmoid junction—IMA branches (last sigmoid arterial branch and superior rectal artery)

| **Nutcracker syndrome** | Compression of left renal vein between superior mesenteric artery and aorta. May cause abdominal (flank) pain, gross hematuria (from rupture of thin-walled renal varicosities), left-sided varicocele. | 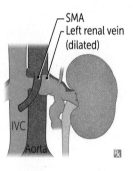 |

| **Superior mesenteric artery syndrome** | Characterized by intermittent intestinal obstruction symptoms (primarily postprandial pain) when SMA and aorta compress transverse (third) portion of duodenum. Typically occurs in conditions associated with diminished mesenteric fat (eg, rapid weight loss, low body weight, malnutrition, gastric bypass surgeries). | 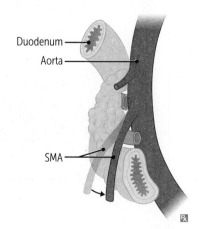 |

Gastrointestinal blood supply and innervation

EMBRYONIC GUT REGION	ARTERY	PARASYMPATHETIC INNERVATION	VERTEBRAL LEVEL	STRUCTURES SUPPLIED
Foregut	Celiac	Vagus	T12/L1	Pharynx (vagus nerve only) and lower esophagus (celiac artery only) to proximal duodenum; liver, gallbladder, pancreas, spleen (mesoderm)
Midgut	SMA	Vagus	L1	Distal duodenum to proximal 2/3 of transverse colon
Hindgut	IMA	Pelvic splanchnic	L3	Distal 1/3 of transverse colon to upper portion of anal canal

Sympathetic innervation arises from abdominal prevertebral ganglia: celiac, superior mesenteric, and inferior mesenteric.

Celiac trunk

Branches of celiac trunk: common hepatic, splenic, and left gastric. These constitute the main blood supply of the foregut.
Strong anastomoses exist between:
- Left and right gastroepiploics
- Left and right gastrics

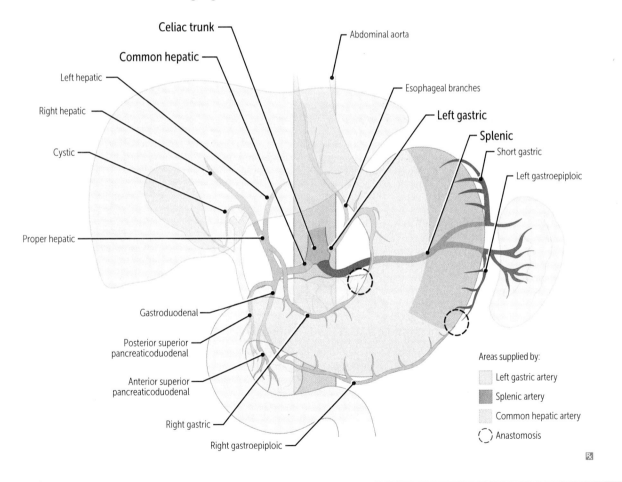

Areas supplied by:
- Left gastric artery
- Splenic artery
- Common hepatic artery
- Anastomosis

Portosystemic anastomoses

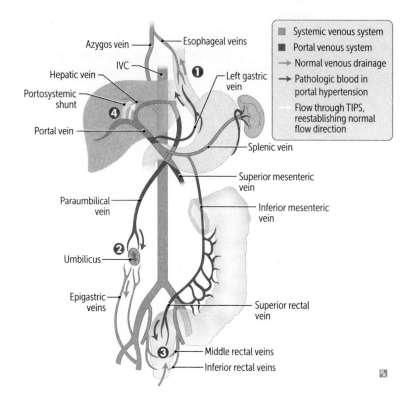

SITE OF ANASTOMOSIS	CLINICAL SIGN	PORTAL ↔ SYSTEMIC
❶ Esophagus	Esophageal varices	Left gastric ↔ esophageal (drains into azygos)
❷ Umbilicus	Caput medusae	Paraumbilical ↔ small epigastric veins (branches of inferior and superficial epigastric veins) of the anterior abdominal wall
❸ Rectum	Anorectal varices	Superior rectal ↔ middle and inferior rectal

Varices of **gut**, **butt**, and **caput** (medusae) are commonly seen with portal hypertension.

❹ Transjugular Intrahepatic Portosystemic Shunt (**TIPS**) treatment creates an anastomosis between portal vein and hepatic vein, relieving portal hypertension by shunting blood to the systemic circulation, bypassing the liver. TIPS can precipitate hepatic encephalopathy due to ↓ clearance of ammonia from shunting.

Pectinate line

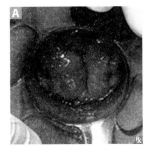

Also called dentate line. Formed where endoderm (hindgut) meets ectoderm.

Internal hemorrhoids—abnormal distention of anal venous plexus Ⓐ. Risk factors include older age and chronic constipation. Receive visceral innervation and are therefore **not painful**.

External hemorrhoids—receive somatic innervation (inferior rectal branch of pudendal nerve) and are therefore **painful** if thrombosed.

Anal fissure—tear in anoderm below pectinate line. Pain while pooping; blood on toilet paper. Located in the posterior midline because this area is poorly perfused. Associated with low-fiber diets and constipation.

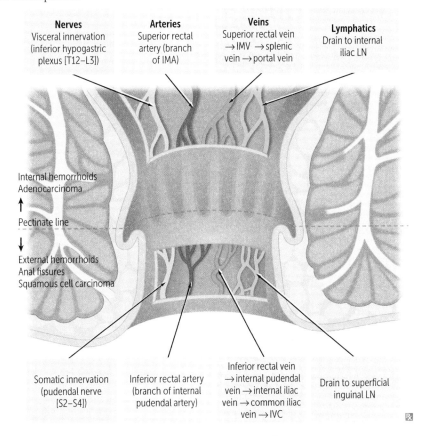

Nerves
Visceral innervation (inferior hypogastric plexus [T12–L3])

Arteries
Superior rectal artery (branch of IMA)

Veins
Superior rectal vein → IMV → splenic vein → portal vein

Lymphatics
Drain to internal iliac LN

Internal hemorrhoids
Adenocarcinoma

↑

Pectinate line

↓

External hemorrhoids
Anal fissures
Squamous cell carcinoma

Somatic innervation (pudendal nerve [S2–S4])

Inferior rectal artery (branch of internal pudendal artery)

Inferior rectal vein → internal pudendal vein → internal iliac vein → common iliac vein → IVC

Drain to superficial inguinal LN

Liver tissue architecture

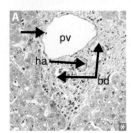

The functional unit of the liver is made up of hexagonally arranged lobules surrounding the central vein with portal triads on the edges (consisting of a portal vein, hepatic artery, bile ducts, as well as lymphatics) A.

Apical surface of hepatocytes faces bile canaliculi. Basolateral surface faces sinusoids.

Kupffer cells (specialized macrophages) located in sinusoids clear bacteria and damaged or senescent RBCs.

Hepatic stellate (Ito) cells in space of Disse store vitamin A (when quiescent) and produce extracellular matrix (when activated). Responsible for hepatic fibrosis.

Dual blood supply to liver: portal vein (~80%) and hepatic artery (~20%).

Zone I—periportal zone:
- Affected 1st by viral hepatitis
- Best oxygenated, most resistant to circulatory compromise
- Ingested toxins (eg, cocaine)

Zone II—intermediate zone:
- Yellow fever

Zone III—pericentral (centrilobular) zone:
- Affected 1st by ischemia as least oxygenated (eg, congestive hepatopathy)
- High concentration of cytochrome P-450
- Most sensitive to metabolic toxins (eg, ethanol, CCl_4, rifampin, acetaminophen)
- Site of alcoholic hepatitis

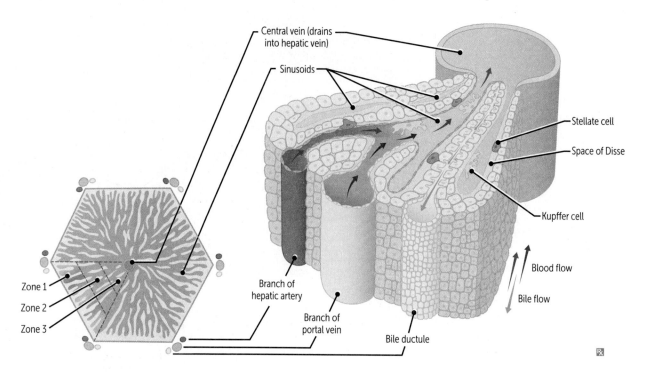

Central vein (drains into hepatic vein)
Sinusoids
Stellate cell
Space of Disse
Kupffer cell
Zone 1
Zone 2
Zone 3
Branch of hepatic artery
Branch of portal vein
Bile ductule
Blood flow
Bile flow

Biliary structures

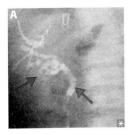

Cholangiography shows filling defects in gallbladder (blue arrow in A) and common bile duct (red arrow in A).

Gallstones that reach the confluence of the common bile and pancreatic ducts at the ampulla of Vater can block both the common bile and pancreatic ducts (double duct sign), causing both cholangitis and pancreatitis, respectively.

Tumors that arise in head of pancreas (usually ductal adenocarcinoma) can cause obstruction of common bile duct → enlarged nontender gallbladder with jaundice (Courvoisier sign).

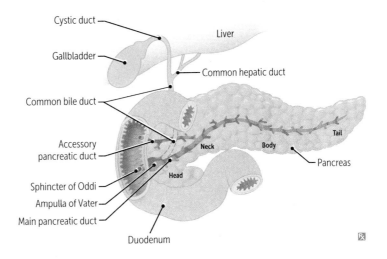

Femoral region

ORGANIZATION	Lateral to medial: nerve-artery-vein-lymphatics.	You go from **lateral to medial** to find your navel.
Femoral triangle	Contains femoral nerve, artery, vein.	Venous near the **penis.**
Femoral sheath	Fascial tube 3–4 cm below inguinal ligament. Contains femoral vein, artery, and canal (deep inguinal lymph nodes) but not femoral nerve.	

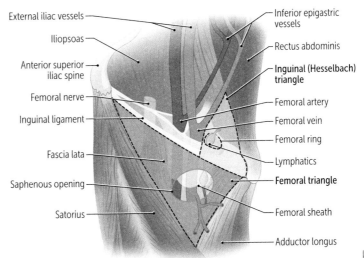

Inguinal canal

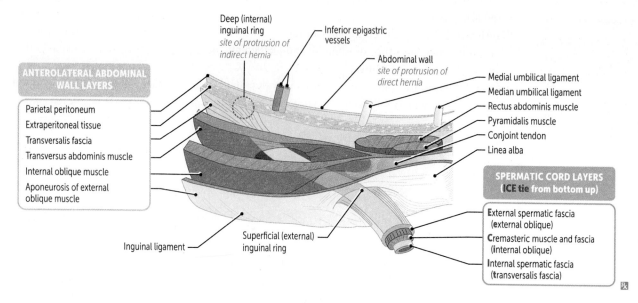

ANTEROLATERAL ABDOMINAL WALL LAYERS

Parietal peritoneum
Extraperitoneal tissue
Transversalis fascia
Transversus abdominis muscle
Internal oblique muscle
Aponeurosis of external oblique muscle

Deep (internal) inguinal ring
site of protrusion of indirect hernia

Inferior epigastric vessels

Abdominal wall
site of protrusion of direct hernia

Medial umbilical ligament
Median umbilical ligament
Rectus abdominis muscle
Pyramidalis muscle
Conjoint tendon
Linea alba

Inguinal ligament

Superficial (external) inguinal ring

SPERMATIC CORD LAYERS
(**ICE tie** from bottom up)

External spermatic fascia (**e**xternal oblique)
Cremasteric muscle and fascia (**i**nternal oblique)
Internal spermatic fascia (**t**ransversalis fascia)

Myopectineal orifice

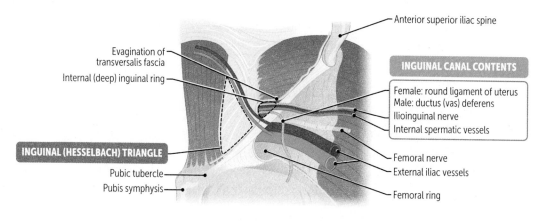

Evagination of transversalis fascia
Internal (deep) inguinal ring

Anterior superior iliac spine

INGUINAL CANAL CONTENTS

Female: round ligament of uterus
Male: ductus (vas) deferens
Ilioinguinal nerve
Internal spermatic vessels

INGUINAL (HESSELBACH) TRIANGLE

Pubic tubercle
Pubis symphysis

Femoral nerve
External iliac vessels

Femoral ring

Anterior abdominal wall
(viewed from inside)

Hernias	Protrusion of peritoneum through an opening, usually at a site of weakness. Contents may be at risk for incarceration (not reducible back into abdomen/pelvis) and strangulation (ischemia and necrosis). Complicated hernias can present with tenderness, erythema, fever.
Spigelian hernia	Also called spontaneous lateral ventral hernia or hernia of semilunar line. Occurs through defects between the rectus abdominis and the semilunar line in the Spigelian aponeurosis. Most occur in the lower abdomen due to lack of the posterior rectus sheath. Presentation is variable but may include abdominal pain and a palpable lump along the Spigelian fascia. Diagnosis: ultrasound and CT scan.

Hernias (continued)

Diaphragmatic hernia

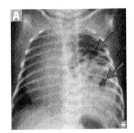

Abdominal structures enter the thorax. Bowel sounds may be heard on chest auscultation. Most common causes:
- Infants—congenital defect of pleuroperitoneal membrane → left-sided herniation (right hemidiaphragm is relatively protected by liver) .
- Adults—laxity/defect of phrenoesophageal membrane → hiatal hernia (herniation of stomach through esophageal hiatus).

Sliding hiatal hernia—gastroesophageal junction is displaced upward as gastric cardia slides into hiatus; "hourglass stomach." Most common type. Associated with GERD.

Paraesophageal hiatal hernia— gastroesophageal junction is usually normal but gastric fundus protrudes into the thorax.

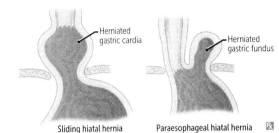

Herniated gastric cardia

Herniated gastric fundus

Sliding hiatal hernia   Paraesophageal hiatal hernia

Indirect inguinal hernia

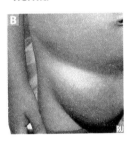

Protrudes through the internal (deep) inguinal ring, external (superficial) inguinal ring, and into the groin. Enters internal inguinal ring lateral to inferior epigastric vessels. Caused by failure of processus vaginalis to close (can form hydrocele). May be noticed in **infants** or discovered in adulthood. Much more common in males .

Follows the pathway of testicular descent. Covered by all 3 layers of spermatic fascia.

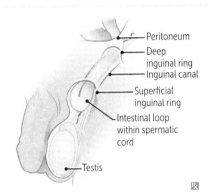

Peritoneum
Deep inguinal ring
Inguinal canal
Superficial inguinal ring
Intestinal loop within spermatic cord
Testis

Direct inguinal hernia

Protrudes through inguinal (Hesselbach) triangle. Bulges directly through parietal peritoneum medial to the inferior epigastric vessels but lateral to the rectus abdominis. Goes through external (superficial) inguinal ring only. Covered by external spermatic fascia. Usually occurs in older males due to acquired weakness of transversalis fascia.

MDs don't **lie**:
  Medial to inferior epigastric vessels = **D**irect hernia.
  Lateral to inferior epigastric vessels = **i**ndirect hernia.

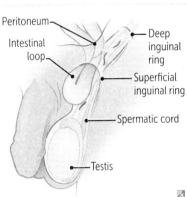

Peritoneum
Intestinal loop
Deep inguinal ring
Superficial inguinal ring
Spermatic cord
Testis

Femoral hernia

Protrudes below inguinal ligament through femoral canal below and lateral to pubic tubercle. More common in **fem**ales, but overall inguinal hernias are the most common. More likely to present with incarceration or strangulation (vs inguinal hernia).

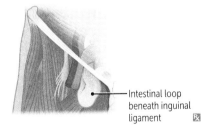

Intestinal loop beneath inguinal ligament

▶ **GASTROINTESTINAL—PHYSIOLOGY**

Gastrointestinal regulatory substances

REGULATORY SUBSTANCE	SOURCE	ACTION	REGULATION	NOTES
Gastrin	G cells (antrum of stomach, duodenum)	↑ gastric H^+ secretion ↑ growth of gastric mucosa ↑ gastric motility	↑ by stomach distention/ alkalinization, amino acids, peptides, vagal stimulation via gastrin-releasing peptide (GRP) ↓ by pH < 1.5	↑ by chronic PPI use ↑ in chronic atrophic gastritis (eg, *H pylori*) ↑↑ in Zollinger-Ellison syndrome (gastrinoma)
Ghrelin	Stomach	↑ appetite ("**ghrowlin'** stomach")	↑ in fasting state ↓ by food	↑ in Prader-Willi syndrome ↓ after gastric bypass surgery
Somatostatin	D cells (pancreatic islets, GI mucosa)	↓ gastric acid and pepsinogen secretion ↓ pancreatic and small intestine fluid secretion ↓ gallbladder contraction ↓ insulin and glucagon release	↑ by acid ↓ by vagal stimulation	Inhibits secretion of various hormones (encourages **somato-stasis**) Octreotide is an analog used to treat acromegaly, carcinoid syndrome, VIPoma, and variceal bleeding
Cholecystokinin	I cells (duodenum, jejunum)	↑ pancreatic secretion ↑ gallbladder contraction ↓ gastric emptying ↑ sphincter of Oddi relaxation	↑ by fatty acids, amino acids	Acts on neural muscarinic pathways to cause pancreatic secretion
Secretin	S cells (duodenum)	↑ pancreatic HCO_3^- secretion ↓ gastric acid secretion ↑ bile secretion	↑ by acid, fatty acids in lumen of duodenum	↑ HCO_3^- neutralizes gastric acid in duodenum, allowing pancreatic enzymes to function
Glucose-dependent insulinotropic peptide	K cells (duodenum, jejunum)	Exocrine: ↓ gastric H^+ secretion Endocrine: ↑ insulin release	↑ by fatty acids, amino acids, oral glucose	Also called gastric inhibitory peptide (GIP) Oral glucose load ↑ insulin compared to IV equivalent due to GIP secretion
Motilin	Small intestine	Produces migrating motor complexes (MMCs)	↑ in fasting state	Motilin receptor agonists (eg, erythromycin) are used to stimulate intestinal peristalsis.
Vasoactive intestinal polypeptide	Parasympathetic ganglia in sphincters, gallbladder, small intestine	↑ intestinal water and electrolyte secretion ↑ relaxation of intestinal smooth muscle and sphincters ↓ gastric acid secretion	↑ by distention and vagal stimulation ↓ by adrenergic input	VIPoma—non-α, non-β islet cell pancreatic tumor that secretes VIP; associated with **Watery Diarrhea, Hypokalemia, Achlorhydria** (**WDHA** syndrome)
Nitric oxide		↑ smooth muscle relaxation, including lower esophageal sphincter (LES)		Loss of NO secretion is implicated in ↑ LES tone of achalasia

Gastrointestinal secretory products

PRODUCT	SOURCE	ACTION	REGULATION	NOTES
Gastric acid	Parietal cells (stomach 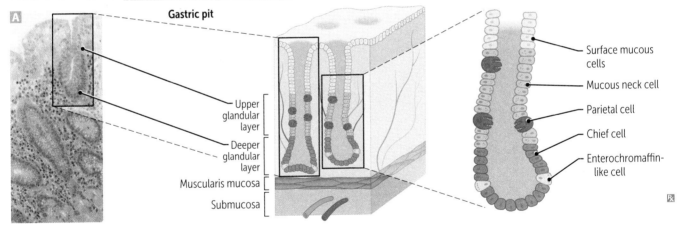)	↓ stomach pH	↑ by histamine, vagal stimulation (ACh), gastrin ↓ by somatostatin, GIP, prostaglandin, secretin	Autoimmune destruction of parietal cells (pink/eosinophilic histology) → chronic gastritis and pernicious anemia
Intrinsic factor	Parietal cells (stomach)	Vitamin B_{12}–binding protein (required for B_{12} uptake in terminal ileum)		
Pepsin	Chief cells (stomach)	Protein digestion	↑ by vagal stimulation (ACh), local acid	Pepsinogen (inactive) is converted to pepsin (active) in the presence of H^+
Bicarbonate	Mucosal cells (stomach, duodenum, salivary glands, pancreas) and Brunner glands (duodenum)	Neutralizes acid	↑ by pancreatic and biliary secretion with secretin	Trapped in mucus that covers the gastric epithelium

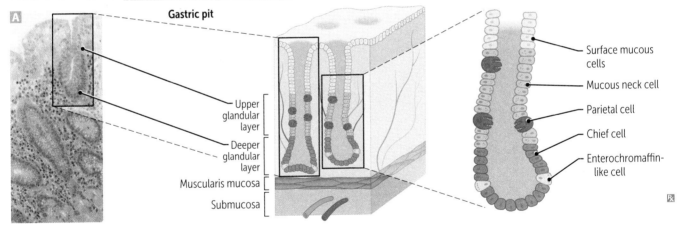

A

Gastric pit

Upper glandular layer
Deeper glandular layer
Muscularis mucosa
Submucosa

Surface mucous cells
Mucous neck cell
Parietal cell
Chief cell
Enterochromaffin-like cell

Locations of gastrointestinal secretory cells

Gastrin ↑ acid secretion primarily through its effects on enterochromaffin-like (ECL) cells (leading to histamine release) rather than through its direct effect on parietal cells.

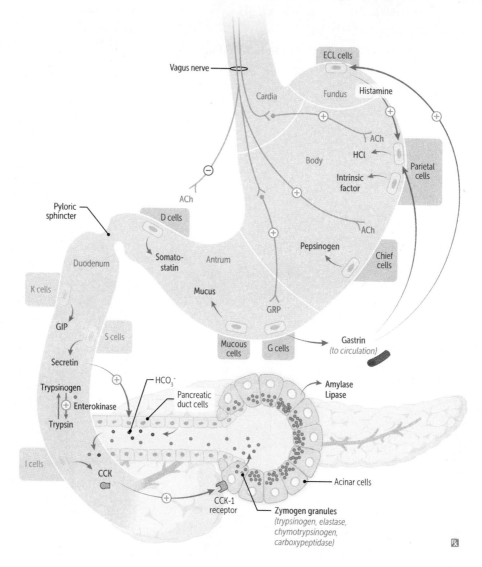

Pancreatic secretions   Isotonic fluid; low flow → high Cl⁻, high flow → high HCO_3^-.

ENZYME	ROLE	NOTES
α-amylase	Starch digestion	Secreted in active form
Lipases	Lipid digestion	
Proteases	Protein digestion	Includes trypsin, chymotrypsin, elastase, carboxypeptidases Secreted as proenzymes also called zymogens Dipeptides and tripeptides degraded within intestinal mucosa via intracellular process
Trypsinogen	Converted to active enzyme trypsin → activation of other proenzymes and cleaving of additional trypsinogen molecules into active trypsin (positive feedback loop)	Converted to trypsin by enterokinase/enteropeptidase, a brush-border enzyme on duodenal and jejunal mucosa

Carbohydrate absorption

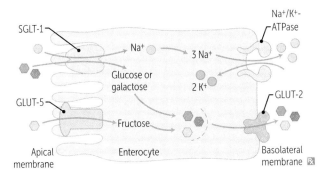

Only monosaccharides (glucose, galactose, fructose) are absorbed by enterocytes. Glucose and galactose are taken up by SGLT1 (Na^+ dependent). Fructose is taken up via facilitated diffusion by GLUT5. All are transported to blood by GLUT2.

D-xylose test: simple sugar that is passively absorbed in proximal small intestine; blood and urine levels ↓ with mucosal damage, normal in pancreatic insufficiency.

Vitamin and mineral absorption

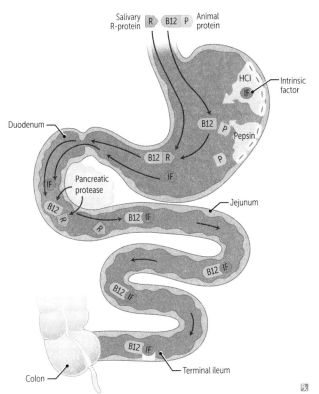

Vitamin and mineral deficiencies may develop in patients with small bowel disease, bowel resection, intestinal failure (also called short bowel syndrome), or bariatric surgery (eg, vitamin B_{12} deficiency complicating terminal ileum resection requires supplementation).

Iron absorbed as Fe^{2+} in duodenum.

Folates absorbed in duodenum and jejunum.

Vitamin B_{12} absorbed in terminal ileum along with bile salts, requires intrinsic factor.

Iron fist, Bro

Dumping syndrome—hyperosmolar food (often sugary) moves too quickly from the stomach to small intestine. Typically occurs after stomach or esophageal surgery.

Peyer patches

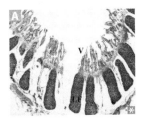

Unencapsulated lymphoid tissue **A** found in lamina propria and submucosa of ileum. Contain specialized Microfold (**M**) cells that sample and present antigens to iMmune cells. B cells stimulated in germinal centers of Peyer patches differentiate into IgA-secreting plasma cells, which ultimately reside in lamina propria. IgA receives protective secretory component and is then transported across the epithelium to the gut to deal with intraluminal antigen.

Think of **IgA**, the Intra-gut Antibody

Bile

Composed of bile salts (bile acids conjugated to glycine or taurine, making them water soluble), phospholipids, cholesterol, bilirubin, water, and ions. Cholesterol 7α-hydroxylase catalyzes rate-limiting step of bile acid synthesis.
Functions:

- Digestion and absorption of lipids and fat-soluble vitamins
- Bilirubin and cholesterol excretion (body's 1° means of elimination)
- Antimicrobial activity (via membrane disruption)

↓ absorption of enteric bile salts at distal ileum (as in short bowel syndrome, Crohn disease) prevents normal fat absorption and may cause bile acid diarrhea.
Calcium, which normally binds oxalate, binds fat instead, so free oxalate is absorbed by gut → ↑ frequency of calcium oxalate kidney stones.

Bilirubin

Heme is metabolized by heme oxygenase to biliverdin (green), which is subsequently reduced to bilirubin (yellow-brown). Unconjugated bilirubin is removed from blood by liver, conjugated with glucuronate, and excreted in bile.
Direct bilirubin: conjugated with glucuronic acid; water soluble (dissolves in water).
Indirect bilirubin: unconjugated; water insoluble.

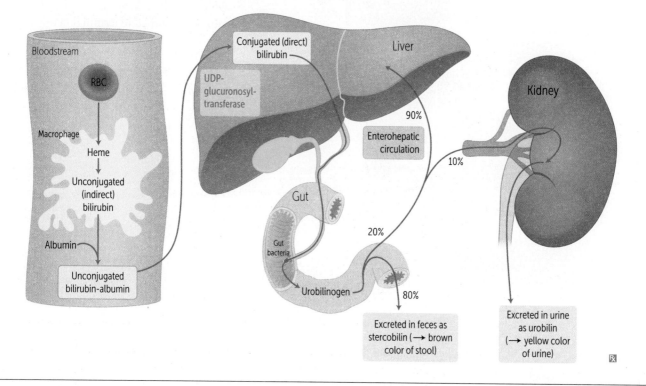

▶ GASTROINTESTINAL—PATHOLOGY

Oral pathologies

Aphthous ulcers	Also called canker sores. Common oral lesions that appear as painful, shallow, round to oval ulcers covered by yellowish exudate **A**. Recurrent aphthous stomatitis is associated with celiac disease, IBD, SLE, Behçet syndrome, HIV infection.
Squamous cell carcinoma	Most common malignancy of oral cavity. Usually affects the tongue. Associated with tobacco, alcohol, HPV-16. Presents as nonhealing ulcer with irregular margins and raised borders. Leukoplakia (white patch **B**) and erythroplakia (red patch) are precursor lesions.
Sialolithiasis	Stone formation in major salivary gland ducts (parotid **C**, submandibular, or sublingual). Associated with salivary stasis (eg, dehydration) and trauma. Presents as recurrent pre-/periprandial pain and swelling in affected gland.
Sialadenitis	Inflammation of salivary gland due to obstruction, infection (eg, S aureus, mumps virus), or immune-mediated mechanisms (eg, Sjögren syndrome).
Salivary gland tumors	Usually benign and most commonly affect the parotid gland. Submandibular, sublingual, and minor salivary gland tumors are more likely to be malignant. Typically present as painless mass/ swelling. Facial paralysis or pain suggests malignant involvement. ▪ Pleomorphic adenoma (benign mixed tumor)—most common salivary gland tumor **D**. Composed of chondromyxoid stroma and epithelium and recurs if incompletely excised or ruptured intraoperatively. May undergo malignant transformation. ▪ **War**thin tumor (papillary cystadenoma lymphomatosum)—benign cystic tumor with **germinal** centers. May be bilateral or multifocal. Typically found in people who **smoke**. "**War**riors from **Germany** love **smoking**." ▪ Mucoepidermoid carcinoma—most common malignant tumor. Mucinous and squamous components.

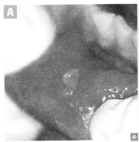 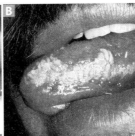 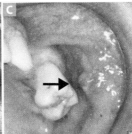 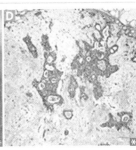

Achalasia

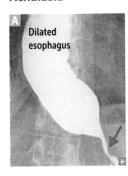

Dilated esophagus

Failure of LES to relax due to degeneration of inhibitory neurons (containing NO and VIP) in the myenteric (Auerbach) plexus of esophageal wall.

1° idiopathic. 2° from Chagas disease (*T cruzi* infection) or extraesophageal malignancies (mass effect or paraneoplastic). Chagas disease can cause achalasia.

Presents with progressive dysphagia to solids and liquids (vs obstruction—primarily solids).

Associated with ↑ risk of esophageal cancer.

Manometry findings include uncoordinated or absent peristalsis with ↑ LES resting pressure.

Barium swallow shows dilated esophagus with area of distal stenosis ("bird's beak" **A**).

Treatment: surgery, endoscopic procedures (eg, botulinum toxin injection).

Other esophageal pathologies

Gastroesophageal reflux disease	Transient decreases in LES tone. Commonly presents as heartburn, regurgitation, dysphagia. May also present as chronic cough, hoarseness (laryngopharyngeal reflux). Associated with asthma. Complications include erosive esophagitis, strictures, and Barrett esophagus.
Esophagitis	Inflammation of esophageal mucosa. Presents with odynophagia and/or dysphagia. Types: ▪ Reflux (erosive) esophagitis—most common type. 2° to GERD. ▪ Medication-induced esophagitis—2° to bisphosphonates, tetracyclines, NSAIDs, ferrous sulfate, potassium chloride. ▪ Eosinophilic esophagitis—chronic, immune-mediated, eosinophil-predominant. Associated with atopic disorders (eg, asthma). Esophageal rings and linear furrows on endoscopy. ▪ Infectious esophagitis—*Candida* (most common; white pseudomembranes 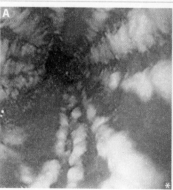), HSV-1 (punched-out ulcers), CMV (linear ulcers). Associated with immunosuppression. ▪ Corrosive esophagitis—2° to caustic ingestion.
Plummer-Vinson syndrome	Triad of dysphagia, iron deficiency anemia, esophageal webs. ↑ risk of esophageal squamous cell carcinoma ("**Plum**ber **dies**"). May be associated with glossitis.
Mallory-Weiss syndrome	Partial thickness, longitudinal lacerations of gastroesophageal junction, confined to mucosa/submucosa, due to severe vomiting. Often presents with hematemesis +/– abdominal/back pain. Usually found in patients with alcohol use disorder, bulimia nervosa.
Esophageal varices	Dilated submucosal veins (red arrows in 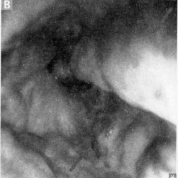) in lower 1/3 of esophagus 2° to portal hypertension. Common in patients with cirrhosis, may be source of life-threatening hematemesis.
Distal esophageal spasm	Formerly called diffuse esophageal spasm. Spontaneous, nonperistaltic (uncoordinated) contractions of the esophagus with normal LES pressure. Presents with dysphagia and anginalike chest pain. Barium swallow may reveal "corkscrew" esophagus. Manometry is diagnostic. Treatment includes nitrates and CCBs.
Scleroderma esophageal involvement	Esophageal smooth muscle atrophy and fibrosis → ↓ LES pressure and distal esophageal dysmotility → acid reflux and dysphagia → stricture, Barrett esophagus, and aspiration. Part of CREST syndrome.
Esophageal perforation	Most commonly iatrogenic following esophageal instrumentation. Noniatrogenic causes include spontaneous rupture, foreign body ingestion, trauma, malignancy. Pneumomediastinum (arrows in 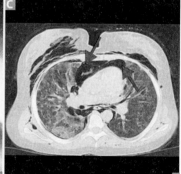) and subcutaneous emphysema (signs include crepitus in the neck region or chest wall) can indicate dissecting air. Boerhaave syndrome—transmural, usually distal esophageal rupture due to violent retching.

Barrett esophagus

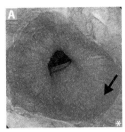
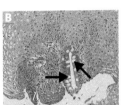

Specialized intestinal metaplasia (arrow in 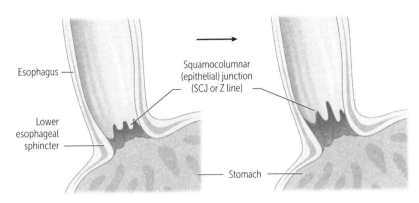)—replacement of nonkeratinized stratified squamous epithelium with intestinal epithelium (nonciliated columnar with goblet cells [arrows in B]) in distal esophagus. Due to chronic gastroesophageal reflux disease (GERD). Associated with ↑ risk of esophageal adenocarcinoma.

Esophagus

Lower esophageal sphincter

Squamocolumnar (epithelial) junction (SCJ or Z line)

Stomach

Esophageal cancer

Typically presents with progressive dysphagia (first solids, then liquids) and weight loss. Aggressive course due to lack of serosa in esophageal wall, allowing rapid extension. Poor prognosis due to advanced disease at presentation.

CANCER	PART OF ESOPHAGUS AFFECTED	RISK FACTORS	PREVALENCE
Squamous cell carcinoma	Upper 2/3	Alcohol, hot liquids, caustic strictures, smoking, achalasia, nitrosamine-rich foods	More common worldwide
Adenocarcinoma	Lower 1/3	Chronic GERD, Barrett esophagus, obesity, tobacco smoking	More common in America

Gastritis

Acute gastritis	Erosions can be caused by: ▪ NSAIDs—↓ PGE$_2$ → ↓ gastric mucosa protection ▪ **Burns** (**Curling** ulcer)—hypovolemia → mucosal ischemia ▪ **Brain** injury (**Cushing** ulcer)—↑ vagal stimulation → ↑ ACh → ↑ H$^+$ production	Especially common among patients with alcohol use disorder and those taking daily NSAIDs (eg, for rheumatoid arthritis) **Burned** by the **Curling** iron Always **Cushion** the **brain**
Chronic gastritis	Mucosal inflammation, often leading to atrophy (hypochlorhydria → hypergastrinemia) and intestinal metaplasia (↑ risk of gastric cancers)	
H pylori	Most common. ↑ risk of peptic ulcer disease, MALT lymphoma	Affects antrum first and spreads to body of stomach
Autoimmune	Autoantibodies (T-cell induced) to the H$^+$/K$^+$-ATPase on parietal cells and to intrinsic factor. ↑ risk of pernicious anemia	Affects body/fundus of stomach

Ménétrier disease 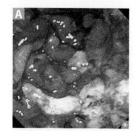	Hyperplasia of gastric mucosa → hypertrophied rugae ("**wavy**" like brain gyri 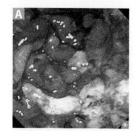). Causes excess mucus production with resultant protein loss and parietal cell atrophy with ↓ acid production. Precancerous. Presents with **W**eight loss, **A**norexia, **V**omiting, **E**pigastric pain, **E**dema (due to protein loss; pronounce "**WAVEE**").

Gastric cancer 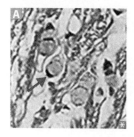	Most commonly gastric adenocarcinoma; lymphoma, GI stromal tumor (common mutations include *KIT* or *PDGFRA*), carcinoid (rare). Early aggressive local spread with node/liver metastases. Often presents late, with **W**eight loss, **E**arly satiety, **A**bdominal **P**ain, **O**bstruction, and in some cases acanthosis **N**igricans or Leser-Trélat sign (**WEAPON**). ▪ Intestinal—associated with *H pylori*, dietary nitrosamines (smoked foods common in East Asian countries), tobacco smoking, achlorhydria, chronic gastritis. Commonly on lesser curvature; looks like ulcer with raised margins. ▪ Diffuse—not associated with *H pylori*; most cases due to E-cadherin mutation; signet ring cells (mucin-filled cells with peripheral nuclei) 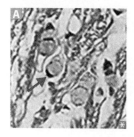; stomach wall grossly thickened and leathery (linitis plastica).	Virchow node—involvement of left supraclavicular node by metastasis from stomach. Krukenberg tumor—metastasis to ovaries (typically bilateral). Abundant mucin-secreting, signet ring cells. Sister Mary Joseph nodule—subcutaneous periumbilical metastasis. Blumer shelf—palpable mass on digital rectal exam suggesting metastasis to rectouterine pouch (pouch of Douglas).

Peptic ulcer disease

	Gastric ulcer	Duodenal ulcer
PAIN	Can be greater with meals—weight loss	Decreases with meals—weight gain
H PYLORI INFECTION	~ 70%	~ 90%
MECHANISM	↓ mucosal protection against gastric acid	↓ mucosal protection or ↑ gastric acid secretion
OTHER CAUSES	NSAIDs	Zollinger-Ellison syndrome
RISK OF CARCINOMA	↑ Biopsy margins to rule out malignancy	Generally benign Not routinely biopsied

Ulcer complications

Hemorrhage	Gastric, duodenal (posterior > anterior). Most common complication. Ruptured gastric ulcer on the lesser curvature of stomach → bleeding from left gastric artery. An ulcer on the posterior wall of duodenum → bleeding from gastroduodenal artery.
Obstruction	Pyloric channel, duodenal.
Perforation	Duodenal (anterior > posterior). Anterior duodenal ulcers can perforate into the anterior abdominal cavity, potentially leading to pneumoperitoneum. May see free air under diaphragm (pneumoperitoneum) 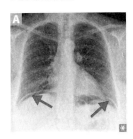 with referred pain to the shoulder via irritation of phrenic nerve.

Acute gastrointestinal bleeding	Upper GI bleeding—originates **proximal** to ligament of Treitz (suspensory ligament of duodenum). Usually presents with hematemesis and/or melena. Associated with peptic ulcer disease, variceal hemorrhage. Lower GI bleeding—originates **distal** to ligament of Treitz. Usually presents with hematochezia. Associated with IBD, diverticulosis, angiodysplasia, hemorrhoids, anal fissure, cancer.	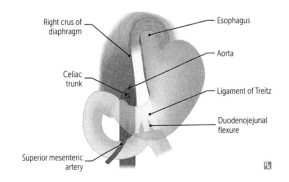

Malabsorption syndromes	Can cause diarrhea, steatorrhea, weight loss, weakness, vitamin and mineral deficiencies. Screen for fecal fat (eg, Sudan stain).	
Celiac disease 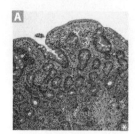	Also called gluten-sensitive enteropathy, celiac sprue. Autoimmune-mediated intolerance of gliadin (gluten protein found in wheat, barley, rye). Associated with HLA-DQ2, HLA-DQ8 (I ate [8] too [2] much gluten at **D**airy **Q**ueen), northern European descent. Primarily affects distal duodenum and/or proximal jejunum → malabsorption and steatorrhea. Treatment: gluten-free diet.	Associated with dermatitis herpetiformis, ↓ bone density, iron deficiency anemia, moderately ↑ risk of malignancy (eg, T-cell lymphoma). D-xylose test: abnormal. Serology: ⊕ IgA anti-tissue transglutaminase (IgA tTG), anti-endomysial, and anti-deamidated gliadin peptide antibodies. Histology: Loss of villi, mucosal atrophy, crypt hyperplasia A, intraepithelial lymphocytosis.

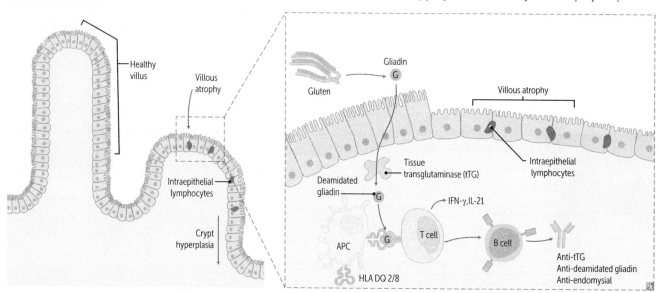

Lactose intolerance	Lactase deficiency. Normal-appearing villi, except when 2° to injury at tips of villi (eg, viral enteritis). Osmotic diarrhea, ↓ stool pH (colonic bacteria ferment lactose).	Lactose hydrogen breath test: ⊕ for lactose malabsorption if post-lactose breath hydrogen value increases > 20 ppm compared with baseline.
Pancreatic insufficiency	Due to chronic pancreatitis, cystic fibrosis, obstructing cancer. Causes malabsorption of fat and fat-soluble vitamins (A, D, E, K) as well as vitamin B_{12}.	↓ duodenal bicarbonate (and pH) and fecal elastase. D-xylose test: normal.
Tropical sprue	Similar findings as celiac sprue (affects small bowel), but responds to antibiotics. Cause is unknown, but seen in residents of or recent visitors to tropics.	↓ mucosal absorption affecting duodenum and jejunum but can involve ileum with time. Associated with megaloblastic anemia due to folate deficiency and, later, B_{12} deficiency.
Whipple disease 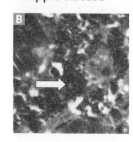	Infection with *Tropheryma whipplei* (intracellular gram ⊕); **PAS** ⊕ **foamy** macrophages in intestinal lamina propria B. **C**ardiac symptoms, **A**rthralgias, and **N**eurologic symptoms are common. Diarrhea/ steatorrhea occur later in disease course. Most common in older males.	**PAS**s the foamy **Whip**ped cream in a **CAN**.

Inflammatory bowel diseases

	Crohn disease	Ulcerative colitis
LOCATION	Any portion of the GI tract, usually the terminal ileum and colon. Skip lesions, rectal sparing.	Colitis = colon inflammation. Continuous colonic lesions, always with rectal involvement.
GROSS MORPHOLOGY	Transmural inflammation → fistulas. Cobblestone mucosa, creeping fat, bowel wall thickening 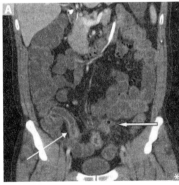 ("string sign" on small bowel follow-through), linear ulcers, fissures.	Mucosal and submucosal inflammation only. Friable mucosa with superficial and/or deep ulcerations (compare normal B with diseased C). Loss of haustra → "lead pipe" appearance on imaging.
MICROSCOPIC MORPHOLOGY	Noncaseating granulomas, lymphoid aggregates.	Crypt abscesses/ulcers, bleeding, no granulomas.
COMPLICATIONS	Malabsorption/malnutrition, colorectal cancer (↑ risk with pancolitis).	
	Fistulas (eg, enterovesical fistulae, which can cause recurrent UTI and pneumaturia), phlegmon/abscess, strictures (causing obstruction), perianal disease.	Fulminant colitis, toxic megacolon, perforation.
INTESTINAL MANIFESTATION	Diarrhea that may or may not be bloody.	Bloody diarrhea (usually painful).
EXTRAINTESTINAL MANIFESTATIONS	Rash (pyoderma gangrenosum, erythema nodosum), eye inflammation (episcleritis, uveitis), oral ulcerations (aphthous stomatitis), arthritis (peripheral, spondylitis).	
	Calcium oxalate kidney stones—inflamed intestines → malabsorption of fat → fat binds calcium in intestine → excess free oxalate in intestines → ↑ oxalate reabsorption → combines with calcium in kidneys; gallstones. May be ⊕ for anti-*Saccharomyces cerevisiae* antibodies (ASCA).	1° sclerosing cholangitis. Associated with MPO-ANCA/p-ANCA.
TREATMENT	Glucocorticoids, azathioprine, antibiotics (eg, ciprofloxacin, metronidazole), biologics (eg, infliximab, adalimumab).	5-aminosalicylic acid preparations (eg, mesalamine), 6-mercaptopurine, infliximab, colectomy.
DISEASE ACTIVITY	Fecal calprotectin used to monitor activity and distinguish from noninflammatory diseases (irritable bowel).	

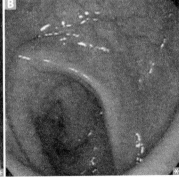
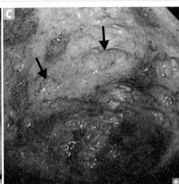

Microscopic colitis

Inflammatory disease of colon that causes chronic watery diarrhea. Most common in older females. Colonic mucosa appears normal on endoscopy. Histology shows lymphocytic infiltrate in lamina propria with intraepithelial lymphocytosis or thickened subepithelial collagen band.

Irritable bowel syndrome	Recurrent abdominal pain associated with ≥ 2 of the following:

- Related to defecation
- Change in stool frequency
- Change in form (consistency) of stool

No structural abnormalities. Most common in middle-aged females. Chronic symptoms may be diarrhea-predominant, constipation-predominant, or mixed. Pathophysiology is multifaceted. May be associated with fibromyalgia and mood disorders (anxiety, depression).
First-line treatment is lifestyle modification and dietary changes.

Appendicitis	

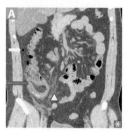

Acute inflammation of the appendix (blue arrow in A), can be due to obstruction by fecalith (in adults) or lymphoid hyperplasia (in children).
Proximal appendiceal lumen obstruction → closed-loop obstruction → ↑ intraluminal pressure → stimulation of visceral afferent nerve fibers at T8-T10 → initial diffuse periumbilical pain → inflammation extends to serosa and irritates parietal peritoneum. Pain localized to RLQ/McBurney point (1/3 the distance from right anterior superior iliac spine to umbilicus). Nausea, fever; may perforate → peritonitis. May elicit psoas, obturator, and Rovsing (severe RLQ pain with palpation of LLQ) signs; guarding and rebound tenderness on exam.
Treatment: appendectomy.

Diverticula of the GI tract

Diverticulum	Blind pouch A protruding from the alimentary tract that communicates with the lumen of the gut. Most diverticula (esophagus, stomach, duodenum, colon) are acquired and are termed "false diverticula."	"True" diverticulum—all gut wall layers outpouch (eg, Meckel). "False" diverticulum or pseudodiverticulum—only mucosa and submucosa outpouch. Occur especially where vasa recta penetrate muscularis externa layer (eg, Zenker).
Diverticulosis	Many false diverticula of the colon B, commonly sigmoid. Common (in ~ 50% of people > 60 years). Caused by ↑ intraluminal pressure and focal weakness in colonic wall. Associated with obesity and diets low in fiber, high in total fat/red meat.	Often asymptomatic or associated with vague discomfort. Complications include diverticular bleeding (painless hematochezia), diverticulitis.
Diverticulitis	Inflammation of diverticula with wall thickening (red arrows in C) classically causing LLQ pain, fever, leukocytosis. Treat with supportive care (uncomplicated) or antibiotics (complicated).	Complications: abscess, fistula (colovesical fistula → pneumaturia), obstruction (inflammatory stenosis), perforation (white arrows in C) (→ peritonitis). Hematochezia is rare.

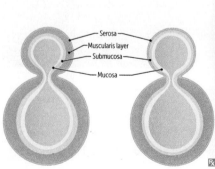

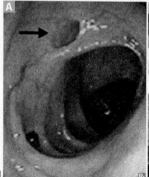

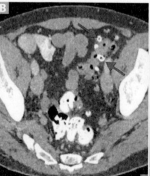

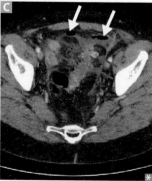

Zenker diverticulum

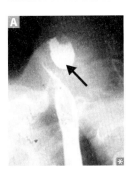

Pharyngoesophageal **false** diverticulum 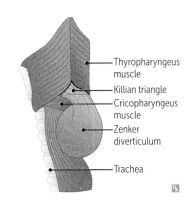. Esophageal dysmotility causes herniation of mucosal tissue at an area of weakness between the thyropharyngeal and cricopharyngeal parts of the inferior pharyngeal constrictor (Killian triangle). Presenting symptoms: dysphagia, obstruction, gurgling, aspiration, foul breath, neck mass. Most common in older males.

Meckel diverticulum

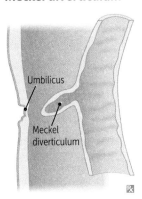

True diverticulum. Persistence of the vitelline (omphalomesenteric) duct. May contain ectopic acid–secreting gastric mucosa and/or pancreatic tissue. Most common congenital anomaly of GI tract. Can cause painless hematochezia/melena (less common), RLQ pain, intussusception, volvulus, or obstruction near terminal ileum.

Diagnosis: ^{99m}Tc-pertechnetate scan (also called Meckel scan) for uptake by heterotopic gastric mucosa.

The rule of 2's:
  2 times as likely in males.
  2 inches long.
  2 feet from the ileocecal valve.
  2% of population.
  Commonly presents in first 2 years of life.
  May have 2 types of epithelia (gastric/
    pancreatic).

Hirschsprung disease

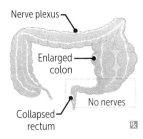

Congenital megacolon characterized by lack of ganglion cells/enteric nervous plexuses (Auerbach and Meissner plexuses) in distal segment of colon. Due to failure of neural crest cell migration. Associated with loss of function mutations in *RET*.

Presents with bilious emesis, abdominal distention, and failure to pass meconium within 48 hours → chronic constipation. Normal portion of the colon proximal to the aganglionic segment is dilated, resulting in a "transition zone."

Risk ↑ with Down syndrome.
Explosive expulsion of feces (squirt sign) → empty rectum on digital exam.
Diagnosed by absence of ganglion cells on rectal suction biopsy.
Treatment: resection.
RET mutation in the **RE**c**T**um.

Malrotation

Anomaly of midgut rotation during fetal development → improper positioning of bowel (small bowel clumped on the right side and colon on the left), formation of fibrous bands (Ladd bands).

Can lead to volvulus, duodenal obstruction.

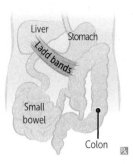

Intussusception

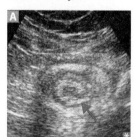

Telescoping of a proximal bowel segment into a distal segment, most commonly at ileocecal junction. Typically seen in infants.

Usually idiopathic in children, less frequently due to an identifiable lead point. Idiopathic form is associated with recent viral infections (eg, adenovirus), rotavirus vaccine → Peyer patch hypertrophy may act as a lead point. Common lead points:

- Children—Meckel diverticulum, small bowel wall hematoma (IgA vasculitis).
- Adults—intraluminal mass/tumor.

Causes small bowel obstruction and vascular compromise → intermittent abdominal pain, vomiting, bloody "currant jelly" stools.

Sausage-shaped mass in right abdomen on exam. Patient may draw their legs to chest to ease pain.

Ultrasound/CT may show "target sign" A.

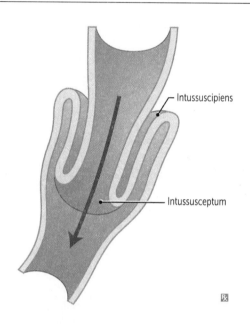

Volvulus

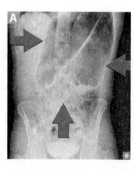

Twisting of portion of bowel around its mesentery; can lead to obstruction and infarction. Can occur throughout the GI tract.

- Gastric volvulus more common with abnormalities (paraesophageal hernia) in adults, and presents with severe abdominal pain, dry heaving, and inability to pass nasogastric tube
- Midgut volvulus more common in infants and children (minors)
- Sigmoid volvulus (coffee bean sign on x-ray A) more common in older adults (seniors)

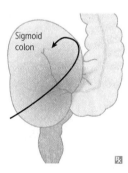

Short bowel syndrome

Inability to adequately absorb nutrients in the small intestine 2° to significant surgical resection (eg, Crohn disease, malignancy, trauma). Malabsorption of bile salts and fat at the distal ileum → postprandial voluminous diarrhea, dehydration, weight loss, anemia, calcium oxalate kidney stones.

Other intestinal disorders

Acute mesenteric ischemia	Critical blockage of intestinal blood flow (often embolic occlusion of SMA) → small bowel necrosis → abdominal pain out of proportion to physical findings. May see red "currant jelly" stools. Risk factors: atrial fibrillation, peripheral arterial disease, recent MI, CHF.
Angiodysplasia	Tortuous dilation of vessels → hematochezia. Most often found in the right-sided colon. More common in older patients. Confirmed by angiography. Associated with end-stage renal disease, von Willebrand disease, aortic stenosis.
Chronic mesenteric ischemia	"Intestinal angina": atherosclerosis of celiac artery, SMA (most commonly affected), or IMA → intestinal hypoperfusion → postprandial epigastric pain → food aversion and weight loss.
Colonic ischemia	Crampy abdominal pain followed by hematochezia. Commonly occurs at watershed areas (splenic flexure, rectosigmoid junction). Typically affects older adults. Thumbprint sign on imaging due to mucosal edema/hemorrhage.
Ileus	Intestinal hypomotility without obstruction → constipation and ↓ flatus; distended/tympanic abdomen with ↓ bowel sounds. Associated with abdominal surgeries, opiates, hypokalemia, sepsis. No transition zone on imaging. Treatment: bowel rest, electrolyte correction, cholinergic drugs (stimulate intestinal motility).
Necrotizing enterocolitis	Seen in premature, formula-fed infants with immature immune system. Necrosis of intestinal mucosa (most commonly terminal ileum and proximal colon), which can lead to pneumatosis intestinalis (arrows in), pneumoperitoneum, portal venous gas.
Proctitis	Inflammation of rectal mucosa, usually associated with infection (*N gonorrhea*, *Chlamydia*, *Campylobacter*, *Shigella*, *Salmonella*, HSV, CMV), IBD, or radiation. Patients report tenesmus, rectal bleeding, and rectal pain. Proctoscopy reveals inflamed rectal mucosa (ulcers/vesicles in the case of HSV). Rectal swabs are used to detect other infectious etiologies.
Small bowel obstruction	Normal flow of intraluminal contents is interrupted → fluid accumulation and intestinal dilation proximal to blockage and intestinal decompression distal to blockage. Presents with abrupt onset of abdominal pain, nausea, vomiting, abdominal distension. Compromised blood flow due to excessive dilation or strangulation may lead to ischemia, necrosis, or perforation. Most commonly caused by intraperitoneal adhesions (fibrous band of scar tissue), tumors, and hernias (in rare cases, meconium plug in newborns → meconium ileus). Upright abdominal x-ray shows air-fluid levels . Management: gastrointestinal decompression, volume resuscitation, bowel rest.
Small intestinal bacterial overgrowth	Abnormal bacterial overgrowth in the small intestine (normally low bacterial colony count). Risk factors: altered pH (eg, achlorhydria, PPI use), anatomical (eg, small bowel obstruction, adhesions, fistula, gastric bypass surgery, blind loop), dysmotility (eg, gastroparesis), immune mediated (IgA deficiency, HIV). Presents with bloating, flatulence, abdominal pain, chronic watery diarrhea, malabsorption (vitamin B_{12}) in severe cases. Diagnosis: carbohydrate breath test or small bowel culture.

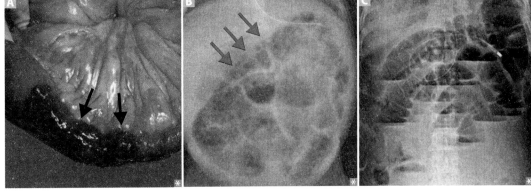

Colonic polyps

Growths of tissue within the colon . Grossly characterized as flat, sessile, or pedunculated on the basis of protrusion into colonic lumen. Generally classified by histologic type.

HISTOLOGIC TYPE	CHARACTERISTICS
Generally nonneoplastic	
Hamartomatous polyps	Solitary lesions do not have significant risk of transformation. Growths of normal colonic tissue with distorted architecture. Associated with Peutz-Jeghers syndrome and juvenile polyposis.
Hyperplastic polyps	Most common; generally smaller and predominantly located in rectosigmoid region. Occasionally evolve into serrated polyps and more advanced lesions.
Inflammatory pseudopolyps	Due to mucosal erosion in inflammatory bowel disease.
Mucosal polyps	Small, usually < 5 mm. Look similar to normal mucosa. Clinically insignificant.
Submucosal polyps	May include lipomas, leiomyomas, fibromas, and other lesions.
Potentially malignant	
Adenomatous polyps	Neoplastic, via chromosomal instability pathway with mutations in *APC* and *KRAS*. Tubular histology has less malignant potential than villous ("**villous** histology is **villainous**"); tubulovillous has intermediate malignant potential. Usually asymptomatic; may present with occult bleeding.
Serrated polyps	Neoplastic. Characterized by CpG island methylator phenotype (CIMP; cytosine base followed by guanine, linked by a phosphodiester bond). Defect may silence mismatch repair gene (eg, *MLH1*) expression. Mutations lead to microsatellite instability and mutations in *BRAF*. "Saw-tooth" pattern of crypts on biopsy. Up to 20% of cases of sporadic CRC.

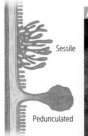
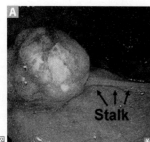
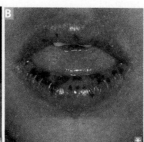
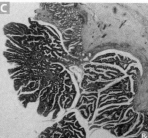
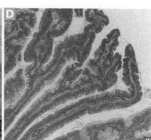

Sessile

Pedunculated

Stalk

Polyposis syndromes

Familial adenomatous polyposis	Autosomal dominant mutation of *APC* tumor suppressor gene on chromosome 5q21-q22. 2-hit hypothesis. Thousands of polyps arise starting after puberty; pancolonic; always involves rectum. Prophylactic colectomy or else 100% progress to CRC.
Gardner syndrome	FAP + osseous and soft tissue tumors (eg, osteomas of skull or mandible), congenital hypertrophy of retinal pigment epithelium, impacted/supernumerary teeth.
Turcot syndrome	FAP or Lynch syndrome + malignant CNS tumor (eg, medulloblastoma, glioma). Turcot = Turban.
Peutz-Jeghers syndrome	Autosomal dominant syndrome featuring numerous hamartomatous polyps throughout GI tract, along with hyperpigmented macules on mouth, lips, hands, genitalia. Associated with ↑ risk of breast and GI cancers (eg, colorectal, stomach, small bowel, pancreatic).
Juvenile polyposis syndrome	Autosomal dominant syndrome in children (typically < 5 years old) featuring numerous hamartomatous polyps in the colon, stomach, small bowel. Associated with ↑ risk of CRC.
***MUTYH*-associated polyposis syndrome**	Autosomal recessive disorder of the *MUTYH* gene responsible for DNA repair. Associated with significantly ↑ risk of CRC, polyps (adenomatous; may be hyperplastic or serrated), and serrated adenomas. Also associated with duodenal adenomas, ovarian and bladder cancers.

Lynch syndrome	Also called hereditary nonpolyposis colorectal cancer (HNPCC). Autosomal dominant mutation of mismatch repair genes (eg, *MLH1*, *MSH2*) with subsequent microsatellite instability. ~ 80% progress to CRC. Proximal Colon is always involved. Associated with Endometrial, Ovarian, and Skin cancers. Merrill **Lynch** has **CEOS**.

Colorectal cancer

EPIDEMIOLOGY	Most patients are > 50 years old. ~ 25% have a family history.
RISK FACTORS	Adenomatous and serrated polyps, familial cancer syndromes, IBD, tobacco use, diet of processed meat with low fiber.
PRESENTATION	Rectosigmoid > ascending > descending. Most are asymptomatic. Right side (cecal, ascending) associated with occult bleeding; left side (rectosigmoid) associated with hematochezia and obstruction (narrower lumen → ↓ stool caliber). Ascending—exophytic mass, iron deficiency anemia, weight loss. Descending—infiltrating mass, partial obstruction, colicky pain, hematochezia. Can present with S *bovis* (*gallolyticus*) bacteremia/endocarditis or as an episode of diverticulitis.
DIAGNOSIS 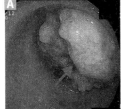 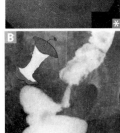	Iron deficiency anemia in males (especially > 50 years old) and postmenopausal females raises suspicion. Screening: <ul><li>Average risk: screen at age 45 with colonoscopy (polyp seen in **A**); alternatives include flexible sigmoidoscopy, fecal occult blood testing (FOBT), fecal immunochemical testing (FIT), FIT-fecal DNA, CT colonography.</li><li>Patients with a first-degree relative who has colon cancer: screen at age 40 with colonoscopy, or 10 years prior to the relative's presentation.</li><li>Patients with IBD: screen 8 years after onset.</li></ul>"Apple core" lesion seen on barium enema x-ray **B**. CEA tumor marker: good for monitoring recurrence, should not be used for screening.

Molecular pathogenesis of colorectal cancer	Chromosomal instability pathway: mutations in *APC* cause FAP and most sporadic cases of CRC (commonly left-sided) via adenoma-carcinoma sequence. Microsatellite instability pathway: mutations or methylation of mismatch repair genes (eg, *MLH1*) cause Lynch syndrome and some sporadic CRC (commonly right sided) via serrated polyp pathway. Overexpression of COX-2 has been linked to CRC, NSAIDs may be chemopreventive.

Chromosomal instability pathway

Always kill polyps

Normal colon	Loss of *APC* gene →	Colon at risk	*KRAS* mutation →	Adenoma	Loss of tumor suppressor gene(s) *(TP53, DCC)* →	Carcinoma
	↓ Intercellular adhesion ↑ Proliferation		Unregulated intracellular signaling		↑ Tumorigenesis	

Cirrhosis and portal hypertension

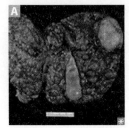

Cirrhosis—diffuse bridging fibrosis (via stellate cells) and regenerative nodules disrupt normal architecture of liver 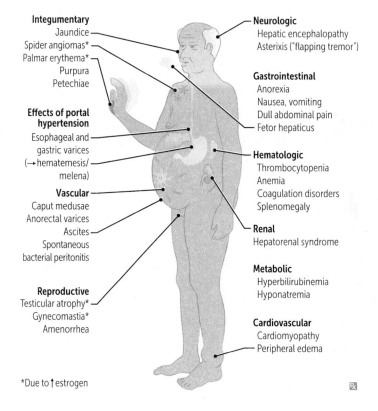; ↑ risk for hepatocellular carcinoma. Can lead to various systemic changes. Etiologies include alcohol, nonalcoholic steatohepatitis, chronic viral hepatitis, autoimmune hepatitis, biliary disease, genetic/metabolic disorders.

Portal hypertension—↑ pressure in portal vein system → new collateral circulation → collateral vessels → varices (ie, esophageal, gastric, and rectal). Causes: cirrhosis (most common), schistosomiasis, portal vein thrombosis.

Ascites—pathological fluid accumulation in the peritoneal cavity due to portal hypertension or portal vein thrombosis. ↑ hepatic sinusoidal pressure → ascites. Serum-to-ascites albumin gradient (SAAG) analysis of ascitic fluid sample determines between etiologies of ascites. SAAG ≥ 1.1 = portal hypertension.

Integumentary
Jaundice
Spider angiomas*
Palmar erythema*
Purpura
Petechiae

Effects of portal hypertension
Esophageal and gastric varices (→hematemesis/ melena)

Vascular
Caput medusae
Anorectal varices
Ascites
Spontaneous bacterial peritonitis

Reproductive
Testicular atrophy*
Gynecomastia*
Amenorrhea

*Due to ↑estrogen

Neurologic
Hepatic encephalopathy
Asterixis ("flapping tremor")

Gastrointestinal
Anorexia
Nausea, vomiting
Dull abdominal pain
Fetor hepaticus

Hematologic
Thrombocytopenia
Anemia
Coagulation disorders
Splenomegaly

Renal
Hepatorenal syndrome

Metabolic
Hyperbilirubinemia
Hyponatremia

Cardiovascular
Cardiomyopathy
Peripheral edema

Budd-Chiari syndrome
Hepatic venous outflow tract obstruction (eg, due to thrombosis, compression) with centrilobular congestion and necrosis → congestive liver disease (hepatomegaly, ascites, varices, abdominal pain, liver failure). Absence of JVD. Associated with hypercoagulable states, polycythemia vera, postpartum state, HCC. May cause nutmeg liver (mottled appearance).

Portal vein thrombosis—thrombosis in portal vein proximal to liver. Usually asymptomatic in the majority of patients, but associated with portal hypertension, abdominal pain, fever. May lead to bowel ischemia if extension to superior mesenteric vein. Etiologies include cirrhosis, malignancy, pancreatitis, and sepsis.

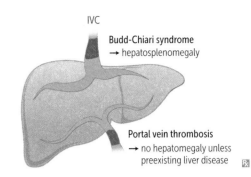

IVC

Budd-Chiari syndrome
→ hepatosplenomegaly

Portal vein thrombosis
→ no hepatomegaly unless preexisting liver disease

Spontaneous bacterial peritonitis
Also called 1° bacterial peritonitis. Common and potentially fatal bacterial infection in patients with cirrhosis and ascites. Often asymptomatic, but can cause fevers, chills, abdominal pain, ileus, or worsening encephalopathy. Commonly caused by gram ⊖ organisms (eg, *E coli*, *Klebsiella*) or less commonly gram ⊕ *Streptococcus*.
Diagnosis: paracentesis with ascitic fluid absolute neutrophil count (ANC) > 250 cells/mm³.
Empiric first-line treatment is 3rd generation cephalosporin (eg, ceftriaxone).

Serum markers of liver pathology

ENZYMES RELEASED IN LIVER DAMAGE	
Aspartate aminotransferase and alanine aminotransferase	↑ in most liver disease: ALT > AST ↑ in **alcoholic** liver disease: **AST > ALT** (ratio usually > 2:1, AST does not typically exceed 500 U/L in alcoholic hepatitis). Make a to**AST** with **alcohol** AST > ALT in nonalcoholic liver disease suggests progression to advanced fibrosis or cirrhosis ↑↑↑ aminotransferases (>1000 U/L): differential includes drug-induced liver injury (eg, acetaminophen toxicity), ischemic hepatitis, acute viral hepatitis, autoimmune hepatitis
Alkaline phosphatase	↑ in cholestasis (eg, biliary obstruction), infiltrative disorders, bone disease
γ-glutamyl transpeptidase	↑ in various liver and biliary diseases (just as ALP can), but not in bone disease (located in canalicular membrane of hepatocytes like ALP); associated with alcohol use
FUNCTIONAL LIVER MARKERS	
Bilirubin	↑ in various liver diseases (eg, biliary obstruction, alcoholic or viral hepatitis, cirrhosis), hemolysis
Albumin	↓ in advanced liver disease (marker of liver's biosynthetic function)
Prothrombin time	↑ in advanced liver disease (↓ production of clotting factors, thereby measuring the liver's biosynthetic function)
Platelets	↓ in advanced liver disease (↓ thrombopoietin, liver sequestration) and portal hypertension (splenomegaly/splenic sequestration)

Reye syndrome	Rare, often fatal childhood hepatic encephalopathy. Associated with viral infection (especially VZV and influenza) that has been treated with aspirin. Aspirin metabolites ↓ β-oxidation by reversible inhibition of mitochondrial enzymes. Findings: mitochondrial abnormalities, fatty liver (microvesicular fatty changes), hyperammonemia, hypoglycemia, vomiting, hepatomegaly, coma. ↑ ICP ↑ morbidity and mortality. Renal and cardiac failure may also occur.	Avoid aspirin (**ASA**) in children, except in Kaw**ASA**ki disease. Salicylates aren't a ray (**Reye**) of sun**SHINEE** for kids: **S**teatosis of liver/hepatocytes **H**ypoglycemia/**H**epatomegaly **I**nfection (VZV, influenza) **N**ot awake (coma) **E**ncephalopathy and diffuse cerebral **E**dema

Alcoholic liver disease

Alcoholic liver disease	Excess NADH production → ↓ fatty acid oxidation and ↑ lipogenesis.
Hepatic steatosis	Macrovesicular fatty change A; may be reversible with alcohol cessation.
Alcoholic hepatitis	Requires sustained, long-term consumption. Swollen and necrotic hepatocytes with neutrophilic infiltration. Mallory bodies B (intracytoplasmic eosinophilic inclusions of damaged keratin filaments).
Alcoholic cirrhosis	Final and usually irreversible form. Sclerosis around central vein may be seen in early disease. Regenerative nodules surrounded by fibrous bands (red arrows in C) in response to chronic liver injury → portal hypertension and end-stage liver disease.

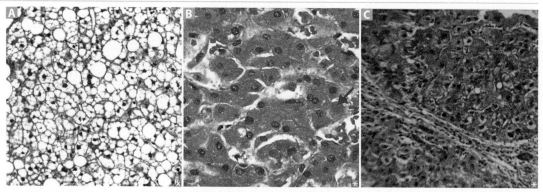

Steatotic liver disease 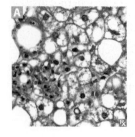	Steatotic liver disease (SLD) encompasses metabolic dysfunction–associated SLD (MASLD; formerly known as nonalcoholic fatty liver disease), MASLD and increased alcohol intake, alcohol-associated liver disease, specific etiology SLD, and cryptogenic SLD. MASLD is associated with metabolic syndrome (obesity, insulin resistance, HTN, hypertriglyceridemia, ↓ HDL); obesity → fatty infiltration of hepatocytes A → cellular "ballooning" and eventual necrosis. Steatosis present without evidence of significant inflammation or fibrosis. May persist or even regress over time. Usually asymptomatic. **Metabolic dysfunction–associated steatohepatitis**—associated with lobular inflammation and hepatocyte ballooning → fibrosis. May progress to cirrhosis and HCC.

Autoimmune hepatitis	Chronic inflammatory liver disease. More common in females. May be asymptomatic or present with fatigue, nausea, pruritus. Often ⊕ for anti-smooth muscle or anti-liver/kidney microsomal-1 antibodies. Labs: ↑ ALT and AST. Histology: portal and periportal lymphoplasmacytic infiltrate.

Hepatic encephalopathy	Cirrhosis → portosystemic shunts → ↓ NH_3 metabolism → neuropsychiatric dysfunction (reversible) ranging from disorientation/asterixis to difficult arousal or coma.
	Triggers:
	  ▪ ↑ NH_3 production and absorption (due to GI bleed, constipation, infection).
	  ▪ ↓ NH_3 removal (due to renal failure, diuretics, bypassed hepatic blood flow post-TIPS).
	Treatment: lactulose (↑ NH_4^+ generation) and rifaximin (↓ NH_3-producing gut bacteria).

Liver tumors

Hepatic hemangioma	Also called cavernous hemangioma. Most common benign liver tumor (venous malformation) 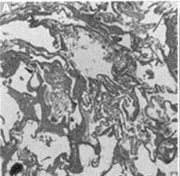; typically occurs at age 30–50 years. Biopsy contraindicated because of risk of hemorrhage.
Focal nodular hyperplasia	Second most common benign liver tumor; occurs predominantly in females aged 35–50 years. Hyperplastic reaction of hepatocytes to an aberrant dystrophic artery. Marked by central stellate scar. Usually asymptomatic and detected incidentally.
Hepatic adenoma	Rare, benign tumor, often related to oral contraceptive or anabolic steroid use; may regress spontaneously or rupture (abdominal pain and shock).
Hepatocellular carcinoma	Also called hepatoma. Most common 1° malignant liver tumor in adults 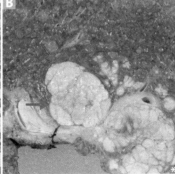. Associated with HBV (+/– cirrhosis) and all other causes of cirrhosis (including HCV, alcoholic and nonalcoholic fatty liver disease, autoimmune disease, hemochromatosis, Wilson disease, α_1-antitrypsin deficiency) and specific carcinogens (eg, aflatoxin from *Aspergillus*). Findings: anorexia, jaundice, tender hepatomegaly. May lead to decompensation of previously stable cirrhosis (eg, ascites) and portal vein thrombosis. Spreads hematogenously. Diagnosis: ultrasound (screening) or contrast CT/MRI 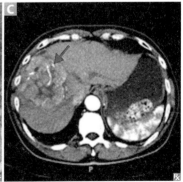 (confirmation); biopsy if diagnosis is uncertain. Recurrence monitored with serum AFP.
Hepatic angiosarcoma	Rare, malignant tumor of endothelial origin; associated with exposure to arsenic, vinyl chloride.
Metastases	Most common malignant liver tumors overall; 1° sources include GI, breast, lung cancers. Metastases are rarely solitary.

α₁-antitrypsin deficiency 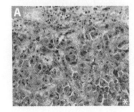	Misfolded gene product protein aggregates in hepatocellular ER → cirrhosis with PAS ⊕ globules 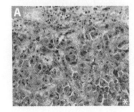 in liver. Codominant trait. Often presents in young patients with liver damage and dyspnea without a history of tobacco smoking.	In lungs, ↓ α₁-antitrypsin → uninhibited elastase in alveoli → ↓ elastic tissue → panacinar emphysema.

Jaundice 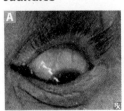	Abnormal yellowing of the skin and/or sclera (icterus) A due to bilirubin deposition. Hyperbilirubinemia 2° to ↑ production or ↓ clearance (impaired hepatic uptake, conjugation, excretion).	**HOT Liver**—common causes of ↑ bilirubin level: **H**emolysis **O**bstruction **T**umor **Liver** disease

Conjugated (direct) hyperbilirubinemia	Biliary tract obstruction: gallstones, cholangiocarcinoma, pancreatic or liver cancer, liver fluke. Biliary tract disease: 1° sclerosing cholangitis, 1° biliary cholangitis Excretion defect: Dubin-Johnson syndrome, Rotor syndrome.
Unconjugated (indirect) hyperbilirubinemia	Hemolytic, benign (neonates), Crigler-Najjar, Gilbert syndrome.
Mixed hyperbilirubinemia	Both direct and indirect hyperbilirubinemia. Hepatitis, cirrhosis.

Benign neonatal hyperbilirubinemia	Formerly called physiologic neonatal jaundice. Mild unconjugated hyperbilirubinemia caused by: ▪ ↑ fetal RBC turnover (↑ hematocrit and ↓ fetal RBC lifespan). ▪ Immature newborn liver (↓ UDP-glucuronosyltransferase activity). ▪ Sterile newborn gut (↓ conversion to urobilinogen → ↑ deconjugation by intestinal brush border β-glucuronidase → ↑ enterohepatic circulation). β-glucuronidase—lysosomal enzyme for direct bilirubin deconjugation. Also found in breast milk. May lead to pigment stone formation. Occurs in nearly all newborns after first 24 hours of life and usually resolves without treatment in 1–2 weeks. Exaggerated forms: Breastfeeding failure jaundice—insufficient breast milk intake → ↓ bilirubin elimination in stool → ↑ enterohepatic circulation. Breast milk jaundice—↑ β-glucuronidase in breast milk → ↑ deconjugation → ↑ enterohepatic circulation. Severe cases may lead to kernicterus (deposition of unconjugated, lipid-soluble bilirubin in the brain, particularly basal ganglia). Treatment: phototherapy (non-UV) isomerizes unconjugated bilirubin to water-soluble form that can be excreted in the bile.

Biliary atresia	Most common reason for pediatric liver transplantation. Fibro-obliterative destruction of bile ducts → cholestasis. Associated with absent/abnormal gallbladder on ultrasonogram. Often presents as a newborn with persistent jaundice after 2 weeks of life, darkening urine, acholic stools, hepatomegaly. Labs: ↑ direct bilirubin and GGT.

Hereditary hyperbilirubinemias

❶ Gilbert syndrome	Mildly ↓ UDP-glucuronosyltransferase conjugation. Asymptomatic or mild jaundice usually with stress, illness, or fasting. ↑ unconjugated bilirubin without overt hemolysis. Relatively common, benign condition.
❷ Crigler-Najjar syndrome, type I	Absent UDP-glucuronosyltransferase. Presents early in life, but some patients may not have neurologic signs until later in life. Findings: jaundice, kernicterus (unconjugated bilirubin deposition in brain), ↑ unconjugated bilirubin. Treatment: plasmapheresis and phototherapy (does not conjugate UCB; but does ↑ polarity and ↑ water solubility to allow excretion). Liver transplant is curative. Type II is less severe and responds to phenobarbital (vs. Type I, more severe), which ↑ liver enzyme synthesis.
❸ Dubin-Johnson syndrome	Conjugated hyperbilirubinemia due to defective liver excretion. Grossly black (**D**ark) liver due to impaired excretion of epinephrine metabolites. Benign.
❹ Rotor syndrome	Phenotypically similar to Dubin-Johnson, but milder in presentation without black (**R**egular) liver. Due to impaired hepatic storage of conjugated bilirubin.

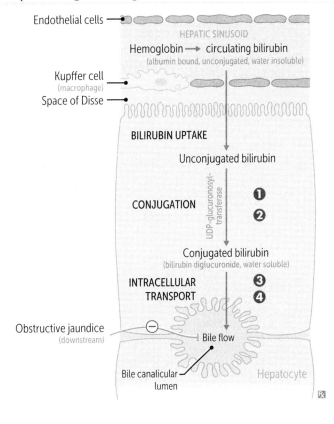

Wilson disease

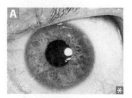

Also called hepatolenticular degeneration. Autosomal recessive mutations in hepatocyte copper-transporting ATPase (*ATP7B* gene; chromosome 13) → ↓ copper incorporation into apoceruloplasmin and excretion into bile → ↓ serum ceruloplasmin. Copper accumulates, especially in liver, brain (eg, basal ganglia), cornea, kidneys; ↑ urine copper.

Presents before age 40 with liver disease (eg, hepatitis, acute liver failure, cirrhosis), neurologic disease (eg, dysarthria, dystonia, tremor, parkinsonism), psychiatric disease, Kayser-Fleischer rings (deposits in Descemet membrane of cornea) **A**, hemolytic anemia, renal disease (eg, Fanconi syndrome).

Treatment: chelation with penicillamine or trientine, oral zinc. Liver transplant in acute liver failure related to Wilson disease.

Hemochromatosis

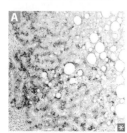

Autosomal recessive. Mutation in *HFE* gene, located on chromosome 6. Leads to abnormal (low) hepcidin production, ↑ intestinal iron absorption. Iron overload can also be 2° to chronic transfusion therapy (eg, β-thalassemia major). Iron accumulates, especially in liver, pancreas, skin, heart, pituitary, joints. Hemosiderin (iron) can be identified on liver MRI or biopsy with Prussian blue stain **A**.

Presents after age 40 when total body iron > 20 g; iron loss through menstruation slows progression in females. Classic triad of cirrhosis, diabetes mellitus, skin pigmentation ("bronze diabetes"). Also causes restrictive cardiomyopathy (classic) or dilated cardiomyopathy (reversible), hypogonadism, arthropathy (calcium pyrophosphate deposition; especially metacarpophalangeal joints). HCC is common cause of death.

Treatment: repeated phlebotomy, iron (Fe) chelation with deferasirox, deferoxamine, deferiprone.

Biliary tract disease

May present with pruritus, jaundice, dark urine, light-colored stool, hepatosplenomegaly. Typically with cholestatic pattern of LFTs (↑ conjugated bilirubin, ↑ cholesterol, ↑ ALP, ↑ GGT).

	PATHOLOGY	EPIDEMIOLOGY	ADDITIONAL FEATURES
Primary sclerosing cholangitis	Unknown cause of concentric "onion skin" bile duct fibrosis → alternating strictures and dilation with "beading" of intra- and extrahepatic bile ducts on ERCP **A**, magnetic resonance cholangiopancreatography (MRCP).	Classically in middle-aged males with ulcerative colitis.	Associated with ulcerative colitis. MPO-ANCA/p-ANCA ⊕. ↑ IgM. Can lead to 2° biliary cirrhosis. ↑ risk of cholangiocarcinoma and gallbladder cancer.
Primary biliary cholangitis	Autoimmune reaction → lymphocytic infiltrate +/– granulomas → destruction of lobular bile ducts.	Classically in middle-aged females.	Antimitochondrial antibody ⊕, ↑ IgM. Associated with other autoimmune conditions (eg, Hashimoto thyroiditis, rheumatoid arthritis, celiac disease). Treatment: ursodiol.
Secondary biliary cirrhosis	Extrahepatic biliary obstruction → ↑ pressure in intrahepatic ducts → injury/ fibrosis and bile stasis.	Patients with known obstructive lesions (gallstones, biliary strictures, pancreatic carcinoma).	May be complicated by acute cholangitis.

Cholelithiasis and related pathologies

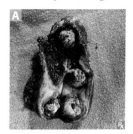

↑ cholesterol and/or bilirubin, ↓ bile salts, and gallbladder stasis all cause sludge or stones.

2 types of stones:

- Cholesterol stones 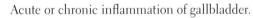 (radiolucent with 10–20% opaque due to calcifications)—80% of stones. Associated with obesity, Crohn disease, advanced age, estrogen therapy, multiparity, rapid weight loss, medications (eg, fibrates), race (↑ incidence in White and Native American populations).
- Pigment stones (black = radiopaque, Ca^{2+} bilirubinate, hemolysis; brown = radiolucent, infection). Associated with Crohn disease, chronic hemolysis, alcoholic cirrhosis, advanced age, biliary infections, total parenteral nutrition (TPN).

Most common complication is cholecystitis; can also cause acute pancreatitis, acute cholangitis.

Diagnose with ultrasound. Treat with elective cholecystectomy if symptomatic.

Risk factors (8 F's): female, fat, fertile, forty, fair, feeds (TPN), fasting (rapid weight loss), fibrates.

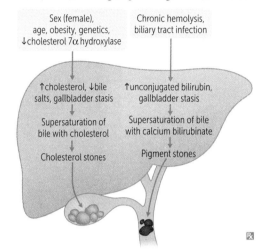

RELATED PATHOLOGIES	CHARACTERISTICS
Biliary colic	Associated with nausea/vomiting and dull RUQ pain. Neurohormonal activation (eg, by CCK after a fatty meal) triggers contraction of gallbladder, forcing stone into cystic duct. Labs are normal, ultrasound shows cholelithiasis.
Choledocholithiasis	Presence of gallstone(s) in common bile duct, often leading to elevated ALP, GGT, direct bilirubin, and/or AST/ALT.
Cholecystitis 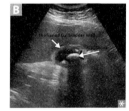	Acute or chronic inflammation of gallbladder. Calculous cholecystitis—most common type; due to gallstone impaction in the cystic duct resulting in inflammation and gallbladder wall thickening (arrows in B); can produce 2° infection. Acalculous cholecystitis—due to gallbladder stasis, hypoperfusion, or infection (CMV); seen in critically ill patients. Murphy sign: inspiratory arrest on RUQ palpation due to pain. Pain may radiate to right shoulder (due to irritation of phrenic nerve). ↑ ALP if bile duct becomes involved (eg, acute cholangitis). Diagnose with ultrasound or cholescintigraphy (HIDA scan). Failure to visualize gallbladder on HIDA scan suggests obstruction. Gallstone ileus—fistula between gallbladder and GI tract → stone enters GI lumen → obstructs at ileocecal valve (narrowest point); can see air in biliary tree (pneumobilia). Rigler triad: radiographic findings of pneumobilia, small bowel obstruction, gallstone (usually in iliac fossa).
Porcelain gallbladder 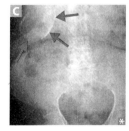	Calcified gallbladder due to chronic cholecystitis; usually found incidentally on imaging C. Treatment: prophylactic cholecystectomy generally recommended due to ↑ risk of gallbladder cancer (mostly adenocarcinoma).
Acute cholangitis	Also called ascending cholangitis. Infection of biliary tree usually due to obstruction that leads to stasis/bacterial overgrowth. Charcot triad of cholangitis includes jaundice, fever, RUQ pain. Reynolds pentad is Charcot triad plus altered mental status and shock (hypotension).

Cholangiocarcinoma	Malignant tumor of bile duct epithelium. Most common location is convergence of right and left hepatic ducts. Risk factors include 1° sclerosing cholangitis, liver fluke infections (eg, *Clonorchis*). Usually presents late with fatigue, weight loss, abdominal pain, jaundice. Imaging may show biliary tract obstruction. Histology: infiltrating neoplastic glands associated with desmoplastic stroma.

Pancreatitis	Refers to inflammation of the pancreas. Usually sterile.
Acute pancreatitis	Autodigestion of pancreas by pancreatic enzymes (**A** shows pancreas [yellow arrows] surrounded by edema [red arrows]). Causes: Idiopathic, Gallstones, Ethanol, Trauma, Steroids, Mumps, Autoimmune disease, Scorpion sting, Hypercalcemia/Hypertriglyceridemia (> 1000 mg/dL), ERCP, Drugs (eg, sulfa drugs, NRTIs, protease inhibitors). **I GET SMASHED.** Diagnosis by 2 of 3 criteria: acute epigastric pain often radiating to the back, serum amylase or lipase (more specific) to 3× upper limit of normal, or characteristic imaging findings. Complications: pancreatic pseudocyst **B** (lined by granulation tissue, not epithelium), abscess, necrosis of parenchymal or peripancreatic tissue, hemorrhage, infection, organ failure (ALI/ARDS, shock, renal failure), hypocalcemia (precipitation of Ca^{2+} soaps).
Chronic pancreatitis	Chronic inflammation, atrophy, calcification of the pancreas **C**. Major risk factors include alcohol use disorder and genetic predisposition (eg, cystic fibrosis, *SPINK1* mutations); can be idiopathic. Complications include pancreatic insufficiency and pseudocysts. Pancreatic insufficiency (typically when <10% pancreatic function) may manifest with steatorrhea, fat-soluble vitamin deficiency, diabetes mellitus. Amylase and lipase may or may not be elevated (almost always elevated in acute pancreatitis).

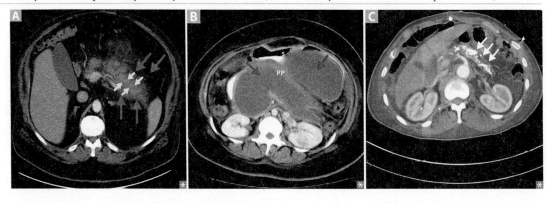

Pancreatic adenocarcinoma

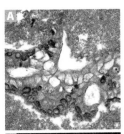
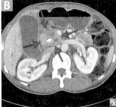

Very aggressive tumor arising from pancreatic ducts (disorganized glandular structure with cellular infiltration **A**); often metastatic at presentation, with average survival ~ 1 year after diagnosis. Tumors more common in pancreatic head **B** (lead to obstructive jaundice). Associated with CA 19-9 tumor marker (also CEA, less specific). Most common genomic abnormality is *KRAS*-activating mutation.

Risk factors:
- Tobacco smoking (strongest risk factor)
- Chronic pancreatitis (especially > 20 years)
- Diabetes
- Age > 50 years

Often presents with:
- Abdominal pain radiating to back
- Weight loss (due to malabsorption and anorexia)
- Migratory thrombophlebitis—redness and tenderness on palpation of extremities (Trousseau syndrome)
- Obstructive jaundice with palpable, nontender gallbladder (Courvoisier sign)

▶ GASTROINTESTINAL—PHARMACOLOGY

Acid suppression therapy

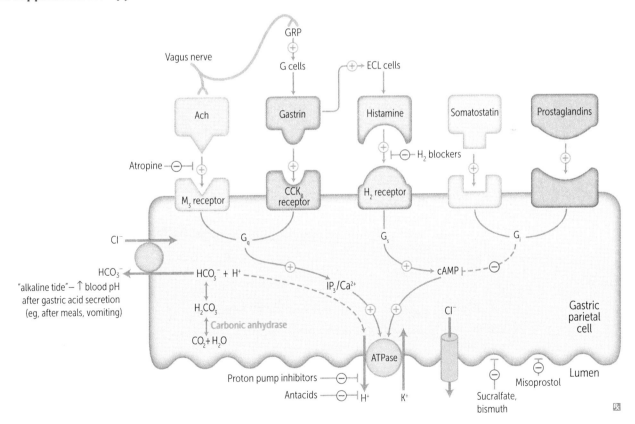

H$_2$-blockers	Cimetidine, famotidine, nizatidine.
	Take H$_2$ blockers before you **dine**. Think "**table for 2**" to remember H$_2$.
MECHANISM	Reversible block of histamine H$_2$-receptors → ↓ H$^+$ secretion by parietal cells.
CLINICAL USE	Peptic ulcer, gastritis, mild esophageal reflux.
ADVERSE EFFECTS	Cimetidine is a potent inhibitor of cytochrome P-450 (multiple drug interactions); it also has antiandrogenic effects (prolactin release, gynecomastia, impotence, ↓ libido in males); can cross blood-brain barrier (confusion, dizziness, headaches) and placenta. Cimetidine ↓ renal excretion of creatinine. Other H$_2$ blockers are relatively free of these effects.

Proton pump inhibitors	Omeprazole, lansoprazole, esomeprazole, pantoprazole, dexlansoprazole.
MECHANISM	Irreversibly inhibit H$^+$/K$^+$-ATPase in stomach parietal cells.
CLINICAL USE	Peptic ulcer, gastritis, esophageal reflux, Zollinger-Ellison syndrome, component of therapy for *H pylori*, stress ulcer prophylaxis.
ADVERSE EFFECTS	↑ risk of *C difficile* infection, pneumonia, acute interstitial nephritis. Vitamin B$_{12}$ malabsorption; ↓ serum Mg^{2+}/Ca^{2+} absorption (potentially leading to increased fracture risk in older adults).

Antacids	Can affect absorption, bioavailability, or urinary excretion of other drugs by altering gastric and urinary pH or by delaying gastric emptying. All can cause hypokalemia.	
Aluminum hydroxide	Constipation, Hypophosphatemia, Osteodystrophy, Proximal muscle weakness, Seizures	Alu**minimum** amount of feces **CHOPS**
Calcium carbonate	Hypercalcemia (milk-alkali syndrome), rebound acid ↑	Can chelate and ↓ effectiveness of other drugs (eg, tetracycline)
Magnesium hydroxide	Diarrhea, hyporeflexia, hypotension, cardiac arrest	Mg^{2+} = Must go 2 the bathroom

Bismuth, sucralfate	
MECHANISM	Bind to ulcer base, providing physical protection and allowing HCO$_3^-$ secretion to reestablish pH gradient in the mucous layer. Sucralfate requires acidic environment, not given with PPIs/H$_2$ blockers.
CLINICAL USE	↑ ulcer healing, travelers' diarrhea (bismuth). Bismuth also used in quadruple therapy for *H pylori*.

Misoprostol	
MECHANISM	PGE$_1$ analog. ↑ production and secretion of gastric mucous barrier, ↓ acid production.
CLINICAL USE	Prevention of NSAID-induced peptic ulcers (NSAIDs block PGE$_1$ production). Also used off-label for induction of labor (ripens cervix).
ADVERSE EFFECTS	Diarrhea. Contraindicated in patients of childbearing potential (abortifacient).

Octreotide

MECHANISM	Long-acting somatostatin analog; inhibits secretion of various splanchnic vasodilatory hormones.
CLINICAL USE	Acute variceal bleeds, acromegaly, VIPoma, carcinoid tumors.
ADVERSE EFFECTS	Nausea, cramps, steatorrhea. ↑ risk of cholelithiasis due to CCK inhibition.

Sulfasalazine

MECHANISM	A combination of sulfapyridine (antibacterial) and 5-aminosalicylic acid (anti-inflammatory). Activated by colonic bacteria.
CLINICAL USE	Ulcerative colitis, Crohn disease (colitis component).
ADVERSE EFFECTS	Malaise, nausea, sulfonamide toxicity, reversible oligospermia.

Loperamide, diphenoxylate

MECHANISM	Agonists at μ-opioid receptors → ↓ gut motility. Poor CNS penetration (low addictive potential).
CLINICAL USE	Diarrhea.
ADVERSE EFFECTS	Constipation, nausea.

Antiemetics

All act centrally in chemoreceptor trigger zone of area postrema.

DRUG	MECHANISM	CLINICAL USE	ADVERSE EFFECTS
Ondansetron, granisetron	5-HT$_3$-receptor antagonists Also act peripherally (↓ vagal stimulation)	Nausea and vomiting after chemotherapy, radiotherapy, or surgery	Headache, constipation, QT interval prolongation, serotonin syndrome
Prochlorperazine, metoclopramide	D$_2$-receptor antagonists Metoclopramide also causes ↑ gastric emptying and ↑ LES tone	Nausea and vomiting Metoclopramide is also used in gastroparesis (eg, diabetic), persistent GERD	Extrapyramidal symptoms, hyperprolactinemia, anxiety, drowsiness, restlessness, depression, GI distress
Aprepitant, fosaprepitant	NK$_1$ (neurokinin-1) receptor antagonists NK$_1$ receptor = substance P receptor	Chemotherapy-induced nausea and vomiting	Fatigue, GI distress

Orlistat

MECHANISM	Inhibits gastric and pancreatic lipase → ↓ breakdown and absorption of dietary fats. Taken with fat-containing meals.
CLINICAL USE	Weight loss.
ADVERSE EFFECTS	Abdominal pain, flatulence, bowel urgency/frequent bowel movements, steatorrhea; ↓ absorption of fat-soluble vitamins.

Anticonstipation drugs

DRUG	MECHANISM	ADVERSE EFFECTS
Bulk-forming laxatives Methylcellulose, psyllium	Soluble fibers that draw water into gut lumen, forming viscous liquid that promotes peristalsis	Bloating
Osmotic laxatives Lactulose, magnesium citrate, magnesium hydroxide, polyethylene glycol	Provide osmotic load to draw water into GI lumen Lactulose also treats hepatic encephalopathy: gut microbiota degrades lactulose into metabolites (lactic acid, acetic acid) that promote nitrogen excretion as NH_4^+ by trapping it in colon	Diarrhea, dehydration; may be misused by patients with bulimia
Stimulant laxatives Bisacodyl, senna	Enteric nerve stimulation → colonic contraction	Diarrhea
Emollient laxatives Docusate	Surfactants that ↓ stool surface tension, promoting water entry into stool	Diarrhea
Lubiprostone	Chloride channel activator → ↑ intestinal fluid secretion	Diarrhea, nausea
Guanylate cyclase-C agonists Linaclotide, plecanatide	Activate intracellular cGMP signaling → ↑ fluid and electrolyte secretion in the intestinal lumen	Diarrhea, bloating, abdominal discomfort, flatulence
Serotonergic agonists Prucalopride	$5HT_4$ agonism → enteric nerve stimulation → ↑ peristalsis, intestinal secretion	Diarrhea, abdominal pain, nausea, headache
NHE_3 inhibitor Tenapanor	Inhibits Na^+/H^+ exchanger → ↓ Na^+ absorption → ↑ H_2O secretion in lumen	Diarrhea, abdominal pain, nausea

Hematology and Oncology

"You're always somebody's type! (blood type, that is)"
—BloodLink

"The best blood will at some time get into a fool or a mosquito."
—Austin O'Malley

"A life touched by cancer is not a life destroyed by cancer."
—Drew Boswell, *Climbing the Cancer Mountain*

"Without hair, a queen is still a queen."
—Prajakta Mhadnak

"Blood can circulate forever if you keep donating it."
—Anonymous

When studying hematology, pay close attention to the many cross connections to immunology. Make sure you master the different types of anemias. Be comfortable interpreting blood smears. When reviewing oncologic drugs, focus on mechanisms and adverse effects rather than details of clinical uses, which may be lower yield.

Please note that solid tumors are covered in their respective organ system chapters.

▶ HEMATOLOGY AND ONCOLOGY—EMBRYOLOGY

Fetal erythropoiesis	Fetal erythropoiesis occurs in: ▪ Yolk sac (3–8 weeks) ▪ Liver (6 weeks–birth) ▪ Spleen (10–28 weeks) ▪ Bone marrow (18 weeks to adult)	Young liver synthesizes blood.
Hemoglobin development	Embryonic globins: ζ and ε. Fetal hemoglobin (HbF) = $\alpha_2\gamma_2$. Adult hemoglobin (HbA$_1$) = $\alpha_2\beta_2$. HbF has higher affinity for O_2 because it binds to 2,3-BPG with relatively lower affinity, allowing HbF to capture O_2 from maternal hemoglobin (HbA$_1$ and HbA$_2$) across the placenta. HbA$_2$ ($\alpha_2\delta_2$) is a form of adult hemoglobin present in small amounts.	From fetal to adult hemoglobin: Alpha always; gamma goes, becomes beta.

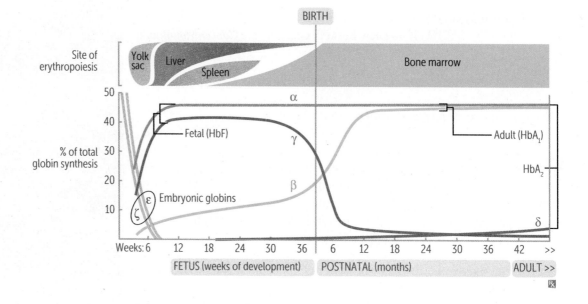

Blood groups

	ABO classification				Rh classification	
	A	**B**	**AB**	**O**	**Rh⊕**	**Rh⊖**
RBC type						
Group antigens on RBC surface	A	B	A & B	NONE	Rh (D)	NONE
Antibodies in plasma	Anti-B IgM	Anti-A IgM	NONE	Anti-A Anti-B IgG, IgM	NONE	Anti-D IgG
Clinical relevance Compatible RBC types to receive	A, O	B, O	AB, A, B, O	O	Rh⊕, Rh⊖	Rh⊖
Compatible RBC types to donate to	A, AB	B, AB	AB	A, B, AB, O	Rh⊕	Rh⊕, Rh⊖

Hemolytic disease of the fetus and newborn

Also called erythroblastosis fetalis. Most commonly involves the antigens of the major blood groups (eg, Rh and ABO), but minor blood group incompatibilities (eg, Kell) can also result in disease, ranging from mild to severe.

	ABO hemolytic disease	Rh hemolytic disease
INTERACTION	Type O pregnant patient; type A or B fetus.	Rh ⊖ pregnant patient; Rh ⊕ fetus.
MECHANISM	Preexisting pregnant patient anti-A and/or anti-B IgG antibodies cross the placenta → attack fetal and newborn RBCs → hemolysis.	First pregnancy: patient exposed to fetal blood (often during delivery) → formation of maternal anti-D IgG. Subsequent pregnancies: anti-D IgG crosses placenta → attacks fetal and newborn RBCs → hemolysis.
PRESENTATION	Mild jaundice in the neonate within 24 hours of birth. Unlike Rh hemolytic disease, can occur in firstborn babies and is usually less severe.	Hydrops fetalis, jaundice shortly after birth, kernicterus.
TREATMENT/PREVENTION	Treatment: phototherapy or exchange transfusion.	Prevent by administration of anti-D IgG to Rh ⊖ pregnant patients during third trimester and early postpartum period as well as in cases of ectopic pregnancy, miscarriage, abdominal trauma, and antepartum hemorrhage (if fetus Rh ⊕). Prevents maternal anti-D IgG production.

▶ HEMATOLOGY AND ONCOLOGY—ANATOMY

Hematopoiesis

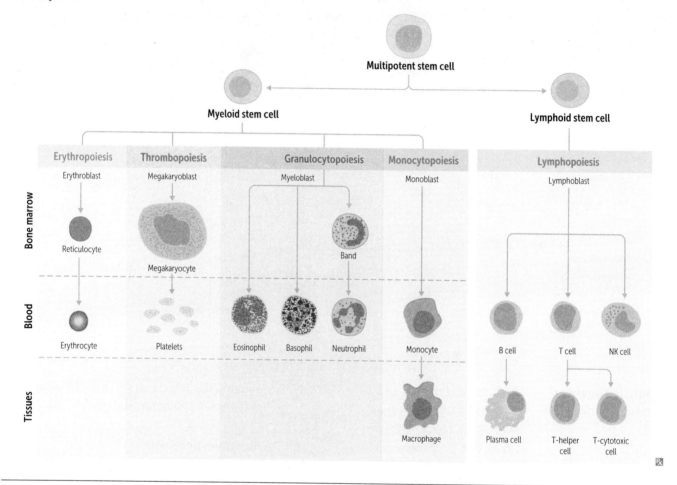

Neutrophils

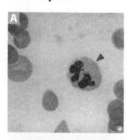

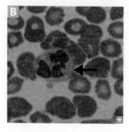

Acute inflammatory response cells. Phagocytic. Multilobed nucleus **A**. Specific granules contain leukocyte alkaline phosphatase (LAP), collagenase, lysozyme, and lactoferrin. Azurophilic granules (lysosomes) contain proteinases, acid phosphatase, myeloperoxidase, and β-glucuronidase.

Inflammatory states (eg, bacterial infection) cause neutrophilia and changes in neutrophil morphology, such as left shift, toxic granulation (dark blue, coarse granules), Döhle bodies (light blue, peripheral inclusions, arrow in **B**), and cytoplasmic vacuoles.

Neutrophil chemotactic agents: C5a, IL-8, LTB_4, 5-HETE (leukotriene precursor), kallikrein, platelet-activating factor, N-formylmethionine (bacterial proteins).

Hypersegmented neutrophils (nucleus has 5–6+ lobes) are seen in vitamin B_{12}/folate deficiency.

Left shift—↑ neutrophil precursors (eg, band cells, metamyelocytes) in peripheral blood. Reflects states of ↑ myeloid proliferation (eg, inflammation, CML).

Leukoerythroblastic reaction—left shift accompanied by immature RBCs. Suggests bone marrow infiltration (eg, myelofibrosis, metastasis).

Erythrocytes

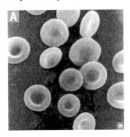

Carry O_2 to tissues and CO_2 to lungs. Anucleate and lack organelles; biconcave , with large surface area-to-volume ratio for rapid gas exchange. Life span of ~120 days in healthy adults; 60–90 days in neonates. Source of energy is glucose (90% used in glycolysis, 10% used in HMP shunt). Membranes contain Cl^-/HCO_3^- antiporter, which allow RBCs to export HCO_3^- and transport CO_2 from the periphery to the lungs for elimination.

Erythro = red; *cyte* = cell.

Erythrocytosis = polycythemia = ↑ Hct.
Anisocytosis = varying sizes.
Poikilocytosis = varying shapes.

Reticulocyte = immature RBC; reflects erythroid proliferation.
Bluish color (polychromasia) on Wright-Giemsa stain of reticulocytes represents residual ribosomal RNA.

Thrombocytes (platelets)

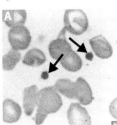

Involved in 1° hemostasis. Anucleate, small cytoplasmic fragments derived from megakaryocytes. Life span of 8–10 days (pl8lets). When activated by endothelial injury, aggregate with other platelets and interact with fibrinogen to form platelet plug. Contain dense granules (Ca^{2+}, ADP, Serotonin, Histamine; CASH) and α granules (vWF, fibrinogen, fibronectin, platelet factor 4). Approximately 1/3 of platelet pool is stored in the spleen.

Thrombocytopenia or ↓ platelet function results in petechiae.
vWF receptor: GpIb.
Fibrinogen receptor: GpIIb/IIIa.
Thrombopoietin stimulates megakaryocyte proliferation.
Alfa granules contain vWF, fibrinogen, fibronectin, platelet factor four.

Monocytes

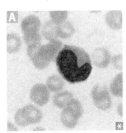

Found in blood, differentiate into macrophages or dendritic cells. in tissues.
Large, kidney-shaped nucleus . Extensive "frosted glass" cytoplasm.

Mono = one (nucleus); *cyte* = cell.

Macrophages

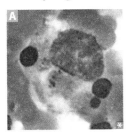

A type of antigen-presenting cell. Phagocytose bacteria, cellular debris, and senescent RBCs. Long life in tissues. Differentiate from circulating blood monocytes . Activated by IFN-γ. Can function as antigen-presenting cell via MHC II. Also engage in antibody-dependent cellular cytotoxicity. Important cellular component of granulomas (eg, TB, sarcoidosis), where they may fuse to form giant cells.

Macro = large; *phage* = eater.
Macrophage naming varies by specific tissue type (eg, Kupffer cells in liver, histiocytes in connective tissue, osteoclasts in bone, microglial cells in brain).
Lipid A from bacterial LPS binds CD14 on macrophages to initiate septic shock.

Dendritic cells

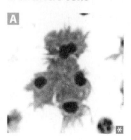

Highly phagocytic antigen-presenting cells (APCs) . Function as link between innate and adaptive immune systems (eg, via T-cell stimulation). Express MHC class II and Fc receptors on surface. Can present exogenous antigens on MHC class I (cross-presentation).

Eosinophils

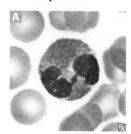

Defend against helminthic infections (major basic protein). Bilobate nucleus. Packed with large eosinophilic granules of uniform size . Highly phagocytic for antigen-antibody complexes.

Produce histaminase, major basic protein (MBP, a helminthotoxin), eosinophil cationic protein, eosinophil-derived neurotoxin, and IL-5, which promotes eosinophilic activation and proliferation.

Eosin = pink dye; *philic* = loving.
Causes of eosinophilia (**PACMAN** Eats):
　Parasites
　Asthma
　Chronic adrenal insufficiency
　Myeloproliferative disorders
　Allergic processes
　Neoplasia (eg, Hodgkin lymphoma)
　Eosinophilic granulomatosis with polyangiitis

Basophils

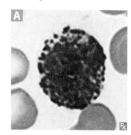

Mediate allergic reaction. Densely basophilic granules contain heparin (anticoagulant) and histamine (vasodilator). Leukotrienes synthesized and released on demand.

Basophilic—stains readily with basic stains.
Basophilia is uncommon, but can be a sign of myeloproliferative disorders, particularly CML.

Mast cells

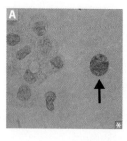

Mediate local tissue allergic reactions. Contain basophilic granules . Originate from same precursor as basophils but are not the same cell type. Can bind the Fc portion of IgE to membrane. Activated by tissue trauma, C3a and C5a, surface IgE cross-linking by antigen (IgE receptor aggregation) → degranulation → release of histamine, heparin, tryptase, and eosinophil chemotactic factors.

Involved in type I hypersensitivity reactions.
Cromolyn sodium prevents mast cell degranulation (used for asthma prophylaxis).
Vancomycin, opioids, and radiocontrast dye can elicit IgE-independent mast cell degranulation.
Mastocytosis—rare; proliferation of mast cells in skin and/or extracutaneous organs. Associated with c-*KIT* mutations and ↑ serum tryptase.
↑ histamine → flushing, pruritus, hypotension, abdominal pain, diarrhea, peptic ulcer disease.

Lymphocytes

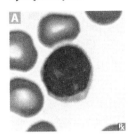

Refer to B cells, T cells, and natural killer (NK) cells. B cells and T cells mediate adaptive immunity. NK cells are part of the innate immune response. Round, densely staining nucleus with small amount of pale cytoplasm A.

Natural killer cells

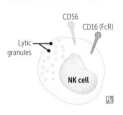

Important in innate immunity, especially against intracellular pathogens. NK cells are larger than B and T cells, with distinctive cytoplasmic lytic granules (containing perforin and granzymes) that, when released, act on target cells to induce apoptosis. Distinguish between healthy and infected cells by identifying cell surface proteins (induced by stress, malignant transformation, or microbial infections). Induce **apoptosis** (natural **killer**) in cells that do not express class I MHC cell surface molecules, eg, virally infected cells in which these molecules are downregulated.

B cells

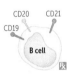

Mediate humoral immune response. Originate from stem cells in bone marrow and matures in marrow. Migrate to peripheral lymphoid tissue (follicles of lymph nodes, white pulp of spleen, unencapsulated lymphoid tissue). When antigen is encountered, B cells differentiate into plasma cells (which produce antibodies) and memory cells. Can function as an APC.

B = bone marrow.

T cells

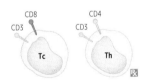

Mediate cellular immune response. Originate from stem cells in the bone marrow, but mature in the thymus. Differentiate into cytotoxic T cells (express CD8, recognize MHC I), helper T cells (express CD4, recognize MHC II), and regulatory T cells. CD28 (costimulatory signal) necessary for T-cell activation. Most circulating lymphocytes are T cells (80%).

T = thymus.
CD4+ helper T cells are the primary target of HIV.

Rule of 8: MHC II × CD4 = 8; MHC I × CD8 = 8.

Plasma cells

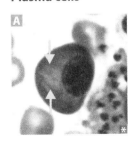

Produce large amounts of antibody specific to a particular antigen. "Clock-face" chromatin distribution and eccentric nucleus, abundant RER, and well-developed Golgi apparatus (arrows in A). Found in bone marrow and normally do not circulate in peripheral blood.

Multiple myeloma is a plasma cell dyscrasia.

▶ HEMATOLOGY AND ONCOLOGY—PHYSIOLOGY

Hemoglobin electrophoresis

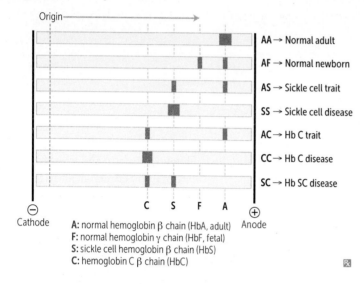

A: normal hemoglobin β chain (HbA, adult)
F: normal hemoglobin γ chain (HbF, fetal)
S: sickle cell hemoglobin β chain (HbS)
C: hemoglobin C β chain (HbC)

During gel electrophoresis, hemoglobin migrates from the negatively charged cathode to the positively charged anode. HbA migrates the farthest, followed by HbF, HbS, and HbC. This is because the missense mutations in HbS and HbC replace glutamic acid ⊖ with valine (neutral) and lysine ⊕, respectively, making HbC and HbS more positively charged than HbA.

A Fat Santa Claus can't go far.
HbC is closest to the Cathode. HbA is closest to the Anode.

Antiglobulin test

Also called Coombs test. Detects the presence of antibodies against circulating RBCs.
Direct antiglobulin test—anti-human globulin (Coombs reagent) added to patient's RBCs. RBCs agglutinate if RBCs are (**directly**) coated with anti-RBC Abs. Used for AIHA diagnosis.
Indirect (**not** direct) antiglobulin test—normal RBCs added to patient's serum. If serum has anti-RBC Abs, RBCs agglutinate when Coombs reagent is added. Used for pretransfusion testing.

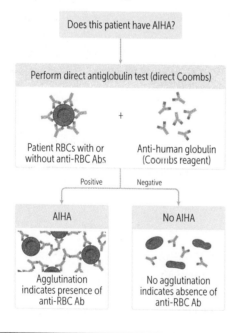

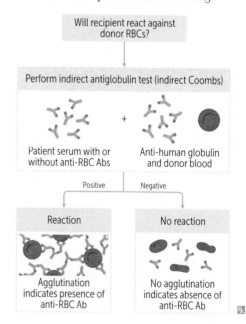

Platelet plug formation (primary hemostasis)

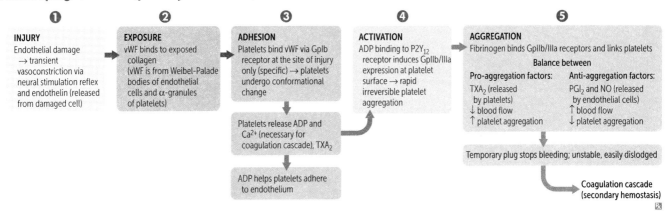

❶ INJURY
Endothelial damage → transient vasoconstriction via neural stimulation reflex and endothelin (released from damaged cell)

❷ EXPOSURE
vWF binds to exposed collagen (vWF is from Weibel-Palade bodies of endothelial cells and α-granules of platelets)

❸ ADHESION
Platelets bind vWF via GpIb receptor at the site of injury only (specific) → platelets undergo conformational change

Platelets release ADP and Ca^{2+} (necessary for coagulation cascade), TXA_2

ADP helps platelets adhere to endothelium

❹ ACTIVATION
ADP binding to $P2Y_{12}$ receptor induces GpIIb/IIIa expression at platelet surface → rapid irreversible platelet aggregation

❺ AGGREGATION
Fibrinogen binds GpIIb/IIIa receptors and links platelets

Balance between

Pro-aggregation factors:
TXA_2 (released by platelets)
↓ blood flow
↑ platelet aggregation

Anti-aggregation factors:
PGI_2 and NO (released by endothelial cells)
↑ blood flow
↓ platelet aggregation

Temporary plug stops bleeding; unstable, easily dislodged

Coagulation cascade (secondary hemostasis)

Thrombogenesis

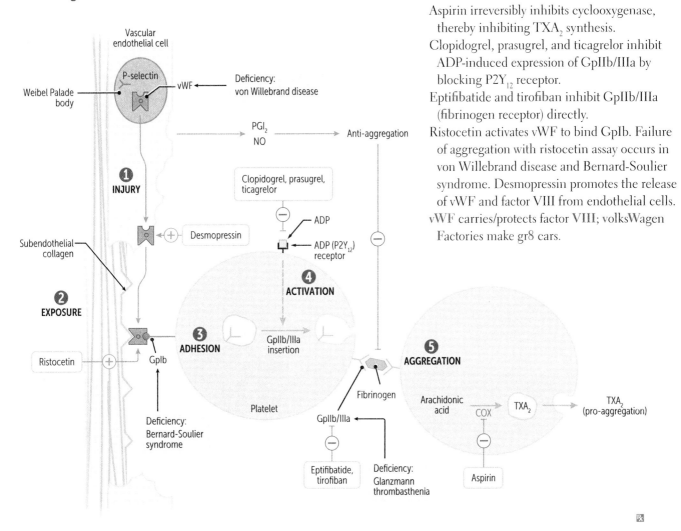

Formation of insoluble fibrin mesh.

Aspirin irreversibly inhibits cyclooxygenase, thereby inhibiting TXA_2 synthesis.

Clopidogrel, prasugrel, and ticagrelor inhibit ADP-induced expression of GpIIb/IIIa by blocking $P2Y_{12}$ receptor.

Eptifibatide and tirofiban inhibit GpIIb/IIIa (fibrinogen receptor) directly.

Ristocetin activates vWF to bind GpIb. Failure of aggregation with ristocetin assay occurs in von Willebrand disease and Bernard-Soulier syndrome. Desmopressin promotes the release of vWF and factor VIII from endothelial cells.

vWF carries/protects factor VIII; volksWagen Factories make gr8 cars.

Coagulation and kinin pathways

PT monitors extrinsic and common pathway, reflecting activity of factors I, II, V, VII, and X. PTT monitors intrinsic and common pathway, reflecting activity of all factors except VII and XIII.

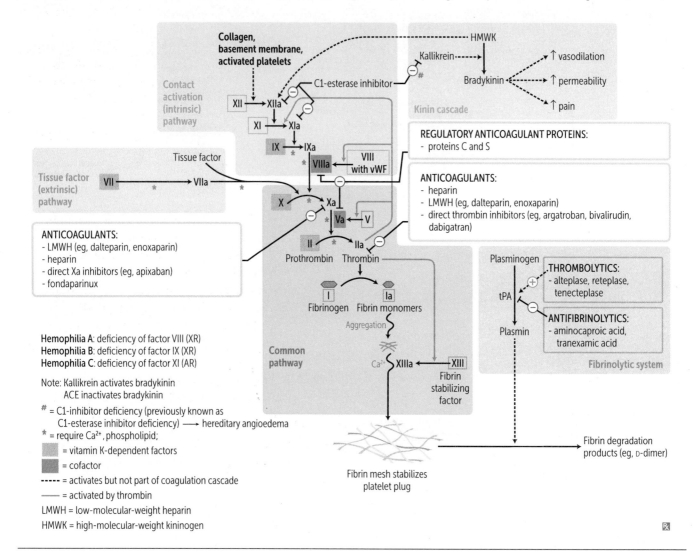

Hemophilia A: deficiency of factor VIII (XR)
Hemophilia B: deficiency of factor IX (XR)
Hemophilia C: deficiency of factor XI (AR)

Note: Kallikrein activates bradykinin
ACE inactivates bradykinin

= C1-inhibitor deficiency (previously known as C1-esterase inhibitor deficiency) ⟶ hereditary angioedema
* = require Ca²⁺, phospholipid;
░ = vitamin K-dependent factors
▓ = cofactor
---- = activates but not part of coagulation cascade
—— = activated by thrombin
LMWH = low-molecular-weight heparin
HMWK = high-molecular-weight kininogen

Vitamin K–dependent coagulation

Procoagulation

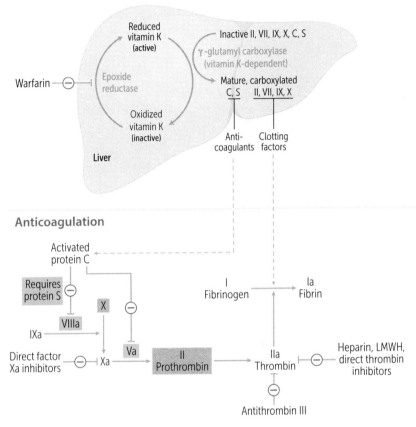

Vitamin K deficiency—↓ carboxylation and maturation of factors II, VII, IX, X, protein C, protein S.

Warfarin inhibits vitamin K epoxide reductase. Vitamin K administration can potentially reverse inhibitory effect of warfarin on clotting factor synthesis (delayed). FFP or PCC administration reverses action of warfarin immediately and can be given with vitamin K in cases of severe bleeding.

Neonates lack enteric ba**K**teria, which produce vitamin **K**. Early administration of vitamin K overcomes neonatal deficiency/coagulopathy. Suppression of gut flora by broad spectrum antibioti**K**s can also contribute to deficiency.

Factor VII (seven)—shortest half-life.

Factor II (**two**)—longest (**too** long) half-life.

Antithrombin inhibits thrombin (factor IIa) and factors VIIa, IXa, Xa, XIa, XIIa.

Heparin enhances the activity of antithrombin.

Principal targets of antithrombin: thrombin and factor Xa.

Factor V Leiden mutation produces a factor V resistant to inhibition by activated protein C.

tPA is used clinically as a thrombolytic.

Anticoagulation

■ = vitamin K-dependent factors   - - - = activates but not part of coagulation cascade

■ = cofactor   LMWH = low-molecular-weight heparin

▶ **HEMATOLOGY AND ONCOLOGY—PATHOLOGY**

RBC morphology

TYPE	ASSOCIATED PATHOLOGY	NOTES
Acanthocytes A ("spur cells")	Liver disease, abetalipoproteinemia, vitamin E deficiency	Projections of varying size at irregular intervals (acanthocytes are asymmetric)
Echinocytes B ("burr cells")	Liver disease, ESRD, pyruvate kinase deficiency	Smaller and more uniform projections than acanthocytes (echinocytes are even)
Dacrocytes C ("teardrop cells")	Bone marrow infiltration (eg, myelofibrosis)	RBC "sheds a **tear**" because it's mechanically squeezed out of its home in the bone marrow
Schistocytes D ("helmet" cells)	Microangiopathic hemolytic anemia (eg, DIC, TTP/HUS, HELLP syndrome), mechanical hemolysis (eg, heart valve prosthesis)	Fragmented RBCs
Degmacytes E ("bite cells")	G6PD deficiency	Due to removal of Heinz bodies by splenic macrophages (they "**deg**" them out of/**bite** them off of RBCs)
Elliptocytes F	Hereditary elliptocytosis	Caused by mutation in genes encoding RBC membrane proteins (eg, spectrin)
Spherocytes G	Hereditary spherocytosis, autoimmune hemolytic anemia	Small, spherical cells without central pallor ↓ surface area-to-volume ratio
Macro-ovalocytes H	Megaloblastic anemia (also hypersegmented PMNs)	
Target cells I	HbC disease, Asplenia, Liver disease, Thalassemia	"HALT," said the hunter to his **target** ↑ surface area-to-volume ratio
Sickle cells J	Sickle cell anemia	Sickling occurs with low O_2 conditions (eg, high altitude, acidosis), high HbS concentration (ie, dehydration)

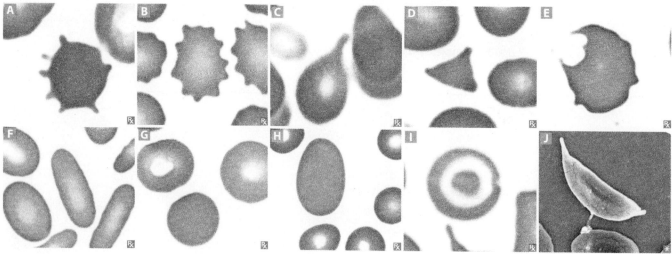

RBC inclusions

TYPE	ASSOCIATED PATHOLOGY	NOTES
Bone marrow		
Iron granules A	Sideroblastic anemias (eg, lead poisoning, myelodysplastic syndromes, chronic alcohol overuse)	Perinuclear mitochondria with excess iron (forming ring in ringed sideroblasts) Require Prussian blue stain to be visualized
Peripheral smear		
Howell-Jolly bodies B	Functional hyposplenia (eg, sickle cell disease), asplenia	Basophilic nuclear remnants (do not contain iron) Usually removed by splenic macrophages
Basophilic stippling C	Sideroblastic anemias, thalassemias	Basophilic ribosomal precipitates (do not contain iron)
Pappenheimer bodies	Sideroblastic anemias	Basophilic granules (contain iron) "Pappen-hammer" bodies
Heinz bodies D	G6PD deficiency	Denatured and precipitated hemoglobin (contain iron) Phagocytic removal of Heinz bodies → bite cells (take a bite of Heinz [ketchup]) Requires supravital stain (eg, crystal violet) to be visualized

Anemias

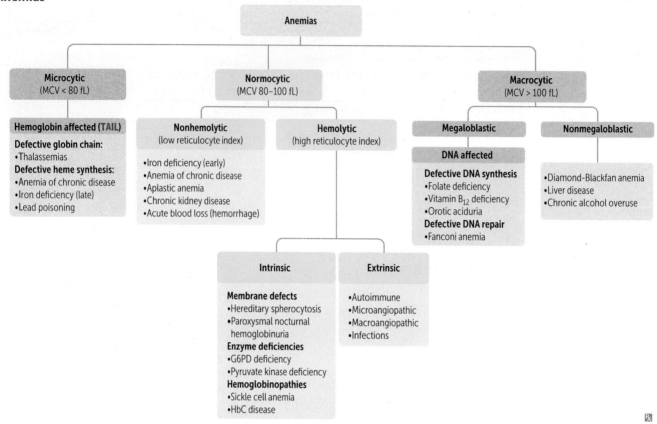

Anemias

Microcytic (MCV < 80 fL)

Normocytic (MCV 80–100 fL)

Macrocytic (MCV > 100 fL)

Hemoglobin affected (TAIL)

Defective globin chain:
• Thalassemias
Defective heme synthesis:
• Anemia of chronic disease
• Iron deficiency (late)
• Lead poisoning

Nonhemolytic (low reticulocyte index)

• Iron deficiency (early)
• Anemia of chronic disease
• Aplastic anemia
• Chronic kidney disease
• Acute blood loss (hemorrhage)

Hemolytic (high reticulocyte index)

Megaloblastic

DNA affected

Defective DNA synthesis
• Folate deficiency
• Vitamin B_{12} deficiency
• Orotic aciduria
Defective DNA repair
• Fanconi anemia

Nonmegaloblastic

• Diamond-Blackfan anemia
• Liver disease
• Chronic alcohol overuse

Intrinsic

Membrane defects
• Hereditary spherocytosis
• Paroxysmal nocturnal hemoglobinuria
Enzyme deficiencies
• G6PD deficiency
• Pyruvate kinase deficiency
Hemoglobinopathies
• Sickle cell anemia
• HbC disease

Extrinsic

• Autoimmune
• Microangiopathic
• Macroangiopathic
• Infections

Reticulocyte production index	Also called corrected reticulocyte count. Used to correct falsely elevated reticulocyte count in anemia. Measures appropriate bone marrow response to anemic conditions (effective erythropoiesis). High RPI (> 3) indicates compensatory RBC production; low RPI (< 2) indicates inadequate response to correct anemia. Calculated as:

$$RPI = \% \text{ reticulocytes} \times \left(\frac{\text{actual Hct}}{\text{normal Hct}} \right) / \text{maturation time}$$

Mentzer index	Used to differentiate between thalassemia trait and iron deficiency anemia. An index of less than 13 suggests thalessemia trait. An increased index (> 13) suggests iron deficiency anemia.

$$\text{Mentzer index} = \frac{\text{MCV}}{\text{RBC count}}$$

Interpretation of iron studies

	Iron deficiency	Chronic disease	Hemochromatosis	Pregnancy/ OCP use
Serum iron	↓	↓	↑	—
Transferrin or TIBC	↑	↓[a]	↓	↑
Ferritin	↓	↑	↑	—
% transferrin saturation (serum iron/TIBC)	↓↓	—/↓	↑↑	↓

↑↓ = 1° disturbance.
Transferrin—transports iron in blood.
TIBC—indirectly measures transferrin.
Ferritin—1° iron storage protein of body.
[a]Evolutionary reasoning—pathogens use circulating iron to thrive. The body has adapted a system in which iron is stored within the cells of the body and prevents pathogens from acquiring circulating iron.

Microcytic, hypochromic anemias	MCV < 80 fL.

Iron deficiency	↓ iron due to chronic bleeding (eg, GI loss, heavy menstrual bleeding), malnutrition, absorption disorders, GI surgery (eg, gastrectomy), or ↑ demand (eg, pregnancy) → ↓ final step in heme synthesis.
	Labs: ↓ iron, ↑ TIBC, ↓ ferritin, ↑ free erythrocyte protoporphyrin, ↑ RDW, ↓ RI. Microcytosis and hypochromasia (↑ central pallor) A.
	Symptoms: fatigue, conjunctival pallor B, restless leg syndrome, pica (persistent craving and compulsive eating of nonfood substances), spoon nails (koilonychia).
	May manifest as glossitis, cheilosis, Plummer-Vinson syndrome (triad of iron deficiency anemia, esophageal webs, and dysphagia).

α-thalassemia	α-globin gene deletions on chromosome 16 → ↓ α-globin synthesis. May have *cis* deletion (deletions occur on same chromosome) or *trans* deletion (deletions occur on separate chromosomes). Normal is αα/αα. Often ↑ RBC count, in contrast to iron deficiency anemia. ↑ prevalence in people of Asian and African descent. Target cells C on peripheral smear.

# OF α-GLOBIN GENES DELETED	DISEASE	CLINICAL OUTCOME
1	α-thalassemia minima	No anemia (silent carrier)
2 Cis or Trans	α-thalassemia minor	Mild microcytic, hypochromic anemia
3	Hemoglobin H disease (HbH); excess β-globin forms β$_4$	Moderate to severe microcytic hypochromic anemia
4	Hemoglobin Barts disease; no α-globin, excess γ-globin forms γ$_4$	Hydrops fetalis; incompatible with life

Microcytic, hypochromic anemias (continued)

β-thalassemia	Point mutation in splice sites or Kozak consensus sequence (promoter) on chromosome 11 → ↓ β-globin synthesis (β^+) or absent β-globin synthesis (β^0). ↑ prevalence in Mediterranean populations.

# OF β-GLOBIN GENES MUTATED	DISEASE	CLINICAL OUTCOME
1 (β^+/β or β^0/β)	β-thalassemia minor	Mild microcytic anemia. ↑ HbA_2.
2 (β^+/β^+ or β^+/β^0)	β-thalassemia intermedia	Variable anemia, ranging from mild/asymptomatic to severe/transfusion-dependent.
2 (β^0/β^0)	β-thalassemia major (Cooley anemia)	Severe microcytic anemia with target cells and ↑ anisopoikilocytosis requiring blood transfusions (↑ risk of 2° hemochromatosis), marrow expansion ("crew cut" on skull x-ray 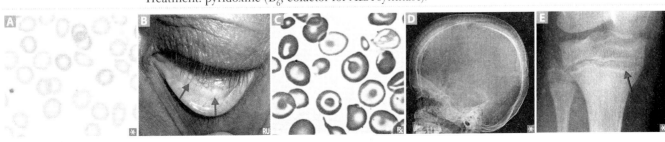) → skeletal deformities, extramedullary hematopoiesis → HSM. ↑ risk of parvovirus B19-induced aplastic crisis. ↑ HbF and HbA_2, becomes symptomatic after 6 months when HbF declines (HbF is protective). Chronic hemolysis → pigmented gallstones.
1 (β^+/HbS or β^0/HbS)	Sickle cell β-thalassemia	Mild to moderate sickle cell disease depending on whether there is ↓ (β^+/HbS) or absent (β^0/HbS) β-globin synthesis.

Lead poisoning	Lead inhibits ferrochelatase and ALA dehydratase → ↓ heme synthesis and ↑ RBC protoporphyrin. Also inhibits rRNA degradation → RBCs retain aggregates of rRNA (basophilic stippling).
	Symptoms of LLEEAAD poisoning:
	▪ Lead Lines on gingivae (Burton lines) and on metaphyses of long bones on x-ray.
	▪ Encephalopathy and Erythrocyte basophilic stippling.
	▪ Abdominal colic and sideroblastic Anemia.
	▪ Drops—wrist and foot drop.
	Treatment: chelation with succimer, EDTA, dimercaprol.
	↑ exposure risk: children—chipped paint in old houses (built before 1978); adults—workplace (eg, batteries, ammunition).

Sideroblastic anemia	Causes: genetic (eg, X-linked defect in ALA synthase gene), acquired (myelodysplastic syndromes), and reversible (alcohol is most common; also lead poisoning, vitamin B_6 deficiency, copper deficiency, drugs [eg, isoniazid, linezolid]).
	Lab findings: ↑ iron, normal/↓ TIBC, ↑ ferritin. Ringed sideroblasts (with iron-laden, Prussian blue–stained mitochondria) seen in bone marrow. Peripheral blood smear: basophilic stippling of RBCs. Some acquired variants may be normocytic or macrocytic.
	Treatment: pyridoxine (B_6, cofactor for ALA synthase).

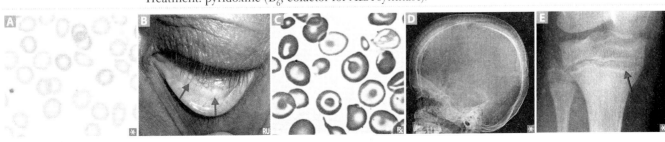

Macrocytic anemias   MCV > 100 fL.

	DESCRIPTION	FINDINGS
Megaloblastic anemia 	Impaired DNA synthesis → maturation of nucleus of precursor cells in bone marrow delayed relative to maturation of cytoplasm. Causes: vitamin B_{12} deficiency, folate deficiency, medications (eg, hydroxyurea, phenytoin, methotrexate, sulfa drugs).	RBC macrocytosis, hypersegmented neutrophils (arrow in A), glossitis.
Folate deficiency	Causes: malnutrition (eg, chronic alcohol overuse), malabsorption, drugs (eg, methotrexate, trimethoprim, phenytoin), ↑ requirement (eg, hemolytic anemia, pregnancy).	↑ homocysteine, normal methylmalonic acid. **No neurologic symptoms** (vs B_{12} deficiency).
Vitamin B_{12} (cobalamin) deficiency	Causes: pernicious anemia, malabsorption (eg, Crohn disease), pancreatic insufficiency, gastrectomy, insufficient intake (eg, veganism), *Diphyllobothrium latum* (fish tapeworm).	↑ homocysteine, ↑ methylmalonic acid. **Neurologic symptoms:** reversible dementia, subacute combined degeneration (due to involvement of B_{12} in fatty acid pathways and myelin synthesis): spinocerebellar tract, lateral corticospinal tract, dorsal column dysfunction. Folate supplementation in vitamin B_{12} deficiency can correct the anemia, but worsens neurologic symptoms. Historically diagnosed with the Schilling test, a test that determines if the cause is dietary insufficiency vs malabsorption. Anemia 2° to insufficient intake may take several years to develop due to liver's ability to store B_{12} (vs folate deficiency, which takes weeks to months).
Orotic aciduria	Inability to convert orotic acid to UMP (de novo pyrimidine synthesis pathway) because of defect in UMP synthase. Autosomal recessive. Presents in children as failure to thrive, developmental delay, and megaloblastic anemia refractory to folate and B_{12}. No hyperammonemia (vs ornithine transcarbamylase deficiency—↑ orotic acid with hyperammonemia).	Orotic acid in urine. Treatment: uridine monophosphate or uridine triacetate to bypass mutated enzyme.
Nonmegaloblastic anemia	Macrocytic anemia in which DNA synthesis is normal. Causes: chronic alcohol overuse, liver disease.	RBC macrocytosis without hypersegmented neutrophils.
Diamond-Blackfan anemia	A congenital form of pure red cell aplasia (vs Fanconi anemia, which causes pancytopenia). Rapid-onset anemia within 1st year of life due to intrinsic defect in erythroid progenitor cells.	↑ % HbF (but ↓ total Hb). Short stature, craniofacial abnormalities, and upper extremity malformations (triphalangeal thumbs) in up to 50% of cases. A **pure Diamond** causes **pure** red cell aplasia.

Normocytic, normochromic anemias	Normocytic, normochromic anemias are classified as nonhemolytic or hemolytic. The hemolytic anemias are further classified according to the cause of the hemolysis (intrinsic vs extrinsic to the RBC) and by the location of hemolysis (intravascular vs extravascular). Hemolysis can lead to ↑ in LDH, reticulocytes, unconjugated bilirubin, pigmented gallstones, and urobilinogen in urine.

Extravascular Hemolysis

Intravascular Hemolysis

Intravascular hemolysis	Findings: ↓ haptoglobin, ↑ schistocytes on blood smear. Characteristic hemoglobinuria, hemosiderinuria, and urobilinogen in urine. Notable causes are mechanical hemolysis (eg, prosthetic valve), paroxysmal nocturnal hemoglobinuria, microangiopathic hemolytic anemias.
Extravascular hemolysis	Mechanism: macrophages in spleen clear RBCs. Findings: splenomegaly, spherocytes in peripheral smear (most commonly due to hereditary spherocytosis and autoimmune hemolytic anemia), no hemoglobinuria/hemosiderinuria. Can present with urobilinogen in urine.

Nonhemolytic, normocytic anemias

	DESCRIPTION	FINDINGS
Anemia of chronic disease	Inflammation (eg, ↑ IL-6) → ↑ hepcidin (released by liver, binds ferroportin on intestinal mucosal cells and macrophages, thus inhibiting iron transport) → ↓ release of iron from macrophages and ↓ iron absorption from gut. Associated with conditions such as chronic infections, neoplastic disorders, chronic kidney disease, and autoimmune diseases (eg, SLE, rheumatoid arthritis).	↓ iron, ↓ TIBC, ↑ ferritin. Normocytic, but can become microcytic. Treatment: address underlying cause of inflammation, judicious use of blood transfusion, consider erythropoiesis-stimulating agents such as EPO (eg, in chronic kidney disease).
Aplastic anemia 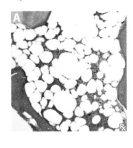	Failure or destruction of hematopoietic stem cells. Causes (reducing volume from inside diaphysis): ▪ Radiation ▪ Viral agents (eg, EBV, HIV, hepatitis viruses) ▪ Fanconi anemia (autosomal recessive DNA repair defect → bone marrow failure); normocytosis or macrocytosis on CBC. Common associated findings include short stature, café-au-lait spots, thumb/radial defects, predisposition to malignancy. ▪ Idiopathic (immune mediated, 1° stem cell defect); may follow acute hepatitis ▪ Drugs (eg, benzene, chloramphenicol, alkylating agents, antimetabolites)	↓ reticulocyte count, ↑ EPO. Pancytopenia characterized by anemia, leukopenia, and thrombocytopenia (vs aplastic crisis, which causes anemia only). Normal cell morphology, but hypocellular bone marrow with fatty infiltration A (↑ adipose tissue in bone marrow in aplastic anemia). Symptoms: fatigue, malaise, pallor, purpura, mucosal bleeding, petechiae, infection. Treatment: withdrawal of offending agent, immunosuppressive regimens (eg, antithymocyte globulin, cyclosporine), bone marrow allograft, RBC/platelet transfusion, bone marrow stimulation (eg, GM-CSF).

Intrinsic hemolytic anemias

	DESCRIPTION	FINDINGS
Hereditary spherocytosis	Primarily autosomal dominant. Due to defect in proteins interacting with RBC membrane skeleton and plasma membrane (eg, ankyrin, band 3, protein 4.2, spectrin). Small, round RBCs with no central pallor. ↓ surface area/dehydration → ↑ MCHC → premature removal by spleen (extravascular hemolysis).	Splenomegaly, pigmented gallstones, aplastic crisis (parvovirus B19 infection). Labs: ↓ mean fluorescence of RBCs in eosin 5-maleimide (EMA) binding test, ↑ fragility in osmotic fragility test (RBC hemolysis with exposure to hypotonic solution). Normal to ↓ MCV with abundance of RBCs. Treatment: splenectomy.
Paroxysmal nocturnal hemoglobinuria	Hematopoietic stem cell mutation → ↑ complement-mediated intravascular hemolysis, especially at night. Acquired *PIGA* mutation → impaired GPI anchor synthesis for decay-accelerating factor (DAF/CD55) and membrane inhibitor of reactive lysis (MIRL/CD59), which protect RBC membrane from complement.	Triad: Coombs ⊖ hemolytic anemia (mainly intravascular), pancytopenia, venous thrombosis (eg, Budd-Chiari syndrome). Pink/red urine in morning. Associated with aplastic anemia, acute leukemias. Labs: CD55/59 ⊖ RBCs on flow cytometry. Treatment: eculizumab (targets terminal complement protein C5).
G6PD deficiency	X-linked recessive. G6PD defect → ↓ NADPH → ↓ reduced glutathione → ↑ RBC susceptibility to oxidative stress (eg, sulfa drugs, antimalarials, **fava beans**) → hemolysis. Causes extravascular and intravascular hemolysis.	Back pain, hemoglobinuria a few days after oxidant **stress**. Labs: ↓ G6PD activity (may be falsely normal during acute hemolysis), blood smear shows RBCs with **Heinz** bodies and **bite** cells. "**Stress** makes me eat **bites** of **fava beans** with **Heinz** ketchup."
Pyruvate kinase deficiency	Autosomal recessive. Pyruvate kinase defect → ↓ ATP → rigid RBCs → extravascular hemolysis. Increases levels of 2,3-BPG → ↓ hemoglobin affinity for O_2.	Hemolytic anemia in a newborn. Labs: blood smear shows burr cells.
Sickle cell anemia	Point mutation in β-globin gene → single amino acid substitution (glutamic acid → valine) alters hydrophobic region on β-globin chain → aggregation of hemoglobin. Causes extravascular and intravascular hemolysis. Pathogenesis: ↓ O_2, ↑ altitude, or acidosis precipitates sickling (deoxygenated HbS polymerizes) → vaso-occlusive disease. Newborns are initially asymptomatic because of ↑ HbF and ↓ HbS. Heterozygotes (sickle cell trait) have resistance to malaria. Sickle cells are crescent-shaped RBCs **A**. "Crew cut" on skull x-ray due to marrow expansion from ↑ erythropoiesis (also seen in thalassemias).	Complications: ▪ Aplastic crisis (transient arrest of erythropoiesis due to parvovirus B19). ▪ Autosplenectomy (Howell-Jolly bodies) → ↑ risk of infection by encapsulated organisms (eg, *Salmonella* osteomyelitis). ▪ Splenic infarct/sequestration crisis. ▪ Painful vaso-occlusive crises: dactylitis (painful swelling of hands/feet), priapism, acute chest syndrome (respiratory distress, new pulmonary infiltrates on CXR, common cause of death), avascular necrosis, stroke. ▪ Sickling in renal medulla (↓ Po_2) → renal papillary necrosis → hematuria (also seen in sickle cell trait). Hb electrophoresis: ↓↓ HbA, ↑ HbF, ↑↑ HbS. Treatment: hydroxyurea (↑ HbF), hydration.
HbC disease	Glutamic acid–to-lycine (lysine) mutation in β-globin. Causes extravascular hemolysis.	HbSC (1 of each mutant gene) milder than HbSS. Blood smear in homozygotes: hemoglobin crystals inside RBCs, target cells.

Extrinsic hemolytic anemias

	DESCRIPTION	FINDINGS
Autoimmune hemolytic anemia	A normocytic anemia that is usually idiopathic and Coombs ⊕. Two types: ▪ **Warm** AIHA–chronic anemia in which primarily Ig**G** causes extravascular >>> intravascular hemolysis. Seen in SLE and CLL and with certain drugs (eg, β-lactams, α-methyldopa). "**Warm** weather is **Good**." ▪ Cold AIHA–acute anemia in which primarily Ig**M** + complement cause RBC agglutination and extravascular >>> intravascular hemolysis upon exposure to cold → painful, blue fingers and toes. Seen in CLL, *Mycoplasma pneumoniae* infections, infectious mononucleosis.	Spherocytes and agglutinated RBCs A on peripheral blood smear. Warm AIHA treatment: steroids, rituximab, splenectomy (if refractory). Cold AIHA treatment: cold avoidance, rituximab.
Drug-induced hemolytic anemia	Most commonly due to antibody-mediated immune destruction of RBCs or oxidant injury via free radical damage (may be exacerbated in G6PD deficiency). Common causes include antibiotics (eg, penicillins, cephalosporins), NSAIDs, immunotherapy, chemotherapy.	Spherocytes suggest immune hemolysis. Bite cells suggest oxidative hemolysis. Can cause both extravascular and intravascular hemolysis.
Microangiopathic hemolytic anemia	RBCs are damaged when passing through obstructed or narrowed vessels. Causes intravascular hemolysis. Seen in DIC, TTP/HUS, SLE, HELLP syndrome, hypertensive emergency.	**Schisto**cytes (eg, "helmet cells") are seen on peripheral blood smear due to mechanical destruction (*schisto* = to split) of RBCs.
Macroangiopathic hemolytic anemia	Prosthetic heart valves and aortic stenosis may also cause hemolytic anemia 2° to mechanical destruction of RBCs.	Schistocytes on peripheral blood smear.
Hemolytic anemia due to infection	↑ destruction of RBCs (eg, malaria, *Babesia*).	

Leukopenias

CELL TYPE	CELL COUNT	CAUSES
Neutropenia	Absolute neutrophil count < 1500 cells/mm³ Severe infections typical when < 500 cells/mm³	Sepsis/postinfection, drugs (including chemotherapy), aplastic anemia, autoimmunity (eg, SLE), radiation, congenital
Lymphopenia	Absolute lymphocyte count < 1500 cells/mm³ (< 3000 cells/mm³ in children)	HIV, DiGeorge syndrome, SCID, SLE, glucocorticoids[a], radiation, sepsis, postoperative
Eosinopenia	Absolute eosinophil count < 30 cells/mm³	Cushing syndrome, glucocorticoids[a]

[a]Glucocorticoids cause neutrophilia, despite causing eosinopenia and lymphopenia. Glucocorticoids ↓ activation of neutrophil adhesion molecules, impairing migration out of the vasculature to sites of inflammation. In contrast, glucocorticoids sequester eosinophils in lymph nodes and cause apoptosis of lymphocytes.

Heme synthesis, porphyrias, and lead poisoning

The porphyrias are hereditary or acquired conditions of defective heme synthesis that lead to the accumulation of heme precursors. Lead inhibits specific enzymes needed in heme synthesis, leading to a similar condition.

CONDITION	AFFECTED ENZYME	ACCUMULATED SUBSTRATE	PRESENTING SYMPTOMS
Lead poisoning 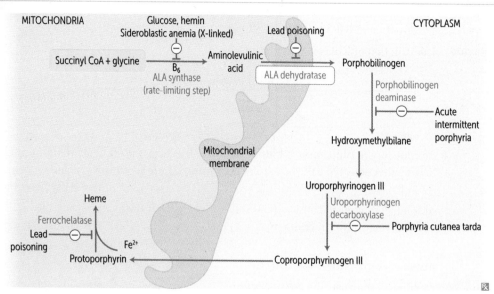	Ferrochelatase and ALA dehydratase	Protoporphyrin, ALA (blood)	Microcytic anemia (basophilic stippling in peripheral smear **A**, ringed sideroblasts in bone marrow), GI and kidney disease.
Acute intermittent porphyria	Porphobilinogen deaminase (autosomal dominant mutation)	Porphobilinogen, ALA	Symptoms (**5 P's**): ▪ Painful abdomen ▪ Port wine–colored **P**ee ▪ Polyneuropathy ▪ Psychological disturbances ▪ Precipitated by factors that ↑ ALA synthase (eg, drugs [CYP450 inducers], alcohol, starvation) Treatment: hemin and glucose.
Porphyria cutanea tarda	Uroporphyrinogen decarboxylase	Uroporphyrin (tea-colored urine)	Blistering cutaneous photosensitivity and hyperpigmentation **B**. Most common porphyria. Exacerbated with alcohol consumption. Causes: familial, hepatitis **C**. Treatment: phlebotomy, sun avoidance, antimalarials (eg, hydroxychloroquine).

Iron poisoning	Occurs via free radical formation and membrane lipid peroxidation → cell death.	
	Acute	**Chronic**
FINDINGS	↑ mortality rate associated with accidental ingestion by children (adult iron tablets may look like candy).	Seen in patients with 1° (hereditary) or 2° (eg, chronic blood transfusions for thalassemia or sickle cell disease) hemochromatosis.
SYMPTOMS/SIGNS	Abdominal pain, vomiting, GI bleeding. Radiopaque pill seen on x-ray. May progress to anion gap metabolic acidosis and multiorgan failure. Leads to scarring with GI obstruction.	Arthropathy, cirrhosis, cardiomyopathy, diabetes mellitus and skin pigmentation ("bronze diabetes"), hypogonadism.
TREATMENT	Chelation (eg, deferoxamine, deferasirox), gastric lavage.	Chelation, regular therapeutic phlebotomy (unless contraindicated, eg, anemia)

Coagulation disorders	PT—tests function of common and extrinsic pathway (factors I, II, V, VII, and X). Defect → ↑ PT (**Play Tennis out**side [**ex**trinsic pathway]).
	INR (international normalized ratio) = patient PT/control PT. 1 = normal, > 1 = prolonged. Most common test used to follow patients on warfarin, which prolongs INR.
	PTT—tests function of common and **in**trinsic pathway (all factors except VII and XIII). Defect → ↑ PTT (**Play Table Tennis in**side).
	TT—measures the rate of conversion of fibrinogen → fibrin. Prolonged by anticoagulants, hypofibrinogenemia, DIC, liver disease.
	Coagulation disorders can be due to clotting factor deficiencies or acquired factor inhibitors (most commonly against factor VIII). Diagnosed with a mixing study, in which normal plasma is added to patient's plasma. Clotting factor deficiencies should correct (the PT or PTT returns to within the appropriate normal range), whereas factor inhibitors will not correct.

DISORDER	PT	PTT	MECHANISM AND COMMENTS
Hemophilia A, B, or C	—	↑	Intrinsic pathway coagulation defect (↑ PTT). ▪ **A**: deficiency of factor **VIII**; X-linked recessive. Pronounce "hemophilia A**te** (**eight**)." ▪ B: deficiency of factor IX; X-linked recessive. ▪ C: deficiency of factor XI; autosomal recessive. Hemorrhage in hemophilia—hemarthroses (bleeding into joints, eg, knee Ⓐ), easy bruising, bleeding after trauma or surgery (eg, dental procedures). Treatment: desmopressin, factor VIII concentrate, emicizumab (A); factor IX concentrate (B); factor XI concentrate (C).
Vitamin K deficiency	↑	↑	General coagulation defect. Bleeding time normal. ↓ activity of factors II, VII, IX, X, protein C, protein S.

Platelet disorders

All platelet disorders have ↑ bleeding time (BT), mucous membrane bleeding, and microhemorrhages (eg, petechiae, epistaxis). Platelet count (PC) is usually low, but may be normal in qualitative disorders.

DISORDER	PC	BT	NOTES
Bernard-Soulier syndrome	–/↓	↑	Autosomal recessive defect in adhesion. ↓ GpIb → ↓ platelet-to-vWF adhesion. Labs: ↓ platelet aggregation, **B**ig platelets.
Glanzmann thrombasthenia	–	↑	Autosomal recessive defect in aggregation. ↓ GpIIb/IIIa (↓ integrin $\alpha_{IIb}\beta_3$) → ↓ platelet-to-platelet aggregation and defective platelet plug formation. Labs: blood smear shows no platelet clumping.
Immune thrombocytopenia	↓	↑	Destruction of platelets in spleen. Most commonly due to anti-GpIIb/IIIa antibodies → splenic macrophages phagocytose platelets. May be idiopathic or 2° to autoimmune disorders (eg, SLE), viral illness (eg, HIV, HCV), malignancy (eg, CLL), or drug reactions. Labs: ↑ megakaryocytes on bone marrow biopsy, ↓ platelet count. Treatment: glucocorticoids, IVIG, rituximab, TPO receptor agonists (eg, eltrombopag, romiplostim), or splenectomy for refractory ITP.
Uremic platelet dysfunction	–	↑	In patients with renal failure, uremic toxins accumulate and interfere with platelet adhesion and aggregation.

Thrombotic microangiopathies

Disorders overlap significantly in symptomatology. May resemble DIC, but do not exhibit lab findings of a consumptive coagulopathy (eg, ↑ PT, ↑ PTT, ↓ fibrinogen), as etiology does not involve widespread clotting factor activation.

	Thrombotic thrombocytopenic purpura	Hemolytic-uremic syndrome
EPIDEMIOLOGY	Typically females	Typically children
PATHOPHYSIOLOGY	Inhibition or deficiency of ADAMTS13 (a vWF metalloprotease) → ↓ degradation of vWF multimers → ↑ large vWF multimers → ↑ platelet adhesion and aggregation (microthrombi formation)	Predominately caused by Shiga toxin–producing *Escherichia coli* (STEC) infection (serotype O157:H7), which causes profound endothelial dysfunction.
PRESENTATION	Triad of thrombocytopenia (↓ platelets), microangiopathic hemolytic anemia (↓ Hb, schistocytes, ↑ LDH), acute kidney injury (↑ Cr)	
DIFFERENTIATING SYMPTOMS	Triad + fever + neurologic symptoms	Triad + bloody diarrhea
LABS	Normal PT and PTT helps distinguish TTP and HUS (coagulation pathway is not activated) from DIC (coagulation pathway is activated)	
TREATMENT	Plasma exchange, glucocorticoids, rituximab	Supportive care

Mixed platelet and coagulation disorders

DISORDER	PC	BT	PT	PTT	NOTES
von Willebrand disease	—	↑	—	—/↑	Intrinsic pathway coagulation defect: ↓ quantity/function of vWF → ↑ PTT (vWF carries/protects factor VIII). Defect in platelet plug formation: ↓ vWF → defect in platelet-to-vWF adhesion. Most are autosomal dominant. Mild but most common inherited bleeding disorder. Commonly presents with menorrhagia or epistaxis. Treatment: vWF concentrates, desmopressin (releases vWF stored in endothelium).
Disseminated intravascular coagulation	↓	↑	↑	↑	Widespread clotting factor activation → thromboembolic state with excessive clotting factor consumption → ↑ thromboses, ↑ hemorrhages (eg, blood oozing from puncture sites). May be acute (life-threatening) or chronic (if clotting factor production can compensate for consumption). Causes: heat Stroke, Snake bites, Sepsis (gram ⊖), Trauma, Obstetric complications, acute Pancreatitis, malignancy, nephrotic syndrome, transfusion (**SSSTOP** making new thrombi). Labs: schistocytes, ↑ fibrin degradation products (D-dimers), ↓ fibrinogen, ↓ factors V and VIII.

Hereditary thrombophilias	Autosomal dominant disorders resulting in hypercoagulable state (↑ tendency to develop thrombosis).
DISEASE	DESCRIPTION
Antithrombin deficiency	Has no direct effect on the PT, PTT, or thrombin time but diminishes the increase in PTT following standard heparin dosing. Can also be acquired: renal failure/nephrotic syndrome → antithrombin loss in urine → ↓ inhibition of factors IIa and Xa.
Factor V Leiden	Production of mutant factor V (guanine → adenine DNA point mutation → Arg506Gln mutation near the cleavage site) that is resistant to degradation by activated protein C. Complications include DVT, cerebral vein thrombosis, recurrent pregnancy loss.
Protein C or S deficiency	↓ ability to inactivate factors Va and VIIIa. ↑ risk of warfarin-induced skin necrosis. Together, protein C Cancels, and protein S Stops, coagulation.
Prothrombin *G20210A* mutation	Point mutation in 3′ untranslated region → ↑ production of prothrombin → ↑ plasma levels and venous clots.

Blood transfusion therapy

COMPONENT	DOSAGE EFFECT	CLINICAL USE
Packed RBCs	↑ Hb and O_2 binding (carrying) capacity, ↑ hemoglobin ~1 g/dL per unit, ↑ hematocrit ~3% per unit	Acute blood loss, severe anemia
Platelets	↑ platelet count ~30,000/microL per unit (↑ ~5000/mm³/unit)	Stop significant bleeding (thrombocytopenia, qualitative platelet defects)
Fresh frozen plasma/ prothrombin complex concentrate	↑ coagulation factor levels; FFP contains all coagulation factors and plasma proteins; PCC generally contains factors II, VII, IX, and X, as well as protein C and S	Cirrhosis, immediate anticoagulation reversal
Cryoprecipitate	Contains fibrinogen, factor VIII, factor XIII, vWF, and fibronectin	Coagulation factor deficiencies involving fibrinogen and factor VIII
Albumin	↑ intravascular volume and oncotic pressure	Post-paracentesis, therapeutic plasmapheresis

Blood transfusion risks include infection transmission (low), transfusion reactions, transfusion-associated circulatory overload (TACO; volume overload → pulmonary edema, hypertension), transfusion-related acute lung injury (TRALI; hypoxia and inflammation → noncardiogenic pulmonary edema, hypotension), iron overload (may lead to 2° hemochromatosis), hypocalcemia (citrate is a Ca^{2+} chelator), and hyperkalemia (RBCs may lyse in old blood units).

Leukemia vs lymphoma

Leukemia	Lymphoid or myeloid neoplasm with widespread involvement of bone marrow. Tumor cells are usually found in peripheral blood.
Lymphoma	Discrete tumor mass arising from lymph nodes. Variable clinical presentation (eg, arising in atypical sites, leukemic presentation).

Hodgkin vs non-Hodgkin lymphoma

Hodgkin	Non-Hodgkin
Both may have constitutional ("B") signs/symptoms: low-grade fever, night sweats, weight loss.	
Localized, single group of nodes with contiguous spread (stage is strongest predictor of prognosis). Better prognosis.	Multiple lymph nodes involved; extranodal involvement common; noncontiguous spread. Worse prognosis.
Characterized by Reed-Sternberg cells.	Majority involve B cells; rarely of T-cell lineage.
Bimodal distribution: young adults, > 55 years.	Can occur in children and adults.
Associated with EBV.	May be associated with autoimmune diseases and viral infections (eg, HIV, EBV, HTLV).

Hodgkin lymphoma

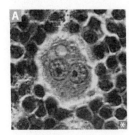

Contains Reed-Sternberg cells: distinctive tumor giant cells; bilobed nucleus with the 2 halves as mirror images ("owl eyes" **A**). RS cells are CD15+ and CD30+ B-cell origin. **2** owl eyes × **15** = **30**.

SUBTYPE	NOTES
Nodular sclerosis	Most common
Mixed cellularity	Eosinophilia; seen in immunocompromised patients
Lymphocyte **rich**	**Best** prognosis (the **rich** have **better** bank accounts)
Lymphocyte **depleted**	**Worst** prognosis (the **poor** have **worse** bank accounts); seen in immunocompromised patients

Non-Hodgkin lymphoma

TYPE	OCCURS IN	GENETICS	COMMENTS
Neoplasms of mature B cells			
Burkitt lymphoma	Adolescents or young adults "Bur**kid**" lymphoma (more common in **kids**)	t(8;14)—translocation of c-*myc* (8) and heavy-chain Ig (14)	"**Starry sky**" appearance (**StarBurst**), sheets of lymphocytes with interspersed "tingible body" macrophages (arrows in 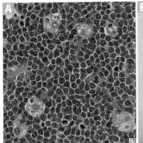). Associated with EBV. Jaw lesion 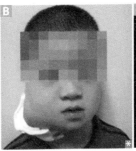 in endemic form in Africa; pelvis or abdomen in sporadic form.
Diffuse large B-cell lymphoma	Usually older adults, but 20% in children	Mutations in *BCL-2*, *BCL-6*	Most common type of non-Hodgkin lymphoma in adults.
Follicular lymphoma	Adults	t(14;18)—translocation of heavy-chain Ig (14) and *BCL-2* (18)	Indolent course with painless "waxing and waning" lymphadenopathy. Bcl-2 normally inhibits apoptosis.
Mantle cell lymphoma	Adult males >> adult females	t(11;14)—translocation of cyclin D1 (11) and heavy-chain Ig (14), CD5+	Very aggressive, patients typically present with late-stage disease.
Marginal zone lymphoma	Adults	t(11;18)	Associated with chronic inflammation (eg, Sjögren syndrome, chronic gastritis [MALT lymphoma; may regress with *H pylori* eradication]).
Primary central nervous system lymphoma	Adults	EBV related; associated with HIV/ AIDS	Considered an AIDS-defining illness. Variable presentation: confusion, memory loss, seizures. CNS mass (often single, ring-enhancing lesion on MRI) in immunocompromised patients 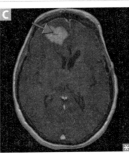, needs to be distinguished from toxoplasmosis via CSF analysis or other lab tests.
Neoplasms of mature T cells			
Adult T-cell lymphoma	Adults	Caused by HTLV (associated with IV drug use)	Adults present with cutaneous lesions; common in Japan (**T**-cell in **T**okyo), West Africa, and the Caribbean. Lytic bone lesions, hypercalcemia.
Cutaneous T-cell lymphoma	Adults		Heterogenous group of T-cell neoplasms affecting the skin ± blood, lymph nodes, or viscera. Most common subtype is mycosis fungoides 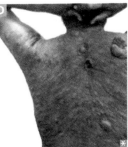 characterized by erythematous patches favoring sun-protected areas that progress to plaques, then eventually tumors.

Plasma cell dyscrasias

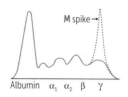

Group of disorders characterized by proliferation of a single plasma cell clone, typically overproducing a monoclonal immunoglobulin (also called paraprotein). Seen in older adults. Screening with serum protein electrophoresis (**M** spike represents overproduction of **M**onoclonal Ig), serum immunofixation, and serum free light chain assay. Urine protein electrophoresis and immunofixation required to confirm urinary involvement (urine dipstick only detects albumin). Diagnostic confirmation with bone marrow biopsy.

Peripheral blood smear may show rouleaux formation 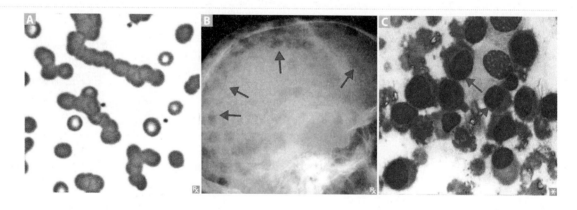 A (RBCs stacked like poker chips).

Multiple myeloma

Overproduction of IgG (most common) > IgA > Ig light chains. Clinical features (**CRAB**): hyper**C**alcemia (↑ cytokine secretion [eg, IL-1, TNF-α, RANK-L] by malignant plasma cells → ↑ osteoclast activity), **R**enal insufficiency, **A**nemia, **B**one lytic lesions ("punched out" on x-ray B → back pain, pathologic fractures). Complications: ↑ infection risk, 1° amyloidosis (AL).

Urinalysis may show Ig light chains (Bence Jones proteinuria) with ⊖ urine dipstick.

Bone marrow biopsy shows >10% monoclonal plasma cells with clock-face chromatin C and intracytoplasmic inclusions containing Ig.

Waldenström macroglobulinemia

Overproduction of IgM (**macro**globulinemia because Ig**M** is the **largest** Ig). Clinical features include anemia, constitutional ("B") signs/symptoms, lymphadenopathy, hepatosplenomegaly, hyperviscosity (eg, headache, bleeding, blurry vision, ataxia), peripheral neuropathy.

Funduscopy shows dilated, segmented, and tortuous retinal veins (sausage link appearance).

Bone marrow biopsy shows >10% monoclonal B lymphocytes with plasma cell features (lymphoplasmacytic lymphoma) and intranuclear pseudoinclusions containing IgM.

Monoclonal gammopathy of undetermined significance

Overproduction of any Ig type (M spike <3 g/dL). Asymptomatic (no CRAB findings). 1%–2% risk per year of progressing to multiple myeloma.

Bone marrow biopsy shows <10% monoclonal plasma cells.

Myelodysplastic syndromes

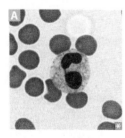

Stem cell disorders involving ineffective hematopoiesis → defects in cell maturation of nonlymphoid lineages. Bone marrow blasts < 20% (vs > 20% in AML). Caused by de novo mutations or environmental exposure (eg, radiation, benzene, chemotherapy). Risk of transformation to AML. More common in older adults.

Pseudo-Pelger-Huët anomaly—neutrophils with bilobed ("**duet**") nuclei A. Associated with myelodysplastic syndromes or drugs (eg, immunosuppressants).

Leukemias	Unregulated growth and differentiation of WBCs in bone marrow → marrow failure → anemia (↓ RBCs), infections (↓ mature WBCs), and hemorrhage (↓ platelets). Usually presents with ↑ circulating WBCs (malignant leukocytes in blood), although some cases present with normal/↓ WBCs. Leukemic cell infiltration of liver, spleen, lymph nodes, and skin (leukemia cutis) possible.

TYPE	NOTES
Lymphoid neoplasms	
Acute lymphoblastic leukemia/lymphoma	Most frequently occurs in children; less common in adults (worse prognosis). T-cell ALL can present as mediastinal mass (presenting as SVC-like syndrome). Associated with Down syndrome. Peripheral blood and bone marrow have ↑↑↑ lymphoblasts A. TdT+ (marker of pre-T and pre-B cells), CD10+ (marker of pre-B cells). Most responsive to therapy. May spread to CNS and testes. t(12;21) → better prognosis; t(9;22) (Philadelphia chromosome) → worse prognosis.
Chronic lymphocytic leukemia/small lymphocytic lymphoma	Age > 60 years. Most common adult leukemia. CD20+, CD23+, CD5+ B-cell neoplasm. Often asymptomatic, progresses slowly; smudge cells B in peripheral blood smear; autoimmune hemolytic anemia. **CLL** = **C**rushed **L**ittle **L**ymphocytes (smudge cells). Richter transformation—CLL/SLL transformation into an aggressive lymphoma, most commonly diffuse large B-cell lymphoma (DLBCL).
Hairy cell leukemia	Adult males. Mature B-cell tumor. Cells have filamentous, hairlike projections (fuzzy appearing on LM C). Peripheral lymphadenopathy is uncommon. Causes marrow fibrosis → dry tap on aspiration. Patients usually present with massive splenomegaly and pancytopenia. Stains **TRAP** (**T**artrate-**R**esistant **A**cid **P**hosphatase) ⊕ (**TRAP**ped in a **hairy** situation). TRAP stain largely replaced with flow cytometry. Associated with *BRAF* mutations. Treatment: purine analogs (cladribine, pentostatin).
Myeloid neoplasms	
Acute myelogenous leukemia	Median onset 65 years. Auer rods D; myeloperoxidase ⊕ cytoplasmic inclusions seen mostly in APL (formerly M3 AML); ↑↑↑ circulating myeloblasts on peripheral smear. May present with leukostasis (capillary occlusion by malignant, nondistensible cells → organ damage). Risk factors: prior exposure to alkylating chemotherapy, radiation, benzene, myeloproliferative disorders, Down syndrome (typically acute megakaryoblastic leukemia [formerly M7 AML]). APL: t(15;17), responds to all-*trans* retinoic acid (vitamin A) and arsenic trioxide, which induce differentiation of promyelocytes; DIC is a common presentation.
Chronic myelogenous leukemia	Peak incidence: 45–85 years; median age: 64 years. Defined by the Philadelphia chromosome (t[9;22], *BCR-ABL*) and myeloid stem cell proliferation. Presents with dysregulated production of mature and maturing granulocytes (eg, neutrophils, metamyelocytes, myelocytes, basophils E) and splenomegaly. May accelerate and transform to AML or ALL ("blast crisis"). Responds to BCR-ABL tyrosine kinase inhibitors (eg, imatinib).

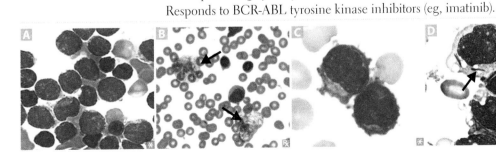
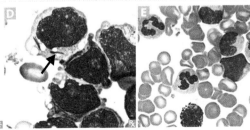

Myeloproliferative neoplasms	Malignant hematopoietic neoplasms with varying impacts on WBCs and myeloid cell lines.
Polycythemia vera	Primary polycythemia. Disorder of ↑ RBCs, usually due to acquired *JAK2* mutation. May present as intense itching after shower (aquagenic pruritus). Rare but classic symptom is erythromelalgia (severe, burning pain and red-blue coloration) due to episodic blood clots in vessels of the extremities A. Associated with hyperviscosity and thrombosis (eg, PE, DVT, Budd-Chiari syndrome). ↓ EPO (vs 2° polycythemia, which presents with endogenous or artificially ↑ EPO). Treatment: phlebotomy, hydroxyurea, ruxolitinib (JAK1/2 inhibitor).
Essential thrombocythemia	Characterized by massive proliferation of megakaryocytes and platelets. Symptoms include bleeding and thrombosis. Blood smear shows markedly increased number of platelets, which may be large or otherwise abnormally formed B. Erythromelalgia may occur.
Myelofibrosis	Atypical megakaryocyte hyperplasia → ↑ TGF-β secretion → ↑ fibroblast activity → obliteration of bone marrow with fibrosis. Associated with massive splenomegaly and "teardrop" RBCs C. "Bone marrow **cries** because it's fibrosed and is a dry tap."

	RBCs	WBCs	PLATELETS	PHILADELPHIA CHROMOSOME	*JAK2* MUTATIONS
Polycythemia vera	↑	↑	↑	⊖	⊕
Essential thrombocythemia	–	–	↑	⊖	⊕ (30–50%)
Myelofibrosis	↓	Variable	Variable	⊖	⊕ (30–50%)
CML	↓	↑	↑	⊕	⊖

Leukemoid reaction vs chronic myelogenous leukemia

	Leukemoid reaction	Chronic myelogenous leukemia
DEFINITION	Reactive neutrophilia > 50,000 cells/mm³	Myeloproliferative neoplasm ⊕ for *BCR-ABL*
NEUTROPHIL MORPHOLOGY	Toxic granulation, Döhle bodies, cytoplasmic vacuoles	Pseudo-Pelger-Huët anomaly
LAP SCORE	↑	↓ (LAP enzyme ↓ in malignant neutrophils)
EOSINOPHILS AND BASOPHILS	Normal	↑

Polycythemia

	PLASMA VOLUME	RBC MASS	O₂ SATURATION	EPO LEVELS	ASSOCIATIONS
Relative	↓	–	–	–	Dehydration, burns.
Appropriate absolute	–	↑	↓	↑	Lung disease, congenital heart disease, high altitude, obstructive sleep apnea.
Inappropriate absolute	–	↑	–	↑	Exogenous EPO (athlete misuse, also called "blood doping"), androgen supplementation. Inappropriate EPO secretion: malignancy (eg, RCC, HCC).
Polycythemia vera	↑	↑↑	–	↓	EPO ↓ in PCV due to negative feedback suppressing renal EPO production.

↑↓ = 1° disturbance

Chromosomal translocations

TRANSLOCATION	ASSOCIATED DISORDER	NOTES
t(8;14)	Burkitt (Burk-8) lymphoma (c-myc activation)	The Ig heavy chain genes on chromosome 14 are constitutively expressed. When other genes (eg, c-myc and BCL-2) are translocated next to this heavy chain gene region, they are overexpressed.
t(11;14)	Mantle cell lymphoma (cyclin D1 activation)	
t(11;18)	Marginal zone lymphoma	
t(14;18)	Follicular lymphoma (BCL-2 activation)	
t(15;17)	APL (formerly M3 type of AML)	
t(9;22) (**Philadelphia** chromosome)	**CML** (BCR-ABL hybrid), ALL (less common); **Philadelphia CreaML** cheese	

Langerhans cell histiocytosis

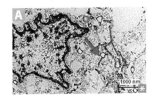

Collective group of proliferative disorders of Langerhans cells (antigen-presenting cells normally found in the skin). Presents in a child as lytic bone lesions and skin rash or as recurrent otitis media with a mass involving the mastoid bone. Cells are functionally immature and do not effectively stimulate primary T cells via antigen presentation. Cells express S-100 and CD1a. Birbeck granules ("tennis rackets" or rod-shaped on EM) are characteristic A.

Tumor lysis syndrome

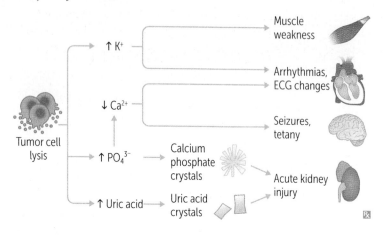

Oncologic emergency triggered by massive tumor cell lysis, seen most often with lymphomas/leukemias. Usually caused by treatment initiation, but can occur spontaneously with fast-growing cancers. Release of K^+ → hyperkalemia, release of PO_4^{3-} → hyperphosphatemia, hypocalcemia due to Ca^{2+} sequestration by PO_4^{3-}. ↑ nucleic acid breakdown → hyperuricemia → acute kidney injury. Prevention and treatment include aggressive hydration, allopurinol, rasburicase. Tumor cell breakdown causes ↑ K^+, ↓ Ca^{2+}, ↑ Uric acid, and ↑ PO_4^{3-} (Brea**K** the **CUP**).

▶ HEMATOLOGY AND ONCOLOGY—PHARMACOLOGY

Heparin

MECHANISM	Activates antithrombin, which ↓ action primarily of factors IIa (thrombin) and Xa. Short half-life.
CLINICAL USE	Immediate anticoagulation for pulmonary embolism (PE), acute coronary syndrome, MI, deep venous thrombosis (DVT). Used during pregnancy (does not cross placenta; low-molecular-weight heparin [eg, enoxaparin] preferred). Monitor PTT.
ADVERSE EFFECTS	Bleeding (reverse with protamine sulfate), heparin-induced thrombocytopenia (HIT), osteoporosis (with long-term use), drug-drug interactions, type 4 renal tubular acidosis. ▪ HIT type 1—mild (platelets > 100,000/mm³), transient, nonimmunologic drop in platelet count that typically occurs within the first 2 days of heparin administration. Not clinically significant. ▪ HIT type 2—development of IgG antibodies against heparin-bound platelet factor 4 (PF4) that typically occurs 5–10 days after heparin administration. Antibody-heparin-PF4 complex binds and activates platelets → removal by splenic macrophages and thrombosis → ↓↓ platelet count. Highest risk with unfractionated heparin. Treatment: discontinue heparin, start alternative anticoagulant (eg, argatroban). Fondaparinux safe to use (does not interact with PF4).
NOTES	Low-molecular-weight heparins (eg, enoxaparin, dalteparin) act mainly on factor Xa. Longer half-life. Fondaparinux acts only on factor Xa. Both are not easily reversible. Unfractionated heparin used in patients with renal insufficiency (low-molecular-weight heparins should be used with caution because they undergo renal clearance).

Warfarin

MECHANISM	Inhibits vitamin K epoxide reductase by competing with vitamin K → inhibition of vitamin K–dependent γ-carboxylation of clotting factors II, VII, IX, and X and proteins C and S. Metabolism affected by polymorphisms in the gene for vitamin K epoxide reductase complex (*VKORC1*). In laboratory assay, has effect on **extrinsic pathway** and ↑ **PT**. Long half-life. "The **ex-PresidenT** went to **war**(farin)."
CLINICAL USE	Chronic anticoagulation (eg, venous thromboembolism prophylaxis and prevention of stroke in atrial fibrillation). Not used in pregnant patients (because warfarin, unlike heparin, crosses placenta). Monitor PT/INR.
ADVERSE EFFECTS	Bleeding, teratogenic effects, skin/tissue necrosis 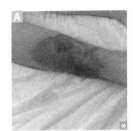, drug-drug interactions (metabolized by cytochrome P-450 [CYP2C9]). Initial risk of hypercoagulation: protein C has shorter half-life than factors II and X. Existing protein C depletes before existing factors II and X deplete, and before warfarin can reduce factors II and X production → hypercoagulation. Skin/tissue necrosis within first few days of large doses believed to be due to small vessel microthrombosis. Heparin "bridging": heparin frequently used when starting warfarin. Heparin's activation of antithrombin enables anticoagulation during initial, transient hypercoagulable state caused by warfarin. Initial heparin therapy reduces risk of recurrent venous thromboembolism and skin/tissue necrosis. For reversal of warfarin, give vitamin K. For rapid reversal, give FFP or PCC.

Heparin vs warfarin

	Heparin	Warfarin
ROUTE OF ADMINISTRATION	Parenteral (IV, SC)	Oral
SITE OF ACTION	Blood	Liver
ONSET OF ACTION	Rapid (seconds)	Slow, limited by half-lives of normal clotting factors
DURATION OF ACTION	Hours	Days
MONITORING	PTT (**intrinsic pathway**)	PT/INR (extrinsic pathway)
CROSSES PLACENTA	No	Yes (teratogenic)

Direct coagulation factor inhibitors

Do not usually require lab monitoring.

DRUG	MECHANISM	CLINICAL USE	ADVERSE EFFECTS
Bivalirudin, argatroban, dabigatran	Directly inhibit thrombin (factor IIa)	Venous thromboembolism, atrial fibrillation. Can be used in HIT, when heparin is **BAD** for the patient	Bleeding (**ida**rucizumab can be used to inhibit **da**bigatran)
Apixaban, edoxaban, rivaroxaban	Directly inhibit (**ban**) factor **Xa**	Oral agents. DVT/PE treatment and prophylaxis; stroke prophylaxis in patients with atrial fibrillation	Bleeding (reverse with andexanet alfa)

Anticoagulation reversal

ANTICOAGULANT	REVERSAL AGENT	NOTES
Heparin	Protamine sulfate	⊕ charged peptide that binds ⊖ charged heparin
Warfarin	Vitamin K (slow) +/– FFP or PCC (rapid)	
Dabigatran	Idarucizumab	Monoclonal antibody Fab fragments
Direct factor Xa inhibitors (eg, apixaban, rivaroxaban)	Andexanet alfa	Recombinant modified factor Xa (inactive)

Antiplatelets

All work by ↓ platelet aggregation.

DRUG	MECHANISM	CLINICAL USE	ADVERSE EFFECTS
Aspirin	Irreversibly blocks COX → ↓ TXA_2 release	Acute coronary syndrome; coronary stenting. ↓ incidence or recurrence of thrombotic stroke	Gastric ulcers, tinnitus, allergic reactions, renal injury, Reye syndrome (in children)
Clopidogrel, prasugrel, ticagrelor	Block ADP ($P2Y_{12}$) receptor → ↓ ADP-induced expression of GpIIb/IIIa	Same as aspirin; dual antiplatelet therapy	Bleeding
Eptifibatide, tirofiban, abciximab	Block GpIIb/IIIa (fibrinogen receptor) on activated platelets	Unstable angina, percutaneous coronary intervention	Bleeding, thrombocytopenia
Cilostazol, dipyridamole	Block phosphodiesterase → ↓ cAMP hydrolysis → ↑ cAMP in platelets	Intermittent claudication, stroke prevention, cardiac stress testing, prevention of coronary stent restenosis	Nausea, headache, facial flushing, hypotension, abdominal pain

Thrombolytics

Alteplase (tPA), reteplase (rPA), tenecteplase (TNK-tPA).

MECHANISM	Directly or indirectly aid conversion of plasminogen to plasmin, which cleaves fibrin clots. ↑ PT, ↑ PTT, no change in platelet count.
CLINICAL USE	Early MI, early ischemic stroke, direct thrombolysis of high-risk PE.
ADVERSE EFFECTS	Bleeding. Contraindicated in patients with active bleeding, history of intracranial bleeding, recent surgery, known bleeding diatheses, or severe hypertension. Nonspecific reversal with antifibrinolytics (eg, aminocaproic acid, tranexamic acid), platelet transfusions, and factor corrections (eg, cryoprecipitate, FFP, PCC).

Cancer therapy—cell cycle

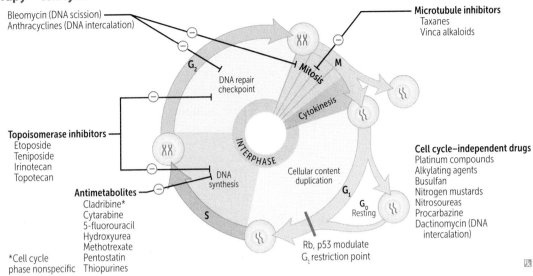

Bleomycin (DNA scission)
Anthracyclines (DNA intercalation)

Microtubule inhibitors
Taxanes
Vinca alkaloids

G_2

DNA repair
checkpoint

M

Mitosis

Cytokinesis

INTERPHASE

Topoisomerase inhibitors
Etoposide
Teniposide
Irinotecan
Topotecan

S

DNA
synthesis

Cellular content
duplication

G_1

G_0
Resting

Cell cycle–independent drugs
Platinum compounds
Alkylating agents
Busulfan
Nitrogen mustards
Nitrosoureas
Procarbazine
Dactinomycin (DNA
intercalation)

Antimetabolites
Cladribine*
Cytarabine
5-fluorouracil
Hydroxyurea
Methotrexate
Pentostatin
Thiopurines

*Cell cycle
phase nonspecific

Rb, p53 modulate
G_1 restriction point

Cancer therapy—targets

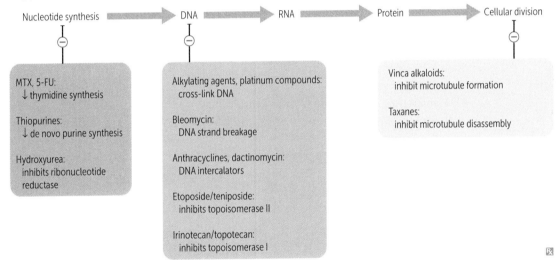

Nucleotide synthesis ⟹ DNA ⟹ RNA ⟹ Protein ⟹ Cellular division

MTX, 5-FU:
↓ thymidine synthesis

Thiopurines:
↓ de novo purine synthesis

Hydroxyurea:
inhibits ribonucleotide
reductase

Alkylating agents, platinum compounds:
cross-link DNA

Bleomycin:
DNA strand breakage

Anthracyclines, dactinomycin:
DNA intercalators

Etoposide/teniposide:
inhibits topoisomerase II

Irinotecan/topotecan:
inhibits topoisomerase I

Vinca alkaloids:
inhibit microtubule formation

Taxanes:
inhibit microtubule disassembly

Antibody-drug conjugates

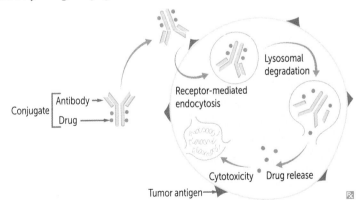

Conjugate [Antibody
Drug]

Receptor-mediated
endocytosis

Lysosomal
degradation

Cytotoxicity

Drug release

Tumor antigen →

Formed by linking monoclonal antibodies
with cytotoxic chemotherapeutic drugs.
Antibody selectivity against tumor antigens
allows targeted drug delivery to tumor cells
while sparing healthy cells → ↑ efficacy and
↓ toxicity.
Example: ado-trastuzumab emtansine (T-DM1)
for HER2 ⊕ breast cancer.

Antitumor antibiotics Dactinomycin is cell cycle nonspecific; bleomycin and anthracycline are G_2/M phase specific.

DRUG	MECHANISM	CLINICAL USE	ADVERSE EFFECTS
Bleomycin	Generates free radicals → DNA strand breaks	Testicular cancer, Hodgkin lymphoma	Pulmonary fibrosis, skin hyperpigmentation
Dactinomycin (actinomycin D)	Intercalates into DNA, preventing RNA synthesis	Wilms tumor, Ewing sarcoma, rhabdomyosarcoma	Myelosuppression
Anthracyclines Doxorubicin, daunorubicin	Generate free radicals Intercalate into DNA → DNA strand breaks → ↓ replication Inhibit topoisomerase II	Solid tumors, leukemias, lymphomas	Dilated cardiomyopathy (often irreversible; prevent with dexrazoxane), myelosuppression

Antimetabolites All are S-phase specific except cladribine, which is cell cycle nonspecific.

DRUG	MECHANISM	CLINICAL USE	ADVERSE EFFECTS
Thiopurines Azathioprine, 6-mercaptopurine	Purine (thiol) analogs → ↓ de novo purine synthesis AZA is converted to 6-MP, which is then activated by HGPRT	Rheumatoid arthritis, IBD, SLE, ALL; steroid-refractory disease Prevention of organ rejection Weaning from glucocorticoids	Myelosuppression; GI, liver toxicity 6-MP is inactivated by thiopurine S-methyl-transferase (genetic polymorphism) and xanthine oxidase (↑ toxicity with allopurinol or febuxostat)
Cladribine, pentostatin	Purine nucleoside analogs → unable to be processed by ADA, interfering with DNA synthesis	Hairy cell leukemia	Myelosuppression
Cytarabine (arabinofuranosyl cytidine)	Pyrimidine nucleoside analog → DNA chain termination Inhibits DNA polymerase	Leukemias (AML), lymphomas	Myelosuppression
5-Fluorouracil	Pyrimidine analog bioactivated to 5-FdUMP → thymidylate synthase inhibition → ↓ dTMP → ↓ DNA synthesis Capecitabine is a prodrug	Colon cancer, pancreatic cancer, actinic keratosis, basal cell carcinoma (topical) Effects enhanced with the addition of leucovorin	Myelosuppression, palmar-plantar erythrodysesthesia (hand-foot syndrome)
Hydroxyurea	Inhibits ribonucleotide reductase → ↓ DNA synthesis	Myeloproliferative disorders (eg, CML, polycythemia vera), sickle cell disease (↑ HbF)	Severe myelosuppression, megaloblastic anemia
Methotrexate	Folic acid analog that competitively inhibits dihydrofolate reductase → ↓ dTMP → ↓ DNA synthesis	Cancers: leukemias (ALL), lymphomas, choriocarcinoma, sarcomas Nonneoplastic: ectopic pregnancy, medical abortion (with misoprostol), rheumatoid arthritis, psoriasis, IBD, vasculitis	Myelosuppression (reversible with leucovorin "rescue"), hepatotoxicity, mucositis (eg, mouth ulcers), pulmonary fibrosis, folate deficiency (teratogenic), nephrotoxicity

Alkylating agents

All are cell cycle nonspecific.

DRUG	MECHANISM	CLINICAL USE	ADVERSE EFFECTS
Busulfan	Cross-links DNA	Used to ablate patient's bone marrow before bone marrow transplantation	Severe myelosuppression (in almost all cases), pulmonary fibrosis, hyperpigmentation
Nitrogen mustards Cyclophosphamide, ifosfamide	Cross-link DNA Require bioactivation by liver	Solid tumors, leukemia, lymphomas, rheumatic disease (eg, SLE, granulomatosis with polyangiitis)	Myelosuppression, SIADH, Fanconi syndrome (ifosfamide), hemorrhagic cystitis and bladder cancer (prevent with mesna)
Nitrosoureas Carmustine, lomustine	Cross-link DNA Require bioactivation by liver Cross blood-brain barrier → CNS entry	Brain tumors (including **glio**blastoma multiforme) Put **nitro** in your **Must**ang and travel the **globe**	CNS toxicity (convulsions, dizziness, ataxia)
Procarbazine	Mechanism unknown Weak MAO inhibitor (risk of hypertensive crisis with tyramine ingestion)	Hodgkin lymphoma, brain tumors	Myelosuppression, pulmonary toxicity, leukemia, disulfiram-like reaction

Platinum compounds

Cisplatin, carboplatin, oxaliplatin.

MECHANISM	Cross-link DNA. Cell cycle nonspecific.
CLINICAL USE	Solid tumors (eg, testicular, bladder, ovarian, GI, lung), lymphomas.
ADVERSE EFFECTS	Nephrotoxicity (eg, Fanconi syndrome; prevent with amifostine), peripheral neuropathy, ototoxicity.

Microtubule inhibitors

All are M-phase specific.

DRUG	MECHANISM	CLINICAL USE	ADVERSE EFFECTS
Taxanes Docetaxel, paclitaxel	Hyper**stabilize** polymerized microtubules → prevent mitotic spindle breakdown	Various tumors (eg, ovarian and breast carcinomas)	Myelosuppression, neuropathy, hypersensitivity **Taxes stabilize** society
Vinca alkaloids Vincristine, vinblastine	Bind β-tubulin and inhibit its polymerization into microtubules → prevent mitotic spindle formation	Solid tumors, leukemias, Hodgkin and non-Hodgkin lymphomas	Vin**cris**tine (**crisps** the nerves): neurotoxicity (axonal neuropathy), constipation (including ileus) Vin**blast**ine (**blasts** the marrow): myelosuppression

Topoisomerase inhibitors

All cause ↑ DNA strand breaks, resulting in cell cycle arrest in S and G_2 phases.

DRUG	MECHANISM	CLINICAL USE	ADVERSE EFFECTS
Irinotecan, topotecan	Inhibit topoisomerase **I** "-tecone"	Colon, ovarian, small cell lung cancer	Severe myelosuppression, diarrhea
Etoposide, teniposide	Inhibit topoisomerase **II** "-bothside"	Testicular, small cell lung cancer, leukemia, lymphoma	Myelosuppression, alopecia

Tamoxifen

MECHANISM	Selective estrogen receptor modulator with complex mode of action: antagonist in breast tissue, partial agonist in endometrium and bone. Blocks the binding of estrogen to ER in ER ⊕ cells.
CLINICAL USE	Prevention and treatment of breast cancer, prevention of gynecomastia in patients undergoing prostate cancer therapy.
ADVERSE EFFECTS	Hot flashes, ↑ risk of thromboembolic events (eg, DVT, PE), endometrial cancer, uterine sarcoma.

Anticancer monoclonal antibodies

Work against extracellular targets to neutralize them or to promote immune system recognition (eg, ADCC by NK cells). Eliminated by macrophages (not cleared by kidneys or liver).

AGENT	TARGET	CLINICAL USE	ADVERSE EFFECTS
Alemtuzumab	CD52	Chronic **lymphocytic** leukemia (CLL), multiple sclerosis.	↑ risk of infections and autoimmunity (eg, ITP)
Bevacizumab	VEGF (inhibits blood vessel formation)	Colorectal cancer (CRC), renal cell carcinoma (RCC), non–small cell lung cancer (NSCLC), angioproliferative retinopathy	Hemorrhage, blood clots, impaired wound healing
Cetuximab, panitumumab	EGFR	Metastatic CRC (wild-type RAS), head and neck cancer	Rash, elevated LFTs, diarrhea
Rituximab	CD20	Non-Hodgkin lymphoma, CLL, rheumatoid arthritis, ITP, TTP, AIHA, multiple sclerosis	Infusion reaction due to cytokine release following interaction of rituximab with its target on B cells
Trastuzumab	HER2 Don't **Trast HER**, she will break your heart	Breast cancer, gastric cancer	Dilated **cardiomyopathy** (often reversible)
Pembrolizumab, nivolumab, cemiplimab	PD-1	Various tumors (eg, NSCLC, RCC, melanoma, urothelial carcinoma)	↑ risk of autoimmunity (eg, dermatitis, enterocolitis, hepatitis, pneumonitis, endocrinopathies)
Atezolizumab, durvalumab, avelumab	PD-L1		
Ipilimumab	CTLA-4		

Anticancer small molecule inhibitors

AGENT	TARGET	CLINICAL USE	ADVERSE EFFECTS
Alectinib, crizotinib	ALK	Non–small cell lung cancer	Edema, rash, diarrhea
Erlotinib, gefitinib, afatinib	EGFR	Non–small cell lung cancer	Rash, diarrhea
Imatinib, dasatinib, nilotinib	BCR-ABL (also other tyrosine kinases [eg, c-KIT])	CML, ALL, GISTs	Myelosuppression, ↑ LFTs, edema, myalgias
Ruxolitinib	JAK1/2	Polycythemia vera	Bruises, ↑ LFTs
Bortezomib, ixazomib, carfilzomib	Proteasome (induce arrest at G2-M phase via accumulation of abnormal proteins → apoptosis)	Multiple myeloma, mantle cell lymphoma	Peripheral neuropathy, herpes zoster reactivation (↓ T-cell activation → ↓ cell-mediated immunity)
Vemurafenib, encorafenib, dabrafenib	BRAF	Melanoma Often co-administered with MEK inhibitors (eg, trametinib)	Rash, fatigue, nausea, diarrhea
Palbociclib	Cyclin-dependent kinase 4/6 (induces arrest at G1-S phase → apoptosis)	Breast cancer	Myelosuppression, pneumonitis
Olaparib	Poly(ADP-ribose) polymerase (↓ DNA repair)	Breast, ovarian, pancreatic, and prostate cancers	Myelosuppression, edema, diarrhea

Chemotoxicity amelioration

DRUG	MECHANISM	CLINICAL USE
Amifostine	Free radical scavenger	Nephrotoxicity from platinum compounds
Dexrazoxane	Iron chelator	Cardiotoxicity from anthracyclines
Leucovorin (folinic acid)	Tetrahydrofolate precursor	Myelosuppression from methotrexate (leucovorin "rescue"); also enhances the effects of 5-FU
Mesna	Sulfhydryl compound that binds acrolein (toxic metabolite of cyclophosphamide/ifosfamide)	Hemorrhagic cystitis from cyclophosphamide/ ifosfamide
Rasburicase	Recombinant uricase that catalyzes metabolism of uric acid to allantoin	Tumor lysis syndrome
Ondansetron, granisetron	5-HT$_3$ receptor antagonists	Acute nausea and vomiting (usually within 1-2 hr after chemotherapy)
Prochlorperazine, metoclopramide	D$_2$ receptor antagonists	
Aprepitant, fosaprepitant	NK$_1$ receptor antagonists	Delayed nausea and vomiting (>24 hr after chemotherapy)
Filgrastim, sargramostim	Recombinant G(M)-CSF	Neutropenia
Epoetin alfa	Recombinant erythropoietin	Anemia

Key chemotoxicities

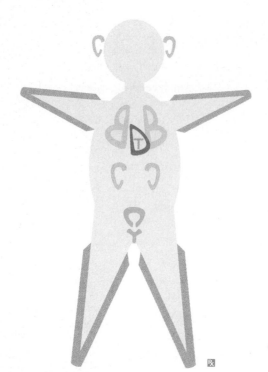

Cisplatin, Carboplatin → ototoxicity

Vincristine → peripheral neuropathy
Bleomycin, Busulfan → pulmonary fibrosis
Doxorubicin, Daunorubicin → cardiotoxicity
Trastuzumab → cardiotoxicity
Cisplatin, Carboplatin → nephrotoxicity

CYclophosphamide → hemorrhagic cystitis

Nonspecific common toxicities of nearly all cytotoxic chemotherapies include myelosuppression (neutropenia, anemia, thrombocytopenia), GI toxicity (nausea, vomiting, mucositis), alopecia.

Musculoskeletal, Skin, and Connective Tissue

"Rigid, the skeleton of habit alone upholds the human frame."
—Virginia Woolf, *Mrs. Dalloway*

"Beauty may be skin deep, but ugly goes clear to the bone."
—Redd Foxx

"The finest clothing made is a person's own skin, but, of course, society demands something more than this."
—Mark Twain

"To thrive in life you need three bones. A wishbone. A backbone. And a funny bone."
—Reba McEntire

This chapter provides information you will need to understand common anatomic dysfunctions, orthopedic conditions, rheumatic diseases, and dermatologic conditions. Be able to interpret 3D anatomy in the context of radiologic imaging. For the rheumatic diseases, create instructional cases that include the most likely presentation and symptoms: risk factors, gender, important markers (eg, autoantibodies), and other epidemiologic factors. Doing so will allow you to answer higher order questions that are likely to be asked on the exam.

▸ MUSCULOSKELETAL, SKIN, AND CONNECTIVE TISSUE—ANATOMY AND PHYSIOLOGY

Upper extremity nerves

NERVE	CAUSES OF INJURY	PRESENTATION
Axillary (C5-C6)	Fractured surgical neck of humerus Anterior dislocation of humerus	Flattened deltoid Loss of arm abduction at shoulder (> 15°) Loss of sensation over deltoid and lateral arm
Musculocutaneous (C5-C7)	Upper trunk compression	↓ biceps (C5-C6) reflex Loss of forearm flexion and supination Loss of sensation over radial and dorsal forearm
Radial (C5-T1)	Compression of axilla, eg, due to crutches or sleeping with arm over chair ("Saturday night palsy") Midshaft fracture of humerus Repetitive pronation/supination of forearm, eg, due to screwdriver use ("finger drop")	Injuries above the elbow cause loss of sensation over posterior arm/forearm and dorsal hand, wrist drop (loss of elbow, wrist, and finger extension) with ↓ grip strength (wrist extension necessary for maximal action of flexors) Injuries below the elbow can cause paresthesias of the dorsal hand (superficial radial nerve) or wrist drop (posterior interosseus nerve) Tricep function and posterior arm sensation spared in midshaft fracture
Median (C5-T1)	Supracondylar fracture of humerus → proximal lesion of the nerve Carpal tunnel syndrome and wrist laceration → distal lesion of the nerve	"Ape hand" and "Hand of benediction" Loss of wrist flexion and function of the lateral two **L**umbricals, **O**pponens pollicis, **A**bductor pollicis brevis, **F**lexor pollicis brevis (**LOAF**) Loss of sensation over thenar eminence and dorsal and palmar aspects of lateral 3 1/2 fingers with proximal lesion
Ulnar (C8-T1)	Fracture of medial epicondyle of humerus (proximal lesion) Fractured hook of hamate (distal lesion) from fall on outstretched hand Compression of nerve against hamate as the wrist rests on handlebar during cycling	"Ulnar claw" on digit extension Radial deviation of wrist upon flexion (proximal lesion) ↓ flexion of ulnar fingers, abduction and adduction of fingers (interossei), thumb adduction, actions of ulnar 2 lumbrical muscles Loss of sensation over ulnar 1 1/2 fingers including hypothenar eminence
Recurrent branch of median nerve (C5-T1)	Superficial laceration of palm	"Ape hand" Loss of thenar muscle group: opposition, abduction, and flexion of thumb No loss of sensation

Humerus fractures, proximally to distally, follow the **ARM** (**A**xillary → **R**adial → **M**edian) nerves

Upper extremity nerves (continued)

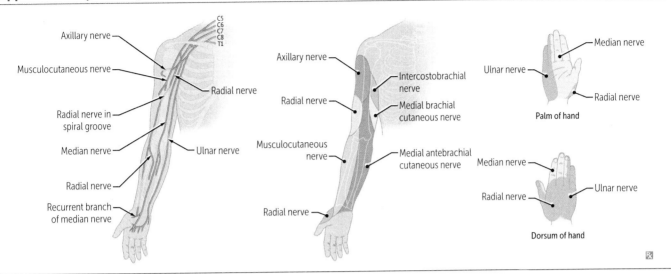

Rotator cuff muscles

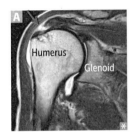

Shoulder muscles that form the rotator cuff:

- Supraspinatus (suprascapular nerve)—abducts arm initially (before the action of the deltoid); most common rotator cuff injury (trauma or degeneration and impingement → tendinopathy or tear [arrow in A]), assessed by "empty/full can" test
- Infraspinatus (suprascapular nerve)—externally rotates arm; pitching injury
- teres minor (axillary nerve)—adducts and externally rotates arm
- Subscapularis (upper and lower subscapular nerves)—internally rotates and adducts arm

Innervated primarily by C5-C6.

SItS (small t is for teres minor).

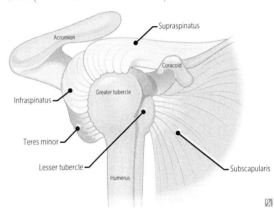

Arm abduction

DEGREE	MUSCLE	NERVE
0°–15°	Supraspinatus	Suprascapular
15°–90°	Deltoid	Axillary
> 90°	Trapezius	Accessory
> 90°	Serratus Anterior	Long Thoracic (SALT)

Brachial plexus lesions

❶ Erb palsy ("waiter's tip")
❷ Klumpke palsy (claw hand)
❸ Wrist drop
❹ Winged scapula
❺ Deltoid paralysis
❻ "Saturday night palsy" (wrist drop)
❼ Difficulty flexing elbow, variable sensory loss
❽ Decreased thumb function, "hand of benediction"
❾ Intrinsic muscles of hand, claw hand

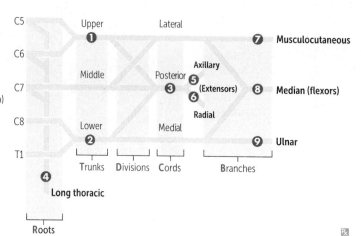

Divisions of brachial plexus:
Remember
To
Drink
Cold
Beer
Trunks of brachial plexus and the subclavian artery pass between anterior and middle scalene muscles. Subclavian vein passes anteromedial to the scalene triangle.

CONDITION	INJURY	CAUSES	MUSCLE DEFICIT	FUNCTIONAL DEFICIT	PRESENTATION
Erb palsy ("waiter's tip")	Traction or tear of **upper** trunk: C5-C6 roots	Infants—lateral traction on neck during delivery Adults—trauma leading to neck traction (eg, falling on head and shoulder in motorcycle accident)	Deltoid, supraspinatus	Abduction (arm hangs by side)	
			Infraspinatus, supraspinatus	Lateral rotation (arm medially rotated)	
			Biceps brachii Herb gets **DIBs** on **tips**	Flexion, supination (arm extended and pronated)	
Klumpke palsy	Traction or tear of **lower** trunk: C8-T1 roots	Infants—upward force on arm during delivery Adults—trauma (eg, grabbing a tree branch to break a fall)	Intrinsic hand muscles: lumbricals, interossei, thenar, hypothenar	Claw hand ("**Claw**mpke" palsy): lumbricals normally flex MCP joints and extend DIP and PIP joints	
Thoracic outlet syndrome	Compression of **lower** trunk and subclavian vessels, most commonly within the scalene triangle	Cervical/anomalous first ribs (arrows in Ⓐ), Pancoast tumor	Same as Klumpke palsy	Atrophy of intrinsic hand muscles; ischemia, pain, and edema due to vascular compression	
Winged scapula	Lesion of long thoracic nerve, roots C5-C7 ("wings of heaven")	Axillary node dissection after mastectomy, stab wounds	Serratus anterior	Inability to anchor scapula to thoracic cage → cannot abduct arm above horizontal position Ⓑ	

Wrist region

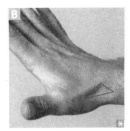

Scaphoid, lunate, triquetrum, pisiform, hamate, capitate, trapezoid, trapezium **A**. (So long to pinky, here comes the thumb)

Scaphoid (palpable in anatomic snuff box **B**) is the most commonly fractured carpal bone, typically due to a fall on an outstretched hand. Complications of proximal scaphoid fractures include avascular necrosis and nonunion due to retrograde blood supply from a branch of the radial artery. Occult fracture not always seen on initial x-ray.

Dislocation of lunate may impinge median nerve and cause carpal tunnel syndrome.

Fracture of the hook of the hamate can cause ulnar nerve compression—**Guyon canal syndrome**.

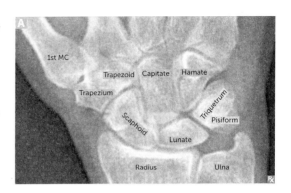

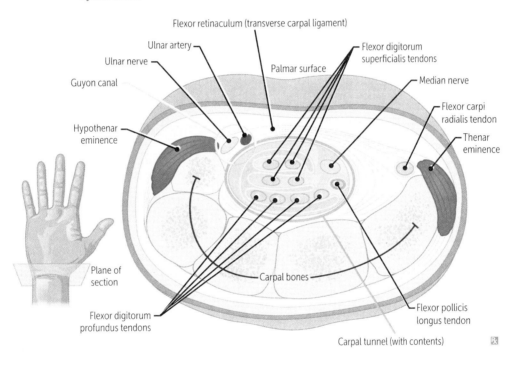

Hand muscles

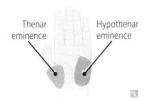

Thenar (median)—Opponens pollicis, Abductor pollicis brevis, Flexor pollicis brevis: superficial and deep (by ulnar nerve) heads, adductor pollicis (by ulnar nerve).

Hypothenar (ulnar)—Opponens digiti minimi, Abductor digiti minimi, Flexor digiti minimi brevis.

Dorsal interossei (ulnar)—abduct the fingers.
Palmar interossei (ulnar)—adduct the fingers.
Lumbricals (1st/2nd, median; 3rd/4th, ulnar)—flex at the MCP joint, extend PIP and DIP joints.

Both groups perform the same functions: Oppose, Abduct, and Flex (OAF).

DAB = Dorsals ABduct.
PAD = Palmars ADduct.

Distortions of the hand

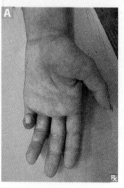

At rest, a balance exists between the extrinsic flexors and extensors of the hand, as well as the intrinsic muscles of the hand—particularly the lumbrical muscles (flexion of MCP, extension of DIP and PIP joints).

"Clawing" A—seen best with **distal** lesions of median or ulnar nerves. Remaining extrinsic flexors of the digits exaggerate the loss of the lumbricals → fingers extend at MCP, flex at DIP and PIP joints.

Deficits less pronounced in **proximal** lesions; deficits present during voluntary flexion of the digits.

SIGN	"Ulnar claw"	"Hand of benediction"	"Median claw"	"Trouble making a fist"
PRESENTATION				
CONTEXT	Extending fingers/at rest	Making a fist	Extending fingers/at rest	Making a fist
LOCATION OF LESION	Distal ulnar nerve	Proximal median nerve	Distal median nerve	Proximal ulnar nerve

Note: Atrophy of the thenar eminence can be seen in median nerve lesions, while atrophy of the hypothenar eminence can be seen in ulnar nerve lesions.

Knee exam

Lateral femoral condyle to anterior tibia: ACL. Medial femoral condyle to posterior tibia: PCL. **LAMP.**

TEST	PROCEDURE
Anterior drawer sign	Positive in ACL tear. Tibia glides anteriorly (relative to femur) when knee is at 90° angle. Alternatively, Lachman test can be done by placing the knee at a 30° angle.
Posterior drawer sign	Bending knee at 90° angle, ↑ posterior gliding of tibia due to PCL injury.
Valgus stress test	Abnormal passive abduction. Knee extended or at ~ 30° angle, lateral (valgus) force → medial space widening of tibia → MCL injury.
Varus stress test	Abnormal passive adduction. Knee extended or at ~ 30° angle, medial (varus) force → lateral space widening of tibia → LCL injury.
McMurray test	During flexion and extension of knee with rotation of tibia/foot (**LIME**): ▪ Pain, "popping" on internal rotation and varus force → Lateral meniscal tear (Internal rotation stresses lateral meniscus) ▪ Pain, "popping" on external rotation and valgus force → Medial meniscal tear (External rotation stresses medial meniscus)

Femur

Lateral condyle — Medial condyle

ACL — PCL

LCL — MCL

Lateral meniscus — Medial meniscus

Fibula — Tibia

Actions of hip muscles

ACTION	MUSCLES	PRESENTATION
Abductors	Gluteus medius, gluteus minimus	
Adductors	Adductor magnus, adductor longus, adductor brevis	
Extensors	Gluteus maximus, semitendinosus, semimembranosus, long head of biceps femoris	
Flexors	Iliopsoas (iliacus and psoas), rectus femoris, tensor fascia lata, pectineus, sartorius	
Internal rotation	Gluteus medius, gluteus minimus, tensor fascia latae	
External rotation	Iliopsoas, gluteus maximus, piriformis, obturator internus, obturator externus	

Lower extremity nerves

NERVE	INNERVATION	CAUSE OF INJURY	PRESENTATION/COMMENTS
Iliohypogastric (T12-L1)	Sensory—suprapubic region Motor—transversus abdominis and internal oblique	Abdominal surgery (commonly inguinal hernia repair)	Neuropathic pain (burning or tingling) in surgical incision site radiating to inguinal and suprapubic region
Genitofemoral nerve (L1-L2)	Sensory—scrotum/labia majora, medial thigh Motor—cremaster	Laparoscopic surgery	↓ upper medial thigh and anterior thigh sensation beneath the inguinal ligament (lateral part of the femoral triangle); absent cremasteric reflex
Lateral femoral cutaneous (L2-L3)	Sensory—anterior and lateral thigh	Tight clothing, obesity, pregnancy, pelvic procedures	↓ thigh sensation (anterior and lateral) Meralgia paresthetica— compression of lateral femoral cutaneous nerve → tingling, numbness, burning pain in anterolateral thigh
Obturator (L2-L4)	Sensory—medial thigh Motor—obturator externus, adductor longus, adductor brevis, gracilis, pectineus, adductor magnus	Pelvic operation	↓ thigh sensation (medial) and adduction
Femoral (L2-L4)	Sensory—anterior thigh, medial leg Motor—quadriceps, iliacus, pectineus, sartorius	Pelvic fracture, compression from retroperitoneal hematoma or psoas abscess	↓ leg extension (↓ patellar reflex)
Sciatic (L4-S3)	Sensory—posterior thigh, posterior knee, and all below knee (except narrow band on medial lower leg) Motor—semitendinosus, semimembranosus, biceps femoris, adductor magnus	Herniated disc, posterior hip dislocation, piriformis syndrome	Splits into common peroneal and tibial nerves

Lower extremity nerves *(continued)*

NERVE	INNERVATION	CAUSE OF INJURY	PRESENTATION/COMMENTS
Common (fibular) peroneal (L4-S2)	Superficial peroneal nerve: ▪ Sensory—dorsum of foot (except webspace between hallux and 2nd digit) ▪ Motor—peroneus longus and brevis Deep peroneal nerve: ▪ Sensory—webspace between hallux and 2nd digit ▪ Motor—tibialis anterior	Trauma or compression of lateral aspect of leg, fibular neck fracture	**PED** = **P**eroneal **E**verts and **D**orsiflexes; if injured, foot drop**PED** Loss of sensation on dorsum of foot Foot drop—inverted and plantarflexed at rest, loss of eversion and dorsiflexion; "steppage gait"
Tibial (L4-S3)	Sensory—sole of foot Motor—biceps femoris (long head), triceps surae, plantaris, popliteus, flexor muscles of foot	Knee trauma, Baker cyst (proximal lesion); tarsal tunnel syndrome (distal lesion)	**TIP** = **T**ibial **I**nverts and **P**lantarflexes; if injured, can't stand on **TIP**toes Inability to curl toes and loss of sensation on sole; in proximal lesions, foot everted at rest with weakened inversion and plantar flexion
Superior gluteal (L4-S1)	Motor—gluteus medius, gluteus minimus, tensor fascia latae	Iatrogenic injury during intramuscular injection to superomedial gluteal region (prevent by choosing superolateral quadrant, preferably anterolateral region)	Trendelenburg sign/gait—pelvis tilts because weight-bearing leg cannot maintain alignment of pelvis through hip abduction Lesion located on side of raised hip, ipsilateral to standing leg
Inferior gluteal (L5-S2)	Motor—gluteus maximus	Posterior hip dislocation	Difficulty climbing stairs, rising from seated position; loss of hip extension
Pudendal (S2-S4)	Sensory—perineum Motor—external urethral and anal sphincters	Stretch injury during childbirth, prolonged cycling, horseback riding	↓ sensation in perineum and genital area; can cause fecal and/or urinary incontinence Can be blocked with local anesthetic during childbirth using ischial spine as a landmark for injection

Normal   Trendelenburg sign

Ankle sprains

Anterior talofibular ligament—most common ankle sprain overall, classified as a **low** ankle sprain. Due to overinversion/supination of foot. Anterior inferior **ti**biofibular ligament—most common **high** ankle sprain. **High tide.**

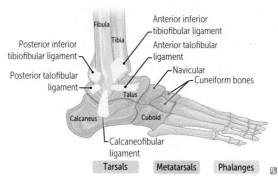

Signs of lumbosacral radiculopathy

Paresthesia and weakness related to specific lumbosacral spinal nerves. Intervertebral disc (nucleus pulposus) herniates posterolaterally through annulus fibrosus (outer ring) into spinal canal due to thin posterior longitudinal ligament and thicker anterior longitudinal ligament along midline of vertebral bodies. Nerve affected is usually below the level of herniation. ⊕ straight leg raise, ⊕ contralateral straight leg raise, ⊕ reverse straight leg raise (femoral stretch).

Disc level herniation	L3-L4	L4-L5	L5-S1
Nerve root affected	L4	L5	S1
Dermatome affected			
Clinical findings	Weakness of knee extension ↓ patellar reflex	Weakness of dorsiflexion Difficulty in heel walking	Weakness of plantar flexion Difficulty in toe walking ↓ Achilles reflex

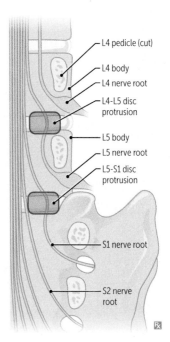

Neurovascular pairing

Nerves and arteries are frequently named together by the bones/regions with which they are associated. The following are exceptions to this naming convention.

LOCATION	NERVE	ARTERY
Axilla/lateral thorax	Long thoracic	Lateral thoracic
Surgical neck of humerus	Axillary	Posterior circumflex
Midshaft of humerus	Radial	Deep brachial
Distal humerus/cubital fossa	Median	Brachial
Popliteal fossa	Tibial	Popliteal
Posterior to medial malleolus	Tibial	Posterior tibial

Motor neuron action potential to muscle contraction

T-tubules are extensions of plasma membrane in contact with the sarcoplasmic reticulum, allowing for coordinated contraction of striated muscles.

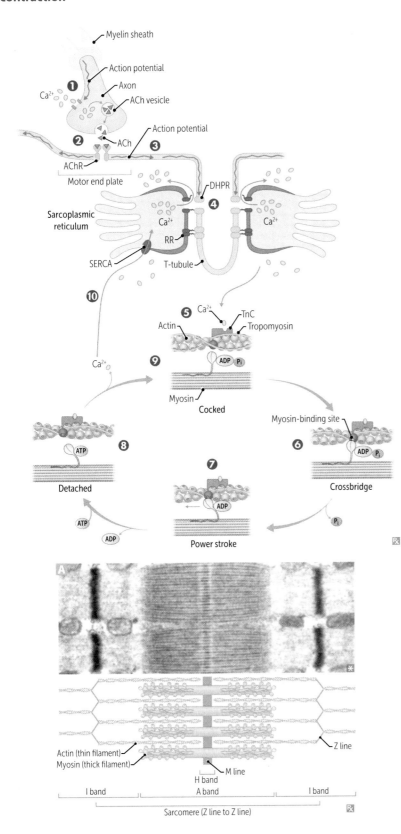

❶ Action potential opens presynaptic voltage-gated Ca^{2+} channels, inducing acetylcholine (ACh) release.

❷ Postsynaptic ACh binding leads to muscle cell depolarization at the motor end plate.

❸ Depolarization travels over the entire muscle cell and deep into the muscle via the T-tubules.

❹ Membrane depolarization induces conformational changes in the voltage-sensitive dihydropyridine receptor (DHPR) and its mechanically coupled ryanodine receptor (RR) → Ca^{2+} release from the sarcoplasmic reticulum (buffered by calsequestrin) into the cytoplasm.

❺ Tropomyosin is blocking myosin-binding sites on the actin filament. Released Ca^{2+} binds to troponin C (TnC), shifting tropomyosin to expose the myosin-binding sites.

❻ Myosin head binds strongly to actin (crossbridge). P_i released, initiating power stroke.

❼ During the power stroke, force is produced as myosin pulls on the thin filament **A**. Muscle shortening occurs, with shortening of **H** and **I** bands and between **Z** lines (**HI**, I'm wearing short **Z**). The **A** band remains the same length (**A** band is **A**lways the same length). ADP is released at the end of the power stroke.

❽ Binding of new ATP molecule causes detachment of myosin head from actin filament. Ca^{2+} is resequestered.

❾ ATP hydrolysis into ADP and P_i results in myosin head returning to high-energy position (cocked). The myosin head can bind to a new site on actin to form a crossbridge if Ca^{2+} remains available.

❿ Reuptake of calcium by sarco(endo)plasmic reticulum Ca^{2+} ATPase (SERCA) → muscle relaxation.

Types of skeletal muscle fibers

Two types, normally distributed randomly within muscle. Muscle fiber type grouping commonly occurs due to reinnervation of denervated muscle fibers in peripheral nerve damage.

	Type I	Type II
CONTRACTION VELOCITY	Slow	Fast
FIBER COLOR	Red	White
PREDOMINANT METABOLISM	Oxidative phosphorylation → sustained contraction	Anaerobic glycolysis
MITOCHONDRIA, MYOGLOBIN	↑	↓
TYPE OF TRAINING	Endurance training	Weight/resistance training, sprinting
NOTES	Think "**1** slow red ox"	Think "**2** fast white antelopes"

Skeletal muscle adaptations

	Atrophy	Hypertrophy
MYOFIBRILS	↓ (removal via ubiquitin-proteasome system)	↑ (addition of sarcomeres in parallel)
MYONUCLEI	↓ (selective apoptosis)	↑ (fusion of satellite cells, which repair damaged myofibrils; absent in cardiac muscles)

Vascular smooth muscle contraction and relaxation

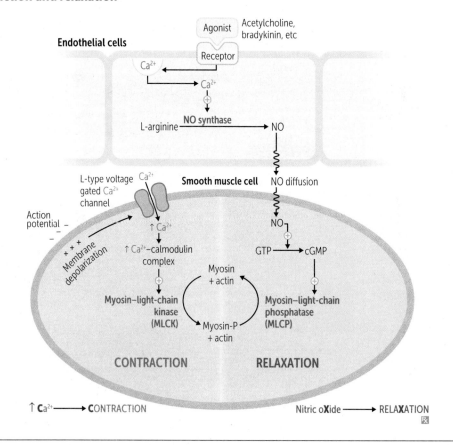

Muscle proprioceptors	Specialized sensory receptors that relay information about muscle dynamics.	
	Muscle stretch receptors	**Golgi tendon organ**
PATHWAY	❶ ↑ length and speed of stretch → ❷ via dorsal root ganglion (DRG) → ❸ activation of inhibitory interneuron and α motor neuron → ❹ simultaneous inhibition of antagonist muscle (prevents overstretching) and activation of agonist muscle (contraction).	❶ ↑ tension → ❷ via DRG → ❸ activation of inhibitory interneuron → ❹ inhibition of agonist muscle (reduced tension within muscle and tendon)
LOCATION/INNERVATION	Body of muscle/type Ia and II sensory axons	Tendons/type Ib sensory axons
ACTIVATION BY	↑ muscle stretch. Responsible for deep tendon reflexes	↑ muscle tension

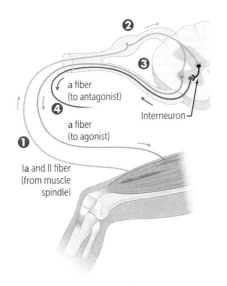 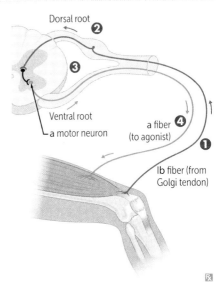

Bone formation

Endochondral ossification	Bones of axial skeleton, appendicular skeleton, and base of skull. Cartilaginous model of bone is first made by chondrocytes. Osteoclasts and osteoblasts later replace with woven bone and then remodel to lamellar bone. In adults, woven bone occurs after fractures and in Paget disease. Defective in achondroplasia.
Membranous ossification	Bones of calvarium, facial bones, and clavicle. Woven bone formed directly without cartilage. Later remodeled to lamellar bone.

Cell biology of bone

Osteoblast	Builds bone by secreting collagen and catalyzing mineralization in alkaline environment via ALP. Differentiates from mesenchymal stem cells in periosteum. Osteoblastic activity measured by bone ALP, osteocalcin, propeptides of type I procollagen.
Osteoclast	Dissolves ("crushes") bone by secreting H^+ and collagenases. Differentiates from a fusion of monocyte/macrophage lineage precursors. RANK receptors on osteoclasts are stimulated by RANKL (RANK ligand, expressed on osteoblasts). OPG (osteoprotegerin, a RANKL decoy receptor) binds RANKL to prevent RANK-RANKL interaction → ↓ osteoclast activity.
Parathyroid hormone	At low, intermittent levels, exerts anabolic effects (building bone) on osteoblasts and osteoclasts (indirect). Chronically ↑ PTH levels (1° hyperparathyroidism) cause catabolic effects (osteitis fibrosa cystica).
Estrogen	Inhibits apoptosis in bone-forming osteoblasts and induces apoptosis in bone-resorbing osteoclasts. Causes closure of epiphyseal plate during puberty. Estrogen deficiency (surgical or postmenopausal) → ↑ cycles of remodeling and bone resorption → ↑ risk of osteoporosis.

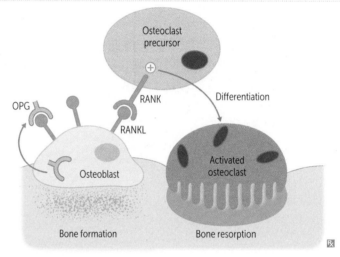

Overuse injuries of the elbow

Medial (golfer's) elbow tendinopathy	Repetitive wrist flexion or idiopathic → pain near medial epicondyle.
Lateral (tennis) elbow tendinopathy	Repetitive wrist extension (backhand shots) or idiopathic → pain near lateral epicondyle.

Clavicle fractures

Common in children and as birth trauma. Usually caused by a fall on outstretched hand or by direct trauma to shoulder. Weakest point at the junction of middle and lateral thirds 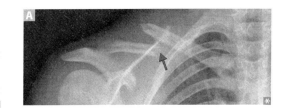; fractures at the middle third segment are most common. Presents as shoulder drop, shortened clavicle (lateral fragment is depressed due to arm weight and medially rotated by arm adductors [eg, pectoralis major]).

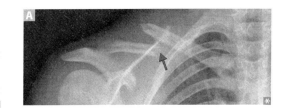

Wrist and hand injuries

Guyon canal syndrome	Compression of ulnar nerve at wrist. Classically seen in cyclists due to pressure from handlebars.	May also be seen with fracture/dislocation of the hook of hamate.
Carpal tunnel syndrome	Entrapment of median nerve in carpal tunnel (between transverse carpal ligament and carpal bones) → nerve compression → paresthesia, pain, and numbness in distribution of median nerve. Thenar eminence atrophies but sensation spared, because palmar cutaneous branch enters hand external to carpal tunnel.	Suggested by ⊕ Tinel sign (percussion of wrist causes tingling) and Phalen maneuver (90° flexion of wrist causes tingling). Associated with pregnancy (due to edema), rheumatoid arthritis, hypothyroidism, diabetes, acromegaly, dialysis-related amyloidosis; may be associated with repetitive use.

Metacarpal neck fracture

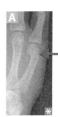

Most commonly the 5th metacarpal 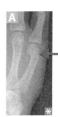 ("boxer's fracture"). Typically occurs in young males due to direct trauma (eg, punching a wall). Presents with pain, swelling, and tenderness over the affected metacarpal; reduced grip strength; possible deformity.

Psoas abscess

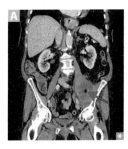

Collection of pus in iliopsoas compartment. May spread from blood (hematogenous) or from adjacent structures (eg, vertebral osteomyelitis, tuberculous spondylitis [also called Pott disease], pyelonephritis). Associated with Crohn disease, diabetes, and immunocompromised states.

Staphylococcus aureus most commonly isolated, but may also occur 2° to tuberculosis.

Findings: flank pain, fever, inguinal mass, ⊕ psoas sign (hip extension exacerbates lower abdominal pain).

Labs: leukocytosis. Imaging (CT/MRI) will show focal hypodense lesion within the muscle plane (red arrow in).

Treatment: abscess drainage, antibiotics.

Common knee conditions

"Unhappy triad"	Common injury in contact sports due to lateral force impacting the knee when foot is planted on the ground. Consists of damage to the ACL **A**, MCL, and medial meniscus (attached to MCL). However, lateral meniscus involvement is more common than medial meniscus involvement in conjunction with ACL and MCL injury. Presents with acute pain and signs of joint instability.	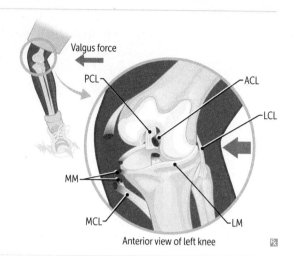
Prepatellar bursitis	Inflammation of the prepatellar bursa in front of the kneecap (red arrow in **B**). Can be caused by repeated trauma or pressure from excessive kneeling (also called "housemaid's knee").	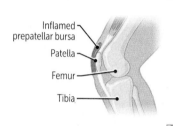
Popliteal cyst	Also called Baker cyst. Popliteal fluid collection (red arrow in **C**) in gastrocnemius-semimembranosus bursa commonly communicating with synovial space and related to chronic joint disease (eg, osteoarthritis, rheumatoid arthritis).	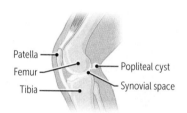

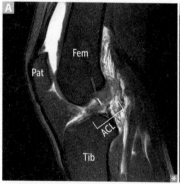
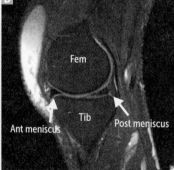
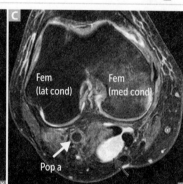

Common musculoskeletal conditions

Costochondritis	Inflammation of costochondral or costosternal junctions. Presents with focal tenderness to palpation and sharp, positional chest pain that may worsen with deep inspiration. More common in younger female patients. May mimic cardiac (eg, MI) or pulmonary (eg, pulmonary embolism) diseases.
De Quervain tenosynovitis	Noninflammatory thickening of abductor pollicis longus and extensor pollicis brevis tendons → pain or tenderness at radial styloid. ⊕ Finkelstein test (pain at radial styloid with active or passive stretch of thumb tendons). ↑ risk in new mothers (lifting baby), golfers, racquet sport players, "thumb" texters.
Dupuytren contracture	Caused by fibroblastic proliferation and thickening of superficial palmar fascia. Typically involves the fascia at the base of the ring and little fingers. Unknown etiology; most frequently seen in males > 50 years old of Northern European descent.
Ganglion cyst	Mucin-filled swelling overlying joint or tendon sheath, most commonly at dorsal side of wrist. Transilluminates with shining light (tumors lack transillumination). Usually resolves spontaneously.
Iliotibial band syndrome	Overuse injury of lateral knee that occurs primarily in runners. Pain develops 2° to friction of iliotibial band against lateral femoral epicondyle.
Limb compartment syndrome	↑ pressure within fascial compartment of a limb → venous outflow obstruction and arteriolar collapse → anoxia, necrosis, rhabdomyolysis → acute tubular necrosis. Causes include significant long bone fractures (eg, tibia), reperfusion injury, animal venoms. Presents with severe pain and tense, swollen compartments with passive stretch of muscles in the affected compartment. Increased serum creatine kinase and motor deficits are late signs of irreversible muscle and nerve damage. **5 P's:** **p**ain, **p**allor, **p**aresthesia, **p**ulselessness, **p**aralysis.
Medial tibial stress syndrome	Also called shin splints. Common cause of shin pain and diffuse tenderness in runners and military recruits. Caused by bone resorption that outpaces bone formation in tibial cortex.
Plantar fasciitis	Inflammation of plantar aponeurosis characterized by heel pain (worse with first steps in the morning or after period of inactivity) and tenderness. Associated with obesity, prolonged standing or jumping (eg, dancers, runners), and flat feet. Heel spurs often coexist.
Temporomandibular disorders	Group of disorders that involve the temporomandibular joint (TMJ) and muscles of mastication. Multifactorial etiology; associated with TMJ trauma, poor head and neck posture, abnormal trigeminal nerve pain processing, psychological factors. Present with dull, constant unilateral facial pain that worsens with jaw movement, otalgia, headache, TMJ dysfunction (eg, limited range of motion).

Childhood musculoskeletal conditions

Radial head subluxation 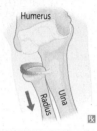	Also called nursemaid's elbow. Common elbow injury in children < 5 years. Caused by a sudden pull on the arm → immature annular ligament slips over head of radius. Injured arm held in slightly flexed and pronated position.
Osgood-Schlatter disease 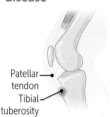	Also called traction apophysitis. Overuse injury caused by repetitive strain and chronic avulsion of the secondary ossification center of the tibial tuberosity. Occurs in adolescents after growth spurt. Common in athletes who run and jump. Presents with progressive anterior knee pain.
Patellofemoral syndrome 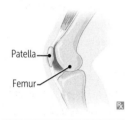	Overuse injury that commonly presents in young, female athletes as anterior knee pain. Exacerbated by prolonged sitting or weight-bearing on a flexed knee.
Developmental dysplasia of the hip	Abnormal acetabulum development in newborns. Risk factor is breech presentation. Results in hip instability/dislocation. Commonly tested with Ortolani and Barlow maneuvers (manipulation of newborn hip reveals a "clunk"). Confirmed via ultrasound (x-ray not used until ~4–6 months because cartilage is not ossified).
Legg-Calvé-Perthes disease	Idiopathic avascular necrosis of femoral head. Commonly presents between 5–7 years with insidious onset of hip pain that may cause child to limp. More common in males (4:1 ratio). Initial x-ray often normal.
Slipped capital femoral epiphysis 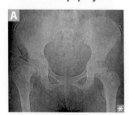	Classically presents in an obese young adolescent with hip/knee pain and altered gait. Increased axial force on femoral head → epiphysis displaces relative to femoral neck (like a scoop of ice cream slipping off a cone). Diagnosed via x-ray A.

Common pediatric fractures

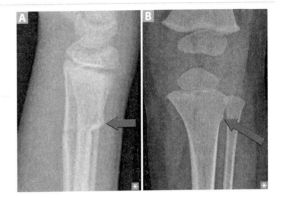

Greenstick fracture	Incomplete fracture extending partway through width of bone A following bending stress; bone fails on tension side; compression side intact (compare to torus fracture). Bone is bent like a **green twig**.
Torus (buckle) fracture	Axial force applied to immature bone → cortex buckles on compression (concave) side and fractures B. Tension (convex) side remains solid (intact).

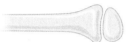
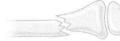

Normal   Complete fracture   Greenstick fracture   Torus fracture

Achondroplasia

Failure of longitudinal bone growth (endochondral ossification) → short limbs. Membranous ossification is not affected → large head relative to limbs. Constitutive activation of fibroblast growth factor receptor (FGFR3) actually inhibits chondrocyte proliferation. > 85% of mutations occur sporadically; autosomal dominant with full penetrance (homozygosity is lethal). Associated with ↑ paternal age. Most common cause of short-limbed dwarfism.

Osteoporosis

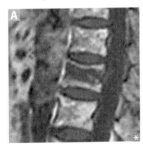

Trabecular (spongy) and cortical bone lose mass despite normal bone mineralization and lab values (serum Ca^{2+} and PO_4^{3-}).

Most commonly due to ↑ bone resorption (↑ osteoclast number and activity) related to ↓ estrogen levels, old age, and cigarette smoking. Can be 2° to drugs (eg, steroids, alcohol, anticonvulsants, anticoagulants, thyroid replacement therapy) or other conditions (eg, hyperparathyroidism, hyperthyroidism, multiple myeloma, malabsorption syndromes, anorexia), low BMI (or weight), and prolonged microgravity exposure (eg, space travel).

Diagnosed by bone mineral density measurement by DEXA (dual-energy x-ray absorptiometry) at the lumbar spine, total hip, and femoral neck, with a T-score of ≤ −2.5 or by a fragility fracture (eg, fall from standing height, minimal trauma) at hip or vertebra. One-time screening recommended in females ≥ 65 years old.

Prophylaxis: regular weight-bearing exercise and adequate Ca^{2+} and vitamin D intake throughout adulthood.

Treatment: bisphosphonates, teriparatide/ abaloparatide, SERMs, denosumab (monoclonal antibody against RANKL), romosozumab (sclerostin inhibitor).

Can lead to vertebral compression fractures A—acute back pain, loss of height, kyphosis. Also can present with fractures of femoral neck, distal radius (Colles fracture).

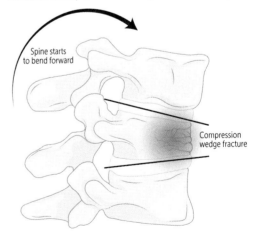

Spine starts to bend forward

Compression wedge fracture

Osteopetrosis

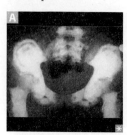

Failure of normal bone resorption due to defective osteoclasts → thickened, dense bones that are prone to fracture. Mutations (eg, carbonic anhydrase II) impair ability of osteoclast to generate acidic environment necessary for bone resorption. Overgrowth of cortical bone fills marrow space → pancytopenia, extramedullary hematopoiesis. Can result in cranial nerve impingement and palsies due to narrowed foramina.

X-rays show diffuse symmetric sclerosis (bone-in-bone, "stone bone" A). Bone marrow transplant is potentially curative as osteoclasts are derived from monocytes.

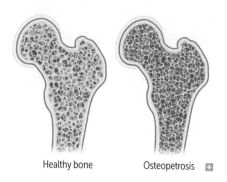

Healthy bone   Osteopetrosis ✦

Osteomalacia/rickets

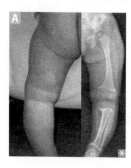

Defective mineralization of osteoid (osteomalacia) or cartilaginous growth plates (rickets, only in children). Most commonly due to vitamin D deficiency.

X-rays show osteopenia and pseudofractures in osteomalacia, epiphyseal widening and metaphyseal cupping/fraying in rickets. Children with rickets have pathologic bow legs (genu varum A), beadlike costochondral junctions (rachitic rosary B), craniotabes (soft skull).

↓ vitamin D → ↓ serum Ca^{2+} → ↑ PTH secretion → ↓ serum PO_4^{3-}.

Hyperactivity of osteoblasts → ↑ ALP.

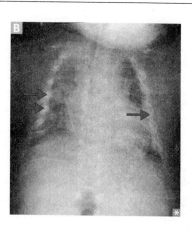

Osteitis deformans

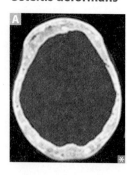

Also called Paget disease of bone. Common, localized disorder of bone remodeling caused by ↑ osteoclastic activity followed by ↑ osteoblastic activity that forms poor-quality bone. Serum Ca^{2+}, phosphorus, and PTH levels are normal. ↑ ALP. Mosaic pattern of woven and lamellar bone (osteocytes within lacunae in chaotic juxtapositions); long bone chalk-stick fractures. ↑ blood flow from ↑ arteriovenous shunts may cause high-output heart failure. ↑ risk of osteosarcoma.

Hat size can be increased due to skull thickening A ; hearing loss is common due to skull deformity.

Stages of Paget disease:
- Early destructive (lytic): osteoclasts
- Intermediate (mixed): osteoclasts + osteoblasts
- Late (sclerotic/blastic): osteoblasts

May enter quiescent phase.

Treatment: bisphosphonates.

Avascular necrosis of bone

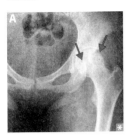

Infarction of bone and marrow, usually very painful. Most common site is femoral head (watershed area) 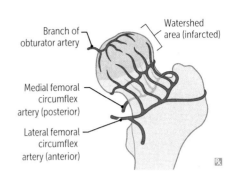 (due to insufficiency of medial circumflex femoral artery). Causes include glucoCorticoids, chronic Alcohol overuse, Sickle cell disease, Trauma, SLE, "the Bends" (caisson/decompression disease), LEgg-Calvé-Perthes disease (idiopathic), Gaucher disease, Slipped capital femoral epiphysis— CASTS Bend LEGS.

Lab values in bone disorders

DISORDER	SERUM Ca^{2+}	PO_4^{3-}	ALP	PTH	COMMENTS
Osteoporosis	—	—	—	—	↓ bone mass; if concurrent ↓ vitamin D → ↑ PTH with normal Ca^{2+}
Osteopetrosis	—/↓	—	—	—	Dense, brittle bones. Ca^{2+} ↓ in severe, malignant disease
Paget disease of bone	—	—	↑	—	Abnormal "mosaic" bone architecture
Osteitis fibrosa cystica					
Primary hyperparathyroidism	↑	↓	↑	↑	"Brown tumors" due to fibrous replacement of bone, subperiosteal thinning Idiopathic or parathyroid hyperplasia, adenoma, carcinoma
Secondary hyperparathyroidism	↓	↑	↑	↑	Often as compensation for CKD (↓ PO_4^{3-} excretion and production of activated vitamin D)
Osteomalacia/rickets	↓	↓	↑	↑	Soft bones; vitamin D deficiency also causes 2° hyperparathyroidism
Hypervitaminosis D	↑	↑	—	↓	Caused by oversupplementation or granulomatous disease (eg, sarcoidosis)

↑ ↓ = 1° change.

Primary bone tumors   Metastatic disease is more common than 1° bone tumors. Benign bone tumors end with -oma, those that start with a c and o are more common in boys. Malignant tumors usually have the ending "-sarcoma".

TUMOR TYPE	EPIDEMIOLOGY	LOCATION	CHARACTERISTICS
Benign tumors			
Osteochondroma (exostosis)	Most common benign bone tumor. Males < 25 years old.	Metaphysis of long bones (most common around knee—distal femur).	Lateral bony projection of growth plate (continuous with marrow space) covered by cartilaginous cap **A**; points away from joint. *EXT1* or *EXT2* gene mutation—hereditary multiple exostoses. Rarely transforms to chondrosarcoma.
Osteoma	Middle age.	Surface of facial bones.	Associated with Gardner syndrome.
Osteoid osteoma	Adults < 25 years old. Males > females.	Cortex of long bones.	Classically presents as bone pain (worse at night) caused by prostaglandins; thus relieved by NSAIDs (vs osteoblastoma). Bony mass (< 1.5 cm) with radiolucent osteoid core **B**.
Osteoblastoma	Males > females.	Vertebrae.	Similar histology to osteoid osteoma Larger size (> 2 cm); pain unresponsive to NSAIDs. X-ray similar to aneurysmal bone cyst.
Giant cell tumor	20–40 years old. Females > males.	Epiphysis of long bones after skeletal maturation (often in knee region), radiographic epicenter is metaphysis.	Locally aggressive benign tumor neoplastic mononuclear cells that express RANKL and reactive multinucleated giant (osteoclastlike) cells; "osteoclastoma". "Soap bubble" appearance on x-ray **C**.
Chondroblastoma	Adolescents. Males > females.	Epiphysis of long bones before skeletal maturation (often in knee region).	May complain of joint pain. Cross physis on x-ray.

Primary bone tumors (continued)

TUMOR TYPE	EPIDEMIOLOGY	LOCATION	CHARACTERISTICS
Malignant tumors			
Osteosarcoma (osteogenic sarcoma)	Accounts for 20% of 1° bone cancers. Peak incidence of 1° tumor in males < 20 years. Less common in older adults; usually 2° to predisposing factors, such as Paget disease of bone, bone infarcts, radiation, familial retinoblastoma, Li-Fraumeni syndrome.	Metaphysis of long bones (often in knee region).	Pleomorphic osteoid-producing cells (malignant osteoblasts). Presents as painful enlarging mass or pathologic fractures. Codman triangle **D** (from elevation of periosteum) or **sun**burst pattern on x-ray **E** (think of an **osteocod** [bone fish] swimming in the **sun**). Aggressive. 1° usually responsive to treatment (surgery, chemotherapy), poor prognosis for 2°.
Chondrosarcoma	Most common in adults > 50 years old.	Medulla of pelvis, proximal femur and humerus.	Tumor of malignant chondrocytes. Lytic (> 50%) cases with intralesional calcifications, endosteal erosion, cortex breach.
Ewing sarcoma	Most common in White patients, generally males < 15 years old.	Diaphysis of long bones (especially femur), pelvic flat bones.	Anaplastic small blue cells of neuroectodermal (mesenchymal) origin (resemble lymphocytes) **F**. Differentiate from conditions with similar morphology (eg, lymphoma, chronic osteomyelitis) by testing for t(11;22) (fusion protein EWS-FLI1). "Onion skin" periosteal reaction. Aggressive with early metastases, but responsive to chemotherapy. 11 + 22 = 33 (Patrick **Ewing**'s jersey number).

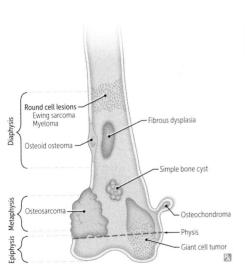

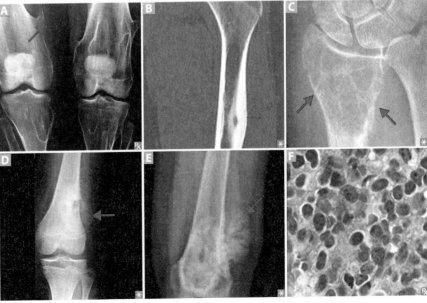

Osteoarthritis vs rheumatoid arthritis

	Osteoarthritis A	Rheumatoid arthritis B
PATHOGENESIS	Chronic mechanical stress destroys articular cartilage → inflammation with inadequate repair (mediated by chondrocytes).	Autoimmune—inflammation C induces formation of proliferative granulation tissue, eroding articular cartilage and bone.
PREDISPOSING FACTORS	Age, female, obesity, joint trauma.	Female, HLA-DR4 (**4**-walled "**rheum**"), HLA-DRB1, smoking. ⊕ rheumatoid factor (IgM antibody that targets IgG Fc; in 80%), anti-cyclic citrullinated peptide antibody (more specific).
PRESENTATION	Pain in weight-bearing joints after use, improving with rest. Asymmetric involvement. No systemic symptoms.	Pain, swelling, and morning stiffness lasting > 1 hour, improving with use. Symmetric involvement. Systemic symptoms (fever, fatigue, weight loss). Extraarticular manifestations.*
JOINT FINDINGS	Osteophytes (bone spurs), joint space narrowing (asymmetric), subchondral sclerosis and cysts, loose bodies. Synovial fluid noninflammatory (WBC < 2000/mm³). Development of Heberden nodes D (at DIP) and Bouchard nodes E (at PIP), and 1st CMC.	Erosions, juxta-articular osteopenia, soft tissue swelling, subchondral cysts, joint space narrowing (symmetric). Deformities: cervical subluxation, ulnar finger deviation, swan neck F, boutonniere G. Involves MCP, PIP, wrist.
TREATMENT	Activity modification, NSAIDs, intra-articular glucocorticoids (use for short-term relief in symptomatic patients; long-term therapy associated with many adverse effects).	NSAIDs, glucocorticoids, disease-modifying agents (eg, methotrexate, sulfasalazine), biologic agents (eg, TNF-α inhibitors).

*Cervical subluxation, rheumatoid nodules (fibrinoid necrosis with palisading histiocytes) in subcutaneous tissue and lung (+ pneumoconiosis = Caplan syndrome), interstitial lung disease, pleuritis, pericarditis, anemia of chronic disease, neutropenia + splenomegaly (Felty syndrome: **SANTA**—**S**plenomegaly, **A**nemia, **N**eutropenia, **T**hrombocytopenia, **A**rthritis [Rheumatoid]), AA amyloidosis, Sjögren syndrome, scleritis, carpal tunnel syndrome.

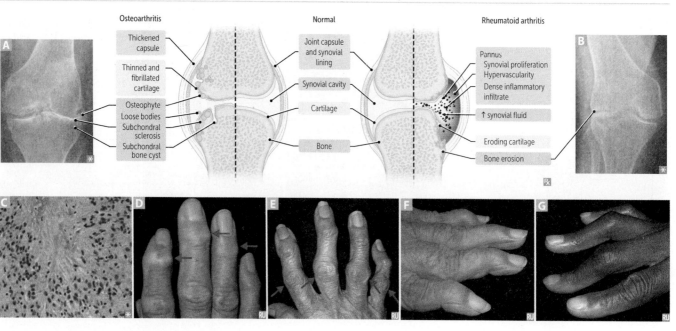

Gout

FINDINGS

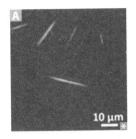

Acute inflammatory monoarthritis caused by precipitation of monosodium urate crystals in joints. Risk factors: male sex, hypertension, obesity, diabetes, dyslipidemia, alcohol use. Strongest risk factor is hyperuricemia, which can be caused by:

- Underexcretion of uric acid (90% of patients)—largely idiopathic, potentiated by renal failure; can be exacerbated by certain medications (eg, thiazide diuretics).
- Overproduction of uric acid (10% of patients)—Lesch-Nyhan syndrome, PRPP excess, ↑ cell turnover (eg, tumor lysis syndrome).
- Combined mechanism—alcohol use and von Gierke disease.

Crystals are needle shaped and ⊖ birefringent under polarized light (yellow under parallel light, blue under perpendicular light). Serum uric acid levels may be normal during an acute attack.

SYMPTOMS

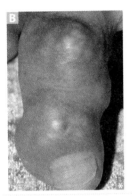

Asymmetric joint distribution. Joint is swollen, red, and painful. Classic manifestation is painful MTP joint of big toe (podagra). Tophus formation B (often on external ear, olecranon bursa, or Achilles tendon). Acute attack tends to occur after a large meal with foods rich in purines (eg, red meat, seafood), trauma, surgery, dehydration, diuresis, or alcohol consumption (↑ blood lactate from metabolism → ↑ resorption of uric acid → hyperuricemia).

TREATMENT

Acute: NSAIDs (eg, indomethacin), glucocorticoids, colchicine.

Chronic (preventive): allopurinol, probenecid.

For overproducers: urate lowering therapies such as xanthine oxidase inhibitors (eg, allopurinol, febuxostat).

Calcium pyrophosphate deposition disease

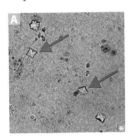

Formerly called pseudogout. Deposition of calcium pyrophosphate crystals within the joint space. Occurs in patients > 50 years old; both sexes affected equally. Usually idiopathic, sometimes associated with hemochromatosis, hyperparathyroidism, joint trauma.

Pain and swelling with acute inflammation (pseudogout) and/or chronic degeneration (pseudo-osteoarthritis). Most commonly affected joint is the knee.

Chondrocalcinosis (cartilage calcification) on x-ray.

Crystals are rhomboid and weakly ⊕ birefringent under polarized light (blue when parallel to light) A.

Acute treatment: NSAIDs, colchicine, glucocorticoids.

Prophylaxis: colchicine.

The **blue P's** of CPPD—**blue** (when parallel), positive birefringence, calcium pyrophosphate, pseudogout.

Systemic juvenile idiopathic arthritis	Systemic arthritis seen in < 16 years of age. Usually presents with daily spiking fevers, salmon-pink macular rash, arthritis (commonly 2+ joints). Associated with anterior uveitis. Frequently presents with leukocytosis, thrombocytosis, anemia, ↑ ESR, ↑ CRP.

Sjögren syndrome 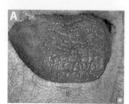	Autoimmune disorder characterized by destruction of exocrine glands (especially lacrimal and salivary) by lymphocytic infiltrates. Predominantly affects females 40–60 years old. Findings: ◦ Inflammatory joint pain ◦ Keratoconjunctivitis sicca (decreased tear production and subsequent corneal damage) → gritty or sandy feeling in eyes ◦ Xerostomia (↓ saliva production) → mucosal atrophy, fissuring of the tongue 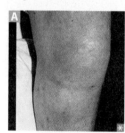 ◦ Presence of antinuclear antibodies, rheumatoid factor (can be positive in the absence of rheumatoid arthritis), antiribonucleoprotein antibodies: SS-A (anti-Ro) and/or SS-B (anti-La) ◦ Dyspareunia ◦ Bilateral parotid enlargement Anti-SSA and anti-SSB may also be seen in SLE.

A common 1° disorder or a 2° syndrome associated with other autoimmune disorders (eg, rheumatoid arthritis, SLE, systemic sclerosis).

Complications: dental caries; mucosa-associated lymphoid tissue (MALT) lymphoma (may present as parotid enlargement); ↑ risk of giving birth to baby with neonatal lupus.

Focal lymphocytic sialadenitis on labial salivary gland biopsy can confirm diagnosis.

Septic arthritis	*S aureus*, *Streptococcus*, and *Neisseria gonorrhoeae* are common causes. Usually monoarticular. Affected joint is often swollen, red, and painful. Synovial fluid purulent (WBC > 50,000/mm³). Complications: osteomyelitis, chronic pain, irreversible joint damage, sepsis. Treatment: antibiotics, aspiration, and drainage (+/– debridement) to prevent irreversible joint damage. Disseminated gonococcal infection—STI that presents as either purulent arthritis (eg, knee) or triad of polyarthralgia, tenosynovitis (eg, hand), dermatitis (eg, pustules).

Osteomyelitis	Chronic or acute infection of the bone; *S aureus* most common (overall), *S epidermidis* (prosthetics), *Salmonella* (sickle cell anemia), *P aeruginosa* (plantar puncture wounds). Spread is commonly hematogenous (usually in children, affecting the metaphysis of the long bones) or exogenous (usually in adults, post-traumatic, iatrogenic, or spread from nearby tissues). Pain, redness, swelling, fever, limping are common. Diagnosis: x-ray (bone destruction and periosteal elevation if chronic), MRI, bone biopsy with cultures and blood cultures. Treatment: antibiotics (+/– surgery).

Seronegative spondyloarthritis	Arthritis without rheumatoid factor (no anti-IgG antibody). Strong association with HLA-B27 (MHC class I serotype). Subtypes (**PAIR**) share variable occurrence of inflammatory back pain (associated with morning stiffness, improves with exercise), peripheral arthritis, enthesitis (inflamed insertion sites of tendons, eg, Achilles), dactylitis ("sausage fingers"), uveitis.	
Psoriatic arthritis	Associated with skin psoriasis and nail lesions. Asymmetric and patchy involvement A. Dactylitis and "pencil-in-cup" deformity of DIP on x-ray B.	Seen in fewer than 1/3 of patients with psoriasis.
Ankylosing spondylitis	Symmetric involvement of spine and sacroiliac joints → ankylosis (joint fusion), uveitis, aortic regurgitation.	Bamboo spine (vertebral fusion) C. Costovertebral and costosternal ankylosis may cause restrictive lung disease. More common in males, with age of onset usually 20–40 years.
Inflammatory bowel disease	Crohn disease and ulcerative colitis are often associated with spondyloarthritis.	
Reactive arthritis	Classic triad: <ul><li>Conjunctivitis</li><li>Urethritis</li><li>Arthritis</li></ul> Commonly associated with hyperkeratotic skin lesions in the palms and soles (keratoderma blennorrhagica).	"Can't see, can't pee, can't bend my knee." Associated with infections by *Shigella*, *Campylobacter*, *Salmonella*, *Chlamydia*, *Yersinia*. "She Caught Students Cheating Yesterday and overreacted."

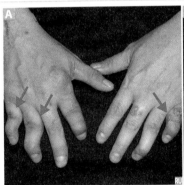
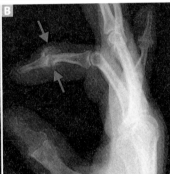
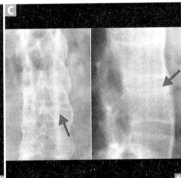

Systemic lupus erythematosus

Systemic, remitting, and relapsing autoimmune disease. Organ damage primarily due to a type III hypersensitivity reaction and, to a lesser degree, a type II hypersensitivity reaction. Associated with deficiency of early complement proteins (eg, C1q, C4, C2) → ↓ clearance of immune complexes. Classic presentation: facial rash (spares nasolabial folds), joint pain, and fever in a female of reproductive age. ↑ prevalence in Black, Caribbean, Asian, and Hispanic populations in the US.

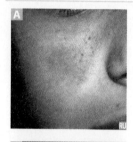

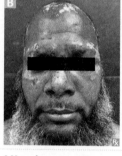

Libman-Sacks Endocarditis (**LSE** in **SLE**).

Lupus nephritis (glomerular deposition of DNA-anti-DNA immune complexes) can be nephritic or nephrotic (causing hematuria or proteinuria). Most common and severe type is diffuse proliferative.

Common causes of death in SLE: renal disease, infections, cardiovascular disease (accelerated CAD). Lupus patients die with redness in their cheeks.

In an anti-SSA ⊕ pregnant patient, ↑ risk of newborn developing neonatal lupus → congenital heart block, periorbital/diffuse rash, transaminitis, and cytopenias at birth.

RASH OR PAIN:
Rash (malar 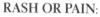 or discoid B)
Arthritis (nonerosive)
Serositis (eg, pleuritis, pericarditis)
Hematologic disorders (eg, cytopenias)
Oral/nasopharyngeal ulcers (usually painless)
Renal disease
Photosensitivity
Antinuclear antibodies
Immunologic disorder (anti-dsDNA, anti-Sm, antiphospholipid)
Neurologic disorders (eg, seizures, psychosis)

Mixed connective tissue disease

Features of SLE, systemic sclerosis, and/or polymyositis. Associated with anti-U1 RNP antibodies (speckled ANA).

Antiphospholipid syndrome

1° or 2° autoimmune disorder (most commonly in SLE).

Diagnosed based on clinical criteria including history of thrombosis (arterial or venous) or recurrent abortion along with laboratory findings of lupus anticoagulant, anticardiolipin, anti-β_2 glycoprotein I antibodies.

Treatment: systemic anticoagulation.

Anticardiolipin antibodies can cause false-positive VDRL/RPR.

Lupus anticoagulant can cause prolonged PTT that is not corrected by the addition of normal platelet-free plasma.

Polymyalgia rheumatica

SYMPTOMS	Pain and stiffness in proximal muscles (eg, shoulders, hips), often with fever, malaise, weight loss. Does not cause muscular weakness. More common in females > 50 years old; associated with giant cell (temporal) arteritis.
FINDINGS	↑ ESR, ↑ CRP, normal CK.
TREATMENT	Rapid response to low-dose glucocorticoids.

Fibromyalgia

Most common in females 20–50 years old. Chronic, widespread musculoskeletal pain associated with "tender points," stiffness, paresthesias, poor sleep, fatigue, cognitive disturbance ("fibro fog"). Normal inflammatory markers like ESR. Treatment: regular exercise, antidepressants (TCAs, SNRIs), neuropathic pain agents (eg, gabapentinoids).

Polymyositis/dermatomyositis

Nonspecific: ⊕ ANA, ↑ CK. Specific: ⊕ anti-Jo-1 (histidyl-tRNA synthetase), ⊕ anti-SRP (signal recognition particle), ⊕ anti-Mi-2 (helicase).

Polymyositis

Progressive symmetric proximal muscle weakness, characterized by endomysial inflammation with CD8+ T cells. Most often involves shoulders.

Dermatomyositis

Clinically similar to polymyositis, but also involves Gottron papules A, photodistributed facial erythema (eg, heliotrope [violaceous] edema of the eyelids B), "shawl and face" rash C, mechanic's hands (thickening, cracking, irregular "dirty"-appearing marks due to hyperkeratosis of digital skin D. ↑ risk of occult malignancy. Perimysial inflammation and atrophy with CD4+ T cells.

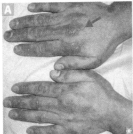 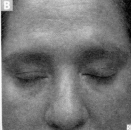 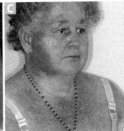 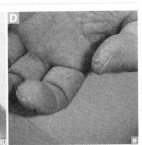

Myositis ossificans

Heterotopic ossification involving skeletal muscle (eg, quadriceps). Associated with blunt muscle trauma. Presents as painful soft tissue mass. Imaging: eggshell calcification. Histology: metaplastic bone surrounding area of fibroblastic proliferation. Benign, but may be mistaken for sarcoma.

IgG4-related disease

Immune-mediated spectrum of conditions, characterized by fibrosis and lymphoplasmacytic infiltrate, that can affect multiple organs. Patients usually have elevated serum IgG4 levels.
Most common IgG4-related conditions are:
- Sialadenitis and dacryoadenitis
- Riedel thyroiditis
- Autoimmune pancreatitis
- Autoimmune aortitis (may lead to TAA, AAA)
- Retroperitoneal fibrosis (may affect the ureters and present with signs of acute kidney injury/CKD and/or hydronephrosis)

Vasculitides	Inflammation and necrosis of blood vessels; either idiopathic or immune mediated (type III hypersensitivity).		
	EPIDEMIOLOGY	PRESENTATION/PATHOPHYSIOLOGY	NOTES
Large-vessel vasculitis			
Giant cell (temporal) arteritis	Females > 50 years old.	Unilateral headache, jaw claudication, temporal artery tenderness, blindness risk (due to anterior ischemic optic neuropathy). Granulomatous inflammation Ⓐ; affects temporal, vertebral, and ophthalmic arteries.	Associated with polymyalgia rheumatica. ↑↑ ESR/CRP; temporal artery biopsy. Treatment: high-dose glucocorticoids before biopsy.
Takayasu arteritis	Asian females < 40 years old.	"Pulseless disease" (weak upper extremity pulses), fever, night sweats, arthritis, myalgias. Granulomatous thickening and narrowing of aortic arch and proximal great vessels Ⓑ.	↑ ESR. Treatment: glucocorticoids.
Medium-vessel vasculitis			
Buerger disease (thromboangiitis obliterans)	Heavy tobacco smoking history, males < 40 years old.	Leading to intermittent claudication, risk of gangrene Ⓒ, Raynaud phenomenon, autoamputation of digits, or superficial nodular phlebitis.	Segmental thrombosing vasculitis with vein and nerve involvement. Treatment: smoking cessation.
Kawasaki disease	Asian children < 4 years old.	Bilateral nonexudative **C**onjunctivitis, **R**ash (polymorphous → desquamating), **A**denopathy (cervical), **S**trawberry tongue (oral mucositis) Ⓓ, **H**and-foot changes (edema, erythema), **fever** (≥ 5 days).	**CRASH** and **burn** on a **Kawasaki**. Complications: coronary artery aneurysms Ⓔ; thrombosis or rupture can cause death. Treatment: IV immunoglobulin and aspirin.
Polyarteritis nodosa	Middle-aged males; 30% with hepatitis B seropositivity.	Fever, weight loss, abdominal pain, melena, hypertension, neurologic dysfunction, cutaneous eruptions, renal damage. Involves renal and visceral vessels, spares lungs; transmural inflammation with fibrinoid necrosis.	"String of pearls" appearance due to microaneurysms on arteriogram Ⓕ. Treatment: glucocorticoids, cyclophosphamide. PAN usually affects the **SKIN**: Skin, Kidneys, Intestines (GI), Nerves.
Small-vessel vasculitis (MPO-ANCA/p-ANCA)			
Microscopic polyangiitis	Typically affects middle-aged adults.	Necrotizing vasculitis involving lungs, kidneys, and skin. Pauci-immune glomerulonephritis (GN) Ⓖ and palpable purpura.	MPO-ANCA/p-ANCA (anti-myeloperoxidase). Treatment: cyclophosphamide, glucocorticoids.
Eosinophilic granulomatosis with polyangiitis		Combination of asthma, eosinophilia, and systemic vasculitis. Eosinophilic infiltration → inflammation → peripheral neuropathy.	Formerly called Churg-Strauss syndrome. Granulomatous, necrotizing vasculitis with eosinophilia Ⓗ. ↑ IgE level.

Vasculitides (continued)

	EPIDEMIOLOGY	PRESENTATION/PATHOPHYSIOLOGY	NOTES
Small-vessel vasculitis (c-ANCA)			
Granulomatosis with polyangiitis	Affects males and females equally, typically middle-aged adults.	Triad: lung, vessels, and renal involvement. Upper respiratory (nasal septum perforation, chronic sinusitis, otitis media, mastoiditis), lower respiratory (hemoptysis, dyspnea), renal (pauci-immune rapidly progressive GN).	c-ANCA ▉ (PR3-ANCA). Treatment: glucocorticoids combined with rituximab, cyclophosphamide.
Small-vessel vasculitis (immune complex mediated)			
Hypocomplementemic urticarial vasculitis (anti-C1q vasculitis)	Often associated with SLE.	Presents as urticaria, purpuric rash, arthralgias, stomach pain, lung or ocular manifestations.	Labs show ↓ C1q complement and ↑ anti-C1q antibodies.
Mixed cryoglobulinemia	Often due to viral infections, especially HCV.	Triad of palpable purpura, weakness, arthralgias. May involve peripheral neuropathy and renal disease (eg, GN).	Cryoglobulins precipitate in the cold (mixed IgG and IgM immune complex deposition).
Immunoglobulin A vasculitis	Most common childhood vasculitis often follows URI.	Vasculitis 2° to IgA immune complex deposition. Classic triad: Hinge pain (arthralgias), stomach pain (abdominal pain associated with intussusception, palpable purpura on buttocks/legs ▉.	Formerly called Henoch-Schönlein purpura. Associated with IgA nephropathy (Berger disease). Treatment: supportive care, glucocorticoids.
Cutaneous small-vessel vasculitis		Palpable purpura, no visceral involvement. Immune complex–mediated leukocytoclastic vasculitis; late involvement indicates systemic.	Occurs 7–10 days after medication use (penicillins, cephalosporins, sulfonamides, phenytoin, allopurinol) or infections (eg, HCV, HIV).
All-vessel vasculitis			
Behçet syndrome	↑ incidence in Turkish, Eastern Mediterranean descent.	Recurrent oral and genital ulcers, uveitis, erythema nodosum. Triggered by HSV or parvovirus. Flares last 1–4 weeks.	Associated with HLA-B51.

Neuromuscular junction diseases

	Myasthenia gravis	Lambert-Eaton myasthenic syndrome
FREQUENCY	Most common NMJ disorder	Uncommon
PATHOPHYSIOLOGY	Autoantibodies to **post**synaptic ACh receptor	Autoantibodies to **pre**synaptic Ca^{2+} channel → ↓ ACh release; **L** comes before **M**
CLINICAL	Fatigable muscle weakness—ptosis; diplopia; proximal weakness; respiratory muscle involvement → dyspnea; bulbar muscle involvement → dysphagia, difficulty chewing Spared reflexes Worsens with muscle use	Proximal muscle weakness, autonomic symptoms (dry mouth, constipation, impotence) Hyporeflexia Improves with muscle use
ASSOCIATED WITH	Thymoma, thymic hyperplasia	Small cell lung cancer
AChE INHIBITOR ADMINISTRATION	Reverses symptoms (pyridostigmine for treatment)	Minimal effect

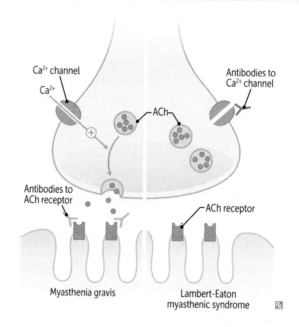

Raynaud phenomenon

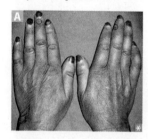

↓ blood flow to skin due to arteriolar (small vessel) vasospasm in response to cold or stress: color change from white (ischemia) to blue (hypoxia) to red (reperfusion). Most often in the fingers A and toes. Called Raynaud disease when 1° (idiopathic), Raynaud syndrome when 2° to a disease process such as mixed connective tissue disease, SLE, or CREST syndrome (limited form of systemic sclerosis). Digital ulceration (critical ischemia) seen in 2° Raynaud syndrome. Treat with calcium channel blockers.

Scleroderma

Systemic sclerosis. Triad of autoimmunity, noninflammatory vasculopathy, and collagen deposition with fibrosis. Commonly sclerosis of skin, manifesting as puffy, taut skin 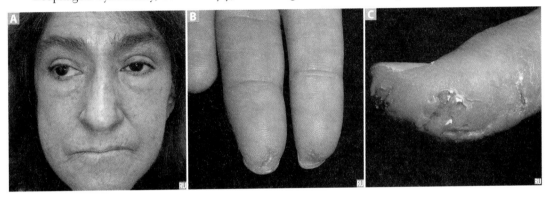 without wrinkles, fingertip pitting B. Can involve other systems, eg, renal (scleroderma renal crisis; treat with ACE inhibitors), pulmonary (interstitial fibrosis, pulmonary HTN), GI (↓ peristalsis and LES tone → dysphagia, heartburn), cardiovascular. 75% female. 2 major types:

- **Diffuse scleroderma**—widespread skin involvement, rapid progression, early visceral involvement. Associated with anti-Scl-70 antibody (anti-DNA topoisomerase-I antibody) and anti-RNA polymerase III.

- **Limited scleroderma**—limited skin involvement confined to fingers and face. Also with CREST syndrome: Calcinosis cutis C, anti-Centromere antibody, Raynaud phenomenon, Esophageal dysmotility, Sclerodactyly, and Telangiectasia. More benign clinical course.

▶ MUSCULOSKELETAL, SKIN, AND CONNECTIVE TISSUE—DERMATOLOGY

Skin layers

Skin has 3 layers: epidermis, dermis, subcutaneous fat (hypodermis, subcutis).
Epidermal layers: come, let's get sunburned.

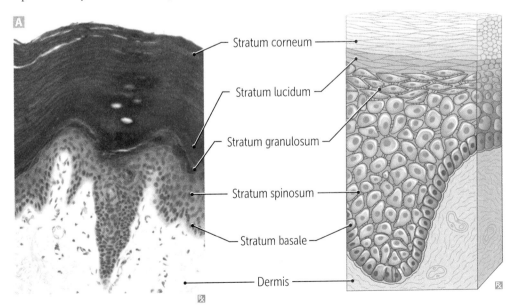

- Stratum corneum
- Stratum lucidum
- Stratum granulosum
- Stratum spinosum
- Stratum basale
- Dermis

Epithelial cell junctions

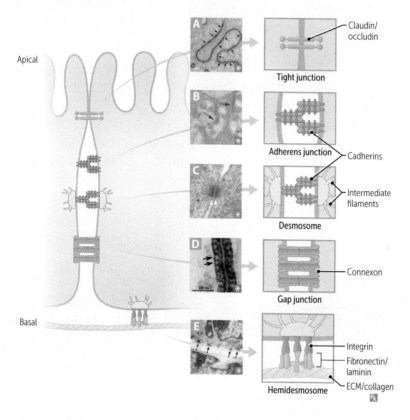

Tight junctions (zonula occludens) **A**–prevents paracellular movement of solutes; composed of claudins and occludins.

Adherens junction (belt desmosome, zonula adherens) **B**–forms "belt" connecting actin cytoskeletons of adjacent cells with **cadherins** (Ca^{2+}-dependent **adhesion** proteins). Loss of E-cadherin promotes metastasis.

Desmosome (spot desmosome, macula adherens) **C**–structural support via intermediate filament interactions. Autoantibodies to desmoglein 3 +/– desmoglein 1 → pemphigus vulgaris.

Gap junction **D**–channel proteins called connexons permit electrical and chemical communication between cells.

Hemidesmosome **E**–connects keratin in basal cells to underlying basement membrane. Autoantibodies → **bullous** pemphigoid. (Hemidesmosomes are down "**bullow**.")

Integrins–membrane proteins that maintain **integrity** of basolateral membrane by binding to collagen, laminin, and fibronectin in basement membrane.

Exocrine glands

Glands that produce substances other than hormones (vs endocrine glands, which secrete hormones) that are released through ducts to the exterior of the body. Can be merocrine (eg, salivary and sweat glands), apocrine (eg, mammary glands), or holocrine (eg, sebaceous glands).

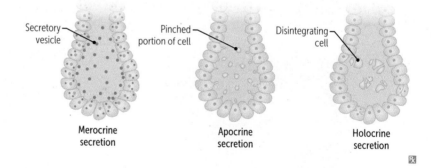

Dermatologic macroscopic terms

LESION	CHARACTERISTICS	EXAMPLES
Macule	Flat lesion with well-circumscribed change in skin color < 1 cm	Freckle (ephelis), labial macule **A**
Patch	Macule > 1 cm	Vitiligo **B**
Papule	Elevated solid skin lesion < 1 cm	Neurofibroma **C**, acne
Plaque	Papule > 1 cm	Psoriasis **D**
Vesicle	Small fluid-containing blister < 1 cm	Chickenpox (varicella), shingles (zoster) **E**
Bulla	Large fluid-containing blister > 1 cm	Bullous pemphigoid **F**
Pustule	Vesicle containing pus	Pustular psoriasis **G**
Wheal	Transient smooth papule or plaque	Hives (urticaria) **H**
Scale	Flaking off of stratum corneum	Eczema, psoriasis, SCC **I**
Crust	Dry exudate	Impetigo **J**
Ulcer	Epidermal loss leading to exposure of the basement membrane and underlying structures (ie, dermis, muscle, bone, or tendon)	Arterial ulcer, decubitus ulcer, leprosy
Erosion	Partial or full loss of epidermis without exposure of the basement membrane	Can be seen in GERD; erosive esophagitis

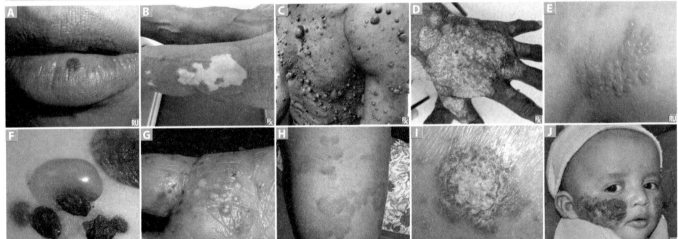

Dermatologic microscopic terms

LESION	CHARACTERISTICS	EXAMPLES
Dyskeratosis	Abnormal premature keratinization	Squamous cell carcinoma
Hyperkeratosis	↑ thickness of stratum corneum	Psoriasis, calluses
Parakeratosis	Retention of nuclei in stratum corneum	Psoriasis, actinic keratosis
Hypergranulosis	↑ thickness of stratum granulosum	Lichen planus
Spongiosis	Epidermal accumulation of edematous fluid in intercellular spaces	Eczematous dermatitis
Acantholysis	Separation of epidermal cells	Pemphigus vulgaris
Acanthosis	Epidermal hyperplasia (↑ spinosum)	Acanthosis nigricans, psoriasis

Pigmented skin disorders

Albinism	Normal melanocyte number with ↓ melanin production 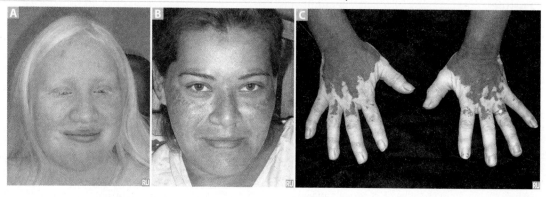 due to ↓ tyrosinase activity or defective tyrosine transport. ↑ risk of skin cancer.
Melasma (chloasma)	Acquired hyperpigmentation associated with pregnancy ("mask of pregnancy" 🅱) or OCP use. More common in patients with darker skin tones.
Vitiligo	Irregular patches of complete depigmentation 🅲. Caused by destruction of melanocytes (believed to be autoimmune). Associated with other autoimmune disorders.
Waardenburg syndrome	Patchy depigmentation of skin, hair, and irises that can be associated with deafness. Caused by defects in the differentiation of neural crest cells into melanocytes.

Seborrheic dermatitis

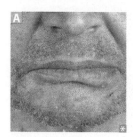

Erythematous, well-demarcated plaques 🄰 with greasy yellow scales in areas rich in sebaceous glands, such as scalp, face, and periocular region. Common in both infants (cradle cap) and adults. Extensive disease may be associated with HIV infection and Parkinson disease. Sebaceous glands are not inflamed, but play a role in disease development. Possibly associated with *Malassezia* spp. Treatment: topical antifungals and glucocorticoids.

Common skin disorders

Acne	Multifactorial etiology—↑ sebum/androgen production, abnormal keratinocyte desquamation, *Cutibacterium acnes* colonization of the pilosebaceous unit (comedones), and inflammation (papules/pustules A, nodules, cysts). Treatment: retinoids, benzoyl peroxide, and antibiotics.
Atopic dermatitis (eczema)	Pruritic eruption associated with ichthyosis vulgaris and other atopic diseases (asthma, allergic rhinitis, food allergies); ↑ serum IgE. Often appears on face in infancy B and then on flexural surfaces C in children and adults.
Allergic contact dermatitis	Type IV hypersensitivity reaction secondary to contact allergen (eg, nickel D, poison ivy E, neomycin).
Keratosis pilaris	Follicular-based papules F from keratin plugging, most often on extensor surfaces of arms and thighs.
Melanocytic nevus	Common mole. Benign, but melanoma can arise in congenital or atypical moles. Intradermal nevi are papular G. Junctional nevi are flat macules H.
Pseudofolliculitis barbae	Inflammatory reaction to hair penetrating the skin characterized by firm papules and pustules that are painful and pruritic. Commonly occurs near jawline as a result of shaving ("razor bumps"), more common with naturally curly hair.
Psoriasis	Papules and plaques with silvery scaling, especially on knees and elbows. Acanthosis with parakeratotic scaling (nuclei still in stratum corneum), Munro microabscesses. ↑ stratum spinosum, ↓ stratum granulosum. Auspitz sign (I)—pinpoint bleeding spots from exposure of dermal papillae when scales are scraped off. Associated with nail pitting and psoriatic arthritis.
Rosacea	Inflammatory facial skin disorder characterized by erythematous papules and pustules J, but no comedones. May be associated with facial flushing in response to external stimuli (eg, alcohol, heat). Complications include ocular involvement, rhinophyma (bulbous deformation of nose).
Seborrheic keratosis	Well-demarcated, verrucous, benign squamous epithelial proliferation of immature keratinocytes with keratin-filled cysts (horn cysts) K. Looks "stuck on." Leser-Trélat sign L—rapid onset of multiple seborrheic keratoses, indicates possible malignancy (eg, GI adenocarcinoma).
Verrucae	Warts; caused by low-risk HPV strains. Soft, tan-colored, cauliflowerlike papules M. Epidermal hyperplasia, hyperkeratosis, koilocytosis. Condyloma acuminatum on anus or genitals N.
Urticaria	Hives. Pruritic wheals that form after mast cell degranulation O. Characterized by superficial dermal edema and lymphatic channel dilation.

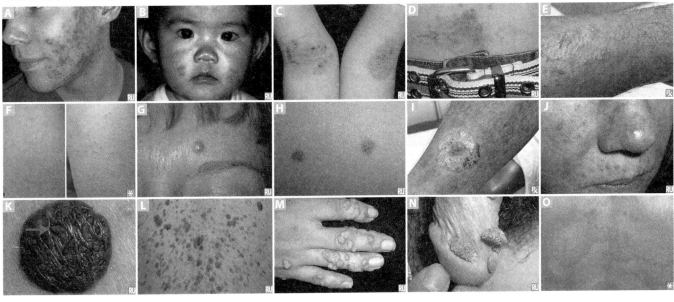

Vascular tumors of skin

Angiosarcoma	Rare blood vessel malignancy typically occurring in the head, neck, and breast areas. Usually in older adults, on sun-exposed areas. Associated with radiation therapy and chronic postmastectomy lymphedema. Stewart-Treves syndrome—cutaneous angiosarcoma developing after chronic lymphedema. Hepatic angiosarcoma associated with vinyl chloride and arsenic exposures. Very aggressive and difficult to resect due to delay in diagnosis.
Bacillary angiomatosis	Benign capillary skin papules **A** found in patients with AIDS. Caused by *Bartonella* infections. Frequently mistaken for Kaposi sarcoma, but has neutrophilic infiltrate.
Cherry angioma	Benign capillary hemangioma **B** commonly appearing in middle-aged adults. Does not regress. Frequency ↑ with age.
Glomus tumor	Benign, painful, red-blue tumor, commonly under fingernails **C**. Arises from modified smooth muscle cells of the thermoregulatory glomus body.
Kaposi sarcoma	Endothelial malignancy most commonly affecting the skin, mouth, GI tract, respiratory tract. Classically seen in older Eastern European males, patients with AIDS, and organ transplant patients. Associated with HHV-8 and HIV. Lymphocytic infiltrate, unlike bacillary angiomatosis.
Pyogenic granuloma	Polypoid lobulated capillary hemangioma **D** that can ulcerate and bleed. Associated with trauma and pregnancy.
Infantile hemangioma	Benign capillary hemangioma of infancy **E**. Appears in first few weeks of life (1/200 births); initially grows rapidly, then involutes starting at age 1. Infantile hemangiomas spontaneously involute; cherry angiomas cannot.

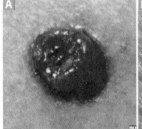 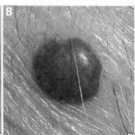 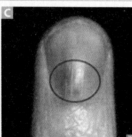 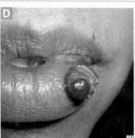 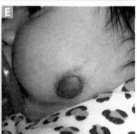

Skin infections

Bacterial infections

Impetigo	Skin infection involving superficial epidermis. Usually from S aureus or S pyogenes. Highly contagious. Honey-colored crusting A. Bullous impetigo B has bullae and is usually caused by S aureus.
Erysipelas	Infection involving upper dermis and superficial lymphatics, usually from S pyogenes. Presents with well-defined, raised demarcation between infected and normal skin C.
Cellulitis	Acute, painful, spreading infection of deeper dermis and subcutaneous tissues. Usually from S pyogenes or S aureus. Often starts with a break in skin from trauma or another infection D.
Abscess	Collection of pus from a walled-off infection within deeper layers of skin E. Offending organism is almost always S aureus.
Necrotizing fasciitis	Deeper tissue injury, usually from anaerobic bacteria or S pyogenes. Pain may be out of proportion to exam findings. Results in crepitus from methane and CO_2 production. "Flesh-eating bacteria." Causes bullae and skin necrosis → violaceous color of bullae, surrounding skin F. Surgical emergency.
Staphylococcal scalded skin syndrome	Exotoxin destroys keratinocyte attachments in stratum granulosum only (vs toxic epidermal necrolysis, which destroys epidermal-dermal junction). No mucosal involvement. Characterized by fever and generalized erythematous rash with sloughing of the upper layers of the epidermis G that heals completely. ⊕ Nikolsky sign (separation of epidermis upon manual stroking of skin). Commonly seen in newborns and children/adults with renal insufficiency.

Viral infections

Herpes	Herpes virus infections (HSV-1 and HSV-2) of skin can occur anywhere from mucosal surfaces to normal skin. These include herpes labialis, herpes genitalis, herpetic whitlow H (finger).
Molluscum contagiosum	Umbilicated papules I caused by a poxvirus. While frequently seen in children, it may be sexually transmitted in adults.
Varicella zoster	Causes varicella (chickenpox) and zoster (shingles). Varicella presents with multiple crops of lesions in various stages from vesicles to crusts. Zoster is a reactivation of the virus in dermatomal distribution (unless it is disseminated).
Hairy leukoplakia	Irregular, white, painless plaques on lateral tongue that cannot be scraped off J. EBV mediated. Occurs in patients living with HIV, organ transplant recipients. Contrast with thrush (scrapable) and leukoplakia (precancerous).

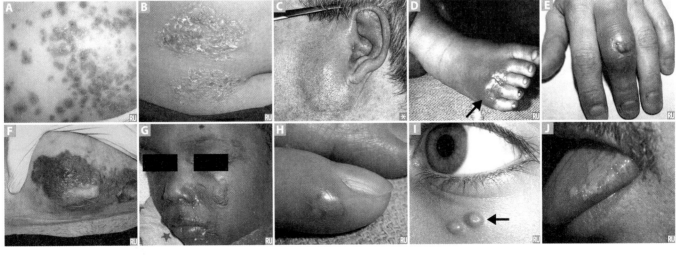

Cutaneous mycoses

Tinea (dermatophytes)	Clinical name for dermatophyte (cutaneous fungal) infections. Dermatophytes include *Microsporum*, *Trichophyton*, and *Epidermophyton*. Branching septate hyphae visible on KOH preparation with blue fungal stain **A**. Associated with pruritus.
Tinea capitis	Occurs on head, scalp. Associated with lymphadenopathy, alopecia, scaling **B**.
Tinea corporis	Occurs on body (usually torso). Characterized by enlarging erythematous, scaly rings ("ringworm") with central clearing **C**. Can be acquired from contact with infected pets or farm animals.
Tinea cruris	Occurs in inguinal area ("jock itch") **D**. Often does not show the central clearing seen in tinea corporis.
Tinea pedis	Three varieties ("athlete's foot"): ▪ Interdigital **E**; most common ▪ Moccasin distribution **F** ▪ Vesicular type
Tinea unguium	Onychomycosis; occurs on nails.
Tinea (pityriasis) versicolor	Caused by *Malassezia* spp. (*Pityrosporum* spp.), a yeastlike fungus (not a dermatophyte despite being called tinea). Degradation of lipids produces acids that inhibit tyrosinase (involved in melanin synthesis) → hypopigmentation **G**; hyperpigmentation and/or pink patches can also occur due to inflammatory response. Less pruritic than dermatophytes. Can occur any time of year, but more common in summer (hot, humid weather). "Spaghetti and meatballs" appearance on microscopy **H**. Treatment: selenium sulfide, topical and/or oral antifungal medications.

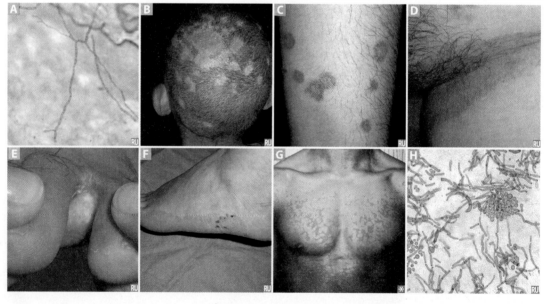

Autoimmune blistering skin disorders

	Pemphigus vulgaris	Bullous pemphigoid
PATHOPHYSIOLOGY	Potentially fatal. Most commonly seen in older adults. Type II hypersensitivity reaction. IgG antibodies against desmoglein 3 +/− desmoglein 1 (component of desmosomes, which connect keratinocytes in the stratum spinosum).	Less severe than pemphigus vulgaris. Most commonly seen in older adults. Type II hypersensitivity reaction. IgG antibodies against hemidesmosomes (epidermal basement membrane; antibodies are "bullow" the epidermis).
GROSS MORPHOLOGY	Flaccid intraepidermal bullae A caused by acantholysis (separation of keratinocytes, "row of tombstones" on H&E stain); oral mucosa is involved. Nikolsky sign ⊕.	Tense blisters C containing eosinophils; oral mucosa spared. Nikolsky sign ⊖.
IMMUNOFLUORESCENCE	Reticular pattern around epidermal cells B.	Linear pattern at epidermal-dermal junction D.

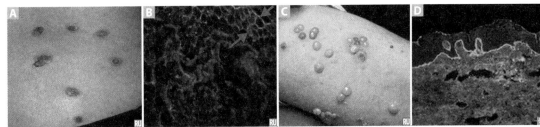

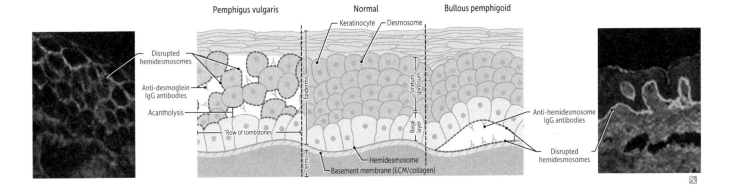

Other blistering skin disorders

Dermatitis herpetiformis	Pruritic papules, vesicles, and bullae (often found on elbows, knees, buttocks) **A**. Deposits of IgA at tips of dermal papillae. Associated with celiac disease. Treatment: dapsone, gluten-free diet.
Erythema multiforme	Associated with infections (eg, *Mycoplasma pneumoniae*, HSV), drugs (eg, sulfa drugs, β-lactams, phenytoin). Presents with multiple types of lesions—macules, papules, vesicles, target lesions (look like targets with multiple rings and dusky center showing epithelial disruption) **B**.
Stevens-Johnson syndrome	Characterized by fever, bullae formation and necrosis, sloughing of skin at dermal-epidermal junction (⊕ Nikolsky), high mortality rate. Typically mucous membranes are involved **C**. Targetoid skin lesions may appear, as seen in erythema multiforme. Usually associated with adverse drug reaction. Toxic epidermal necrolysis (TEN) **D** **E** is more severe form of SJS involving > 30% body surface area. 10–30% involvement denotes SJS-TEN.
Inherited Epidermolysis Bullosa	Group of inherited skin disorders characterized by bullae, erosions, and ulcers triggered by minor trauma. Presents with blisters early in life and oral blisters with bottle feeding. Most commonly caused by mutations in keratin genes.

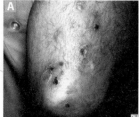 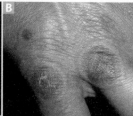 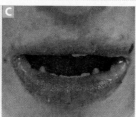 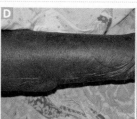 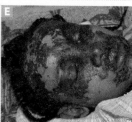

Cutaneous ulcers

	Venous ulcer	Arterial ulcer	Neuropathic ulcer	Pressure injury
ETIOLOGY	Chronic venous insufficiency; most common ulcer type	Peripheral artery disease (eg, atherosclerotic stenosis)	Peripheral neuropathy (eg, diabetic foot)	Prolonged unrelieved pressure (eg, immobility)
LOCATION	Gaiter area (ankle to midcalf), typically over malleoli	Distal toes, anterior shin, pressure points	Bony prominences (eg, metatarsal heads, heel)	Weightbearing points (eg, sacrum, ischium, calcaneus)
APPEARANCE	Irregular border, shallow, exudative A	Symmetric with well-defined punched-out appearance B	Hyperkeratotic edge with undermined borders C	Varies based on stage from non-blanchable erythema to full-thickness skin loss D
PAIN	Mild to moderate	Severe	Absent	Present
ASSOCIATED SIGNS	Telangiectasias, varicose veins, edema, stasis dermatitis (erythematous eczematous patches)	Arterial insufficiency, cold and pale atrophic skin, hair loss, absent pulses	Claw toes, Charcot joints, absent reflexes	Soft tissue infection and osteomyelitis are frequent complications

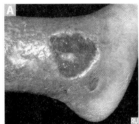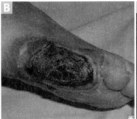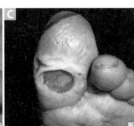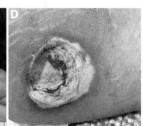

Miscellaneous skin disorders

Acanthosis nigricans	Epidermal hyperplasia causing symmetric, hyperpigmented thickening of skin, especially in axilla or on neck 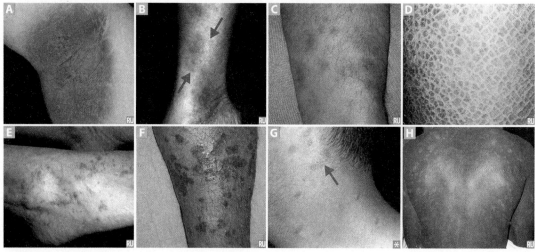. Associated with insulin resistance (eg, diabetes, obesity, Cushing syndrome, PCOS), visceral malignancy (eg, gastric adenocarcinoma).
Erythema nodosum	Painful, raised inflammatory lesions of subcutaneous fat (panniculitis), usually on anterior shins. Often idiopathic, but can be associated with sarcoidosis, coccidioidomycosis, histoplasmosis, TB, streptococcal infections B, leprosy C, inflammatory bowel disease.
Ichthyosis vulgaris	Disorder of defective keratinocyte desquamation due to filaggrin gene mutations resulting in diffuse scaling of the skin D most commonly on the extensor side of extremities and the trunk. Manifests in infancy or early childhood. Strong association with atopic dermatitis.
Lichen Planus	Pruritic, purple, polygonal planar papules and plaques are the 6 P's of lichen Planus E F. Mucosal involvement manifests as Wickham striae (reticular white lines) and hypergranulosis. Sawtooth infiltrate of lymphocytes at dermal-epidermal junction. Associated with hepatitis C.
Pityriasis rosea	"Herald patch" G followed days later by other scaly erythematous plaques, often in a "Christmas tree" distribution on trunk H. Multiple pink plaques with collarette scale. Self-resolving in 6–8 weeks.
Sunburn	Acute cutaneous inflammatory reaction due to excessive UV irradiation. Causes DNA mutations, inducing apoptosis of keratinocytes. UVB is dominant in sunBurn, UVA in tAnning and photoAging. Exposure to UVA and UVB ↑ risk of skin cancer.
Radiation dermatitis	Can be acute or late. Acute occurs ≤ 90 days after radiotherapy due to apoptosis of basal keratinocytes and epidermal edema. Presents with erythema, desquamation, superficial ulceration, and blistering. Late occurs months to years after radiotherapy due to fibrosis with homogenization of dermal collagen fibers on histology, vascular damage, and telangiectasias.

Estimation of body surface area

Approximated by the rule of 9's. Used to assess the extent of burn injuries.

Inhalation injury—complication of inhalation of noxious stimuli (eg, smoke). Heat, particulates (< 1 µm diameter), or irritants (eg, NH_3) → chemical tracheobronchitis, edema, pneumonia, acute respiratory distress syndrome. Singed nasal hairs or soot in oropharynx common on exam. Bronchoscopy shows severe edema, congestion of bronchus, and soot deposition (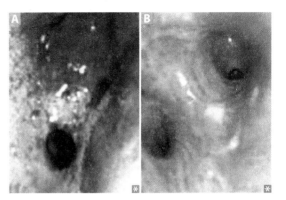 A, 18 hours after inhalation injury; B, resolution at 11 days after injury).

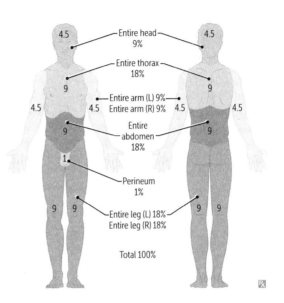

Entire head 9%
Entire thorax 18%
Entire arm (L) 9%
Entire arm (R) 9%
Entire abdomen 18%
Perineum 1%
Entire leg (L) 18%
Entire leg (R) 18%

Total 100%

Burn classification

DEPTH	INVOLVEMENT	APPEARANCE	SENSATION
Superficial burn	Epidermis only	Similar to sunburn; histamine release causes localized, dry, blanching redness without blisters	Painful
Superficial partial-thickness burn	Epidermis and papillary dermis	Blisters, blanches with pressure, swollen, warm	Painful to temperature and air
Deep partial-thickness burn	Epidermis and reticular dermis	Blisters (easily unroofed), does not blanch with pressure	Painless; perception of pressure only
Full-thickness burn	Epidermis and full-thickness dermis	White, waxy, dry, inelastic, leathery, does not blanch with pressure	Painless; perception of deep pressure only
Deeper injury burn	Epidermis, dermis, and involvement of underlying tissue (eg, fascia, muscle)	White, dry, inelastic, does not blanch with pressure	Painless; some perception of deep pressure

Skin cancer	Basal cell carcinoma (BCC) more common above **upper lip**. Squamous cell carcinoma (SCC) more common below **lower lip**. Sun exposure strongly predisposes to skin cancer. 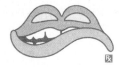

Basal cell carcinoma	Most common skin cancer. Found in sun-exposed areas of body (eg, face). Locally invasive, but rarely metastasizes. Waxy, pink, pearly nodules, commonly with telangiectasias, rolled borders A, central crusting or ulceration. BCCs also appear as a scaling plaque (superficial BCC) B.
Squamous cell carcinoma	Second most common skin cancer. Associated with immunosuppression, chronic nonhealing wounds, and occasionally arsenic exposure. Marjolin ulcer—SCC arising in chronic wounds or scars; usually develops > 20 years after insult. Commonly appears on face C, lower lip D, ears, hands. Locally invasive, may spread to lymph nodes, and will rarely metastasize. Ulcerative red lesions. Histopathology: keratin "pearls" E. Actinic keratosis—Premalignant lesions caused by sun exposure. Small, rough, erythematous or brownish papules or plaques F. Risk of squamous cell carcinoma is proportional to degree of epithelial dysplasia.
Melanoma	Common tumor with significant risk of metastasis. S-100 tumor marker. Associated with dysplastic nevi; people with lighter skin tones are at ↑ risk. Depth of tumor (Breslow thickness) correlates with risk of metastasis. Look for the **ABCDE**s: **A**symmetry, **B**order irregularity, **C**olor variation, **D**iameter > 6 mm, and **E**volution over time. At least 4 different types of melanoma, including superficial spreading G, nodular H, lentigo maligna I, and acral lentiginous (highest prevalence in people with darker skin tones) J. Often driven by activating mutation in BRAF kinase. Primary treatment is excision with appropriately wide margins. Advanced melanoma also treated with immunotherapy (eg, ipilimumab) and/or BRAF inhibitors (eg, vemurafenib).

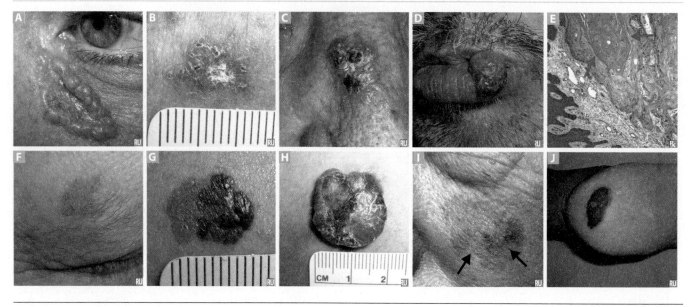

▶ MUSCULOSKELETAL, SKIN, AND CONNECTIVE TISSUE—PHARMACOLOGY

Arachidonic acid pathways

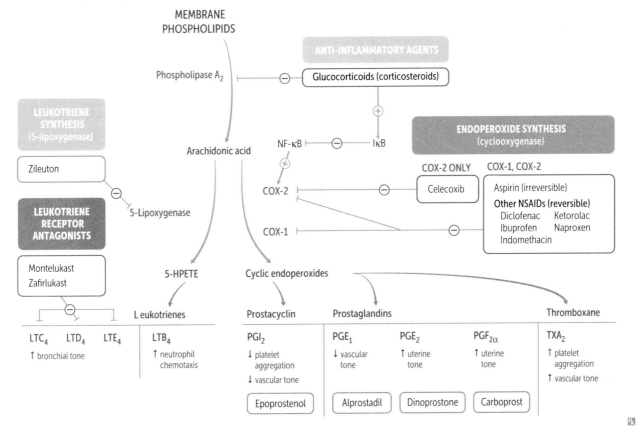

LTB$_4$ is a **neutrophil** chemotactic agent.
PGI$_2$ is a vasodilator and platelet aggregation inhibitor.

Neutrophils arrive "B4" others.
Platelet-**G**athering **I**nhibitor.

Acetaminophen

MECHANISM	Reversibly inhibits cyclooxygenase, mostly in CNS. Inactivated peripherally.
CLINICAL USE	Antipyretic, analgesic, but not anti-inflammatory. Used instead of aspirin to avoid Reye syndrome in children with viral infection.
ADVERSE EFFECTS	Overdose produces hepatic necrosis; acetaminophen metabolite (NAPQI) depletes glutathione and forms toxic tissue byproducts in liver. N-acetylcysteine is antidote—regenerates glutathione.

Aspirin

MECHANISM	NSAID that **ir**reversibly (aspirin) inhibits cyclooxygenase (both COX-1 and COX-2) by covalent acetylation → ↓ synthesis of TXA_2 and prostaglandins. ↑ bleeding time. No effect on PT, PTT. Effect lasts until new platelets are produced.
CLINICAL USE	Low dose (< 300 mg/day): ↓ platelet aggregation. Intermediate dose (300–2400 mg/day): antipyretic and analgesic. High dose (2400–4000 mg/day): anti-inflammatory.
ADVERSE EFFECTS	Gastric ulceration, tinnitus (CN VIII), allergic reactions (especially in patients with asthma or nasal polyps). Chronic use can lead to acute kidney injury, interstitial nephritis, GI bleeding. Risk of Reye syndrome in children treated for viral infection. Toxic doses cause respiratory alkalosis early, but transitions to mixed metabolic acidosis-respiratory alkalosis. Overdose treatment: $NaHCO_3$.

Celecoxib

MECHANISM	Reversibly and **select**ively inh**ib**its the cyclooxygenase (**COX**) isoform 2 ("**Selecoxib**"), which is found in inflammatory cells and vascular endothelium and mediates inflammation and pain; spares COX-1, which helps maintain gastric mucosa. Thus, does not have the corrosive effects of other NSAIDs on the GI lining. Spares platelet function as TXA_2 production is dependent on COX-1.
CLINICAL USE	Rheumatoid arthritis, osteoarthritis.
ADVERSE EFFECTS	↑ risk of thrombosis, sulfa allergy.

Nonsteroidal anti-inflammatory drugs

Ibuprofen, naproxen, indomethacin, ketorolac, diclofenac, meloxicam, piroxicam.

MECHANISM	Reversibly inhibit cyclooxygenase (both COX-1 and COX-2). Block prostaglandin synthesis.
CLINICAL USE	Antipyretic, analgesic, anti-inflammatory. Indomethacin is used to close a PDA.
ADVERSE EFFECTS	Interstitial nephritis, gastric ulcer (prostaglandins protect gastric mucosa), renal ischemia (prostaglandins vasodilate afferent arteriole), aplastic anemia.

Leflunomide

MECHANISM	Reversibly inhibits dihydroorotate dehydrogenase, preventing pyrimidine synthesis. Suppresses T-cell proliferation.
CLINICAL USE	Rheumatoid arthritis, psoriatic arthritis.
ADVERSE EFFECTS	Diarrhea, hypertension, hepatotoxicity, teratogenicity.

Bisphosphonates

Alendronate, ibandronate, risedronate, zoledronate.

MECHANISM	Pyrophosphate analogs; bind hydroxyapatite in bone, inhibiting osteoclast activity and promoting osteoclast apoptosis.
CLINICAL USE	Osteoporosis, hypercalcemia, Paget disease of bone, metastatic bone disease, osteogenesis imperfecta.
ADVERSE EFFECTS	Esophagitis, osteonecrosis of jaw, atypical femoral stress fractures.

Recombinant parathyroid hormone	Teriparatide, abaloparatide.
MECHANISM	Recombinant PTH analog. ↑ osteoblastic activity when administered in pulsatile fashion.
CLINICAL USE	Osteoporosis. Causes ↑ bone growth compared to antiresorptive therapies (eg, bisphosphonates).
ADVERSE EFFECTS	Dizziness, tachycardia, transient hypercalcemia, muscle spasms.

Gout drugs

Chronic gout drugs (preventive)

Allopurinol	Competitive inhibitor of xanthine oxidase → ↓ conversion of hypoxanthine and xanthine to urate. Also used in lymphoma and leukemia to prevent tumor lysis–associated urate nephropathy. ↑ concentrations of xanthine oxidase active metabolites, azathioprine, and 6-MP.	All painful flares are preventable.
Pegloticase	Recombinant uricase catalyzing uric acid to allantoin (a more water-soluble product).	
Febuxostat	Inhibits xanthine oxidase. Think, "febu-**xo-stat** makes **X**anthine **O**xidase **stat**ic."	
Probenecid	Inhibits reabsorption of uric acid in proximal convoluted tubule (also inhibits secretion of penicillin). Can precipitate uric acid calculi or lead to sulfa allergy.	

Acute gout drugs

NSAIDs	Any NSAID. Use salicylates with caution (may decrease uric acid excretion, particularly at low doses).
Glucocorticoids	Oral, intra-articular, or parenteral.
Colchicine	Binds and stabilizes tubulin to inhibit microtubule polymerization, impairing neutrophil chemotaxis and degranulation. Acute and prophylactic value. GI, neuromyopathic adverse effects. Can also cause myelosuppression, nephrotoxicity.

Purines
↓
Hypoxanthine
↓ Xanthine oxidase
Xanthine ⊖⊖ Allopurinol, Febuxostat
↓ Xanthine oxidase
Plasma uric acid

Tubular secretion | Tubular reabsorption
⊖ | ⊖
Diuretics, low-dose salicylates | Probenecid, high-dose salicylates

Urine

TNF-α inhibitors

DRUG	MECHANISM	CLINICAL USE	ADVERSE EFFECTS
Etanercept	Fusion protein (decoy receptor for TNF-α + IgG1 Fc), produced by recombinant DNA. Etanercept intercepts TNF.	Rheumatoid arthritis, psoriasis, ankylosing spondylitis.	Predisposition to infection, including reactivation of latent TB, since TNF is important in granuloma formation and stabilization. Can also lead to drug-induced lupus.
Adalimumab, infliximab	Anti-TNF-α monoclonal antibody.	Inflammatory bowel disease, rheumatoid arthritis, ankylosing spondylitis, psoriasis.	

Psoriasis biologics

DRUG	TARGET
Ustekinumab	IL-12/IL-23
Ixekizumab Secukinumab	IL-17
Brodalumab	IL-17 receptor
Guselkumab Risankizumab Tildrakizumab	IL-23

Imiquimod

MECHANISM	Binds toll-like receptor 7 (TLR-7) of macrophages, monocytes, and dendritic cells to activate them → topical antitumor immune response modifier.
CLINICAL USE	Anogenital warts, actinic keratosis.
ADVERSE EFFECTS	Itching, burning pain at site of application, rashes.

Neurology and Special Senses

"We are all now connected by the Internet, like neurons in a giant brain."
—Stephen Hawking

"Exactly how [the brain] operates remains one of the biggest unsolved mysteries, and it seems the more we probe its secrets, the more surprises we find."
—Neil deGrasse Tyson

"It's not enough to be nice in life. You've got to have nerve."
—Georgia O'Keeffe

"I not only use all the brains that I have, but all that I can borrow."
—Woodrow Wilson

"The chief function of the body is to carry the brain around."
—Thomas Edison

"I opened two gifts this morning. They were my eyes."
—Zig Ziglar

Understand the difference between the findings and underlying anatomy of upper motor neuron and lower motor neuron lesions. Know the major motor, sensory, cerebellar, and visual pathways and their respective locations in the CNS. Connect key neurological associations with certain pathologies (eg, cerebellar lesions, stroke manifestations, Brown-Séquard syndrome). Recognize common findings on MRI/CT (eg, ischemic and hemorrhagic stroke) and on neuropathology (eg, neurofibrillary tangles and Lewy bodies). High-yield medications include those used to treat epilepsy, Parkinson disease, migraine, and pain (eg, opioids).

▶ NEUROLOGY—EMBRYOLOGY

Neural development

Notochord (precursor to nucleus pulposus of intervertebral discs) induces ectoderm to form neuroectoderm → neural plate.

Neural plate gives rise to neural tube and neural crest cells.

Lateral walls of neural tube are divided into alar and basal plates.

Alar plate (dorsal): sensory; induced by bone morphogenetic proteins (BMPs)

Basal plate (ventral): motor; induced by sonic hedgehog (SHH)

] Same orientation as spinal cord

Homeobox (*HOX*) genes regulate neural tube segmentation, cranial-caudal differentiation. Mutations → syndactyly (limbs), hypospadias (urogenital).

Neural plate — Notochord; Neural fold; Neural tube — Neural crest cells

---

Regionalization of neural tube

Telencephalon is the 1st part. **Diencephalon** is the **2nd** part. The rest are arranged alphabetically: **m**esencephalon, **m**etencephalon, **m**yelencephalon.

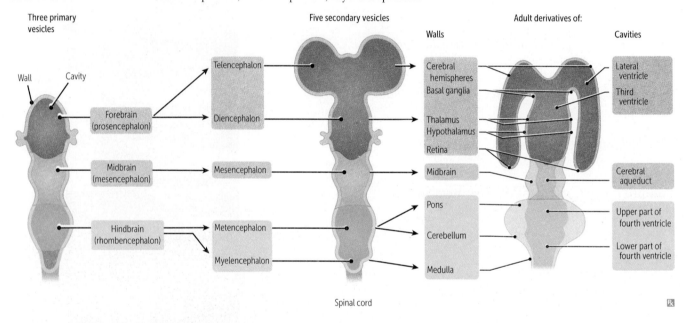

Three primary vesicles	Five secondary vesicles	Adult derivatives of: Walls	Cavities
Forebrain (prosencephalon)	Telencephalon	Cerebral hemispheres / Basal ganglia	Lateral ventricle
	Diencephalon	Thalamus / Hypothalamus / Retina	Third ventricle
Midbrain (mesencephalon)	Mesencephalon	Midbrain	Cerebral aqueduct
Hindbrain (rhombencephalon)	Metencephalon	Pons / Cerebellum	Upper part of fourth ventricle
	Myelencephalon	Medulla	Lower part of fourth ventricle

Wall / Cavity

Spinal cord

Central and peripheral nervous systems origins

Neuroepithelia in neural tube—CNS neurons, CNS glial cells (astrocytes, oligodendrocytes, ependymal cells).

Neural crest—PNS neurons (dorsal root ganglia, autonomic ganglia [sympathetic, parasympathetic, enteric]), PNS glial cells (Schwann cells, satellite cells), adrenal medulla.

Mesoderm—microglia (specialized macrophages).

Neural tube defects	Failure of the neural tube to close completely by week 4 of development, associated with maternal folate deficiency or exposure to teratogens such as valproate and carbamazepine during pregnancy. Diagnosis: ultrasound, maternal serum AFP and/or amniotic fluid AChE (↑ in open NTDs).
Spinal dysraphism	
Spina bifida occulta	Closed NTD. Failure of caudal neural tube to close, but no herniation. Dura is intact. Usually seen at lower vertebral levels. Associated with tuft of hair or skin dimple at level of bony defect.
Meningocele	Open NTD. Meninges (but no neural tissue) herniate through bony defect.
Myelomeningocele	Open NTD. Meninges and neural tissue (eg, cauda equina) herniate through bony defect.
Myeloschisis	Open NTD. Exposed, unfused neural tissue without skin/meningeal covering.
Cranial dysraphism	
Anencephaly	Open NTD. Failure of rostral neuropore to close → no forebrain, open calvarium. Often presents with polyhydramnios (↓ fetal swallowing due to lack of neural control).

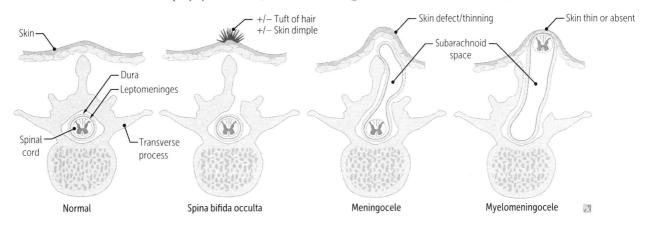

Brain malformations	Often incompatible with postnatal life. Survivors may be profoundly disabled.
Holoprosencephaly	Failure of forebrain (prosencephalon) to divide into 2 cerebral hemispheres; developmental field defect usually occurring at weeks 3–4 of development. Associated with *SHH* mutations. May be seen in Patau syndrome (trisomy 13), fetal alcohol syndrome. Presents with midline defects: monoventricle 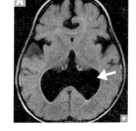, fused basal ganglia, cleft lip/palate, hypotelorism, cyclopia, proboscis. ↑ risk for pituitary dysfunction (eg, diabetes insipidus).
Lissencephaly	Failure of neuronal migration → smooth brain surface that lacks sulci and gyri 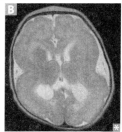. Presents with dysphagia, seizures, microcephaly, facial anomalies.

Posterior fossa malformations

Chiari I malformation	Downward displacement of cerebellar **tonsils** through foramen magnum (**1** structure) **A**. Usually asymptomatic in childhood, manifests in adulthood with headaches and cerebellar symptoms. Associated with spinal cord cavitations (eg, syringomyelia).
Chiari II malformation	Downward displacement of **cerebellum** (vermis and tonsils) and **medulla** (**2** structures) through foramen magnum → noncommunicating hydrocephalus. More severe than Chiari I, usually presents early in life with dysphagia, stridor, apnea, limb weakness. Associated with myelomeningocele (usually lumbosacral).
Dandy-Walker malformation	Agenesis of cerebellar vermis → cystic enlargement of 4th ventricle (arrow in **B**) that fills the enlarged posterior fossa. Associated with noncommunicating hydrocephalus, spina bifida.

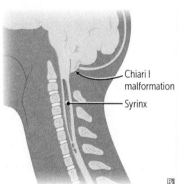

Chiari I malformation

Syrinx

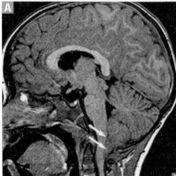

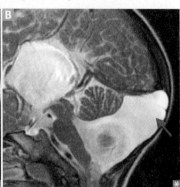

Syringomyelia

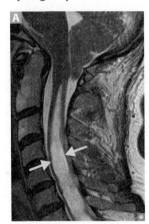

Fluid-filled, gliosis-lined cavity within spinal cord (yellow arrows in **A**). Fibers crossing in anterior white commissure (spinothalamic tract) are typically damaged first → "cape-like" loss of pain and temperature sensation in bilateral upper extremities. As lesion expands it may damage anterior horns → lower motor neuron (LMN) findings.

Syrinx (Greek) = tube, as in "syringe." Most lesions occur between C2 and T9. Usually associated with Chiari I malformation (red arrow in **A**). Less commonly associated with other malformations, infections, tumors, trauma.

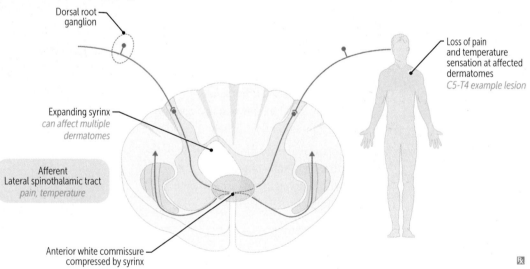

Dorsal root ganglion

Expanding syrinx
can affect multiple dermatomes

Afferent
Lateral spinothalamic tract
pain, temperature

Anterior white commissure
compressed by syrinx

Loss of pain and temperature sensation at affected dermatomes
C5-T4 example lesion

▶ **NEUROLOGY—ANATOMY AND PHYSIOLOGY**

Cells of the nervous system	Neurons and nonneuronal (glial) cells. Neurons—permanent, signal-transmitting cells of the nervous system composed of dendrites (receive input), cell bodies, and axons (send output). Dendrites and cell bodies can be seen on Nissl staining (stains rough endoplasmic reticulum [RER]; not present in axons). Markers: neurofilament protein, synaptophysin.	CNS glial cells—neuroectoderm (except microglia, which derive from mesoderm). PNS glial cells—neural crest ectoderm. Myelin is a multilayer wrapping of electrical insulation formed around axons → ↑ conduction velocity of transmitted signals via saltatory conduction of action potentials at nodes of Ranvier (↑↑ Na⁺ channel density).

CNS glial cells

Astrocytes	Physical support, repair, removal of excess neurotransmitters, component of blood-brain barrier, glycogen fuel reserve buffer. GFAP ⊕.	Largest and most abundant glial cell in CNS. Reactive gliosis in response to neural injury.
Oligodendrocytes	Myelinate axons in CNS (including CN II). "Fried **egg**" appearance histologically ("ol**egg**odendrocytes").	Each myelinates many axons (~ 30). Predominant type of glial cell in white matter. Injured in multiple sclerosis, leukodystrophies, progressive multifocal leukoencephalopathy.
Ependymal cells	Ciliated simple columnar glial cells lining ventricles and central canal of spinal cord. Apical surfaces are covered with cilia (which circulate CSF) and microvilli (which help with CSF absorption).	Specialized ependymal cells (choroid plexus) produce CSF.
Microglia	Activation in response to tissue damage → release of inflammatory mediators (eg, nitric oxide, glutamate). Not readily discernible by Nissl stain.	Phagocytic scavenger cells of CNS. HIV-infected microglia fuse to form multinucleated giant cells in CNS in HIV-associated dementia.

PNS glial cells

Satellite cells	Surround neuronal cell bodies in ganglia.	Similar supportive role to astrocytes.
Schwann cells	Myelinate axons in PNS (including CN III-XII). S100 ⊕.	Each myelinates a **single** axon ("**Schw**one"). Injured in Guillain-Barré syndrome.

Central nervous system   Peripheral nervous system

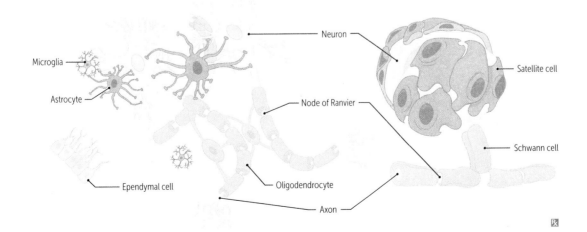

Microglia · Astrocyte · Ependymal cell · Oligodendrocyte · Axon · Neuron · Node of Ranvier · Satellite cell · Schwann cell

Neuron action potential

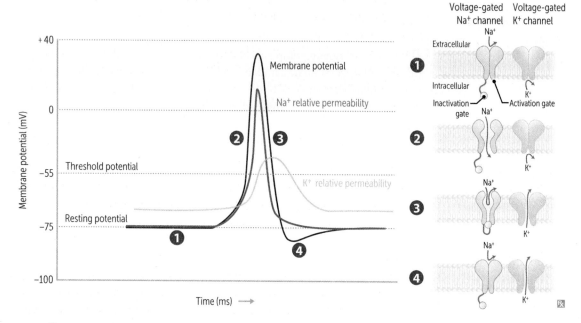

❶ Resting membrane potential: membrane is more permeable to K⁺ than Na⁺ at rest. Voltage-gated Na⁺ and K⁺ channels are closed.

❷ Membrane depolarization: Na⁺ activation gate opens → Na⁺ flows inward.

❸ Membrane repolarization: Na⁺ inactivation gate closes at peak potential, thus stopping Na⁺ inflow. K⁺ activation gate opens → K⁺ flows outward.

❹ Membrane hyperpolarization: K⁺ activation gates are slow to close → excess K⁺ efflux and brief period of hyperpolarization. Voltage-gated Na⁺ channels switch back to resting state. Na⁺/K⁺ pump restores ions concentration.

Sensory receptors

RECEPTOR TYPE	SENSORY NEURON FIBER TYPE	LOCATION	SENSES
Free nerve endings	Aδ—**fast**, myelinated fibers C—**slow**, unmyelinated **A Delta** plane is **fast**, but a tax**C** is **slow**	All tissues except cartilage and eye lens; numerous in skin	Pain, temperature
Meissner corpuscles	Large, myelinated fibers; adapt quickly	Glabrous (hairless) skin (eg, palms, soles, lips)	Dynamic, fine/light touch, low-frequency vibration, skin indentation
Pacinian corpuscles	Large, myelinated fibers; adapt quickly	Deep skin layers, ligaments, joints	High-frequency vibration, pressure (**pressure cooker**)
Merkel discs	Large, myelinated fibers; adapt slowly	Finger tips, superficial skin	Pressure, deep static touch (eg, shapes, edges)
Ruffini corpuscles	Large, myelinated fiber intertwined among collagen fiber bundles; adapt slowly	Finger tips, joints	Stretch, joint angle change

Peripheral nerve

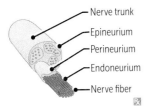

- Nerve trunk
- Epineurium
- Perineurium
- Endoneurium
- Nerve fiber

Endoneurium—thin, supportive connective tissue that ensheathes and supports individual myelinated nerve fibers. May be affected in Guillain-Barré syndrome.

Perineurium (blood-nerve permeability barrier)—surrounds a fascicle of nerve fibers.

Epineurium—dense connective tissue that surrounds entire nerve (fascicles and blood vessels).

Endo = inner
Peri = around
Epi = outer

Neuronal response to axonal injury

Chromatolysis—dispersion of Nissl substance throughout cytoplasm (RER no longer visible on staining). Neuronal cell body reaction reflecting ↑ protein synthesis in effort to repair damaged axon. Accompanied by round cellular swelling and displacement of nucleus to periphery.

Axonal retraction—proximal axon segment retracts and sprouts new protrusions that grow toward other neurons for potential reinnervation. In PNS, Schwann cells create a tract that guides axonal regeneration.

Wallerian degeneration—distal axon segment and associated myelin sheath disintegrates with macrophages removing debris. In CNS, persistence of myelin debris and reactive gliosis prevent axonal regeneration. Facilitate axonal regeneration in response to neural injury.

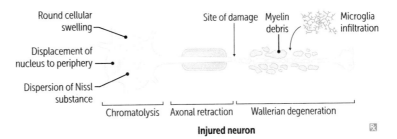

Round cellular swelling · Displacement of nucleus to periphery · Dispersion of Nissl substance · Chromatolysis · Axonal retraction · Site of damage · Myelin debris · Microglia infiltration · Wallerian degeneration

Injured neuron

Neurotransmitter changes with disease

	LOCATION OF SYNTHESIS	ANXIETY	DEPRESSION	SCHIZOPHRENIA	ALZHEIMER DISEASE	HUNTINGTON DISEASE	PARKINSON DISEASE
Acetylcholine	Basal nucleus of Meynert (forebrain)				↓	↓	↑
Dopamine	Ventral tegmentum, SNc (midbrain)		↓	↑		↑	↓
GABA	Nucleus accumbens (basal ganglia)	↓				↓	
Norepinephrine	Locus ceruleus (pons)	↑	↓				
Serotonin	Raphe nuclei (brainstem)	↓	↓				↓

Meninges

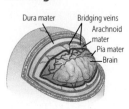

Three membranes that surround and protect the brain and spinal cord. Derived from both neural crest and mesoderm:

- Dura mater—thick outer layer closest to skull.
- Arachnoid mater—middle layer, contains weblike connections.
- Pia mater—thin, fibrous inner layer that firmly adheres to brain and spinal cord.

CSF flows in the subarachnoid space, located between arachnoid and pia mater.

Epidural space—potential space between dura mater and skull/vertebral column containing fat and blood vessels. Site of blood collection associated with middle meningeal artery injury.

Blood-brain barrier

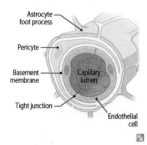

Prevents circulating blood substances (eg, bacteria, drugs) from reaching the CSF/CNS. Formed by 4 structures:

- Tight junctions between nonfenestrated capillary endothelial cells
- Basement membrane
- Pericytes
- Astrocyte foot processes

Glucose and amino acids cross slowly by carrier-mediated transport mechanisms.

Nonpolar/lipid-soluble substances cross rapidly via diffusion.

Circumventricular organs with fenestrated capillaries and no blood-brain barrier allow molecules in blood to affect brain function (eg, area postrema—vomiting after chemotherapy; OVLT [organum vasculosum lamina terminalis]—osmoreceptors) or neurosecretory products to enter circulation (eg, neurohypophysis—ADH release).

BBB disruption (eg, stroke) → vasogenic edema.

Hyperosmolar agents (eg, mannitol) can disrupt the BBB → ↑ permeability of medications.

Vomiting center

Coordinated by NTS in the medulla, which receives information from the chemoreceptor trigger zone (CTZ, located within area postrema (pronounce "puke"-strema) at the base of the 4th ventricle), GI tract (via vagus nerve), vestibular system, and CNS.

CTZ and adjacent vomiting center nuclei receive input through 5 major receptors: histamine (H_1), muscarinic (M_1), neurokinin (NK-1), dopamine (D_2), and serotonin ($5\text{-}HT_3$).

- $5\text{-}HT_3$, D_2, and NK-1 antagonists treat chemotherapy-induced vomiting.
- H_1 and M_1 antagonists treat motion sickness; H_1 antagonists treat hyperemesis gravidarum.

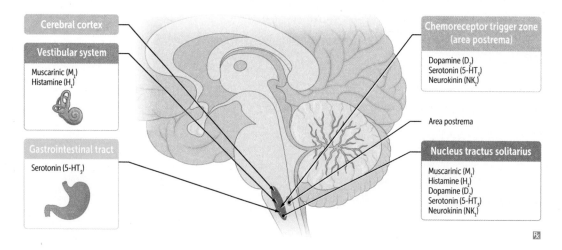

Sleep physiology

Sleep occurs in 4-6 cycles per night, each lasting ~90 mins and consisting of 2 main stages:
- Non-rapid eye movement (NREM) sleep
- Rapid-eye movement (REM) sleep; duration of REM sleep ↑ through the night

Sleep-wake cycle is regulated by circadian rhythm in the suprachiasmatic nucleus (SCN). ↓ light → ↓ SCN activity → ↑ NE from superior cervical ganglion → ↑ melatonin from pineal gland.

EEG waveforms: **B**eta, **A**lpha, **T**heta, **S**leep spindle, **D**elta, **B**eta. At night, **BATS** Drink **B**lood.

SLEEP STAGE (% OF TOTAL SLEEP)	DESCRIPTION	EEG WAVEFORM
Awake	Alert, active mental concentration. Eyes open—beta waves (highest frequency, lowest amplitude). Eyes closed—alpha waves.	
NREM sleep		
Stage N1 (5%)	Light sleep; theta waves.	
Stage N2 (45%)	Deeper sleep; sleep spindles and K complexes. When bruxism occurs ("**twoth**" grinding in N2).	
Stage N3 (25%)	Deepest NREM sleep (slow-wave sleep); delta waves (lowest frequency, highest amplitude). When **bedwetting**, **sleepwalking**, and night terrors occur (**wee** and **flee** in N3).	
REM sleep (25%)	Loss of muscle tone (atonia) except in diaphragm and extraocular muscles, ↑ brain O_2 use, variable pulse/BP. When **dreaming**, nightmares, and penile/clitoral tumescence occur (**REM**ember dreams).	

REM sleep behavior disorder

Loss of atonia leading to dream enactment (often violent) and vocalization. Most commonly associated with Lewy body dementia and Parkinson disease.

Factors affecting sleep architecture

Alcohol, benzodiazepines, barbiturates: ↓ N3 and REM sleep (benzodiazepines are useful for sleepwalking and night terrors).

Aging: ↓ N3 and REM sleep, ↑ sleep-onset latency, early morning awakening.

Depression: ↓ N3 sleep, ↑ REM sleep, ↓ REM latency, repeated nighttime awakenings, early morning awakening (terminal insomnia).

Narcolepsy: ↓ REM latency.

Hypothalamus	Maintains homeostasis by regulating Thirst and water balance, controlling Adenohypophysis (anterior pituitary) and Neurohypophysis (posterior pituitary) release of hormones produced in the hypothalamus, and regulating Hunger, Autonomic nervous system, Temperature, and Sexual urges (**TAN HATS**). Inputs (areas not protected by blood-brain barrier): OVLT (senses change in osmolarity), area postrema (found in dorsal medulla, responds to emetics).	
Lateral nucleus	Hunger. Stimulated by ghrelin, inhibited by leptin.	Lateral injury makes you lean. Destruction → anorexia, failure to thrive (infants).
Ventromedial nucleus	Satiety. Stimulated by leptin.	Ventromedial injury makes you very massive. Destruction (eg, craniopharyngioma) → hyperphagia.
Anterior nucleus	Cooling, parasympathetic.	A/C = Anterior Cooling.
Posterior nucleus	Heating, sympathetic.	Heating controlled by posterior nucleus ("hot pot").
Suprachiasmatic nucleus	Circadian rhythm.	SCN is a Sun-Censing Nucleus.
Supraoptic and paraventricular nuclei	Synthesize ADH and oxytocin.	**SAD POX**: Supraoptic = ADH, Paraventricular = OXytocin. ADH and oxytocin are carried by neurophysins down axons to posterior pituitary, where these hormones are stored and released. Destruction → central diabetes insipidus.
Preoptic nucleus	Thermoregulation, sexual behavior. Releases GnRH.	Failure of GnRH-producing neurons to migrate from olfactory pit → Kallmann syndrome.

Thalamus	Major relay for all ascending sensory information except olfaction.			
NUCLEI	INPUT	SENSES	DESTINATION	MNEMONIC
Ventral posterolateral nucleus	Spinothalamic and dorsal columns/medial lemniscus	Vibration, pain, pressure, proprioception (conscious), light touch, temperature	1° somatosensory cortex (parietal lobe)	
Ventral postero-medial nucleus	Trigeminal and gustatory pathway	Face sensation, taste	1° somatosensory cortex (parietal lobe)	Very pretty makeup goes on the face
Lateral geniculate nucleus	CN II, optic chiasm, optic tract	Vision	1° visual cortex (occipital lobe)	Lateral = light (vision)
Medial geniculate nucleus	Superior olive and inferior colliculus of tectum	Hearing	1° auditory cortex (temporal lobe)	Medial = music (hearing)
Ventral anterior and ventral lateral nuclei	Basal ganglia, cerebellum	Motor	Motor cortices (frontal lobe)	Venus astronauts vow to love moving

Limbic system

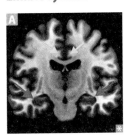

Collection of neural structures involved in emotion, long-term memory, olfaction, behavior modulation, ANS function. Consists of hippocampus (red arrows in Ⓐ), amygdalae, mammillary bodies, anterior thalamic nuclei, cingulate gyrus (yellow arrows in Ⓐ), entorhinal cortex. Responsible for feeding, fleeing, fighting, feeling, and sex.

The famous 5 F's.

Dopaminergic pathways

Commonly altered by drugs (eg, antipsychotics) and movement disorders (eg, Parkinson disease). The mesocortical and mesolimbic pathways are involved in addiction behaviors.

PATHWAY	PROJECTION	FUNCTION	SYMPTOMS OF ALTERED ACTIVITY	NOTES
Mesocortical	Ventral tegmental area → prefrontal cortex	Motivation and reward	↓ activity → negative symptoms	Antipsychotics have limited effect
Mesolimbic	Ventral tegmental area → nucleus accumbens		↑ activity → positive symptoms	1° therapeutic target of antipsychotics
Nigrostriatal	Substantia nigra → dorsal striatum	**Motor** control (pronounce "nigro**stride**atal")	↓ activity → extrapyramidal symptoms	Significantly affected by antipsychotics and in Parkinson disease
Tuberoinfundibular	Hypothalamus → pituitary	Regulation of prolactin secretion	↓ activity → ↑ prolactin	Significantly affected by antipsychotics

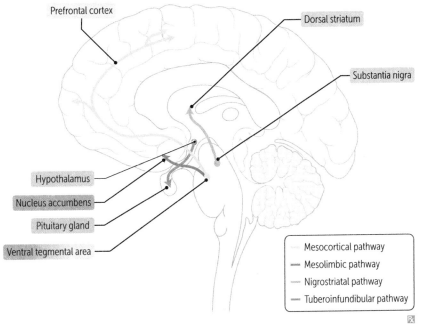

Cerebellum

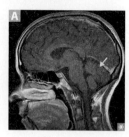

Modulates movement; aids in coordination and balance 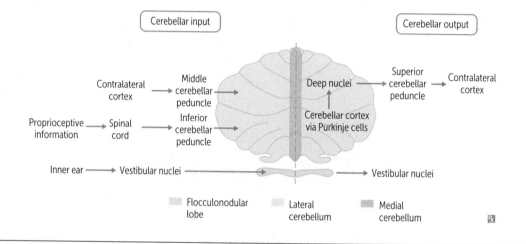.

- Ipsilateral (unconscious) proprioceptive information via inferior cerebellar peduncle from spinal cord
- Deep nuclei (lateral → medial)—dentate, emboliform, globose, fastigial (**d**on't **e**at **g**reasy **f**oods)

Medial cerebellum (eg, vermis) controls axial and proximal limb musculature bilaterally (**medial** structures).

Lateral cerebellum (ie, hemisphere) controls distal limb musculature ipsilaterally (**lateral** structures).

Tests: rapid alternating movements (pronation/supination), finger-to-nose, heel-to-shin, gait, look for intention tremor.

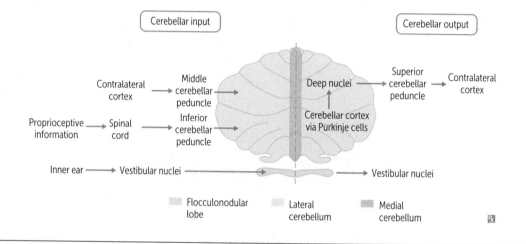

Cerebellar input		Cerebellar output

Contralateral cortex → Middle cerebellar peduncle →

Proprioceptive information → Spinal cord → Inferior cerebellar peduncle →

Deep nuclei → Superior cerebellar peduncle → Contralateral cortex

Cerebellar cortex via Purkinje cells

Inner ear → Vestibular nuclei → → Vestibular nuclei

- Flocculonodular lobe
- Lateral cerebellum
- Medial cerebellum

Basal ganglia

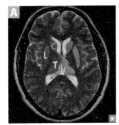

Important in voluntary movements and adjusting posture A.
Receives cortical input, provides negative feedback to cortex to modulate movement.
Striatum = putamen (motor) + Caudate nucleus (cognitive).
Lentiform nucleus = putamen + globus pallidus.

D_1 Receptor = DIRect pathway.
Indirect (D_2) = Inhibitory.

Direct (excitatory) pathway—cortical input (via glutamate) stimulates GABA release from the striatum, which inhibits GABA release from GPi, disinhibiting (activating) the Thalamus → ↑ motion.

Indirect (inhibitory) pathway—cortical input (via glutamate) stimulates GABA release from the striatum, which inhibits GABA release from GPe, disinhibiting (activating) the STN. STN input (via glutamate) stimulates GABA release from GPi, inhibiting the Thalamus → ↓ motion.

Dopamine from SNc (nigrostriatal pathway) stimulates the direct pathway (by binding to D_1 receptor) and inhibits the indirect pathway (by binding to D_2 receptor) → ↑ motion.

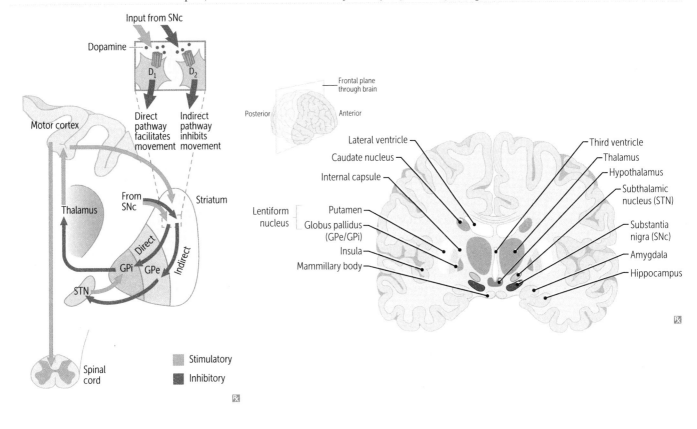

Cerebral cortex regions

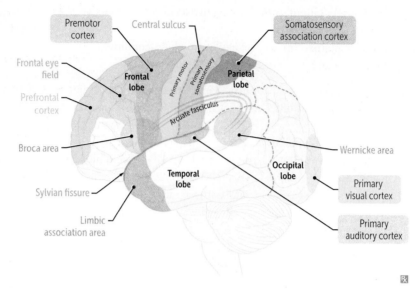

Cerebral perfusion

Relies on tight autoregulation. Primarily driven by P_{CO_2} (P_{O_2} also modulates perfusion in severe hypoxia, eg, mountain sickness—hypoxia → ↑ cerebral vasodilation → ↑ cerebral blood flow → cerebral edema).

Also relies on a pressure gradient between mean arterial pressure (MAP) and intracranial pressure (ICP). ↓ blood pressure or ↑ ICP → ↓ cerebral perfusion pressure (CPP).

Cushing reflex—triad of hypertension, bradycardia, and respiratory depression in response to ↑ ICP.

Therapeutic hyperventilation → ↓ P_{CO_2} → vasoconstriction → ↓ cerebral blood flow → ↓ ICP. May be used to treat acute cerebral edema (eg, 2° to stroke) unresponsive to other interventions.

CPP = MAP – ICP. If CPP = 0, there is no cerebral perfusion → brain death (coma, absent brainstem reflexes, apnea).

Hypoxemia increases CPP only if P_{O_2} < 50 mm Hg.

CPP is directly proportional to P_{CO_2} until P_{CO_2} > 90 mm Hg.

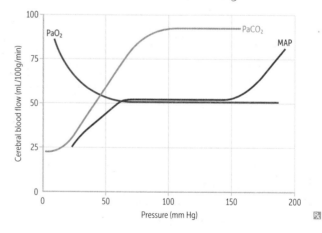

Homunculus

Topographic representation of motor and sensory areas in the cerebral cortex. Distorted appearance is due to certain body regions being more richly innervated and thus having ↑ cortical representation.

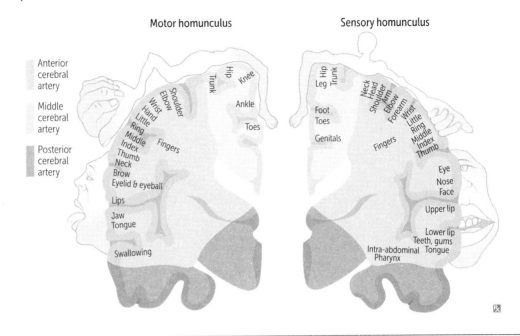

Cerebral arteries—cortical distribution

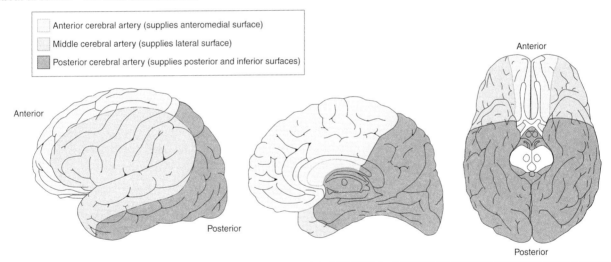

Watershed zones

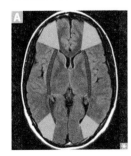

Cortical border zones occur between anterior and middle cerebral arteries and posterior and middle cerebral arteries (blue areas in Ⓐ). Internal border zones occur between the superficial and deep vascular territories of the middle cerebral artery (red areas in Ⓐ).

Common locations for brain metastases. Infarct due to severe hypoperfusion:
- ACA-MCA watershed infarct—proximal upper extremity weakness sparing the lower extremities ("man-in-a-barrel syndrome").
- PCA-MCA watershed infarct—higher-order visual dysfunction.

Circle of Willis

Anastamoses linking anterior and posterior circulations. Maintain cerebral perfusion in cases of occlusion/stenosis of major cranial arteries.

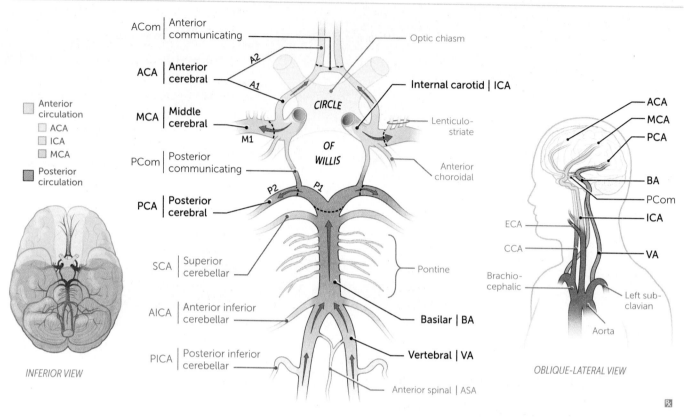

| Anterior circulation |
| ACA |
| ICA |
| MCA |
| Posterior circulation |

ACom | Anterior communicating

ACA | Anterior cerebral

MCA | Middle cerebral

PCom | Posterior communicating

PCA | Posterior cerebral

SCA | Superior cerebellar

AICA | Anterior inferior cerebellar

PICA | Posterior inferior cerebellar

A2
A1
CIRCLE
OF
WILLIS
M1
P2 P1

Optic chiasm
Internal carotid | ICA
Lenticulo-striate
Anterior choroidal
Pontine
Basilar | BA
Vertebral | VA
Anterior spinal | ASA

INFERIOR VIEW

OBLIQUE-LATERAL VIEW

ACA
MCA
PCA
BA
PCom
ICA
VA

ECA
CCA
Brachio-cephalic
Left sub-clavian
Aorta

Dural venous sinuses

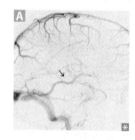

A

Large venous channels **A** that run through the periosteal and meningeal layers of the dura mater. Drain blood from cerebral veins (arrow) and receive CSF from arachnoid granulations. Empty into internal jugular vein.

Venous sinus thrombosis—presents with signs/symptoms of ↑ ICP (eg, headache, seizures, papilledema, focal neurologic deficits). May lead to venous hemorrhage. Associated with hypercoagulable states (eg, pregnancy, OCP use, factor V Leiden).

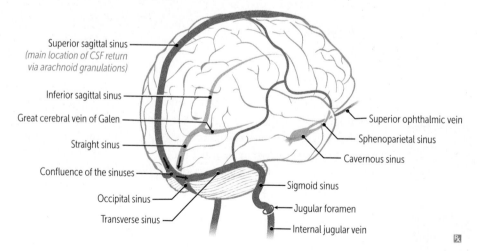

Superior sagittal sinus
(main location of CSF return via arachnoid granulations)

Inferior sagittal sinus

Great cerebral vein of Galen

Straight sinus

Confluence of the sinuses

Occipital sinus

Transverse sinus

Superior ophthalmic vein

Sphenoparietal sinus

Cavernous sinus

Sigmoid sinus

Jugular foramen

Internal jugular vein

Ventricular system

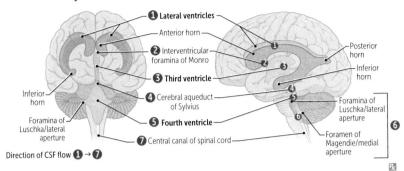

Direction of CSF flow ❶ → ❼

Lateral ventricles → 3rd ventricle via right and left interventricular foramina of Monro.

3rd ventricle → 4th ventricle via cerebral aqueduct of Sylvius.

4th ventricle → subarachnoid space via:
- Foramina of **L**uschka = **l**ateral.
- Foramen of **M**agendie = **m**edial.

CSF made by choroid plexuses located in the lateral, 3rd, and 4th ventricles. Travels to subarachnoid space via foramina of Luschka and Magendie, is reabsorbed by arachnoid granulations, and then drains into dural venous sinuses.

Brainstem—ventral view

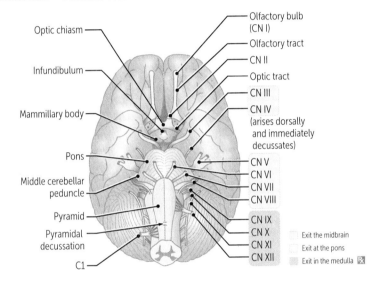

4 CN exit above pons (I, II, III, IV).
4 CN exit the pons (V, VI, VII, VIII).
4 CN exit in medulla (IX, X, XI, XII).
4 CN nuclei are medial (III, IV, VI, XII).
"Factors of 12, except 1 and 2."

Brainstem—dorsal view (cerebellum removed)

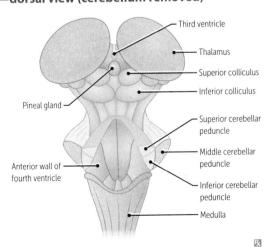

Pineal gland—melatonin secretion, circadian rhythm.

Superior colliculi—process visual stimuli; direct eye and head movements primarily to visual stimuli.

Inferior colliculi—auditory processing; direct eye movements to auditory stimuli.

Eyes **above** ears → superior colliculus (visual) **above** inferior colliculus (auditory).

Cranial nerve nuclei Located in tegmentum portion of brainstem (between dorsal and ventral portions):

- Midbrain—nuclei of CN III, IV
- Pons—nuclei of CN V, VI, VII, VIII
- Medulla—nuclei of CN IX, X, XII
- Spinal cord—nucleus of CN XI

Lateral nuclei = sensory (alar plate).
—Sulcus limitans—
Medial nuclei = motor (basal plate).

Vagal nuclei

NUCLEUS	FUNCTION	CRANIAL NERVES
Nucleus tractus solitarius	Visceral sensory information (eg, taste, baroreceptors, gut distention) May play a role in vomiting	VII, IX, X
Nucleus ambiguus	Motor innervation of pharynx, larynx, upper esophagus (eg, swallowing, palate elevation)	IX, X
Dorsal motor nucleus	Sends autonomic (parasympathetic) fibers to heart, lungs, upper GI	X

Brainstem cross sections

Midbrain

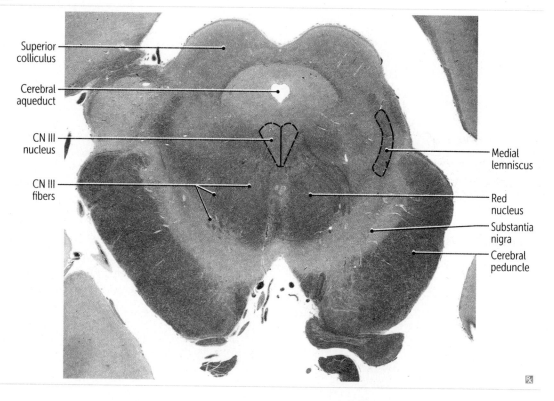

Superior colliculus
Cerebral aqueduct
CN III nucleus
CN III fibers
Medial lemniscus
Red nucleus
Substantia nigra
Cerebral peduncle

Brainstem cross sections (*continued*)

Pons

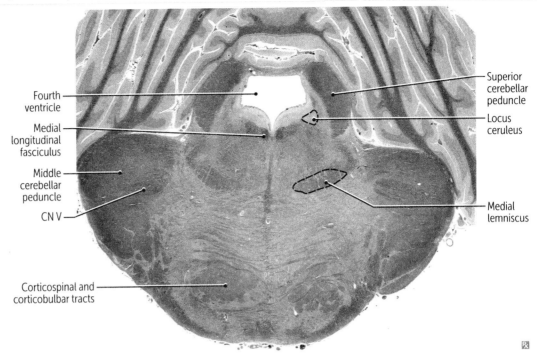

Fourth ventricle

Medial longitudinal fasciculus

Middle cerebellar peduncle

CN V

Corticospinal and corticobulbar tracts

Superior cerebellar peduncle

Locus ceruleus

Medial lemniscus

Medulla

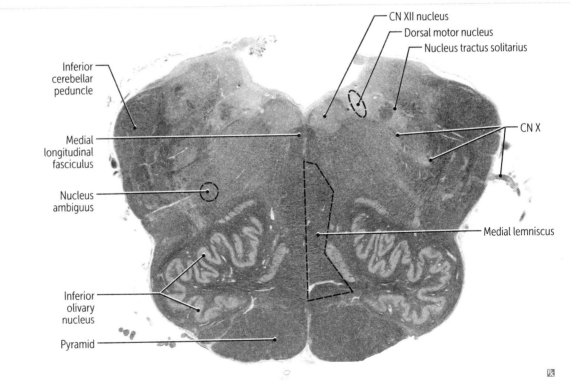

CN XII nucleus

Dorsal motor nucleus

Nucleus tractus solitarius

Inferior cerebellar peduncle

Medial longitudinal fasciculus

Nucleus ambiguus

Inferior olivary nucleus

Pyramid

CN X

Medial lemniscus

Cranial nerves and vessel pathways

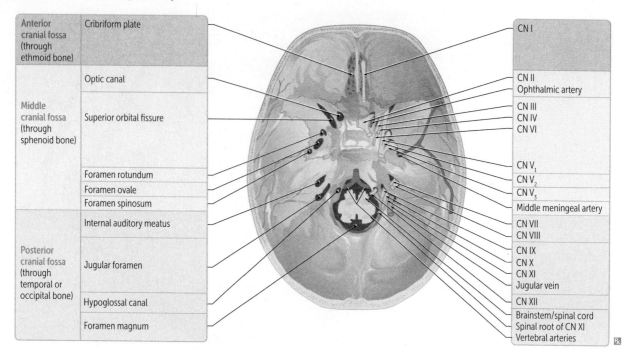

Anterior cranial fossa (through ethmoid bone)	Cribriform plate	
Middle cranial fossa (through sphenoid bone)	Optic canal	
	Superior orbital fissure	
	Foramen rotundum	
	Foramen ovale	
	Foramen spinosum	
Posterior cranial fossa (through temporal or occipital bone)	Internal auditory meatus	
	Jugular foramen	
	Hypoglossal canal	
	Foramen magnum	

CN I
CN II
Ophthalmic artery
CN III
CN IV
CN VI
CN V$_1$
CN V$_2$
CN V$_3$
Middle meningeal artery
CN VII
CN VIII
CN IX
CN X
CN XI
Jugular vein
CN XII
Brainstem/spinal cord
Spinal root of CN XI
Vertebral arteries

Cranial nerves and arteries

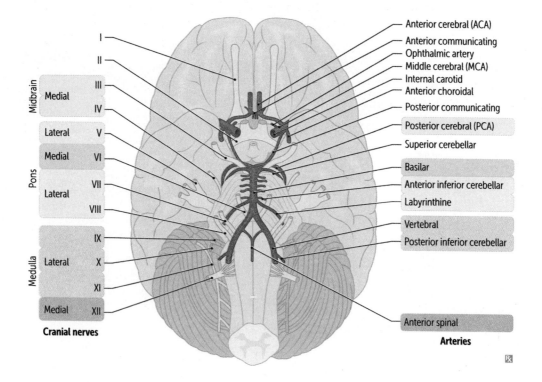

Midbrain — Medial: III, IV; Lateral: V
Pons — Medial: VI; Lateral: VII, VIII
Medulla — Lateral: IX, X, XI; Medial: XII

I
II

Cranial nerves

Anterior cerebral (ACA)
Anterior communicating
Ophthalmic artery
Middle cerebral (MCA)
Internal carotid
Anterior choroidal
Posterior communicating
Posterior cerebral (PCA)
Superior cerebellar
Basilar
Anterior inferior cerebellar
Labyrinthine
Vertebral
Posterior inferior cerebellar
Anterior spinal

Arteries

Cranial nerves

NERVE	CN	FUNCTION	TYPE	MNEMONIC
Olfactory	I	Smell (only CN without thalamic relay to cortex)	Sensory	Some
Optic	II	Sight	Sensory	Say
Oculomotor	III	Eye movement (SR, IR, MR, IO), pupillary constriction (sphincter pupillae), accommodation (ciliary muscle), eyelid opening (levator palpebrae)	Motor	Marry
Trochlear	IV	Eye movement (SO). Crosses midline → only CN with contralateral function	Motor	Money
Trigeminal	V	Mastication, facial sensation (ophthalmic, maxillary, mandibular divisions), somatosensation from anterior 2/3 of tongue, dampening of loud noises (tensor tympani)	Both	But
Abducens	VI	Eye movement (LR)	Motor	My
Facial	VII	Facial movement, eye closing (orbicularis oculi), auditory volume modulation (stapedius), taste from anterior 2/3 of tongue (chorda tympani), lacrimation, salivation (submandibular and sublingual glands are innervated by CN seven)	Both	Brother
Vestibulocochlear	VIII	Hearing, balance	Sensory	Says
Glossopharyngeal	IX	Taste and sensation from posterior 1/3 of tongue, swallowing, salivation (parotid gland), monitoring carotid body and sinus chemo- and baroreceptors, and elevation of pharynx/larynx (stylopharyngeus)	Both	Big
Vagus	X	Taste from supraglottic region, swallowing, soft palate elevation, midline uvula, talking, cough reflex, parasympathetics to thoracoabdominal viscera, monitoring aortic arch chemo- and baroreceptors	Both	Brains
Accessory	XI	Head turning, shoulder shrugging (SCM, trapezius)	Motor	Matter
Hypoglossal	XII	Tongue movement	Motor	Most

Cranial nerve reflexes

REFLEX	AFFERENT	EFFERENT
Accommodation	II	III
Corneal	V_1 ophthalmic (nasociliary branch)	Bilateral VII (temporal and zygomatic branches—orbicularis oculi)
Cough	X	X (also phrenic and spinal nerves)
Gag	IX	X
Jaw jerk	V_3 (sensory—muscle spindle from masseter)	V_3 (motor—masseter)
Lacrimation	V_1 (loss of reflex does not preclude emotional tears)	VII
Pupillary	II	III

Mastication muscles	3 muscles close jaw: **m**asseter, **t**emporalis, medial pterygoid (**my** teeth **m**unch). Lateral pterygoids lower (open) and protrude jaw. All are innervated by mandibular branch of trigeminal nerve (CN V₃).

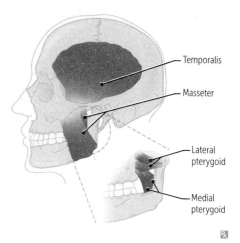

Spinal nerves

There are 31 pairs of spinal nerves: 8 cervical, 12 thoracic, 5 lumbar, 5 sacral, 1 coccygeal.
Nerves C1–C7 exit above the corresponding vertebrae (eg, C3 exits above the 3rd cervical vertebra).
C8 spinal nerve exits below C7 and above T1. All other nerves exit below (eg, L2 exits below the 2nd lumbar vertebra).

Spinal cord—lower extent

In adults, spinal cord ends at lower border of L1–L2 vertebrae. Subarachnoid space (which contains the CSF) extends to lower border of **S2** vertebra. Lumbar puncture (LP) is usually performed between L3–L4 or L4–L5 (level of cauda equina) to obtain sample of CSF while avoiding spinal cord. To **keep** the cord **alive**, keep the spinal needle between **L3** and **L5**.
Needle passes through:
❶ Skin
❷ Fascia and fat
❸ Supraspinous ligament
❹ Interspinous ligament
❺ Ligamentum flavum
❻ Epidural space (epidural anesthesia needle stops here)
❼ Dura mater
❽ Arachnoid mater
❾ Subarachnoid space (CSF collection occurs here)

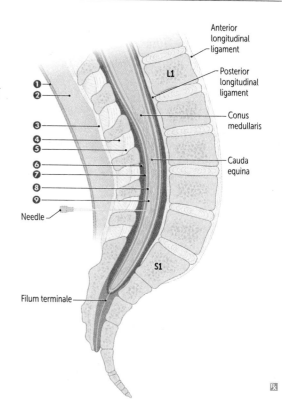

Conus medullaris and cauda equina syndrome

Rare neurosurgical emergencies caused by compression (eg, disc herniation, tumors, trauma) of terminal end of spinal cord (conus medullaris) or lumbosacral spinal nerve roots (cauda equina). Present with radicular low back pain, saddle/perianal anesthesia, bladder and bowel dysfunction, lower limb weakness → symmetric with upper motor neuron (UMN) signs (eg, spastic) in conus medullaris syndrome, asymmetric with LMN signs (eg, flaccid) in cauda equina syndrome.

Spinal cord levels and associated tracts

Legs (lumbosacral) are lateral in lateral corticospinal, spinothalamic tracts.

Dorsal columns are organized as you are, with hands at sides. "Arms outside, legs inside."

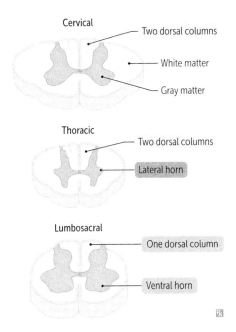

Cervical
— Two dorsal columns
— White matter
— Gray matter

Thoracic
— Two dorsal columns
— Lateral horn

Lumbosacral
— One dorsal column
— Ventral horn

Spinal tract anatomy and functions

Spinothalamic tract and dorsal column (ascending tracts) synapse then cross.
Corticospinal tract (descending tract) crosses then synapses.

	Spinothalamic tract	Dorsal column	Corticospinal tract
FUNCTION	Pain, temperature	Pressure, vibration, fine touch, proprioception (conscious)	Voluntary movement
1ST-ORDER NEURON	Sensory nerve ending (Aδ and C fibers) of pseudounipolar neuron in dorsal root ganglion → enters spinal cord	Sensory nerve ending of pseudounipolar neuron in dorsal root ganglion → enters spinal cord → ascends ipsilaterally in dorsal columns	UMN: 1° motor cortex → descends ipsilaterally (through posterior limb of internal capsule and cerebral peduncle), decussates at caudal medulla (pyramidal decussation) → descends contralaterally
1ST SYNAPSE	Posterior horn (spinal cord)	Nucleus gracilis (medial, lower limbs, below T6) and nucleus cuneatus (lateral, upper limbs, above T6) in the ipsilateral medulla (grass on the ground, clouds in the sky)	Anterior horn (spinal cord)
2ND-ORDER NEURON	Decussates in spinal cord as the anterior white commissure → ascends contralaterally	Decussates in medulla → ascends contralaterally as the medial lemniscus	LMN: leaves spinal cord
2ND SYNAPSE	VPL (thalamus)	VPL (thalamus)	NMJ (skeletal muscle)
3RD-ORDER NEURON	Projects to 1° somatosensory cortex	Projects to 1° somatosensory cortex	

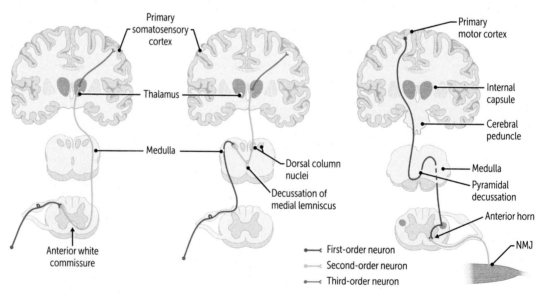

Clinical reflexes

Reflexes count up in order (main nerve root in **bold**):

- Achilles reflex = **S1**, S2 ("buckle my shoe")
- Patellar reflex = **L2-L4** ("kick the door")
- Biceps and brachioradialis reflexes = **C5**, C6 ("pick up sticks")
- Triceps reflex = C6, **C7**, C8 ("lay them straight")

Additional reflexes:
- Cremasteric reflex = L1, L2 ("testicles move")
- Anal wink reflex = S3, S4 ("winks galore")

Reflex grading:
- 0: absent
- 1+: hypoactive
- 2+: normal
- 3+: hyperactive
- 4+: clonus

C5, 6
C6, 7, 8
L2, 3, 4
S1, 2

Primitive reflexes

Primitive CNS reflexes present in healthy infants which disappear within 1st year of life due to inhibition from developing frontal lobe. Absent in neurologically intact adult. May reemerge in adults with frontal lobe lesions → loss of inhibition.

Moro reflex	"Hang on for life" reflex—abduct/extend arms when startled, and then draw together.
Rooting reflex	Movement of head toward one side if cheek or mouth is stroked (nipple seeking).
Sucking reflex	Sucking response when roof of mouth is touched.
Palmar reflex	Curling of fingers if palm is stroked.
Plantar reflex	Dorsiflexion of large toe and fanning of other toes with plantar stimulation. Babinski sign—presence of this reflex in an adult, which may signify a UMN lesion.
Galant reflex	Stroking along one side of the spine while newborn is in ventral suspension (face down) causes lateral flexion of lower body toward stimulated side.

Landmark dermatomes

DERMATOME	CHARACTERISTICS
C2	Posterior half of skull
C3	High turtleneck shirt Diaphragm and gallbladder pain referred to the right shoulder via phrenic nerve C3, 4, 5 keeps the diaphragm **alive**
C4	Low-collar shirt
C6	Includes thumbs **Thumbs up** sign on left hand looks like a 6
T4	At the **nipple** T4 at the teat **pore**
T7	At the xiphoid process 7 letters in xiphoid
T10	At the umbilicus (belly bu**ten**) Point of referred pain in early appendicitis
L1	At the Inguinal Ligament
L4	Includes the kneecaps Down on **ALL** 4's
S2, S3, S4	Sensation of penile and anal zones S2, 3, 4 keep the penis off the **floor**

▶ NEUROLOGY—PATHOLOGY

Common brain lesions

AREA OF LESION	COMPLICATIONS
Prefrontal cortex	Frontal lobe syndrome—disinhibition, hyperphagia, impulsivity, loss of empathy, impaired executive function, akinetic mutism. Seen in frontotemporal dementia.
Frontal eye fields	Eyes look toward brain lesion (ie, away from side of hemiplegia). Seen in MCA stroke.
Paramedian pontine reticular formation	Eyes look away from brain lesion (ie, toward side of hemiplegia).
Dominant parietal cortex	Gerstmann syndrome—agraphia, acalculia, finger agnosia, left-right disorientation.
Nondominant parietal cortex	Hemispatial neglect syndrome—agnosia of the contralateral side of the world.
Basal ganglia	Tremor at rest, chorea, athetosis. Seen in Parkinson disease, Huntington disease.
Subthalamic nucleus	Contralateral hemiballismus.
Mammillary bodies	Bilateral lesions → Wernicke-Korsakoff syndrome (due to thiamine deficiency).
Amygdala	Bilateral lesions → Klüver-Bucy syndrome—disinhibition (eg, hyperphagia, hypersexuality, hyperorality). Seen in HSV-1 encephalitis.
Hippocampus	Bilateral lesions → anterograde amnesia (no new memory formation). Seen in Alzheimer disease.
Dorsal midbrain	Parinaud syndrome (often due to pineal gland tumors).
Reticular activating system	Reduced levels of arousal and wakefulness, coma.
Medial longitudinal fasciculus	Internuclear ophthalmoplegia (impaired adduction of ipsilateral eye; nystagmus of contralateral eye with abduction). Seen in multiple sclerosis.
Cerebellar hemisphere	Intention tremor, limb ataxia, loss of balance; damage to cerebellum → ipsilateral deficits; fall toward side of lesion. Cerebellar hemispheres are **lateral**ly located—affect **lateral** limbs.
Cerebellar vermis	Truncal ataxia (wide-based, "drunken sailor" gait), nystagmus, dysarthria. Degeneration associated with chronic alcohol overuse. Vermis is **central**ly located—affects **central** body.

Abnormal motor posturing

	Decorticate (flexor) posturing	Decerebrate (extensor) posturing
SITE OF LESION	Above red nucleus (often cerebral cortex)	Between red and vestibular nuclei (brainstem)
OVERACTIVE TRACTS	Rubrospinal and vestibulospinal tracts	Vestibulospinal tract
PRESENTATION	Upper limb flexion, lower limb extension	Upper and lower limb extension
NOTES	"Your hands are near the **cor** (heart)"	Worse prognosis

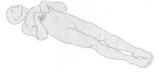

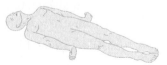

| **Ischemic brain disease/stroke** | Irreversible neuronal injury begins after 5 minutes of hypoxia. Most **vulnerable: hippocampus** (CA1 region), neocortex, cerebellum (**Purkinje cells**), **watershed areas** ("**vulnerable hippos need pure water**"). |

Stroke imaging: noncontrast CT to exclude hemorrhage (before tPA can be given). CT detects ischemic changes in 6–24 hr. Diffusion-weighted MRI can detect ischemia within 3–30 min.

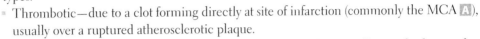

TIME SINCE ISCHEMIC EVENT	12–24 HOURS	24–72 HOURS	3–5 DAYS	1–2 WEEKS	> 2 WEEKS
Histologic features	Eosinophilic cytoplasm + pyknotic nuclei (red neurons)	Necrosis + neutrophils	Macrophages (microglia)	Reactive gliosis (astrocytes) + vascular proliferation	Glial scar

| **Ischemic stroke** | Ischemia → infarction → liquefactive necrosis. |

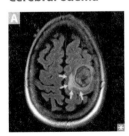

3 types:
- Thrombotic—due to a clot forming directly at site of infarction (commonly the MCA Ⓐ), usually over a ruptured atherosclerotic plaque.
- Embolic—due to an embolus from another part of the body. Can affect multiple vascular territories. Examples: atrial fibrillation, carotid artery stenosis, DVT with patent foramen ovale (paradoxical embolism), infective endocarditis.
- Hypoxic—due to systemic hypoperfusion or hypoxemia. Common during cardiovascular surgeries, tends to affect watershed areas.

Treatment: tPA (if within 3–4.5 hr of onset and no hemorrhage/risk of hemorrhage) and/or thrombectomy (if large artery occlusion). Reduce risk with medical therapy (eg, aspirin, clopidogrel); optimum control of blood pressure, blood sugars, lipids; smoking cessation; and treat conditions that ↑ risk (eg, atrial fibrillation, carotid artery stenosis).

| **Transient ischemic attack** | Brief, reversible episode of focal neurologic dysfunction without acute infarction (⊖ MRI), with the majority resolving in < 15 minutes; ischemia (eg, embolus, small vessel stenosis). May present with amaurosis fugax (transient visual loss) due to retinal artery emboli from carotid artery disease. |

| **Cerebral edema** | Fluid accumulation in brain parenchyma → ↑ ICP. Types: |

- Cytotoxic edema—intracellular fluid accumulation due to osmotic shift (eg, Na^+/K^+-ATPase dysfunction → ↑ intracellular Na^+). Caused by ischemia (early), hyperammonemia, SIADH.
- Vasogenic edema—extracellular fluid accumulation due to disruption of BBB (↑ permeability). Caused by ischemia (late), trauma, hemorrhage, inflammation, tumors (arrows in Ⓐ show surrounding vasogenic edema).

Effects of strokes

ARTERY	AREA OF LESION	SYMPTOMS	NOTES
Anterior circulation			
Anterior cerebral artery	Motor and sensory cortices—lower limb.	Contralateral paralysis and sensory loss—lower limb, urinary incontinence.	
Middle cerebral artery	Motor and sensory cortices A—upper limb and face. Temporal lobe (Wernicke area); frontal lobe (Broca area).	Contralateral paralysis and sensory loss—lower face and upper limb. Aphasia if in dominant (usually left) hemisphere. Hemineglect if lesion affects nondominant (usually right) hemisphere.	Wernicke aphasia is associated with right superior quadrant visual field defect due to temporal lobe involvement.
Lenticulo-striate artery	Striatum, internal capsule.	Contralateral paralysis. Absence of cortical signs (eg, neglect, aphasia, visual field loss).	Pure motor stroke (most common). Common location of lacunar infarcts B, due to microatheroma and hyaline arteriosclerosis (lipohyalinosis) 2° to unmanaged hypertension.
Posterior circulation			
Posterior cerebral artery	Occipital lobe C.	Contralateral hemianopia with macular sparing; alexia without agraphia (dominant hemisphere, extending to splenium of corpus callosum); prosopagnosia (inability to recognize familiar faces; nondominant hemisphere).	Weber syndrome—midbrain stroke due to occlusion of paramedian branches of PCA → ipsilateral CN III palsy and contralateral hemiplegia (damage to ipsilateral cerebral peduncle).
Basilar artery	Pons, medulla, lower midbrain.	If RAS spared, consciousness is preserved.	**Locked-in** syndrome (**locked in the basement**).
	Corticospinal and corticobulbar tracts.	Quadriplegia; loss of voluntary facial (except blinking), mouth, and tongue movements.	
	Ocular cranial nerve nuclei, paramedian pontine reticular formation.	Loss of horizontal, but not vertical, eye movements.	
Anterior inferior cerebellar artery	Facial nerve nuclei.	Paralysis of face (LMN lesion vs UMN lesion in cortical stroke), ↓ lacrimation, ↓ salivation, ↓ taste from anterior 2/3 of tongue.	Lateral pontine syndrome. Facial nerve nuclei effects are specific to AICA lesions.
	Vestibular nuclei. Spinothalamic tract, spinal trigeminal nucleus.	Vomiting, vertigo, nystagmus ↓ pain and temperature sensation from contralateral body, ipsilateral face.	
	Sympathetic fibers. Middle and inferior cerebellar peduncles.	Ipsilateral Horner syndrome. Ipsilateral ataxia, dysmetria.	
	Inner ear.	Ipsilateral sensorineural deafness, vertigo.	Supplied by labyrinthine artery, a branch of AICA.

Effects of strokes *(continued)*

ARTERY	AREA OF LESION	SYMPTOMS	NOTES
Posterior inferior cerebellar artery	Nucleus ambiguus (CN IX, X).	**Dysphagia, hoarseness,** ↓ gag reflex, hiccups.	Lateral medullary (Wallenberg) syndrome.
	Vestibular nuclei.	Vomiting, vertigo, nystagmus	Nucleus ambiguus effects are specific to **PICA** lesions 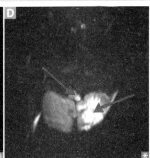.
	Lateral spinothalamic tract, spinal trigeminal nucleus.	↓ pain and temperature sensation from contralateral body, ipsilateral face.	"Don't **pick a** (PICA) **lame** (lateral medullary syndrome) **horse** (hoarseness) that **can't eat** (dysphagia)."
	Sympathetic fibers.	Ipsilateral Horner syndrome.	
	Inferior cerebellar peduncle.	Ipsilateral ataxia, dysmetria.	
Anterior spinal artery	Corticospinal tract.	Contralateral paralysis—upper and lower limbs.	Medial Medullary syndrome— caused by infarct of paramedian branches of ASA and/or vertebral arteries. **Ants** love **M&M's.**
	Medial lemniscus.	↓ contralateral proprioception.	
	Caudal medulla—hypoglossal nerve.	Ipsilateral hypoglossal dysfunction (tongue deviates ipsilaterally).	

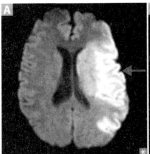 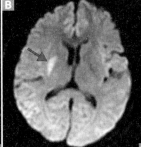 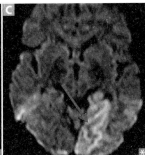

Neonatal intraventricular hemorrhage

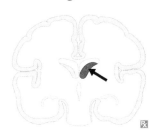

Bleeding into ventricles (arrow in illustration shows blood in intraventricular space). ↑ risk in premature and low-birth-weight infants. Originates in germinal matrix, a highly vascularized layer within the subventricular zone. Due to reduced glial fiber support and impaired autoregulation of BP in premature infants. Can present with altered level of consciousness, bulging fontanelle, hypotension, seizures, coma.

Extracranial injuries

Occur during birth leading to blood accumulation within the scalp and skull. Commonly seen in vacuum-assisted delivery.

DISORDER	PRESENTATION
Caput succedaneum	Self-limited, benign, edematous swelling above periosteum; crosses suture lines. May be caused by prolonged fetal–birth canal engagement. Resolves spontaneously.
Subgaleal hemorrhage	Serious, life-threatening damage of fetal emissary veins → blood accumulation between periosteum and gala aponeurosis. Presents as diffuse, fluctuant scalp swelling extending posteriorly and laterally. May lead to anemia and hypovolemic shock.
Cephalohematoma	Blood accumulation between skull and periosteum; does not cross suture lines. May be caused by forcep delivery. Presents with firm, localized swelling over parietal or occipital lobe. May lead to indirect hyperbilirubinemia.

Intracranial hemorrhage

Epidural hematoma	Rupture of middle meningeal artery (branch of maxillary artery), often 2° to skull fracture (circle in **A**) involving the pterion (thinnest area of the lateral skull). Might present with transient loss of consciousness → recovery ("lucid interval") → rapid deterioration due to hematoma expansion. Scalp hematoma (arrows in **A**) and rapid intracranial expansion (arrows in **B**) under systemic arterial pressure → transtentorial herniation, CN III palsy. CT shows biconvex (lentiform), hyperdense blood collection **B** **not crossing suture lines**.
Subdural hematoma	Rupture of bridging veins. Can be acute (traumatic, high-energy impact → brighter, or hyperdense, on CT) or chronic (associated with mild trauma, cerebral atrophy, ↑ age, chronic alcohol overuse → darker, or hypodense, on CT). Also seen in shaken babies. Crescent-shaped hemorrhage (red arrows in **C** and **D**) that **crosses suture lines**. Can cause midline shift, findings of acute (hyperdense border) on chronic (hypodense crescent) hemorrhage (blue arrows in **D**).
Subarachnoid hemorrhage	Bleeding **E** **F** due to trauma, or rupture of an aneurysm (such as a saccular aneurysm) or arteriovenous malformation. Rapid time course. Patients complain of "worst headache of my life." Bloody or yellow (xanthochromic) LP. Vasospasm can occur due to blood breakdown or rebleed 3–10 days after hemorrhage → ischemic infarct; nimodipine used to prevent/reduce vasospasm. ↑ risk of developing communicating and/ or noncommunicating hydrocephalus.
Intraparenchymal hemorrhage	Most commonly caused by systemic hypertension. Also seen with amyloid angiopathy (recurrent lobar hemorrhagic stroke in older adults), arteriovenous malformations, vasculitis, neoplasm. May be 2° to reperfusion injury in ischemic stroke. Hypertensive hemorrhages (Charcot-Bouchard microaneurysm) most often occur in putamen/ globus pallidus of basal ganglia (lenticulostriate vessels **G**), followed by internal capsule, thalamus, pons, and cerebellum **H**.

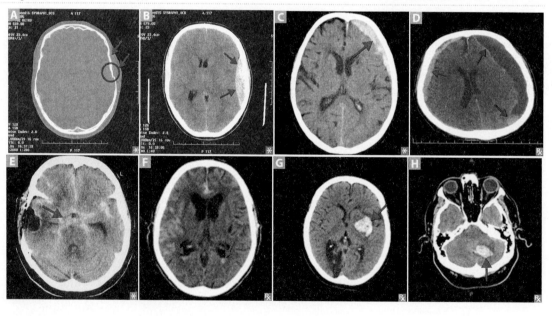

Thalamic pain syndrome	Severe, treatment-resistant neuropathic pain following thalamic lesions; may be due to occlusion of a lenticulostriate artery. Initial paresthesias followed in weeks to months by allodynia (ordinarily painless stimuli cause pain), hyperalgesia (hypersensitivity to pain), and dysesthesia (altered sensation) on the contralateral side.
Phantom limb pain	Sensation of burning, aching, or electric shock–like pain in a limb that is no longer present. Common after amputation. Associated with reorganization of the 1° somatosensory cortex.
Diffuse axonal injury 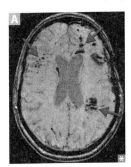	Traumatic shearing of white matter tracts during rapid acceleration and/or deceleration of the brain (eg, motor vehicle accident). Usually results in devastating neurologic injury, often causing coma or persistent vegetative state. MRI shows multiple lesions (punctate hemorrhages) involving white matter tracts A.

Aphasia

Higher-order language deficit (inability to understand/produce/use language appropriately); caused by pathology in dominant cerebral hemisphere (usually left).
Distinguish from dysarthria—motor inability to produce speech (movement deficit).

TYPE	COMMENTS
Broca (expressive)	Broca area in inferior frontal gyrus of frontal lobe. Nonfluent speech with intact language comprehension. Patients appear frustrated, insight intact. Broca = broken boca (*boca* = mouth in Spanish).
Wernicke (receptive)	Wernicke area in superior temporal gyrus of temporal lobe. Fluent speech with impaired language comprehension. Patients do not have insight. Wernicke is a word salad and makes no sense.
Conduction	Can be caused by damage to arcuate fasciculus. Impaired speech repetition.
Global	Broca and Wernicke areas affected. Nonfluent speech with impaired language comprehension.

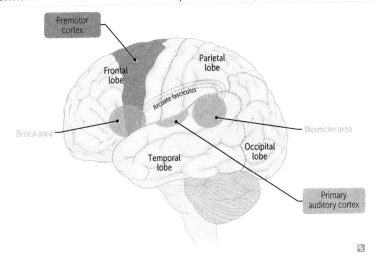

Aneurysms	Abnormal dilation of an artery due to weakening of vessel wall.

Saccular aneurysm

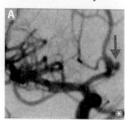

Also called berry aneurysm A. Occurs at bifurcations in the circle of Willis. Most common site is junction of ACom and ACA. Associated with ADPKD, Ehlers-Danlos syndrome. Other risk factors: advanced age, hypertension, tobacco smoking.

Usually clinically silent until rupture (most common complication) → subarachnoid hemorrhage ("worst headache of my life" or "thunderclap headache") → focal neurologic deficits. Can also cause symptoms via direct compression of surrounding structures by growing aneurysm.

- ACom—compression → bitemporal hemianopia (compression of optic chiasm); visual acuity deficits; rupture → ischemia in ACA distribution → contralateral lower extremity hemiparesis, sensory deficits.
- MCA—rupture → ischemia in MCA distribution → contralateral upper extremity and lower facial hemiparesis, sensory deficits.
- PCom—compression → ipsilateral CN III palsy → mydriasis ("blown pupil"); may also see ptosis, "down and out" eye.

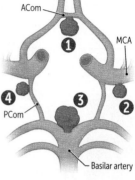

Circle of Willis

1. Anterior communicating artery (ACom) aneurysm
2. Middle cerebral artery (MCA) aneurysm
3. Basilar tip aneurysm
4. Posterior communicating artery (PCom) aneurysm

Charcot-Bouchard microaneurysm

Common, associated with chronic hypertension; affects small vessels (eg, lenticulostriate arteries in basal ganglia, thalamus) and can cause hemorrhagic intraparenchymal strokes. Not visible on angiography.

Fever vs heat stroke

	Fever	Heat stroke
PATHOPHYSIOLOGY	Cytokine activation during inflammation (eg, infection)	Inability of body to dissipate heat (eg, exertion)
TEMPERATURE	Usually < 40°C (104°F)	Usually > 40°C (104°F)
COMPLICATIONS	Febrile seizure (benign, usually self-limiting)	CNS dysfunction (eg, confusion), rhabdomyolysis, acute kidney injury, ARDS, DIC
MANAGEMENT	Acetaminophen or ibuprofen for comfort (does not prevent future febrile seizures), antibiotic therapy if indicated	Rapid external cooling, rehydration and electrolyte correction

Seizures	Characterized by synchronized, high-frequency neuronal firing. Consist of 3 phases: ▪ Aura—early part of a seizure, may include odd smells or tastes. ▪ Ictal—time from first symptom to end of seizure activity. ▪ Postictal—period of gradual recovery back to preseizure baseline level of function/awareness.

Focal seizures	Originate in a single area of the brain, most commonly the medial temporal lobe. Types: ▪ Focal aware (formerly called simple partial)—consciousness intact; motor, sensory, autonomic, psychic symptoms ▪ Focal impaired awareness (formerly called complex partial)—impaired consciousness, automatisms	Epilepsy—disorder of recurrent, unprovoked seizures (febrile seizures are not epilepsy). Convulsive status epilepticus—continuous (≥ 5 min) or recurring seizures without interictal return to baseline consciousness that may result in brain injury. Causes of seizures by age: ▪ Children < 18—genetic, infection (febrile), trauma, congenital, metabolic ▪ Adults 18–65—tumor, trauma, stroke, infection ▪ Adults > 65—stroke, tumor, trauma, metabolic, infection
Generalized seizures	Diffuse. Types: ▪ Absence (petit mal)—3 Hz spike-and-wave discharges on EEG; short (usually 10 seconds), frequent episodes of blank stare, possible automatisms; no postictal confusion. Can be triggered by hyperventilation ▪ Myoclonic—quick, repetitive jerks; no loss of consciousness or postictal confusion ▪ Tonic-clonic (grand mal)—alternating stiffening and movement, postictal confusion, urinary incontinence, tongue biting ▪ Tonic—stiffening ▪ Atonic—"drop" seizures (falls to floor); commonly mistaken for fainting	Psychogenic nonepileptic events—resemble prolonged (> 1 minute) syncopal or tonic-clonic episodes without postictal phase, autonomic disturbances, or tongue biting. Often witnessed with vocalizations and preceding aura. Female sex predominance. Risk factors: history of psychiatric disorders, substance use. Normal video EEG.

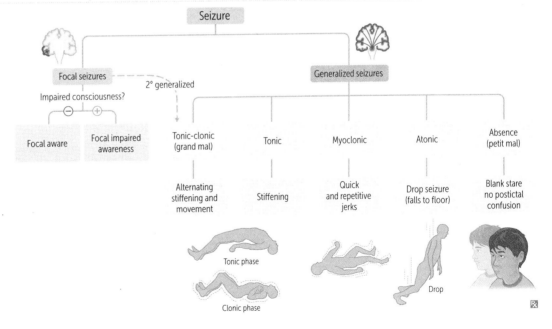

Headaches

Pain due to irritation of intra- or extracranial structures (eg, meninges, blood vessels). Primary headaches include tension-type, migraine, and cluster. Secondary headaches include medication overuse, meningitis, subarachnoid hemorrhage, hydrocephalus, neoplasia, giant cell arteritis.

CLASSIFICATION	LOCALIZATION	DURATION	DESCRIPTION	TREATMENT
Tension-type	Bilateral	> 30 min (typically 4–6 hr); constant	Steady, "bandlike" pain. No nausea or vomiting. No more than one of photophobia or phonophobia. No aura. Most common primary headache; more common in females.	Acute: analgesics, NSAIDs, acetaminophen. Prophylaxis: TCAs (eg, amitriptyline), behavioral therapy.
Migraine	Unilateral	4–72 hr	Pulsating pain with nausea, photophobia, and/or phonophobia. May have "aura." Due to irritation of CN V, meninges, or blood vessels (release of vasoactive neuropeptides [eg, substance P, calcitonin gene-related peptide]). More common in females. POUND–Pulsatile, One-day duration, Unilateral, Nausea, Disabling.	Acute: NSAIDs, triptans, dihydroergotamine, antiemetics (eg, prochlorperazine, metoclopramide). Prophylaxis: lifestyle changes (eg, sleep, exercise, diet), β-blockers, amitriptyline, topiramate, valproate, botulinum toxin, anti-CGRP monoclonal antibodies.
Cluster	Unilateral	15 min–3 hr; repetitive	Excruciating periorbital pain with autonomic symptoms (eg, lacrimation, rhinorrhea, conjunctival injection). May present with Horner syndrome. More common in males.	Acute: sumatriptan, 100% O_2. Prophylaxis: verapamil.

Trigeminal neuralgia

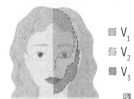

V₁
V₂
V₃

Recurrent brief episodes of intense unilateral pain in CN V distribution (usually V_2 and/or V_3). Most cases are due to compression of CN V root by an aberrant vascular loop. Pain is described as electric shock–like or stabbing and usually lasts seconds. Typically triggered by light facial touch or facial movements (eg, chewing, talking). Treatment: carbamazepine, oxcarbazepine.

Dyskinesias

DISORDER	PRESENTATION	NOTES
Akathisia	Restlessness and intense urge to move	Can be seen with neuroleptic use or as an adverse effect of Parkinson disease treatment
Asterixis	"Flapping" motion upon extension of wrists	Associated with hepatic encephalopathy, Wilson disease, and other metabolic derangements
Athetosis	Slow, snakelike, writhing movements; especially seen in the fingers	Caused by lesion to basal ganglia Seen in Huntington disease
Chorea	Sudden, jerky, purposeless movements	*Chorea* (Greek) = dancing Caused by lesion to basal ganglia Seen in Huntington disease and acute rheumatic fever (Sydenham chorea).
Dystonia	Sustained, involuntary muscle contractions	Writers cramp, blepharospasm, torticollis Treatment: botulinum toxin injection
Essential tremor	High-frequency tremor with sustained posture (eg, outstretched arms); worsened with movement or anxiety	Often familial Patients often self-medicate with alcohol, which ↓ tremor amplitude Treatment: nonselective β-blockers (eg, propranolol), barbiturates (primidone)
Intention tremor	Slow, zigzag motion when pointing/extending toward a target	Caused by cerebellar dysfunction
Resting tremor	Uncontrolled movement of distal appendages (most noticeable in hands); tremor alleviated by intentional movement	Caused by lesion to substantia nigra Occurs at **rest**; "pill-rolling tremor" of **Park**inson disease; when you **park** your car, it is at **rest**
Hemiballismus	Sudden, wild flailing of one side of the body	Caused by lesion to contralateral subthalamic nucleus (eg, due to lacunar stroke) In **hemi**ballismus, **half**-of-body is going **ballistic**
Myoclonus	Sudden, brief, uncontrolled muscle contraction	Jerks; hiccups; common in metabolic abnormalities (eg, renal and liver failure), Creutzfeldt-Jakob disease

Restless legs syndrome	Uncomfortable sensations in legs causing irresistible urge to move them. Emerge during periods of inactivity; most prominent in the evening or at night. Transiently relieved by movement (eg, walking). Usually idiopathic (often with genetic predisposition), but may be associated with iron deficiency, CKD, diabetes mellitus (especially with neuropathy). Treatment: gabapentinoids, dopamine agonists.

Neurodegenerative movement disorders

Parkinson disease

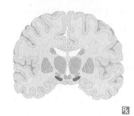

Loss of dopaminergic neurons in substantia nigra pars compacta (depigmentation in **A**).
Symptoms typically manifest after age 60 ("body **TRAP**"):

- Tremor (pill-rolling tremor at rest)
- Rigidity (cogwheel or leadpipe)
- Akinesia/bradykinesia → shuffling gait, small handwriting (micrographia)
- Postural instability (tendency to fall)

Dementia is usually a late finding.
Affected neurons contain Lewy bodies: intracellular eosinophilic inclusions composed of α-synuclein **B**. Think "Parkinsynuclein."

Progressive supranuclear palsy—a Parkinson-plus syndrome. Clinical presentation: TRAP features, vertical gaze palsy, and cognitive dysfunction. Associated with "hummingbird sign" on midbrain MRI.

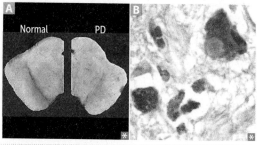

Huntington disease

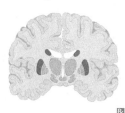

Loss of GABAergic neurons in striatum.
Autosomal dominant trinucleotide (CAG)$_n$ repeat expansion in **huntingtin** (*HTT*) gene on chromosome 4 (**4 letters**) → toxic gain of function.
Symptoms typically manifest between age 30 and 50: chorea, athetosis, aggression, depression, dementia (sometimes initially mistaken for substance use).

Atrophy of caudate and putamen with ex vacuo ventriculomegaly.
↑ dopamine, ↓ GABA, ↓ ACh in brain.
Neuronal death via NMDA receptor binding and glutamate excitotoxicity.
Anticipation results from expansion of **CAG** repeats. Caudate loses **ACh** and **GABA**.

Dementia

Decline in cognitive ability (eg, memory, executive function) with intact consciousness. Reversible causes of dementia include depression (pseudodementia), hypothyroidism, vitamin B$_{12}$ deficiency, neurosyphilis, normal pressure hydrocephalus.

Neurodegenerative

Alzheimer disease

Most common cause of dementia in older adults. Advanced age is the strongest risk factor. Down syndrome patients have ↑ risk of developing early-onset Alzheimer disease, as amyloid precursor protein (APP) is located on chromosome 21. ↓ ACh in brain.
Associated with the following altered proteins:

- ApoE-2: ↓ risk of sporadic form
- ApoE-4: ↑ risk of sporadic form
- APP, presenilin-1, presenilin-2: familial forms (10%) with earlier onset

ApoE-2 is "protwoctive," ApoE-4 is "**four**" Alzheimer disease.
Widespread cortical atrophy, especially in hippocampi. Narrowing of gyri and widening of sulci.
Senile plaques **A** in gray matter: extracellular amyloid-β (Aβ) core; may cause amyloid angiopathy → intraparenchymal hemorrhage; Aβ is derived from cleavage of APP.

Neurofibrillary tangles **B**: intracellular, hyperphosphorylated tau protein = insoluble cytoskeletal elements; number of tangles correlates with degree of dementia.
Hirano bodies: intracellular eosinophilic proteinaceous rods in hippocampus.

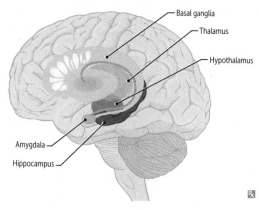

- Basal ganglia
- Thalamus
- Hypothalamus
- Amygdala
- Hippocampus

Dementia (continued)

Frontotemporal dementia	Formerly called Pick disease. Early changes in personality and behavior (behavioral variant), or aphasia (primary progressive aphasia). May have associated movement disorders.	Frontal and/or temporal lobe atrophy. Inclusions of hyperphosphorylated tau (round Pick bodies **C**) or ubiquitinated TDP-43.
Lewy body dementia	Visual hallucinations ("ha**Lewy**cinations"), dementia with fluctuating cognition/alertness, REM sleep behavior disorder, and parkinsonism.	Intracellular **Lewy** bodies primarily in cortex. Called Lewy body dementia if cognitive and motor symptom onset < 1 year apart, otherwise considered dementia 2° to Parkinson disease.

Vascular

Vascular dementia	2nd most common cause of dementia in older adults. Result of multiple arterial infarcts and/or chronic ischemia. Step-wise decline in cognitive ability with late-onset memory impairment.	MRI or CT shows multiple cortical and/or subcortical infarcts **D**.

Infective

Creutzfeldt-Jakob disease	Rapidly progressive (weeks to months) dementia with myoclonus ("startle myoclonus") and ataxia. Fatal. Caused by prions: $PrP^c \rightarrow PrP^{sc}$ (β-pleated sheet resistant to proteases). Typically sporadic, but may be transmitted by contaminated materials (eg, corneal transplant, neurosurgical equipment).	Spongiform cortex **E** (vacuolation without inflammation). Associated with periodic sharp wave complexes on EEG and ↑ 14-3-3 protein in CSF.
HIV-associated dementia	Subcortical dysfunction associated with advanced HIV infection. Characterized by cognitive deficits, gait disturbance, irritability, depressed mood.	Diffuse gray matter and subcortical atrophy. Microglial nodules with multinucleated giant cells.

Idiopathic intracranial hypertension	Also called pseudotumor cerebri. ↑ ICP with no obvious structural findings on imaging. Risk factors include **female** sex, **T**etracyclines, **O**besity, vitamin **A** excess, **D**anazol (**female TOAD**). Associated with dural venous sinus stenosis. Findings: headache (exacerbated when lying down), tinnitus, diplopia (usually from CN VI palsy), no change in mental status. Impaired optic nerve axoplasmic flow → papilledema. Visual field testing shows enlarged blind spot and peripheral constriction. LP reveals ↑ opening pressure and provides temporary headache relief. Treatment: weight loss, acetazolamide, invasive procedures for refractory cases (eg, CSF shunt placement, optic nerve sheath fenestration surgery for visual loss).

Hydrocephalus	↑ CSF volume → ventricular dilation +/− ↑ ICP.

Communicating

Communicating hydrocephalus	↓ CSF absorption by arachnoid granulations (eg, arachnoid scarring post-meningitis) → ↑ ICP, papilledema, herniation. All ventricles are dilated.
Normal pressure hydrocephalus	Affects older adults; idiopathic; CSF pressure elevated only episodically; does not result in increased subarachnoid space volume. Expansion of ventricles **A** distorts the fibers of the corona radiata → triad of **gait apraxia** (magnetic gait), **cognitive dysfunction**, and **urinary incontinence**. "**Wobbly, wacky,** and **wet**." Treatment: CSF drainage via LP or shunt placement.

Noncommunicating (obstructive)

Noncommunicating hydrocephalus	Caused by structural blockage of CSF circulation within ventricular system (eg, stenosis of aqueduct of Sylvius, colloid cyst blocking foramen of Monro, tumor **B**). Ventricles "upstream" of the obstruction are dilated.

Hydrocephalus mimics

Ex vacuo ventriculomegaly	Appearance of ↑ CSF on imaging **C**, but is actually due to ↓ brain tissue and neuronal atrophy (eg, Alzheimer disease, HIV, frontotemporal dementia, Huntington disease). ICP is normal; NPH triad is not seen.

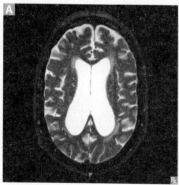 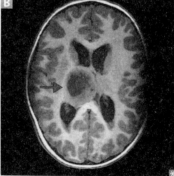 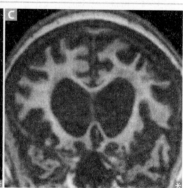

Multiple sclerosis	Autoimmune inflammation and demyelination of CNS (brain and spinal cord) with subsequent axonal damage. Most often affects females aged 20–40; higher prevalence in individuals who grew up farther from equator and have ↓ serum vitamin D levels. Can present with

- Optic neuritis (acute painful monocular visual loss, associated with relative afferent pupillary defect)
- Brainstem/cerebellar syndromes (eg, diplopia, ataxia, vertigo, scanning speech, dysarthria, intention tremor, nystagmus/intranuclear ophthalmoplegia [INO] [bilateral > unilateral])
- Pyramidal tract demyelination (eg, weakness, spasticity)
- Spinal cord syndromes (eg, electric shock–like sensation originating from cervical flexion, transmitted along the spinal cord [Lhermitte sign], neurogenic bladder, paraparesis, sensory manifestations affecting the trunk or one or more extremities)

Symptoms may be exacerbated by stressors (eg, heat [Uhthoff phenomenon], exercise, or infection). Relapsing and remitting is most common clinical course.

FINDINGS	↑ IgG level and myelin basic protein in CSF. Oligoclonal bands in CSF aid in diagnosis. MRI is gold standard. Periventricular plaques 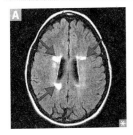 (areas of oligodendrocyte loss and reactive gliosis). Multiple white matter lesions disseminated in space and time.
TREATMENT	Stop relapses and halt/slow progression with disease-modifying therapies (eg, β-interferon, glatiramer, natalizumab). Treat acute flares with IV steroids. Symptomatic treatment for neurogenic bladder (muscarinic antagonists, botulinum toxin injection), spasticity (baclofen, GABA$_B$ receptor agonists), pain (TCAs, anticonvulsants).

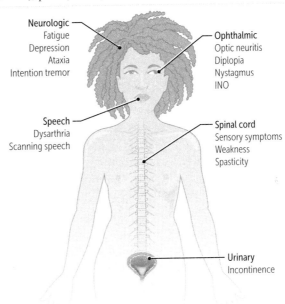

Neurologic
Fatigue
Depression
Ataxia
Intention tremor

Ophthalmic
Optic neuritis
Diplopia
Nystagmus
INO

Speech
Dysarthria
Scanning speech

Spinal cord
Sensory symptoms
Weakness
Spasticity

Urinary
Incontinence

Other demyelinating and dysmyelinating disorders

Osmotic demyelination syndrome 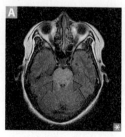	Also called central pontine myelinolysis. Massive axonal demyelination in pontine white matter 🅰 2° to rapid osmotic changes, most commonly iatrogenic correction of hyponatremia but also rapid shifts of other osmolytes (eg, glucose). Acute paralysis, dysarthria, dysphagia, diplopia, loss of consciousness. Can cause altered level of consciousness. Correcting serum Na⁺ too fast: ▪ "From low to high, your pons will die" (osmotic demyelination syndrome) ▪ "From high to low, your brains will blow" (cerebral edema/herniation)
Acute inflammatory demyelinating polyneuropathy	Most common subtype of **Guillain-Barré syndrome**. Autoimmune condition that destroys Schwann cells via inflammation and demyelination of motor fibers, sensory fibers, peripheral nerves (including CN III-XII). Likely facilitated by molecular mimicry and triggered by inoculations or stress. Despite association with infections (eg, *Campylobacter jejuni*, viruses [eg, Zika]), no definitive causal link to any pathogen. Results in symmetric ascending muscle weakness/paralysis and depressed/absent DTRs beginning in lower extremities. Facial paralysis (usually bilateral) and respiratory failure are common. May see autonomic dysregulation (eg, cardiac irregularities, hypertension, hypotension) or sensory abnormalities. Most patients survive with good functional recovery. ↑ CSF protein with normal cell count (albuminocytologic dissociation). Respiratory support is critical until recovery. Disease-modifying treatment: plasma exchange or IV immunoglobulins. No role for steroids.
Acute disseminated (postinfectious) encephalomyelitis	Multifocal inflammation and demyelination after infection or vaccination. Presents with rapidly progressive multifocal neurologic symptoms, altered mental status.
Charcot-Marie-Tooth disease	Also called hereditary motor and sensory neuropathy. Group of progressive hereditary nerve disorders related to the defective production of proteins involved in the structure and function of peripheral nerves or the myelin sheath. Typically autosomal dominant and associated with foot deformities (eg, pes cavus, hammer toe), lower extremity weakness (eg, foot drop), and sensory deficits (eg, decreased vibration, proprioception). Most common type, **CMT1A**, is caused by *PMP22* gene duplication (**C**an't **M**ove **T**oes).
Progressive multifocal leukoencephalopathy 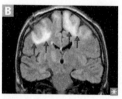	Demyelination of CNS 🅱 due to destruction of oligodendrocytes (2° to reactivation of latent JC virus infection). Associated with severe immunosuppression (eg, lymphomas and leukemias, AIDS, organ transplantation). Rapidly progressive, usually fatal. Predominantly involves parietal and occipital areas; visual symptoms are common. ↑ risk associated with organ transplantation, medications (eg, natalizumab).
Critical illness polyneuropathy	Axonal degeneration (likely from inflammatory mediators and microcirculation injury), ↓ nerve excitability 2° to Na⁺ channel inactivation → symmetric weakness (proximal > distal), ↓ deep tendon reflexes; diaphragmatic weakness may lead to difficulty weaning from mechanical ventilation.
Other disorders	Krabbe disease, metachromatic leukodystrophy, adrenoleukodystrophy.

Neurocutaneous disorders

DISORDER	GENETICS	PRESENTATION	NOTES
Sturge-Weber syndrome	Congenital nonhereditary anomaly of neural crest derivatives. Somatic mosaicism of an activating mutation in one copy of the *GNAQ* gene.	Capillary vascular malformation → port-wine stain A (nevus flammeus or non-neoplastic birthmark) in CN V_1/V_2 distribution; ipsilateral leptomeningeal angioma with calcifications B → seizures/epilepsy; intellectual disability; episcleral hemangioma → ↑ IOP → early-onset glaucoma.	Also called encephalotrigeminal angiomatosis.
Tuberous sclerosis complex	AD, variable expression. Mutation in tumor suppressor genes *TSC1* on chromosome 9 (hamartin), *TSC2* on chromosome 16 (tuberin; pronounce "twoberin").	Hamartomas in CNS and skin, angiofibromas C, mitral regurgitation, ash-leaf spots D, cardiac rhabdomyoma, intellectual disability, renal angiomyolipoma E, seizures, shagreen patches.	↑ incidence of subependymal giant cell astrocytomas and ungual fibromas.
Neurofibromatosis type I	AD, 100% penetrance. Mutation in *NF1* tumor suppressor gene on chromosome 17 (encodes neurofibromin, a negative RAS regulator).	Café-au-lait spots F, Intellectual disability, Cutaneous neurofibromas G, Lisch nodules (pigmented iris hamartomas H), Optic gliomas, Pheochromocytomas, Seizures/focal neurologic Signs (often from meningioma), bone lesions (eg, sphenoid dysplasia).	Also called von Recklinghausen disease. 17 letters in "von Recklinghausen." CICLOPSS.
Neurofibromatosis type II	AD. Mutation in *NF2* tumor suppressor gene (merlin) on chromosome 22.	Bilateral vestibular schwannomas, juvenile cataracts, meningiomas, ependymomas.	NF2 affects 2 ears, 2 eyes.
von Hippel-Lindau disease	AD. Deletion of *VHL* gene on chromosome 3p. pVHL ubiquitinates hypoxia-inducible factor 1a.	Hemangioblastomas (high vascularity with hyperchromatic nuclei I) in retina, brainstem, cerebellum, spine J; Angiomatosis; bilateral Renal cell carcinomas; Pheochromocytoma. HARP.	Numerous tumors, benign and malignant. VHL = 3 letters = chromosome 3; associated with RCC (also 3 letters).

Adult primary brain tumors

TUMOR	DESCRIPTION	HISTOLOGY
Glioblastoma	Common, highly malignant 1° brain tumor with ~ 1-year median survival. Found in cerebral hemispheres. Can cross corpus callosum ("butterfly glioma" A). Associated with *EGFR* amplification.	Astrocyte origin, GFAP ⊕. "Pseudopalisading" pleomorphic tumor cells B border central areas of necrosis, hemorrhage, and/or microvascular proliferation.
Oligodendroglioma	Relatively rare, slow growing. Most often in frontal lobes C. Often calcified.	Oligodendrocyte origin. "Fried egg" cells—round nuclei with clear cytoplasm D. "Chicken-wire" capillary pattern.
Meningioma	Common, typically benign. Females > males. Occurs along surface of brain or spinal cord. Extra-axial (external to brain parenchyma) and may have a dural attachment ("tail" E). Well circumscribed, spherical or lobular shape. Often asymptomatic; may present with seizures or focal neurologic signs. Treatment: resection and/or radiosurgery.	Arachnoid cell origin. Spindle cells concentrically arranged in a whorled pattern; psammoma bodies (laminated calcifications, arrow in F).
Hemangioblastoma	Most often cerebellar G. Associated with von Hippel-Lindau syndrome when found with retinal angiomas. Can produce erythropoietin → 2° polycythemia.	Blood vessel origin. Closely arranged, thin-walled capillaries with minimal intervening parenchyma H.
Pituitary adenoma	May be nonfunctioning (silent) or hyperfunctioning (hormone-producing). Nonfunctional tumors present with mass effect (eg, bitemporal hemianopia [due to pressure on optic chiasm I]). Pituitary apoplexy → hypopituitarism. Prolactinoma classically presents as galactorrhea, amenorrhea, ↓ bone density due to suppression of estrogen in females and as ↓ libido, infertility in males. Treatment: dopamine agonists (eg, bromocriptine, cabergoline), transsphenoidal resection.	Hyperplasia of only one type of endocrine cells found in pituitary. Most commonly from lactotrophs (prolactin) J → hyperprolactinemia. Less commonly, from somatotrophs (GH) → acromegaly, gigantism; corticotrophs (ACTH) → Cushing disease. Rarely, from thyrotrophs (TSH), gonadotrophs (FSH, LH).
Schwannoma	Classically at the cerebellopontine angle K, benign, involving CNs V, VII, and VIII, but can be along any peripheral nerve. Often localized to CN VIII in internal acoustic meatus → vestibular schwannoma (can present as hearing loss, tinnitus, and unsteady gait). Bilateral vestibular schwannomas found in NF-2. Treatment: resection or stereotactic radiosurgery.	Schwann cell origin, S-100 ⊕. Biphasic, dense, hypercellular areas containing spindle cells alternating with hypocellular, myxoid areas L.

Adult primary brain tumors *(continued)*

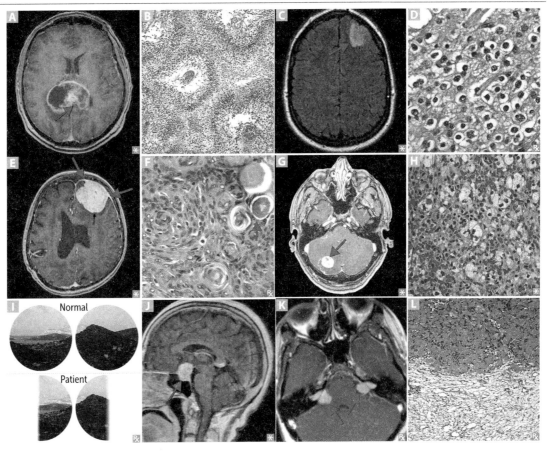

Childhood primary brain tumors

TUMOR	DESCRIPTION	HISTOLOGY
Pilocytic astrocytoma	Most common 1° brain tumor in childhood. Usually well circumscribed. In children, most often found in posterior fossa (eg, cerebellum). May be supratentorial. Cystic appearance with mural nodule **A**. Benign; good prognosis.	Astrocyte origin, GFAP ⊕. Bipolar neoplastic cells with hairlike projections. Associated with microcysts and Rosenthal fibers (eosinophilic, corkscrew fibers **B**).
Medulloblastoma	Most common malignant brain tumor in childhood. Commonly involves cerebellum **C**. Can involve the cerebellar vermis → truncal ataxia. Can compress 4th ventricle → noncommunicating hydrocephalus → headaches, papilledema. Can send "drop metastases" to spinal cord.	Form of primitive neuroectodermal tumor (PNET). Homer-Wright rosettes (small, round, blue cells surrounding central area of neuropil **D**). Synaptophysin ⊕.
Ependymoma	Most commonly found in 4th ventricle **E** → noncommunicating hydrocephalus. Poor prognosis.	Ependymal cell origin. Characteristic perivascular pseudorosettes **F**. Rod-shaped blepharoplasts (basal ciliary bodies) found near the nucleus.
Craniopharyngioma	Most common childhood supratentorial tumor. Calcification is common **G**. Commonly arises along pituitary stalk → compression of optic chiasm → bitemporal hemianopia (may be confused with pituitary adenoma). Associated with a high recurrence rate.	Derived from remnants of Rathke pouch (ectoderm). Anucleate squamous cells ("ghost cells") forming keratinous nodules with dystrophic calcifications **H**. Cholesterol crystals found in "motor oil"-like fluid within tumor.
Pineal gland tumors	Most commonly extragonadal germ cell tumors. ↑ incidence in males. Present with noncommunicating hydrocephalus (compression of cerebral aqueduct), Parinaud syndrome (compression of dorsal midbrain)—triad of upward gaze palsy, convergence-retraction nystagmus, and light-near dissociation.	Similar to testicular seminomas.

Herniation syndromes

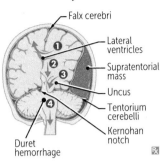

Falx cerebri
Lateral ventricles
Supratentorial mass
Uncus
Tentorium cerebelli
Kernohan notch
Duret hemorrhage

❶ Cingulate (subfalcine) herniation under falx cerebri

Can cause anterior cerebral artery compression → contralateral lower extremity weakness. If affecting the dominant hemisphere, can cause arcuate fasciculus compression → aphasia.

❷ Central/downward transtentorial herniation

Caudal displacement of brainstem → rupture of paramedian basilar artery branches → Duret hemorrhages. Usually fatal.

❸ Uncal transtentorial herniation

Uncus = medial temporal lobe. Early herniation → ipsilateral blown pupil (unilateral CN III compression), contralateral hemiparesis. Late herniation → coma, Kernohan phenomenon (misleading ipsilateral hemiparesis +/– contralateral blown pupil due to contralateral cerebral peduncle +/– CN III compression against Kernohan notch).

❹ Cerebellar tonsillar herniation into the foramen magnum

Coma and death result when these herniations compress the brainstem.

Motor neuron signs

SIGN	UMN LESION	LMN LESION	COMMENTS
Weakness	+	+	**Lower** motor neuron = everything **lowered** (↓ muscle mass, tone, reflexes, toes)
Atrophy	–	+	
Fasciculations	–	+	**Upper** motor neuron = everything **up** (↑ tone, reflexes, toes)
Reflexes	↑	↓	
Tone	↑	↓	Fasciculations = muscle twitching
Babinski	+	–	Positive Babinski is normal in infants
Spastic paresis	+	–	
Flaccid paralysis	–	+	
Clasp knife spasticity	+	–	

Spinal cord lesions

Poliomyelitis 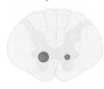	Destruction of anterior horns by poliovirus. Fecal-oral transmission → replication in lymphoid tissue of oropharynx and small intestine → spread to CNS via bloodstream. Acute LMN signs (**asymmetric** weakness) and symptoms of viral meningitis (eg, fever, headache, neck stiffness). Respiratory muscle involvement leads to respiratory failure. CSF shows ↑ WBCs (lymphocytic pleocytosis) and slight ↑ of protein (with no change in CSF glucose). Poliovirus can be isolated from stool or throat secretions.
Spinal muscular atrophy 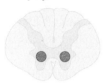	Congenital degeneration of anterior horns. Autosomal recessive *SMN1* mutation (encodes **s**urvival **m**otor **n**euron protein) → defective snRNP assembly → LMN apoptosis. Spinal muscular atrophy type 1 (most common) is also called Werdnig-Hoffmann disease. LMN signs only (**symmetric** weakness). "Floppy baby" with marked hypotonia (flaccid paralysis) and tongue fasciculations.
Amyotrophic lateral sclerosis 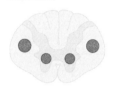	Combined UMN (corticospinal/corticobulbar) and LMN (brainstem/spinal cord) degeneration. Usually idiopathic. Familial form (less common) may be linked to *SOD1* mutations (encodes **s**uper**o**xide **d**ismutase 1). ALS is also called **Lou** Gehrig disease. LMN signs: flaccid limb weakness, fasciculations, atrophy, bulbar palsy (dysarthria, dysphagia, tongue atrophy). UMN signs: spastic limb weakness, hyperreflexia, clonus, pseudobulbar palsy (dysarthria, dysphagia, emotional lability). No sensory or bowel/bladder deficits. Fatal (most often from respiratory failure). Treatment: riluzole ("ri**Lou**zole"), edaravone (free radical scavenger) → slow functional decline.
Tabes dorsalis 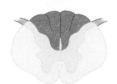	Degeneration/demyelination of dorsal columns and roots by *T pallidum* (3° syphilis). Causes progressive sensory ataxia (impaired proprioception → poor coordination). ⊕ Romberg sign and absent DTRs. Associated with shooting pain, Argyll Robertson pupils, Charcot joints.
Subacute combined degeneration 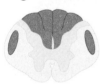	Demyelination of **S**pinocerebellar tracts, lateral **C**orticospinal tracts, and **D**orsal columns (**SCD**) due to vitamin B_{12} deficiency. Ataxic gait, paresthesias, impaired position/vibration sense (⊕ Romberg sign), UMN signs.
Anterior spinal artery occlusion 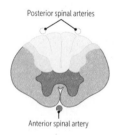 Posterior spinal arteries Anterior spinal artery	Spinal cord infarction sparing dorsal horns and dorsal columns. Watershed area is mid-thoracic ASA territory, as the artery of Adamkiewicz supplies ASA below T8. Can be caused by aortic aneurysm repair. Presents with UMN signs below the lesion (corticospinal tract), LMN signs at the level of the lesion (anterior horn), and loss of pain and temperature sensation below the lesion (spinothalamic tract).

Brown-Séquard syndrome

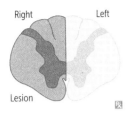

Hemisection of spinal cord. Findings due to deficits in

❶ All sensory pathways—ipsilateral loss of all sensation **at** the lesion level.

❷ Corticospinal tract—ipsilateral LMN signs (eg, flaccid paralysis) **at** lesion level.

❸ Corticospinal tract—ipsilateral UMN signs **below** lesion level.

❹ Dorsal columns—ipsilateral loss of proprioception, vibration, and fine (2-point discrimination) touch **below** lesion level.

❺ Spinothalamic tract—contralateral loss of pain, temperature, and crude (nondiscriminative) touch **below** lesion level.

Oculosympathetic pathway (if lesion occurs above T1)—ipsilateral Horner syndrome.

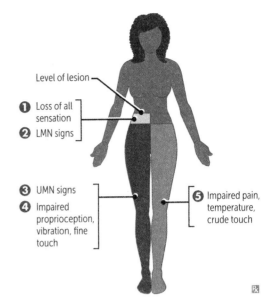

Friedreich ataxia

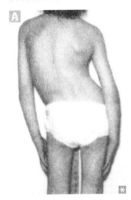

Autosomal recessive trinucleotide repeat disorder (**GAA**)$_n$ on chromosome 9 in gene that encodes frataxin (iron-binding protein). Leads to impairment in mitochondrial functioning. Degeneration of lateral corticospinal tract (spastic paralysis), spinocerebellar tract (ataxia), dorsal columns (↓ vibratory sense, proprioception), and dorsal root ganglia (loss of DTRs). **Staggering** gait, frequent **falling**, nystagmus, dysarthria, pes cavus, hammer toes, **diabetes** mellitus, **hypertrophic cardiomyopathy** (cause of death). Presents in childhood with kyphoscoliosis A.

Friedreich is fratastic (**frataxin**): he's your favorite **frat** brother, always **staggering** and **falling** but has a **sweet**, **big heart**. Ataxic **GAA**it.

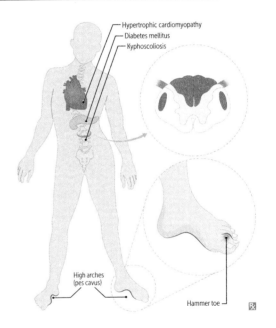

Cerebral palsy

Permanent motor dysfunction resulting from nonprogressive injury to developing fetal/infant brain. Most common movement disorder in children.

Multifactorial etiology; prematurity and low birth weight are the strongest risk factors. Associated with development of periventricular leukomalacia (focal necrosis of white matter tracts).

Presents with UMN signs (eg, spasticity, hyperreflexia) affecting ≥ 1 limbs, persistence of primitive reflexes, abnormal posture, developmental delay in motor skills, neurobehavioral abnormalities (excessive docility, irritability).

Treatment: muscle relaxants (eg, baclofen), botulinum toxin injections, selective dorsal rhizotomy.

Prevention: prenatal magnesium sulfate for high-risk pregnancies ↓ incidence and severity.

Common cranial nerve lesions

CN V motor lesion	Jaw deviates **toward** side of lesion due to unopposed force from the opposite pterygoid muscle.
CN X lesion	Uvula deviates **away** from side of lesion. Weak side collapses and uvula points away.
CN XI lesion	Weakness turning head **away** from side of lesion (SCM). Shoulder droop on side of lesion (trapezius).
CN XII lesion	LMN lesion. Tongue deviates **toward** side of lesion ("lick your wounds") due to weakened tongue muscles on affected side.

Facial nerve lesions

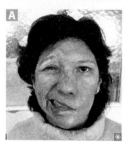

Bell palsy is the most common cause of peripheral facial palsy A. Usually develops after HSV reactivation. Treatment: glucocorticoids +/– acyclovir. Most patients gradually recover function, but aberrant regeneration can occur. Other causes of peripheral facial palsy include Lyme disease, herpes zoster (**Ramsay Hunt syndrome**—triad of ipsilateral facial paralysis, otalgia, and vesicles near the auditory canal), sarcoidosis, tumors (eg, parotid gland), diabetes mellitus.

	Upper motor neuron lesion	Lower motor neuron lesion
LESION LOCATION	Motor cortex, connection from motor cortex to facial nucleus in pons	Facial nucleus, anywhere along CN VII
AFFECTED SIDE	Contralateral	Ipsilateral
MUSCLES INVOLVED	Lower muscles of facial expression	Upper and lower muscles of facial expression
FOREHEAD INVOLVEMENT	Spared, due to bilateral UMN innervation	Affected
OTHER SYMPTOMS	Variable; depends on size of lesion	Incomplete eye closure (dry eyes, corneal ulceration), hyperacusis, loss of taste sensation to anterior tongue

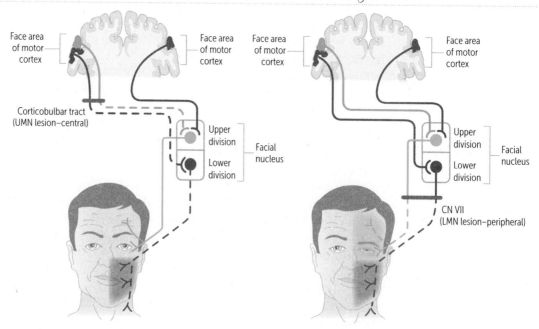

▸ **NEUROLOGY—OTOLOGY**

Auditory anatomy and physiology

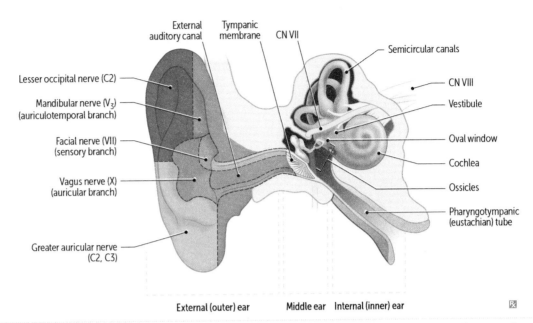

External (outer) ear   Middle ear   Internal (inner) ear

Outer ear	Visible portion of ear (pinna), includes auditory canal and tympanic membrane. Transfers sound waves via vibration of tympanic membrane.
Middle ear	Air-filled space with three bones called the ossicles (malleus, incus, stapes). Ossicles conduct and amplify sound from tympanic membrane to inner ear.
Inner ear	Snail-shaped, fluid-filled cochlea. Contains basilar membrane that vibrates 2° to sound waves. Vibration transduced via specialized hair cells → auditory nerve signaling → brainstem. Each frequency leads to vibration at specific location on basilar membrane (tonotopy): <ul><li>Low frequency heard at apex near helicotrema (wide and flexible).</li><li>High frequency heard best at base of cochlea (thin and rigid).</li></ul>

Otitis externa

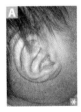

Inflammation of external auditory canal. Most commonly due to *Pseudomonas*. Associated with water exposure (swimmer's ear), ear canal trauma/occlusion (eg, hearing aids).
Presents with otalgia that worsens with ear manipulation, pruritus, hearing loss, discharge Ⓐ.
Malignant (necrotizing) otitis externa—invasive infection causing osteomyelitis. Complication of otitis externa mostly seen in older patients with diabetes. Presents with severe otalgia and otorrhea. May lead to cranial nerve palsies. Physical exam shows granulation tissue in ear canal.

Otitis media

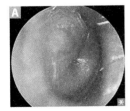

Inflammation of middle ear. Most commonly due to nontypeable *Streptococcus pneumoniae*, *Haemophilus influenzae*, *Moraxella catarrhalis*. Associated with eustachian tube dysfunction, which promotes overgrowth of bacterial colonizers of upper respiratory tract.
Usually seen in children < 2 years old. Presents with fever, otalgia, hearing loss. Physical exam shows bulging, erythematous tympanic membrane Ⓐ that may rupture.
Mastoiditis—infection of mastoid process of temporal bone. Complication of acute otitis media due to continuity of middle ear cavity with mastoid air cells. Presents with postauricular pain, erythema, swelling. May lead to brain abscess.

Common causes of hearing loss

Noise-induced hearing loss	Damage to stereociliated cells in organ of Corti. Loss of high-frequency hearing first. Sudden extremely loud noises can produce hearing loss due to tympanic membrane rupture.
Presbycusis	**Aging**-related progressive bilateral/symmetric sensorineural hearing loss (often of higher frequencies) due to destruction of hair cells at the cochlear base (preserved low-frequency hearing at apex).

Diagnosing hearing loss

	Normal	Conductive	Sensorineural
Weber test Tuning fork on vertex of skull	No localization	Localizes to affected ear ↓ transmission of background noise	Localizes to unaffected ear ↓ transmission of all sound
Rinne test Tuning fork in front of ear (air conduction, AC), Tuning fork on mastoid process (bone conduction, BC)	AC > BC	BC > AC	AC > BC

Cholesteatoma

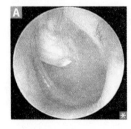

Abnormal growth of keratinized squamous epithelium in middle ear **A** ("skin in wrong place"). Usually acquired, but can be congenital. 1° acquired results from tympanic membrane retraction pockets that form due to eustachian tube dysfunction. 2° acquired results from tympanic membrane perforation (eg, due to otitis media) that permits migration of squamous epithelium to middle ear. Classically presents with painless otorrhea. May erode ossicles → conductive hearing loss.

Vertigo

Sensation of spinning while actually stationary. Subtype of "dizziness," but distinct from "lightheadedness." Peripheral vertigo is more common than central vertigo.

Peripheral vertigo	Due to inner ear pathologies such as vestibular neuritis; benign paroxysmal positional vertigo— semicircular canal debris → episodic vertigo lasting ≤ 1 minute provoked by certain head movements (diagnosed via Dix-Hallpike maneuver, treated via Epley maneuver); and **Mén**ière disease—endolymphatic hydrops (↑ endolymph in inner ear) → triad of **v**ertigo, **s**ensorineural hearing loss, **t**innitus ("**men** wear **vests**"). Findings: mixed horizontal-torsional nystagmus (never purely torsional or vertical) that does not change direction and is suppressible with visual fixation.
Central vertigo	Due to brainstem or cerebellar lesions (eg, stroke affecting vestibular nuclei, demyelinating disease, or posterior fossa tumor). Findings: nystagmus of any direction that is not suppressible with visual fixation, neurologic findings (eg, diplopia, ataxia, dysmetria).

▶ NEUROLOGY—OPHTHALMOLOGY

Normal eye anatomy

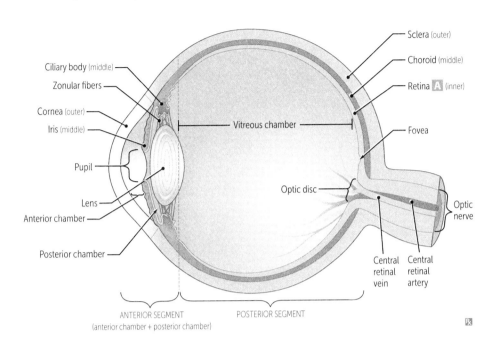

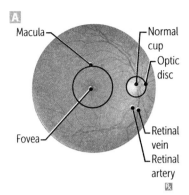

Conjunctivitis 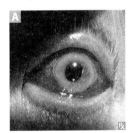	Inflammation of the conjunctiva → red eye A.
	Allergic—itchy eyes, bilateral.
	Bacterial—purulent discharge; treat with antibiotics.
	Viral—most common, often adenovirus; sparse mucous discharge, swollen preauricular node, ↑ lacrimation; self-resolving.
	Neonatal—eyelid swelling, exudative discharge after vaginal birth. Detect bacterial etiologies with NAAT. Maternal prenatal screening and treatment ↓ incidence.
	▪ *C trachomatis* serotypes D-K (most common)—onset 5–14 days after birth; treat with erythromycin or azithromycin.
	▪ *N gonorrhoeae*—onset 2–5 days after birth; prophylaxis: erythromycin eyedrops; treat with ceftriaxone to prevent blindness.
	▪ Other pathogens—HSV, adenovirus.

Refractive errors	Common cause of impaired vision, correctable with glasses. **My cave "hy"-des (hides) vexed cylinders.**
Myopia	Most common. Also called "nearsightedness." Eye too long for refractive power of cornea and lens → light focused in front of retina. Correct with concave (diverging) lens.
Hyperopia	Also called "farsightedness." Eye too short for refractive power of cornea and lens → light focused behind retina. Correct with convex (converging) lens.
Astigmatism	Irregular or asymmetric curvature of the cornea or lens → different refractive power at different axes. Correct with cylindrical lens.

Lens disorders

Presbyopia	Aging-related impairment in accommodation (focusing on near objects). Pathophysiology not fully understood but likely includes ↓ lens elasticity. Patients often need reading glasses or magnifiers.
Cataract 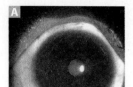	Painless, often bilateral, opacification of lens A. Can result in glare, loss of red reflex, and ↓ vision, especially at night. Acquired risk factors: ↑ age, tobacco smoking, alcohol overuse, excessive sunlight, prolonged glucocorticoid use, diabetes mellitus, trauma, infection. Congenital risk factors: classic galactosemia, galactokinase deficiency, trisomies (13, 18, 21), TORCH infections (eg, rubella), Marfan syndrome, Alport syndrome, myotonic dystrophy, NF-2. Treatment: surgical replacement with an artificial lens.
Lens dislocation	Also called ectopia lentis. Displacement or malposition of lens. Usually due to trauma, but may occur in association with systemic diseases (eg, Marfan syndrome, homocystinuria).

Aqueous humor pathway

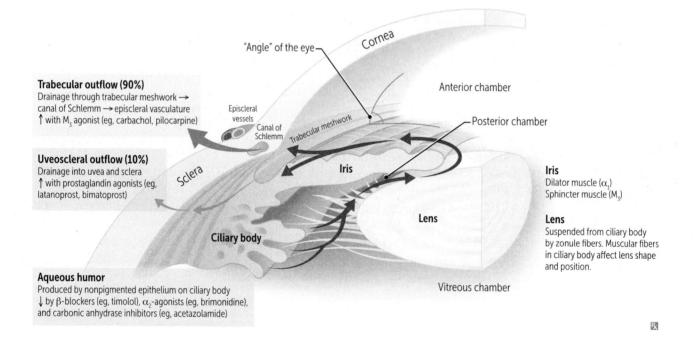

Trabecular outflow (90%)
Drainage through trabecular meshwork → canal of Schlemm → episcleral vasculature
↑ with M₃ agonist (eg, carbachol, pilocarpine)

Uveoscleral outflow (10%)
Drainage into uvea and sclera
↑ with prostaglandin agonists (eg, latanoprost, bimatoprost)

Aqueous humor
Produced by nonpigmented epithelium on ciliary body
↓ by β-blockers (eg, timolol), α₂-agonists (eg, brimonidine), and carbonic anhydrase inhibitors (eg, acetazolamide)

Iris
Dilator muscle (α₁)
Sphincter muscle (M₃)

Lens
Suspended from ciliary body by zonule fibers. Muscular fibers in ciliary body affect lens shape and position.

"Angle" of the eye — Cornea
Anterior chamber
Posterior chamber
Episcleral vessels
Canal of Schlemm
Trabecular meshwork
Iris
Sclera
Lens
Ciliary body
Vitreous chamber

Glaucoma	Optic neuropathy causing progressive vision loss (peripheral → central). Usually, but not always, accompanied by ↑ intraocular pressure (IOP). Etiology is most often 1°, but can be 2° to an identifiable cause (eg, uveitis, glucocorticoids). Funduscopy: optic disc cupping (normal A vs thinning of outer rim of optic disc B). Treatment: pharmacologic or surgical lowering of IOP.
Open-angle glaucoma	Anterior chamber angle is open (normal). Most common type in US. Associated with ↑ resistance to aqueous humor drainage through trabecular meshwork. Risk factors: ↑ age, race (↑ incidence in Black population), family history, diabetes mellitus. Typically asymptomatic and discovered incidentally. Treat with prostaglandins or β-blockers.
Angle-closure glaucoma	Anterior chamber angle is narrowed or closed. Associated with anatomic abnormalities (eg, anteriorly displaced lens resting against central iris) → ↓ aqueous flow through pupil (pupillary block) → pressure buildup in posterior chamber → peripheral iris pushed against cornea → obstruction of drainage pathways by the iris. Usually chronic and asymptomatic, but may develop acutely. Acute angle-closure glaucoma—complete pupillary block causing abrupt angle closure and rapid ↑ IOP. Presents with severe eye pain, conjunctival erythema C, sudden vision loss, halos around lights, headache, fixed and mid-dilated pupil, nausea and vomiting. **H**urts in a **h**urry with **h**alos, a **h**eadache, and a "**h**alf-dilated" pupil. True ophthalmic emergency that requires immediate management to prevent blindness. Mydriatic agents are contraindicated. Treat with β-blocker, α_2-agonist, pilocarpine, acetazolamide, mannitol.

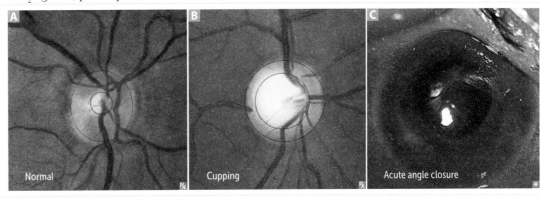

A — Normal
B — Cupping
C — Acute angle closure

Open-angle glaucoma

→ Normal aqueous flow
→ Abnormal aqueous flow

↑ trabecular outflow resistance

Open angle

Angle-closure glaucoma

Obstruction of drainage pathways by the iris

Closed angle

Pupillary block

Retinal disorders

Age-related macular degeneration	Degeneration of macula (central area of retina) → loss of central vision (scotomas). Two types: ▪ **D**ry (most common)—gradual ↓ in vision with subretinal **d**eposits (**d**rusen, arrows in A). ▪ Wet—rapid ↓ in vision due to bleeding 2° to choroidal neovascularization. Distortion of straight lines (metamorphopsia) is an early symptom.
Diabetic retinopathy	Chronic hyperglycemia → ↑ permeability and occlusion of retinal vessels. Two types: ▪ Nonproliferative (most common)—microaneurysms, hemorrhages (arrows in B), cotton-wool spots, hard exudates. Vision loss mainly due to macular edema. ▪ Proliferative—retinal neovascularization due to chronic hypoxia. Abnormal new vessels may cause vitreous hemorrhage and tractional retinal detachment.
Hypertensive retinopathy	Chronic hypertension → spasm, sclerosis, and fibrinoid necrosis of retinal vessels. Funduscopy: arteriovenous nicking, microaneurysms, hemorrhages, cotton-wool spots (blue arrow in C), hard exudates (may form macular "star," red arrow in C). Presence of papilledema is indicative of hypertensive emergency and warrants immediate lowering of blood pressure.
Retinal artery occlusion	Blockage of central or branch retinal artery usually due to embolism (carotid artery atherosclerosis > cardiogenic); less commonly due to giant cell arteritis. Presents with acute, painless monocular vision loss. Funduscopy: cloudy retina with "cherry-red" spot at fovea D, identifiable retinal emboli (eg, cholesterol crystals appear as small, yellow, refractile deposits in arterioles).
Retinal vein occlusion	Central retinal vein occlusion is due to 1° thrombosis; branch retinal vein occlusion is due to 2° thrombosis at arteriovenous crossings (sclerotic arteriole compresses adjacent venule causing turbulent blood flow). Funduscopy: retinal hemorrhage and venous engorgement ("blood and thunder" appearance; arrows in E), retinal edema in affected areas.
Retinal detachment	Separation of neurosensory retina from underlying retinal pigment epithelium → loss of choroidal blood supply → hypoxia and degeneration of photoreceptors. Two types: ▪ Rhegmatogenous (most common)—due to retinal tears; often associated with posterior vitreous detachment (↑ risk with advanced age, high myopia), less frequently traumatic. ▪ Nonrhegmatogenous—tractional or exudative (fluid accumulation). Commonly presents with symptoms of posterior vitreous detachment (eg, floaters, light flashes) followed by painless monocular vision loss ("dark curtain"). Funduscopy: opacification and wrinkling of detached retina F, change in vessel direction. Surgical emergency.
Retinitis pigmentosa	Group of inherited dystrophies causing progressive degeneration of photoreceptors and retinal pigment epithelium. May be associated with abetalipoproteinemia. Early symptoms: night blindness (nyctalopia) and peripheral vision loss. Funduscopy: triad of optic disc pallor, retinal vessel attenuation, and retinal pigmentation with bone spicule-shaped deposits G.
Retinopathy of prematurity	Preterm birth → loss of normal hypoxic environment in utero → relative hyperoxia (↑ with supplemental O_2 for NRDS) → ↓ VEGF → arrest of normal retinal vascularization. As the eyes grow → hypoxia of avascular retina → ↑ VEGF → retinal neovascularization (may cause tractional retinal detachment). Common cause of childhood blindness.
Retinoblastoma	Most common intraocular malignancy in children. Arises from immature retinal cells H. Caused by mutations to both *RB1* tumor suppressor genes on chromosome 13, which normally impede G_1 → S phase progression. Can be sporadic or familial (loss of heterozygosity). Presents with leukocoria, strabismus, nystagmus, eye redness.

Retinal disorders *(continued)*

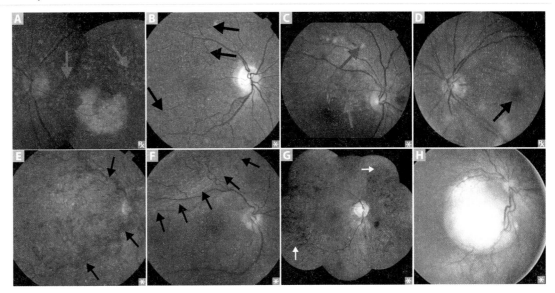

Papilledema	Optic disc swelling (usually bilateral) due to ↑ ICP (eg, 2° to mass effect). Results from impaired axoplasmic flow in optic nerve. Funduscopy: elevated optic disc with blurred margins **A**.

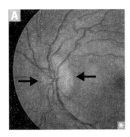

Leukocoria	Loss (whitening) of the red reflex. Important causes in children include retinoblastoma **A**, congenital cataract.

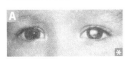

Uveitis	Inflammation of uvea; specific name based on location within affected eye. Anterior uveitis: iritis; posterior uveitis: choroiditis and/or retinitis. May have hypopyon (accumulation of pus in anterior chamber **A**) or conjunctival redness. Associated with systemic inflammatory disorders (eg, sarcoidosis, Behçet syndrome, juvenile idiopathic arthritis, HLA-B27–associated conditions).

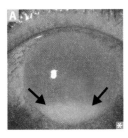

Pupillary control

Miosis	Constriction, parasympathetic: ▪ 1st neuron: Edinger-Westphal nucleus to ciliary ganglion via CN III ▪ 2nd neuron: short ciliary nerves to sphincter pupillae muscles **Short** ciliary nerves **short**en the pupil diameter.

Pupillary light reflex

Light in either retina sends a signal via CN II to pretectal nuclei in midbrain that activates bilateral Edinger-Westphal nuclei; pupils constrict bilaterally (direct and consensual reflex).

Result: illumination of 1 eye results in bilateral pupillary constriction.

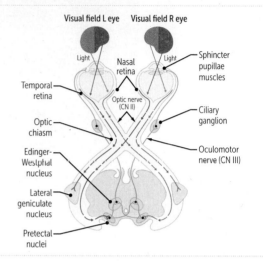

Mydriasis

Dilation, sympathetic:
▪ 1st neuron: hypothalamus to ciliospinal center of Budge (C8–T2)
▪ 2nd neuron: exit at T1 to superior cervical ganglion (travels along cervical sympathetic chain near lung apex, subclavian vessels)
▪ 3rd neuron: plexus along internal carotid, through cavernous sinus; enters orbit as long ciliary nerve to pupillary dilator muscles. Sympathetic fibers also innervate smooth muscle of eyelids (minor retractors) and sweat glands of forehead and face.

Long ciliary nerves make the pupil diameter **long**er.

Relative afferent pupillary defect

Also called Marcus Gunn pupil. Extent of pupillary constriction differs when light is shone in one eye at a time due to unilateral or asymmetric lesions of afferent limb of pupillary reflex (eg, retina, optic nerve). When light shines into a normal eye, constriction of the ipsilateral eye (direct reflex) and contralateral eye (consensual reflex) is observed. When light is swung from a normal eye to an affected eye, both pupils dilate instead of constricting.

Horner syndrome

Sympathetic denervation of face:
- Ptosis (slight drooping of eyelid: superior tarsal muscle)
- Miosis (pupil constriction)
- Anhidrosis (absence of sweating) and absence of flushing of affected side of face

Associated with lesions along the sympathetic chain:
- 1st neuron: pontine hemorrhage, lateral medullary syndrome, spinal cord lesion above T1 (eg, Brown-Séquard syndrome, late-stage syringomyelia)
- 2nd neuron: stellate ganglion compression by Pancoast tumor
- 3rd neuron: carotid dissection (painful); anhidrosis is usually absent

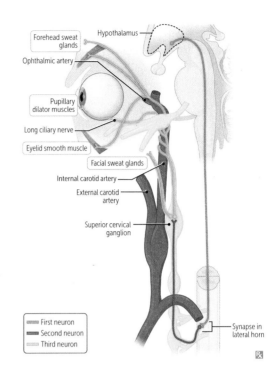

Ocular motility

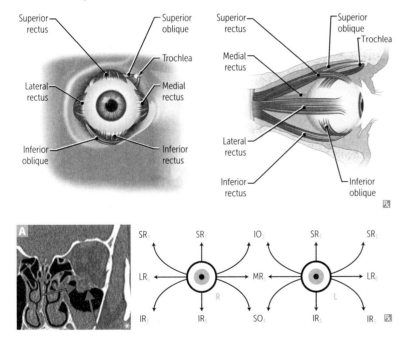

CN **VI** innervates the Lateral Rectus.
CN **IV** innervates the Superior Oblique.
CN **III** innervates the Rest.
The "chemical formula" $LR_6SO_4R_3$.

Arrows in illustration depict direction of gaze with which to test each muscle.
Obliques go Opposite (left SO and IO tested with patient looking right)
IOU: IO tested looking Up

Blowout fracture—orbital floor fracture; usually due to trauma to eyeball or infraorbital rim. ↑ risk of IR muscle A and/or orbital fat entrapment. May lead to infraorbital nerve injury.

Strabismus

Eye misalignment ("crossed eyes"). Deviation of eye toward the nose (esotropia) is the most common type of strabismus in children. Complications include amblyopia, diplopia, adverse psychosocial impact.

Amblyopia ("lazy eye")—↓ visual acuity due to maldevelopment of visual cortex. Caused by abnormal visual experience early in life (eg, due to strabismus). Typically unilateral.

Cranial nerve III, IV, VI palsies

CN III damage	CN III has both motor (central) and parasympathetic (peripheral) components. Common causes include: • Ischemia → pupil sparing (motor fibers affected more than parasympathetic fibers) • Uncal herniation → coma • PCom aneurysm → sudden-onset headache • Cavernous sinus thrombosis → proptosis, involvement of CNs IV, V_1/V_2, VI • Midbrain stroke → contralateral hemiplegia **M**otor output to extraocular muscles—affected primarily by vascular disease (eg, diabetes mellitus: glucose → sorbitol) due to ↓ diffusion of oxygen and nutrients to the interior (**middle**) fibers from compromised vasculature that resides on outside of nerve. Signs: ptosis, "down-and-out" gaze. **P**arasympathetic output—fibers on the **p**eriphery are first affected by compression (eg, PCom aneurysm, uncal herniation). Signs: diminished or absent pupillary light reflex, "blown pupil" often with "down-and-out" gaze.	Motor = **m**iddle (central) Parasympathetic = **p**eripheral 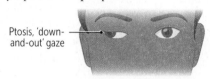 Ptosis, 'down-and-out' gaze CN III (oculomotor) palsy, motor 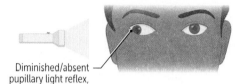 Diminished/absent pupillary light reflex, 'blown pupil', +/– 'down-and-out' gaze CN III (oculomotor) palsy, parasympathetic
CN IV damage	Pupil is higher in the affected eye. Characteristic head tilt to contralateral/unaffected side to compensate for lack of intorsion in affected eye. Can't see the **floor** with CN **IV** damage (eg, difficulty going down stairs, reading).	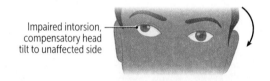 Impaired intorsion, compensatory head tilt to unaffected side CN IV (trochlear) palsy
CN VI damage	Affected eye unable to abduct and is displaced medially in primary position of gaze.	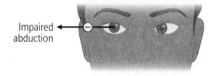 Impaired abduction CN VI (abducens) palsy

CN III

Visual field defects

Ventral optic radiation (Meyer loop)—lower retina; travels through temporal lobe; loops around inferior horn of lateral ventricle.

Dorsal optic radiation—superior retina; travels through parietal lobe.

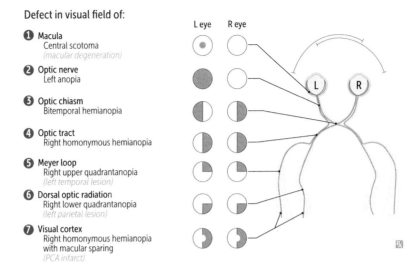

Defect in visual field of:

❶ Macula
Central scotoma
(macular degeneration)

❷ Optic nerve
Left anopia

❸ Optic chiasm
Bitemporal hemianopia

❹ Optic tract
Right homonymous hemianopia

❺ Meyer loop
Right upper quadrantanopia
(left temporal lesion)

❻ Dorsal optic radiation
Right lower quadrantanopia
(left parietal lesion)

❼ Visual cortex
Right homonymous hemianopia
with macular sparing
(PCA infarct)

Note: When an image hits 1° visual cortex, it is upside down and left-right reversed.

Cavernous sinus

Collection of venous sinuses on either side of pituitary. Blood from eye and superficial cortex → cavernous sinus → internal jugular vein.

CNs III, IV, V_1, V_2, and VI plus postganglionic sympathetic pupillary fibers en route to orbit all pass through cavernous sinus. Cavernous portion of internal carotid artery is also here. Internal carotid artery, Trigeminal nerve (Ophthalmic and Maxillary divisions), Abducens nerve, Trochlear nerve, Oculomotor nerve (**I, TOMATO**).

Cavernous sinus syndrome—presents with variable ophthalmoplegia (eg, CN III and CN VI), ↓ corneal sensation, Horner syndrome and occasional ↓ maxillary sensation. 2° to pituitary tumor mass effect, carotid-cavernous fistula, or cavernous sinus thrombosis related to infection (spread due to lack of valves in dural venous sinuses).

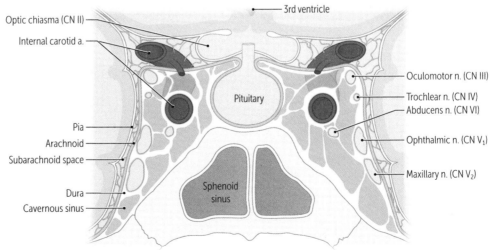

Internuclear ophthalmoplegia

Medial longitudinal fasciculus (MLF): pair of tracts that interconnect CN VI and CN III nuclei. Coordinates both eyes to move in same horizontal direction. Highly myelinated (must communicate quickly so eyes move at same time). Lesions may be unilateral or bilateral (latter classically seen in multiple sclerosis, stroke).

Lesion in MLF = internuclear ophthalmoplegia (INO), a conjugate horizontal gaze palsy. Lack of communication such that when CN VI nucleus activates ipsilateral lateral rectus, contralateral CN III nucleus does not stimulate medial rectus to contract. Abducting eye displays nystagmus (CN VI overfires to stimulate CN III). Convergence normal.

MLF in **MS**.

When looking left, the left nucleus of CN VI fires, which contracts the left lateral rectus and stimulates the contralateral (right) nucleus of CN III via the right MLF to contract the right medial rectus.

Directional term (eg, right INO, left INO) refers to the eye that is unable to adduct.

INO = **I**psilateral adduction failure, **N**ystagmus **O**pposite.

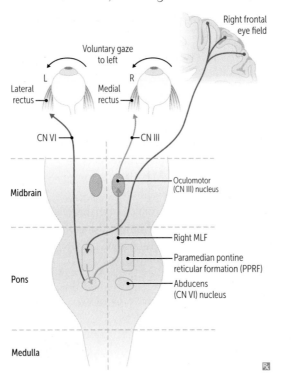

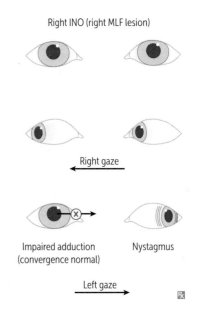

Eyelid disorders

DISORDER	PRESENTATION
Preseptal cellulitis	Anterior soft tissue eyelid infection. Mild presentation with unilateral ocular pain, swelling, and erythema present at rest.
Orbital cellulitis	Posterior eyelid infection affecting orbit contents (fat and muscles). Pain with ocular movement. Infection affecting the orbital contents (fat and muscles), usually secondary to bacterial sinusitis. Pain and double vision (diplopia) with ocular movement. Risk of vision loss, cavernous sinus thrombosis, and intracranial spread. Most commonly caused by S *aureus* and streptococci.
Blepharitis	Eyelid margin and lid inflammation, irritation, and crusting.
Hordeolum (stye)	Acute infection of the sebaceous or sweat glands of the eyelid. Tender, erythematous nodule.
Chalazion	Noninfectious granulomatous inflammation caused by obstruction of a meibomian (modified sebaceous) or Zeis (sebaceous) gland.
Xanthelasma	Yellowish patch on medial eyelid. May be associated with genetic and lifestyle factors, eg, high cholesterol.

▶ NEUROLOGY—PHARMACOLOGY

Anticonvulsants

	MECHANISM	COMMON ADVERSE EFFECTS	RARE BUT SERIOUS ADVERSE EFFECTS
Narrow spectrum (focal seizures)			
Phenytoin	Block Na^+ channel	Sedation, dizziness, diplopia, gingival hypertrophy (preventable with folate supplementation), rash, hirsutism, drug interactions (CYP450 induction)	SJS, DRESS, hepatotoxicity, neuropathy, osteoporosis, folate depletion, teratogenicity
Carbamazepine		Sedation, dizziness, diplopia, vomiting, diarrhea, SIADH, rash, drug interactions (CYP450 induction)	SJS, DRESS, hepatotoxicity, agranulocytosis, aplastic anemia, folate depletion, teratogenicity
Gabapentinoids Gabapentin, pregabalin	Block Ca^{2+} channel	Sedation, dizziness, ataxia, weight gain	
Narrow spectrum (absence seizures only)			
Ethosuximide	Blocks Ca^{2+} channel	Sedation, dizziness, vomiting	
Broad spectrum (focal and generalized seizures)			
Valproate	Blocks Na^+ channel Blocks Ca^{2+} channel Blocks GABA transaminase	Sedation, dizziness, vomiting, weight gain, hair loss, easy bruising, drug interactions (CYP450 inhibition)	Hepatotoxicity, pancreatitis, teratogenicity (highest risk of all anticonvulsants)
Lamotrigine	Blocks Na^+ channel	Sedation, dizziness, rash	SJS, DRESS
Levetiracetam	Blocks Synaptic Vesicle protein 2A (**SV2A**)	Sedation, dizziness, fatigue	Neuropsychiatric (eg, psychosis)
Topiramate	Blocks Na^+ channel Potentiates $GABA_A$ receptor	Sedation, dizziness, mood disturbance (eg, depression), weight loss, paresthesia	Kidney stones, angle-closure glaucoma

Anticonvulsants (continued)

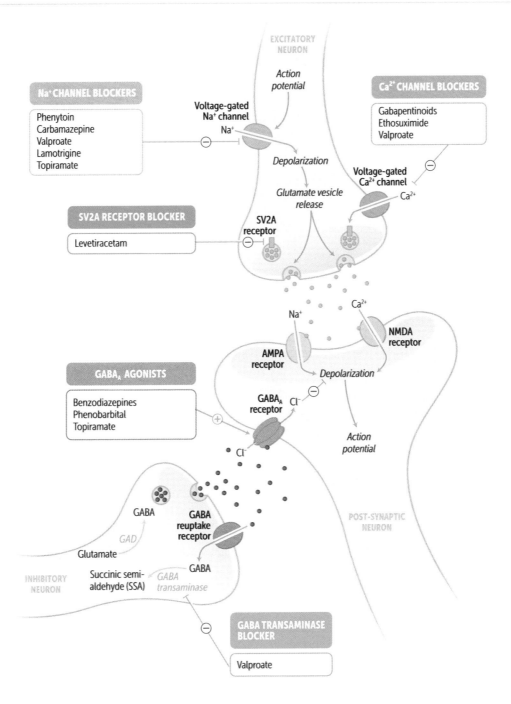

Barbiturates	Phenobarbital, pentobarbital.
MECHANISM	Facilitate GABA$_A$ action by ↑ **duration** of Cl$^-$ channel opening, thus ↓ neuron firing (barbi**dura**tes ↑ **dura**tion).
CLINICAL USE	Sedative for anxiety, seizures, insomnia; alcohol or sedative withdrawal.
ADVERSE EFFECTS	Respiratory and cardiovascular depression (can be fatal); CNS depression (exacerbated by alcohol use); dependence; drug interactions (induces CYP-450). Contraindicated in porphyria. Overdose treatment is supportive (assist respiration and maintain BP).

Benzodiazepines	Diazepam, lorazepam, triazolam, temazepam, oxazepam, midazolam, chlordiazepoxide, alprazolam.
MECHANISM	Facilitate $GABA_A$ action by ↑ **frequency** of Cl^- channel opening ("**frenzo**diazepines" ↑ frequency). ↓ REM sleep. Most have long half-lives and active metabolites (exceptions [**ATOM**]: **A**lprazolam, **T**riazolam, **O**xazepam, and **M**idazolam are short acting → higher addictive potential).
CLINICAL USE	Anxiety, panic disorder, spasticity, status epilepticus (lorazepam, diazepam, midazolam), eclampsia, medically supervised withdrawal (eg, alcohol/DTs; long-acting chlordiazepoxide and diazepam are preferred), night terrors/sleepwalking (↓ N3 and REM sleep), general anesthetic (amnesia, muscle relaxation), hypnotic (insomnia). **L**orazepam, **O**xazepam, and **T**emazepam can be used for those with liver disease who drink a **LOT** due to minimal first-pass metabolism.
ADVERSE EFFECTS	Dependence, additive CNS depression effects with alcohol and barbiturates (all bind the $GABA_A$ receptor). Less risk of respiratory depression and coma than with barbiturates. Treat overdose with flumazenil (competitive antagonist at GABA benzodiazepine receptor). Can precipitate seizures by causing acute benzodiazepine withdrawal.

Insomnia therapy

AGENT	MECHANISM	ADVERSE EFFECTS	NOTES
Nonbenzodiazepine hypnotics	Examples: **Z**olpidem, **Z**aleplon, es**Z**opiclone Act via the BZ_1 subtype of GABA receptor	Ataxia, headaches, confusion Cause only modest day-after psychomotor depression and few amnestic effects (vs older sedative-hypnotics)	These **ZZZ**s put you to sleep Short duration due to rapid metabolism by liver enzymes; effects reversed by flumazenil ↓ dependency risk and ↓ sleep cycle disturbance (vs benzodiazepine hypnotics)
Suvorexant	Orexin (hypocretin) receptor **ant**agonist	CNS depression (somnolence), headache, abnormal sleep-related activities	Contraindications: narcolepsy, combination with strong CYP3A4 inhibitors Not recommended in patients with liver disease Limited risk of dependency
Ramelteon	Melatonin receptor agonist: binds MT1 and MT2 in suprachiasmatic nucleus	Dizziness, nausea, fatigue, headache	No known risk of dependency

Triptans	Sumatriptan
MECHANISM	$5\text{-}HT_{1B/1D}$ agonists. Inhibit trigeminal nerve activation, prevent vasoactive peptide release, induce vasoconstriction.
CLINICAL USE	Acute migraine, cluster **head**ache attacks. A **sumo** wrestler **trip**s and falls on their **head**.
ADVERSE EFFECTS	Coronary vasospasm (contraindicated in patients with CAD or vasospastic angina), mild paresthesia, serotonin syndrome (in combination with other 5-HT agonists).

Parkinson disease therapy	Most effective treatments are non-ergot dopamine agonists (younger patients) and levodopa/carbidopa (older patients). Deep brain stimulation of the STN or GPi aids in advanced disease.
STRATEGY	AGENTS
Dopamine agonists	Non-ergot (preferred)—pramipexole, ropinirole; toxicity includes nausea, impulse control disorder (eg, gambling), postural hypotension, hallucinations, confusion, sleepiness, edema. Ergot—bromocriptine; rarely used due to toxicity.
↑ dopamine availability	Amantadine (↑ dopamine release and ↓ dopamine reuptake); mainly used to reduce levodopa-induced dyskinesias; toxicity = peripheral edema, livedo reticularis, ataxia.
↑ L-DOPA availability	Agents prevent peripheral (pre-BBB) L-DOPA degradation → ↑ L-DOPA entering CNS → ↑ central L-DOPA available for conversion to dopamine. ▪ Levodopa (L-DOPA)/carbidopa—carbidopa blocks peripheral conversion of L-DOPA to dopamine by inhibiting DOPA decarboxylase. Also reduces adverse effects of peripheral L-DOPA conversion into dopamine (eg, nausea, vomiting). ▪ Entacapone and tolcapone prevent peripheral L-DOPA degradation to 3-O-methyldopa (3-OMD) by inhibiting COMT. Used in conjunction with levodopa.
Prevent dopamine breakdown	Agents act centrally (post-BBB) to inhibit breakdown of dopamine. ▪ Selegiline, rasagiline—block dopamine → 3,4-dihydroxyphenylacetic acid (DOPAC) conversion via **selective** inhibition of MAO-B, which is more commonly found in the **B**rain than periphery. Improve symptoms for patients with cyclic fluctuations in levodopa efficacy (on/off phenomenon). ▪ Tolcapone—crosses BBB and blocks conversion of dopamine to 3-methoxytyramine (3-MT) in the brain by inhibiting central COMT. Tolcapone pays the **toll** and can cross the BBB.
Curb excess cholinergic activity	Benztropine, **trihexyphenidyl** (Antimuscarinic; improves tremor and rigidity but has little effect on bradykinesia in **P**arkinson disease). **Tri Parking** my Mercedes-**Benz**.

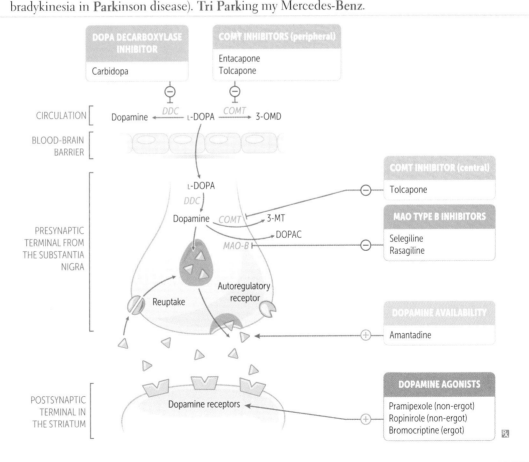

Carbidopa/levodopa

MECHANISM	↑ dopamine in brain. Unlike dopamine, L-DOPA can cross BBB and is converted by DOPA decarboxylase in the CNS to dopamine. Carbidopa, a peripheral DOPA decarboxylase inhibitor that cannot cross BBB, is given with L-DOPA to ↑ bioavailability of L-DOPA in the brain and to limit peripheral adverse effects.
CLINICAL USE	Parkinson disease.
ADVERSE EFFECTS	Nausea, hallucinations, postural hypotension. With progressive disease, L-DOPA can lead to "on-off" phenomenon with improved mobility during "on" periods, then impaired motor function during "off" periods when patient responds poorly to L-DOPA or medication wears off.

Neurodegenerative disease therapy

DISEASE	AGENT	MECHANISM	NOTES
Alzheimer disease	Donepezil, **riva**stigmine, ga**la**ntamine	AChE inhibitor	1st-line treatment Adverse effects: nausea, dizziness, insomnia; contraindicated in patients with cardiac conduction abnormalities **Dona Riva** forgot the **gala**
	Memantine	NMDA receptor antagonist; helps prevent excitotoxicity (mediated by Ca^{2+})	Used for moderate to advanced dementia Adverse effects: dizziness, confusion, hallucinations
Amyotrophic lateral sclerosis	Riluzole	↓ neuron glutamate excitotoxicity	↑ survival Treat **Lou** Gehrig disease with ri**Lou**zole
Huntington disease	Deutetrabenazine, tetrabenazine	Inhibit vesicular monoamine transporter (VMAT) → ↓ dopamine vesicle packaging and release	May be used for Huntington chorea and tardive dyskinesia

Local anesthetics

Esters—benzocaine, chloroprocaine, cocaine, tetracaine.

Amides—bupivacaine, lidocaine, mepivacaine, prilocaine, ropivacaine (amides have **2** i's in name).

MECHANISM

Block neurotransmission via binding to voltage-gated Na⁺ channels on inner portion of the channel along nerve fibers. Most effective in rapidly firing neurons. 3° amine local anesthetics penetrate membrane in uncharged form, then bind to ion channels as charged form.

Can be given with vasoconstrictors (usually epinephrine) to enhance block duration of action by ↓ systemic absorption.

In infected (acidic) tissue, alkaline anesthetics are charged and cannot penetrate membrane effectively → need more anesthetic.

Order of loss: (1) pain, (2) temperature, (3) touch, (4) pressure.

CLINICAL USE

Minor surgical procedures, spinal anesthesia. If allergic to esters, give amides.

ADVERSE EFFECTS

CNS excitation, severe cardiovascular toxicity (bupivacaine), hypertension, hypotension, arrhythmias (cocaine), methemoglobinemia (benzocaine, prilocaine).

General anesthetics

CNS drugs must be lipid soluble (cross the BBB) or be actively transported.

Drugs with ↓ solubility in blood (eg, nitrous oxide [N₂O]) = rapid induction and recovery times.

Drugs with ↑ solubility in lipids (eg, isoflurane) = ↑ potency.

MAC = **M**inimum **A**lveolar **C**oncentration (of inhaled anesthetic) required to prevent 50% of subjects from moving in response to noxious stimulus (eg, skin incision). Potency = 1/MAC.

	MECHANISM	ADVERSE EFFECTS/NOTES
Inhaled anesthetics		
Sevoflurane		Respiratory depression, ↓ cough reflex
Desflurane		Myocardial depression, ↓ BP
Isoflurane	Mechanism unknown	↑ cerebral blood flow (↑ ICP), ↓ metabolic rate
		↓ skeletal and smooth muscle tone
		Postoperative nausea and vomiting
		Malignant hyperthermia
N₂O		Diffusion into and expansion (N₂O) of gas-filled cavities (eg, pneumothorax); very low potency
Intravenous anesthetics		
Propofol	Potentiates GABA_A receptor / Inhibits NMDA receptor	Respiratory depression, ↓ BP; most commonly used IV agent for induction of anesthesia
Etomidate	Potentiates GABA_A receptor	Acute adrenal insufficiency, postoperative nausea and vomiting; hemodynamically neutral
Ketamine	Inhibits NMDA receptor	Sympathomimetic: ↑ BP, ↑ HR, ↑ cerebral blood flow (↑ ICP), bronchodilation / Psychotomimetic: hallucinations, vivid dreams

Neuromuscular blocking drugs	Muscle paralysis in surgery or mechanical ventilation. Selective for N_m nicotinic receptors at neuromuscular junction but not autonomic N_n receptors.
Depolarizing neuromuscular blocking drugs	Succinylcholine—strong N_m nicotinic receptor agonist; produces sustained depolarization and prevents muscle contraction. Reversal of blockade: ▪ Phase I (prolonged depolarization)—no antidote. Block potentiated by cholinesterase inhibitors. ▪ Phase II (repolarized but blocked; N_m nicotinic receptors are available, but desensitized)—may be reversed with cholinesterase inhibitors. Complications include hypercalcemia, hyperkalemia, malignant hyperthermia. ↑ risk of prolonged muscle paralysis in patients with pseudocholinesterase deficiency.
Nondepolarizing neuromuscular blocking drugs	Atracurium, cisatracurium, pancuronium, rocuronium, vecuronium—competitive N_m nicotinic receptor antagonist. Reversal of blockade—sugammadex or cholinesterase inhibitors (eg, neostigmine). Anticholinergics (eg, atropine, glycopyrrolate) are given with cholinesterase inhibitors to prevent muscarinic effects (eg, bradycardia).
Malignant hyperthermia	Rare, life-threatening, hypermetabolic condition caused by the administration of potent inhaled anesthetics (sevoflurane, desflurane, isoflurane) or succinylcholine in susceptible individuals. Susceptibility to malignant hyperthermia is caused by de novo or inherited (autosomal dominant) mutations to ryanodine (*RYR1*) or dihydropyridine receptors (*DHPR*). ↑↑ Ca^{2+} release from sarcoplasmic reticulum → sustained muscle contraction → hypercapnia, tachycardia, masseter/generalized muscle rigidity, rhabdomyolysis, hyperthermia. Treatment: dantrolene (ryanodine receptor antagonist).

Skeletal muscle relaxants

DRUG	MECHANISM	CLINICAL USE	NOTES
Baclofen	$GABA_B$ receptor agonist in spinal cord	Muscle spasticity, dystonia, multiple sclerosis	Acts on the back (spinal cord) May cause sedation
Cyclobenzaprine	Acts within CNS, mainly at the brainstem	Muscle spasms	Centrally acting Structurally related to TCAs May cause anticholinergic adverse effects, sedation
Dantrolene	Prevents release of Ca^{2+} from sarcoplasmic reticulum of skeletal muscle by inhibiting the ryanodine receptor	Malignant hyperthermia (toxicity of inhaled anesthetics and succinylcholine) and neuroleptic malignant syndrome (toxicity of antipsychotics)	Acts directly on muscle
Tizanidine	α_2 agonist, acts centrally	Muscle spasticity, multiple sclerosis, ALS, cerebral palsy	

Opioid analgesics

MECHANISM	Act as agonists at opioid receptors (μ = β-endorphin, δ = enkephalin, κ = dynorphin) to modulate synaptic transmission—close presynaptic Ca^{2+} channels, open postsynaptic K^+ channels → ↓ synaptic transmission. Inhibit release of ACh, norepinephrine, 5-HT, glutamate, substance P.
EFFICACY	Full agonist: morphine, meperidine (long acting), methadone, codeine (prodrug; activated by CYP2D6), fentanyl. Partial agonist: buprenorphine. Mixed agonist/antagonist: butorphanol, nalbuphine. Antagonist: naloxone, naltrexone, methylnaltrexone.
CLINICAL USE	Moderate to severe or refractory pain, diarrhea (loperamide, diphenoxylate), acute pulmonary edema, maintenance programs for opiate use disorder (methadone, buprenorphine + naloxone), neonatal abstinence syndrome (methadone, morphine).
ADVERSE EFFECTS	Nausea, vomiting, pruritus (histamine release), opiate use disorder, respiratory depression, constipation, sphincter of Oddi spasm, miosis (except meperidine → mydriasis), additive CNS depression with other drugs. Tolerance does not develop to miosis and constipation. Treat toxicity with naloxone and prevent relapse with naltrexone once detoxified.

Tramadol

MECHANISM	Very weak opioid agonist; also inhibits the reuptake of norepinephrine and serotonin.
CLINICAL USE	Chronic pain.
ADVERSE EFFECTS	Similar to opioids; decreases seizure threshold; serotonin syndrome.

Butorphanol, nalbuphine

MECHANISM	μ-opioid receptor partial agonists and κ-opioid receptor full agonists.
CLINICAL USE	Analgesia for severe pain (eg, labor).
NOTES	Mixed opioid agonists/antagonists cause less respiratory depression than full opioid agonists. Can cause opioid withdrawal symptoms if patient is also taking full opioid agonist (due to competition for opioid receptors). Not easily reversed with naloxone.

Capsaicin

	Naturally found in hot peppers.
MECHANISM	Excessive stimulation and desensitization of nociceptive fibers → ↓ substance P release → ↓ pain.
CLINICAL USE	Musculoskeletal and neuropathic pain.

Glaucoma therapy

↓ IOP via ↓ amount of aqueous humor (inhibit synthesis/secretion or ↑ drainage).
"βαD humor may not be politically correct."

DRUG CLASS	EXAMPLES	MECHANISM	ADVERSE EFFECTS
β-blockers	Timolol, betaxolol, carteolol	↓ aqueous humor synthesis	No pupillary or vision changes
α-agonists	Epinephrine (α_1), apraclonidine, brimonidine (α_2)	↓ aqueous humor synthesis via vasoconstriction (epinephrine) ↓ aqueous humor synthesis (apraclonidine, brimonidine) ↑ outflow of aqueous humor via uveoscleral pathway	Mydriasis (α_1); do not use in closed-angle glaucoma Blurry vision, ocular hyperemia, foreign body sensation, ocular allergic reactions, ocular pruritus
Diuretics	Acetazolamide	↓ aqueous humor synthesis via inhibition of carbonic anhydrase	No pupillary or vision changes
Prostaglandins	Bimatoprost, latanoprost ($PGF_{2\alpha}$)	↑ outflow of aqueous humor via ↓ resistance of flow through uveoscleral pathway	Darkens color of iris (browning), eyelash growth
Cholinomimetics (M$_3$)	Direct: pilocarpine, carbachol Indirect: physostigmine, echothiophate	↑ outflow of aqueous humor via contraction of ciliary muscle and opening of trabecular meshwork Use pilocarpine in acute angle closure glaucoma—very effective at opening meshwork into canal of Schlemm	Miosis (contraction of pupillary sphincter muscles) and cyclospasm (contraction of ciliary muscle)

Psychiatry

"Words of comfort, skillfully administered, are the oldest therapy known to man."

—Louis Nizer

"Psychiatry at its best is what all medicine needs more of—humanity, art, listening, and sympathy."

—Susannah Cahalan

"It's time to tell everyone who's dealing with a mental health issue that they're not alone, and that getting support and treatment isn't a sign of weakness, it's a sign of strength."

—Michelle Obama

"I have schizophrenia. I am not schizophrenia. I am not my mental illness. My illness is a part of me."

—Jonathan Harnisch

This chapter encompasses overlapping areas in psychiatry, psychology, sociology, and psychopharmacology. High-yield topics include schizophrenia, mood disorders, eating disorders, personality disorders, somatic symptom disorders, substance use disorders, and antipsychotics. Know the DSM-5 criteria for diagnosing common psychiatric disorders. Some questions may focus on the duration of symptoms to identify the underlying disorder.

▶ PSYCHIATRY—PSYCHOLOGY

Classical conditioning	Learning in which a natural response (salivation) is elicited by a conditioned, or learned, stimulus (bell) that previously was presented in conjunction with an unconditioned stimulus (food).	Usually elicits **involuntary** responses. Pavlov's classical experiments with dogs— ringing the bell provoked salivation.

Operant conditioning	Learning in which a particular action is elicited because it produces a punishment or reward. Usually elicits **voluntary** responses.	
Reinforcement	Target behavior (response) is followed by desired reward (positive reinforcement) or removal of aversive stimulus (negative reinforcement).	Skinner operant conditioning quadrants:
Punishment	Repeated application of aversive stimulus (positive punishment) or removal of desired reward (negative punishment) to extinguish unwanted behavior.	
Extinction	Discontinuation of reinforcement (positive or negative) eventually eliminates behavior. Can occur in operant or classical conditioning.	

Skinner operant conditioning quadrants:

	Increase behavior	Decrease behavior
Add a stimulus	Positive reinforcement	Positive punishment
Remove a stimulus	Negative reinforcement	Negative punishment

Transference and countertransference

Transference	Patient projects feelings about formative or other important persons onto physician (eg, psychiatrist is seen as parent).
Countertransference	Physician projects feelings about formative or other important persons onto patient (eg, patient reminds physician of younger sibling).

Ego defenses	Thoughts and behaviors (voluntary or involuntary) used to resolve conflict and prevent undesirable feelings (eg, anxiety, depression).

IMMATURE DEFENSES	DESCRIPTION	EXAMPLE
Acting out	Subconsciously coping with stressors or emotional conflict using actions rather than reflections or feelings.	A patient skips therapy appointments after deep discomfort from dealing with his past.
Denial	Avoiding the awareness of some painful reality.	A patient with cancer plans a full-time work schedule despite being warned of significant fatigue during chemotherapy.
Displacement	Redirection of emotions or impulses to a neutral person or object (vs projection).	After being reprimanded by her principal, a frustrated teacher returns home and criticizes her wife's cooking instead of confronting the principal directly.
Dissociation	Temporary, drastic change in personality, memory, consciousness, or motor behavior to avoid emotional stress. Patient has incomplete or no memory of traumatic event.	A survivor of sexual abuse sees the abuser and suddenly becomes numb and detached.

Ego defenses (continued)

IMMATURE DEFENSES	DESCRIPTION	EXAMPLE
Fixation	Partially remaining at a more childish level of development (vs regression).	A college student continues to suck her thumb when studying for stressful exams.
Idealization	Expressing extremely positive thoughts of self and others while ignoring negative thoughts.	A patient boasts about his physician and his accomplishments while ignoring any flaws.
Identification	Largely unconscious assumption of the characteristics, qualities, or traits of another person or group.	A resident starts putting her stethoscope in her pocket like her favorite attending, instead of wearing it around her neck like before.
Intellectualization	Using facts and logic to emotionally distance oneself from a stressful situation.	A patient diagnosed with cancer discusses the pathophysiology of the disease.
Isolation (of affect)	Separating feelings from ideas and events.	Describing murder in graphic detail with no emotional response.
Passive aggression	Demonstrating hostile feelings in a nonconfrontational manner; showing indirect opposition.	A disgruntled employee is repeatedly late to work, but won't admit it is a way to get back at the manager.
Projection	Attributing an unacceptable internal impulse to an external source (vs displacement).	A man who wants to cheat on his wife accuses his wife of being unfaithful.
Rationalization	Asserting plausible explanations for events that actually occurred for other reasons, usually to avoid self-blame.	An employee who was recently fired claims that the job was not important anyway.
Reaction formation	Replacing a warded-off idea or feeling with an emphasis on its opposite (vs sublimation).	A stepfather treats a child he resents with excessive nurturing and overprotection.
Regression	Involuntarily turning back the maturational clock to behaviors previously demonstrated under stress (vs fixation).	A previously toilet-trained child begins bedwetting again following the birth of a sibling.
Repression	Involuntarily withholding an idea or feeling from conscious awareness (vs suppression).	A 20-year-old does not remember going to counseling during his parents' divorce 10 years earlier.
Splitting	Believing that people are either all good or all bad at different times due to intolerance of ambiguity. Common in **border**line personality disorder. **Borders split** countries.	A patient says that all the nurses are cold and insensitive, but the physicians are warm and friendly.

MATURE DEFENSES		
Sublimation	Replacing an unacceptable wish with a course of action that is similar to the wish but socially acceptable (vs reaction formation).	A teenager's aggression toward her parents because of their high expectations is channeled into excelling in sports.
Altruism	Alleviating negative feelings via unsolicited generosity, which provides gratification (vs reaction formation).	A mafia boss makes a large donation to charity.
Suppression	Intentionally withholding an idea or feeling from conscious awareness (vs repression); temporary.	An athlete focuses on other tasks to prevent worrying about an important upcoming match.
Humor	Lightheartedly expressing uncomfortable feelings to shift the internal focus away from the distress.	A nervous medical student jokes about the boards.
	Mature adults wear a **SASH**.	

Grief   Natural feeling that occurs in response to the death of a loved one. Symptoms and trajectory vary for each individual, are specific to each loss, and do not follow a fixed series of stages. In addition to guilt, sadness, and yearning, patients may experience somatic symptoms, hallucinations of the deceased, and/or transient episodes of wishing they had died with or instead of their loved one. Typical acute grief is time limited (adaptations within 6 months) and is not a disorder.

Prolonged grief disorder—diagnosed if grief remains intense, persistent, and prolonged (at least 6–12 months), significantly impair functioning, is inconsistent with patient's cultural or religious norms, and do not meet criteria for another disorder (eg, major depressive disorder [MDD]).

Normal infant and child development   Milestone dates are ranges that have been approximated and vary by source. Children not meeting milestones may need assessment for potential developmental delay.

AGE	MOTOR	SOCIAL	VERBAL/COGNITIVE
Infant	**Parents**	**Start**	**Observing,**
0–12 mo	Primitive reflexes disappear—Moro, rooting, palmar, Babinski (**Mr. Peanut Butter**) Posture—lifts head up prone (by 1 mo), rolls and sits (by 6 mo), crawls (by 8 mo), stands (by 10 mo), walks (by 12–18 mo) Picks—passes toys hand to hand (by 6–9 mo), Pincer grasp (by 10 mo) Points to objects (by 12 mo)	Social smile (by 2 mo) Stranger anxiety (by 6 mo) Separation anxiety (by 9 mo)	Orients—first to voice (by 4 mo), then to name and gestures (by 9 mo) Object permanence (by 9 mo) Oratory—says "mama" and "dada" (by 10 mo)
Toddler	**Child**	**Rearing**	**Working,**
12–36 mo	Cruises, takes first steps (by 12 mo) Climbs stairs (by 18 mo) Cubes stacked (number) = age (yr) × 3 Cutlery—feeds self with fork and spoon (by 20 mo) Kicks ball (by 24 mo)	Recreation—parallel play (by 24–36 mo) Rapprochement—moves away from and returns to parent (by 24 mo) Realization—core gender identity formed (by 36 mo)	Words—uses 50-200 words (by 2 yr), uses 300+ words (by 3 yr)
Preschool	**Don't**	**Forget, they're still**	**Learning!**
3–5 yr	Drive—tricycle (**3** wheels at **3** yr) Drawings—copies line or circle, stick figure (by 4 yr) Dexterity—hops on one foot by 4 yr ("4 on one foot"), uses buttons or zippers, grooms self (by 5 yr)	Freedom—comfortably spends part of day away from parent (by 3 yr) Friends—cooperative play, has imaginary friends (by 4 yr)	Language—understands 1000 (**3 zeros**) words (by 3 yr), uses complete sentences and prepositions (by 4 yr) Legends—can tell detailed stories (by 4 yr)

▶ **PSYCHIATRY—PATHOLOGY**

Child abuse	All cases of suspected child abuse must be reported to local child protective services.	
	SIGNS	EPIDEMIOLOGY
Neglect	Poor hygiene, malnutrition, withdrawn affect, impaired social/emotional development, failure to thrive due to failure to provide a child with adequate food, shelter, supervision, education, and/or affection.	Most common form of child maltreatment.
Physical abuse	Nonaccidental trauma (eg, fractures, bruises, burns). Injuries often in different stages of healing or in patterns resembling possible implements of injury. Includes abusive head trauma (shaken baby syndrome), characterized by subdural hematomas or retinal hemorrhages. Caregivers may delay seeking medical attention for the child or provide explanations inconsistent with the child's developmental stage or pattern of injury.	40% of deaths related to child abuse or neglect occur in children < 1 year old.
Sexual abuse	STIs, UTIs, and genital, anal, or oral trauma. Most often, there are no physical signs; sexual abuse should not be excluded from a differential diagnosis in the absence of physical trauma. Children often exhibit sexual knowledge or behavior incongruent with their age.	Peak incidence 9–12 years old.
Emotional abuse	Babies or young children may lack a bond with the caregiver but are overly affectionate with less familiar adults. They may be aggressive towards children and animals or unusually anxious. Older children are often emotionally labile and prone to angry outbursts. They may distance themselves from caregivers and other children. They can experience vague somatic symptoms for which a medical cause cannot be found.	~ 80% of young adult victims of child emotional abuse meet the criteria for ≥ 1 psychiatric illness by age 21.

Vulnerable child syndrome	Parents misperceive the child as especially susceptible to illness or injury (vs factitious disorder imposed on another). Usually follows a child's serious illness or life-threatening event. Can result in missed school or overuse of medical services (think kid wrapped in bubble wrap).

Childhood and early-onset disorders

Attention-deficit hyperactivity disorder	Onset before age 12, but diagnosis can only be established after age 4. Characterized by hyperactivity, impulsivity, and/or inattention in ≥ 2 settings (eg, school, home, places of worship). Normal intelligence, but commonly coexists with difficulties in school. Often persists into adulthood. Commonly coexists with other behavioral, cognitive, or developmental disorders. Treatment: stimulants (eg, methylphenidate) +/– behavioral therapy; alternatives include atomoxetine and α_2-agonists (eg, clonidine, guanfacine).
Autism spectrum disorder	Onset in early childhood. Social and communication deficits, repetitive/ritualized behaviors, restricted interests. May be accompanied by intellectual disability and/or above average abilities in specific skills (eg, music). More common in males. Associated with ↑ head and/or brain size.
Conduct disorder	Repetitive, pervasive behavior violating societal norms or the basic rights of others (eg, aggression toward people and animals, destruction of property, theft). After age 18, often reclassified as antisocial personality disorder. Conduct = children, antisocial = adults. Treatment: psychotherapy (eg, cognitive behavioral therapy [CBT]).
Disruptive mood dysregulation disorder	Onset before age 10 and diagnosed after age 6. Severe, recurrent temper outbursts out of proportion to situation. Child is constantly angry and irritable between outbursts. Treatment: CBT, stimulants, antipsychotics.
Intellectual disability	Global cognitive deficits (vs specific learning disorder) that affect reasoning, memory, abstract thinking, judgment, language, learning. Adaptive functioning is impaired, leading to major difficulties with education, employment, communication, socialization, independence. Treatment: psychotherapy, occupational therapy, special education.
Intermittent explosive disorder	Onset after age 6. Recurrent verbal or physical outbursts representing a failure to control aggressive impulses. Outbursts last < 30 minutes and are out of proportion to provocation and may lead to legal, financial, or social consequences. Episodes are not premeditated and may provide an immediate sense of relief, followed by remorse. Treatment: psychotherapy, SSRIs.
Oppositional defiant disorder	Pattern of anger and irritability with argumentative, vindictive, and defiant behavior toward authority figures lasting ≥ 6 months. Treatment: psychotherapy (eg, CBT).
Selective mutism	Onset before age 5. Anxiety disorder lasting ≥ 1 month involving refraining from speech in certain situations despite speaking in other, usually more comfortable situations. Development (eg, speech and language) not typically impaired. Interferes with social, academic, and occupational tasks. Commonly coexists with social anxiety disorder. Treatment: behavioral, family, and play therapy; SSRIs.
Separation anxiety disorder	Overwhelming fear of separation from home or attachment figure lasting ≥ 4 weeks. Can be normal behavior up to age 3–4. May lead to factitious physical complaints to avoid school. Treatment: CBT, play therapy, family therapy.
Specific learning disorder	Onset during school-age years. Inability to acquire or use information from a specific subject (eg, math, reading, writing) near age-expected proficiency for ≥ 6 months despite focused intervention. General functioning and intelligence are normal (vs intellectual disability). Treatment: academic support, counseling, extracurricular activities.
Tourette syndrome	Onset before age 18. Sudden, recurrent, nonrhythmic, stereotyped motor (eg, grimacing, shrugging) and vocal (eg, grunting, throat clearing) tics that persist for > 1 year. Coprolalia (involuntary obscene speech) found in some patients. Associated with OCD and ADHD. Treatment: psychoeducation, behavioral therapy. For intractable and distressing tics: tetrabenazine, antipsychotics, α_2-agonists.

| **Orientation** | Patients' ability to know the date and time, where they are, and who they are (order of loss: time → place → person). Common causes of loss of orientation: alcohol, drugs, fluid/electrolyte imbalance, head trauma, hypoglycemia, infection, nutritional deficiencies, hypoxia. |

Amnesias

Retrograde amnesia	Inability to remember things that occurred **before** a CNS insult.
Anterograde amnesia	Inability to remember things that occurred **after** a CNS insult (↓ acquisition of new memory).
Korsakoff syndrome	Amnesia (anterograde > retrograde) and disorientation caused by vitamin B_1 deficiency. Associated with disruption and destruction of the limbic system, especially mammillary bodies and anterior thalamus. Seen in chronic alcohol use as a late neuropsychiatric manifestation of Wernicke encephalopathy. Confabulations are characteristic.

Dissociative disorders

Depersonalization/ derealization disorder	Persistent feelings of detachment or estrangement from one's own body, thoughts, perceptions, and actions (depersonalization) or one's environment (derealization). Intact reality testing (vs psychosis).
Dissociative amnesia	Inability to recall important personal information, usually following severe trauma or stress. May be accompanied by dissociative fugue (abrupt, unexpected travelling away from home).
Dissociative identity disorder	Formerly called multiple personality disorder. Presence of ≥ 2 distinct identities or personality states, typically with distinct memories and patterns of behavior. More common in females. Associated with history of sexual abuse, PTSD, depression, substance use, borderline personality disorder, somatic symptom disorders.

| **Delirium** | "Waxing and waning" level of consciousness with acute onset, ↓ attention span, ↓ level of arousal. Characterized by disorganized thinking, hallucinations (often visual), misperceptions (eg, illusions), disturbance in sleep-wake cycle, cognitive dysfunction, agitation. Reversible.

 Usually 2° to other identifiable illness (eg, CNS disease, infection, trauma, substance use/ withdrawal, metabolic/electrolyte disturbances, hemorrhage, urinary/fecal retention), or medications (eg, anticholinergics), especially in older adults.

 Most common presentation of altered mental status in inpatient setting, especially in the ICU or during prolonged hospital stays. | Delirium = changes in senso**rium**.
 EEG may show diffuse background rhythm slowing.
 Treatment: identification and management of underlying condition. Orientation protocols (eg, keeping a clock or calendar nearby), ↓ sleep disturbances, and ↑ cognitive stimulation to manage symptoms. Antipsychotics (eg, haloperidol) as needed. Avoid unnecessary restraints and drugs that may worsen delirium (eg, anticholinergics, benzodiazepines, opioids). |

Psychosis

Distorted perception of reality characterized by delusions, hallucinations, and/or disorganized thought/speech. Can occur in patients with psychiatric illness or another medical condition, or secondary to substance or medication use.

Delusions

False, fixed, idiosyncratic beliefs that persist despite evidence to the contrary and are not typical of a patient's culture or religion (eg, a patient who believes that others are reading his thoughts). Types include erotomanic, grandiose, jealous, persecutory, somatic, mixed, and unspecified.

Disorganized thought

Speech may be incoherent ("word salad"), tangential, or derailed ("loose associations").

Hallucinations

Perceptions in the absence of external stimuli (eg, seeing a light that is not actually present). Types include:

- Auditory—more commonly due to psychiatric illness (eg, schizophrenia) than neurologic disease.
- Visual—more commonly due to neurologic disease (eg, dementia), delirium, or drug intoxication than psychiatric illness.
- Tactile—common in alcohol withdrawal and stimulant use (eg, "cocaine crawlies," a type of delusional parasitosis).
- Olfactory—often occur as an aura of temporal lobe epilepsy (eg, burning rubber) and in brain tumors.
- Gustatory—rare, but seen in epilepsy.
- Hypnagogic—occurs while **go**ing to sleep. Sometimes seen in narcolepsy.
- Hypno**pompic**—occurs while waking from sleep ("get **pomp**ed up in the morning"). Sometimes seen in narcolepsy.

Contrast with illusions, which are misperceptions of real external stimuli (eg, mistaking a shadow for a black cat).

Mood disorder

Characterized by an abnormal range of moods or internal emotional states and loss of control over them. Severity of moods causes distress and impairment in social and occupational functioning. Includes major depressive, bipolar, dysthymic, and cyclothymic disorders. Episodic superimposed psychotic features (delusions, hallucinations, disorganized speech/behavior) may be present at any time during mood episodes (other than hypomania).

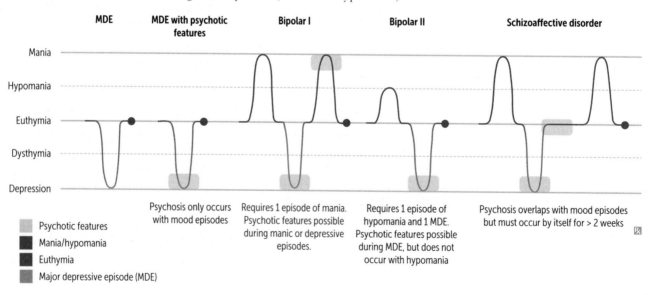

MDE	MDE with psychotic features	Bipolar I	Bipolar II	Schizoaffective disorder
	Psychosis only occurs with mood episodes	Requires 1 episode of mania. Psychotic features possible during manic or depressive episodes.	Requires 1 episode of hypomania and 1 MDE. Psychotic features possible during MDE, but does not occur with hypomania	Psychosis overlaps with mood episodes but must occur by itself for > 2 weeks

Psychotic features
Mania/hypomania
Euthymia
Major depressive episode (MDE)

Schizophrenia spectrum disorders

Schizophrenia	Chronic illness causing profound functional impairment. Symptom categories include:
	• Positive—excessive or distorted functioning (eg, hallucinations, delusions, unusual thought processes, disorganized speech, bizarre behavior)
	• Negative—diminished functioning (eg, blunted affect, apathy, anhedonia, alogia, asocial behavior)
	• Cognitive—reduced ability to understand or make plans, diminished working memory, inattention
	Diagnosis requires ≥ 2 of the following active symptoms, including ≥ 1 from symptoms #1–3:
	  1. Delusions
	  2. Hallucinations, often auditory
	  3. Disorganized speech
	  4. Disorganized or catatonic behavior
	  5. Negative symptoms
	Symptom onset ≥ 6 months prior to diagnosis; requires ≥ 1 month of active symptoms over the past 6 months.
	
	Brief psychotic disorder—≥ 1 positive symptom(s) lasting between 1 day and 1 month, usually stress-related.
	
	Schizophreniform disorder—≥ 2 symptoms lasting 1–6 months.
		Associated with altered dopaminergic activity, ↑ serotonergic activity, and ↓ dendritic branching. Ventriculomegaly on brain imaging. Lifetime prevalence—1.5% (males > females). Presents earlier in males (late teens to early 20s) than in females (late 20s to early 30s). ↑ suicide risk.
		Heavy cannabis use in adolescence is associated with ↑ incidence and worsened course of psychotic, mood, and anxiety disorders.
		Treatment: atypical antipsychotics (eg, risperidone) are first line.
		Negative symptoms often persist after treatment, despite resolution of positive symptoms.

Schizoaffective disorder	Shares symptoms with both schizophrenia and mood disorders (MDD or bipolar disorder). To differentiate from a mood disorder with psychotic features, patient must have ≥ 2 weeks of psychotic symptoms without a manic or depressive episode.	
Delusional disorder	≥ 1 delusion(s) lasting > 1 month, but without a mood disorder or other psychotic symptoms. Daily functioning, including socialization, may be impacted by the pathological, fixed belief but is otherwise unaffected. Can be shared by individuals in close relationships (folie à deux).	
Schizotypal personality disorder	Cluster A personality disorder that also falls on the schizophrenia spectrum. May include brief psychotic episodes (eg, delusions) that are less frequent and severe than in schizophrenia.	

Manic episode	Distinct period of abnormally and persistently elevated, expansive, or irritable mood and ↑ activity or energy. Diagnosis requires marked functional impairment with ≥ 3 of the following for ≥ 1 week, or any duration if hospitalization is required (people with mania **DIG FAST**): <table><tr><td>• Distractibility • Impulsivity/Indiscretion—seeks pleasure without regard to consequences (hedonistic) • Grandiosity—inflated self-esteem</td><td>• Flight of ideas—racing thoughts • ↑ goal-directed Activity/psychomotor Agitation • ↓ need for Sleep • Talkativeness or pressured speech</td></tr></table>

Hypomanic episode	Similar to a manic episode except mood disturbance is not severe enough to cause marked impairment in social and/or occupational functioning or to necessitate hospitalization. Abnormally ↑ activity or energy usually present. No psychotic features. Lasts ≥ 4 consecutive days.
Bipolar disorder	Bipolar I (requires 1 type of episode)—≥ 1 manic episode +/– a hypomanic or depressive episode (may be separated by any length of time).
	Bipolar II (requires 2 types of episodes)—a hypomanic and a depressive episode (no history of manic episodes).
	Patient's mood and functioning usually normalize between episodes. Use of antidepressants can destabilize mood. High suicide risk. Treatment: atypical antipsychotics, mood stabilizers (eg, lithium, lamotrigine, valproate, carbamazepine). A little less variable character.
	Cyclothymic disorder—milder form of bipolar disorder fluctuating between mild depressive and hypomanic symptoms. Must last ≥ 2 years with symptoms present at least half of the time, with any remission lasting ≤ 2 months.
Major depressive disorder	Recurrent episodes lasting ≥ 2 weeks characterized by ≥ 5 of 9 diagnostic symptoms including depressed mood or anhedonia (or irritability in children). **SIG: E CAPS**:
	<ul><li>Sleep disturbances</li><li>↓ Interest in pleasurable activities (anhedonia)</li><li>Guilt or feelings of worthlessness</li><li>↓ Energy</li><li>↓ Concentration</li><li>Appetite/weight changes</li><li>Psychomotor retardation or agitation</li><li>Suicidal ideation</li></ul>
	Screen for previous manic or hypomanic episodes to rule out bipolar disorder.
	Treatment: CBT and SSRIs are first line; alternatives include SNRIs, mirtazapine, bupropion, electroconvulsive therapy (ECT), ketamine.
	Responses to a significant loss (eg, bereavement, natural disaster, disability) may resemble a depressive episode. Diagnosis of MDD is made if criteria are met.
MDD with psychotic features	MDD + hallucinations or delusions. Psychotic features are typically mood congruent (eg, depressive themes of inadequacy, guilt, punishment, nihilism, disease, or death) and occur only in the context of major depressive episode (vs schizoaffective disorder). Treatment: antidepressant with atypical antipsychotic, ECT.
Persistent depressive disorder	Also called dysthymia. Often milder than MDD; ≥ 2 depressive symptoms lasting ≥ 2 years (≥ 1 year in children), with any remission lasting ≤ 2 months.
MDD with seasonal pattern	Formerly called seasonal affective disorder. Major depressive episodes occurring only during a particular season (usually winter) in ≥ 2 consecutive years and in most years across a lifetime. Atypical symptoms common. Treatment: standard MDD therapies + light therapy.
Depression with atypical features	Characterized by mood reactivity (transient improvement in response to a positive event), hypersomnia, hyperphagia, leaden paralysis (heavy feeling in arms and legs), long-standing interpersonal rejection sensitivity. Most common subtype of depression. Treatment: CBT and SSRIs are first line. MAO inhibitors are effective but not first line because of their risk profile.

Peripartum mood disturbances	Onset during pregnancy or within 4 weeks of delivery. ↑ risk with history of mood disorders.
Postpartum blues	50–85% incidence rate. Characterized by depressed affect, tearfulness, and fatigue starting 2–3 days after delivery. Usually resolves within 2 weeks. Treatment: supportive. Follow up to assess for possible MDD with peripartum onset.
MDD with peripartum onset	10–15% incidence rate. Formerly called postpartum depression. Meets MDD criteria with onset either during pregnancy or within 4 weeks after delivery. Treatment: CBT and SSRIs are first line.
Postpartum psychosis	0.1–0.2% incidence rate. Characterized by mood-congruent delusions, hallucinations, and thoughts of harming the baby or self. Risk factors include first pregnancy, family history, bipolar disorder, psychotic disorder, recent medication change. Treatment: hospitalization and initiation of atypical antipsychotic; if insufficient, ECT may be used.

Electroconvulsive therapy	Rapid-acting method to treat refractory depression, depression with psychotic symptoms, catatonia, and acute suicidality. Induces tonic-clonic seizure under anesthesia and neuromuscular blockade. Adverse effects include disorientation, headache, partial anterograde/retrograde amnesia usually resolving in 6 months. No absolute contraindications. Safe in pregnant individuals and older adults.

Risk factors for suicide death	Sex (male)	**SAD PERSONS** are more likely to die from suicide.
	Age (young adult or older adult)	
	Depression	Most common method in US is firearms; access to guns ↑ risk of suicide death.
	Previous attempt (highest risk factor)	
	Ethanol or drug use	Women try more often; men die more often.
	Rational thinking loss (psychosis)	Other risk factors include recent psychiatric hospitalization and family history of suicide death.
	Sickness (medical illness)	
	Organized plan	
	No spouse or other social support	Protective factors include effective care for comorbidities; medical, familial, or community connectedness; cultural/religious beliefs encouraging self-preservation; and strong problem-solving skills.
	Stated future intent	

Anxiety disorders	Inappropriate experiences of fear/worry and their physical manifestations incongruent with the magnitude of the stressors. Symptoms are not attributable to another medical condition (eg, psychiatric disorder, hyperthyroidism) or substance use. Includes panic disorder, phobias, generalized anxiety disorder, selective mutism, illness anxiety disorder, OCD, PTSD.

Panic disorder	Recurrent panic attacks involving intense fear and discomfort +/– a known trigger. Attacks typically peak in 10 minutes with ≥ 4 of the following: palpitations, paresthesias, depersonalization or derealization, abdominal distress or nausea, intense fear of dying, intense fear of losing control, lightheadedness, chest pain, chills, choking, sweating, shaking, shortness of breath. Strong genetic component. ↑ risk of suicide.	Diagnosis requires attack followed by ≥ 1 month of ≥ 1 of the following: ▪ Persistent concern of additional attacks ▪ Worrying about consequences of attack ▪ Behavioral change related to attacks Symptoms are systemic manifestations of fear. Treatment: CBT, SSRIs, and venlafaxine are first line. Benzodiazepines occasionally used in acute setting.

Phobias

Severe, persistent (≥ 6 months) fear or anxiety due to presence or anticipation of a specific object or situation. Person often recognizes fear is excessive. Treatment: CBT with exposure therapy.

Social anxiety disorder—exaggerated fear of embarrassment in social situations (eg, public speaking, using public restrooms). Treatment: CBT, SSRIs, SNRIs. For performance type (eg, anxiety restricted to public speaking), use β-blockers or benzodiazepines as needed.

Agoraphobia—irrational fear, anxiety, and/or avoidance while facing or anticipating ≥ 2 specific situations (eg, public transportation, open/closed spaces, lines/crowds, being outside of home alone). Symptoms stem from the concern that help or escape may be unavailable. Associated with panic disorder. Treatment: CBT, SSRIs.

Generalized anxiety disorder

Excessive anxiety and worry about different aspects of daily life (eg, work, school, children) for most days of ≥ 6 months. Associated with ≥ 3 of the following for adults (≥ 1 for kids): difficulty **C**oncentrating, **R**estlessness, **I**rritability, **M**uscle tension, fatigue (low **E**nergy), **S**leep disturbance (anxiety over **CRIMES**). Treatment: CBT, SSRIs, SNRIs are first line. Buspirone, TCAs, benzodiazepines are second line.

Obsessive-compulsive disorders

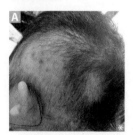

Obsessions (recurring intrusive thoughts or sensations that can cause severe distress), and/or compulsions (repetitive, often time-consuming actions that may relieve distress). Associated with tic disorders. Poor insight into beliefs/actions linked to worse outcomes. Treatment: CBT and SSRIs; clomipramine and venlafaxine are second line.

Body dysmorphic disorder—preoccupation with minor or imagined defects in appearance. Causes significant emotional distress and repetitive appearance-related behaviors (eg, mirror checking, excessive grooming). Common in eating disorders. Treatment: CBT.

Trichotillomania—compulsively pulling out one's hair. Causes significant distress and persists despite attempts to stop. Presents with areas of thinning hair or baldness on any area of the body, most commonly the scalp **A**. Remaining hair shafts are of different lengths (vs alopecia). Incidence highest in childhood but spans all ages. Treatment: CBT and SSRIs.

Trauma and stress-related disorders

Adjustment disorder	Emotional or behavioral symptoms (eg, anxiety, outbursts) that occur within 3 months of an identifiable psychosocial stressor (eg, divorce, illness) lasting < 6 months once the stressor has ended. Symptoms do not meet criteria for another psychiatric illness. If symptoms persist > 6 months after stressor ends, reevaluate for other explanations (eg, MDD, GAD). Treatment: CBT is first line; antidepressants and anxiolytics may be considered.
Post-traumatic stress disorder	Experiencing, witnessing, or discovering that a loved one has experienced a life-threatening situation (eg, serious injury, sexual assault) → persistent **H**yperarousal, **A**voidance of associated stimuli, intrusive **R**e-experiencing of the event (eg, nightmares, flashbacks), changes in cognition or mood (eg, fear, horror, **D**istress) (having PTSD is **HARD**). Disturbance lasts > 1 month with significant distress or impaired functioning. Treatment: CBT, SSRIs, and venlafaxine are first line. Prazosin can reduce nightmares. Acute stress disorder—lasts between 3 days and 1 month. Treatment: CBT; pharmacotherapy is usually not indicated.

Diagnostic criteria by symptom duration

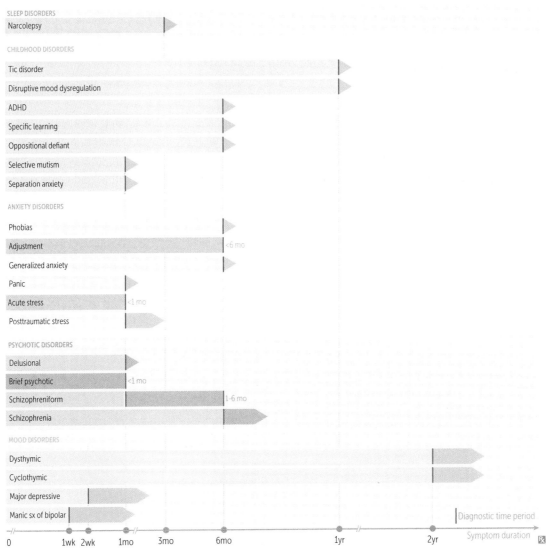

Personality disorders	Inflexible, maladaptive, and rigidly pervasive patterns of behavior causing subjective distress and/or impaired functioning; person is usually not aware of problem (egosyntonic). Usually present by early adulthood. Contrast with **personality traits**—nonpathologic enduring patterns of perception and behavior. Three clusters: <ul><li>Cluster A (remember as "weird")—odd or eccentric; inability to develop meaningful social relationships. No psychosis; genetic association with schizophrenia.</li><li>Cluster B (remember as "wild")—dramatic, emotional, or erratic; genetic association with mood disorders and substance use.</li><li>Cluster C (remember as "worried")—anxious or fearful; genetic association with anxiety disorders.</li></ul>

Cluster A	
Paranoid	Pervasive distrust (accusatory), suspiciousness, hypervigilance, and a profoundly cynical view of the world.
Schizoid	Prefers social withdrawal and solitary activities (vs avoidant), limited emotional expression, indifferent to others' opinions (aloof).
Schizotypal	Eccentric appearance, odd beliefs or magical thinking, interpersonal awkwardness. Included on the schizophrenia spectrum. Pronounce "schizo-type-al" for odd-type thoughts.

Cluster B	
Antisocial	Disregard for the rights of others with lack of remorse (bad). Involves criminality, impulsivity, hostility, and manipulation (sociopath). Males > females. Must be ≥ 18 years old with evidence of conduct disorder onset before age 15. If patient is < 18, diagnosis is conduct disorder.
Borderline	Unstable mood and interpersonal relationships, fear of abandonment, impulsivity, self-mutilation, suicidality, sense of emotional emptiness (borderline). Females > males. Splitting is a major defense mechanism. Treatment: dialectical behavior therapy.
Histrionic	Attention-seeking, dramatic speech and emotional expression, shallow and labile emotions, sexually provocative. May use physical appearance to draw attention (flamboyant).
Narcissistic	Grandiosity, sense of entitlement; lacks empathy and requires excessive admiration; often demands the "best" and reacts to criticism with rage and/or defensiveness (must be the best). Fragile self-esteem. Often envious of others.

Cluster C	
Avoidant	Hypersensitive to rejection and criticism, socially inhibited, timid (cowardly), feelings of inadequacy, desires relationships with others (vs schizoid).
Obsessive-compulsive	Preoccupation with order, perfectionism, and control (obsessive-compulsive); egosyntonic: behavior consistent with one's own beliefs and attitudes (vs OCD).
Dependent	Excessive need for support (clingy), submissive, low self-confidence. Patients often get stuck in abusive relationships.

Malingering	Symptoms are intentional, motivation is intentional. Patient consciously fakes, profoundly exaggerates, or claims to have a disorder in order to attain a specific 2° (external) gain (eg, avoiding work, obtaining compensation). Poor compliance with treatment or follow-up of diagnostic tests. Complaints cease after gain (vs factitious disorder).

Factitious disorders	Symptoms are intentional, motivation is unconscious. Patient consciously creates physical and/or psychological symptoms in order to assume "sick role" and to get medical attention and sympathy (1° [internal] gain).
Factitious disorder imposed on self	Formerly called Munchausen syndrome. Chronic factitious disorder with predominantly physical signs and symptoms. Characterized by a history of multiple hospital admissions and willingness to undergo invasive procedures. More common in females and healthcare workers.
Factitious disorder imposed on another	Formerly called Munchausen syndrome by proxy. Illness in an individual being cared for (most often a child, also seen in disabled or older adults) is directly caused (eg, physically harming a child) or fabricated (eg, lying about a child's symptoms) by the caregiver. Form of child/elder abuse.

Somatic symptom and related disorders	Symptoms are unconscious, motivation is unconscious. Category of disorders characterized by physical symptoms causing significant distress and impairment. Symptoms not intentionally produced or feigned.
Somatic symptom disorder	≥ 1 bodily complaints (eg, abdominal pain, fatigue) lasting months to years. Associated with excessive, persistent thoughts and anxiety about symptoms. May co-occur with medical illness. Treatment: regular office visits with the same physician with the goals of addressing active symptoms, reassuring the patient, and avoiding unnecessary tests or medications.
Conversion disorder	Also called functional neurologic symptom disorder. Unexplained loss of sensory or motor function (eg, psychogenic nonepileptic seizures, paralysis, blindness, mutism), often following an acute stressor; patient may be aware of but indifferent toward symptoms ("la belle indifférence"); more common in females, adolescents, and young adults.
Illness anxiety disorder	Preoccupation with acquiring or having a serious illness, often despite medical evaluation and reassurance; minimal to no somatic symptoms.

Malingering vs factitious disorder vs somatic symptom disorders

	Malingering	Factitious disorder	Somatic symptom disorders
SYMPTOMS	Intentional	Intentional	Unconscious
MOTIVATION	Intentional	Unconscious	Unconscious

Eating disorders	Most common in young women.
Anorexia nervosa	Intense fear of weight gain, overvaluation of thinness, and body image distortion leading to calorie restriction and severe weight loss resulting in inappropriately low body weight (BMI < 18.5 kg/m² for adults). Physiological disturbances may present as bradycardia, hypotension, hypothermia, hypothyroidism, osteoporosis, lanugo, amenorrhea (low calorie intake → ↓ leptin → ↓ GnRH → ↓ LH, FSH → ↓ estrogen → amenorrhea). Binge-eating/purging type—recurring purging behaviors (eg, laxative or diuretic abuse, self-induced vomiting) or binge eating over the last 3 months. Associated with hypokalemia. Restricting type—primary disordered behaviors include dieting, fasting, and/or over-exercising. No recurring purging behaviors or binge eating over the last 3 months. Refeeding syndrome—often occurs in significantly malnourished patients with sudden ↑ calorie intake → ↑ insulin → electrolyte imbalances (↓ PO₄³⁻, ↓ K⁺, ↓ Mg²⁺) → cardiac complications, rhabdomyolysis, seizures. Treatment: nutritional rehabilitation, psychotherapy, olanzapine.
Bulimia nervosa	Recurring episodes of binge eating with compensatory purging behaviors at least weekly over the last 3 months. BMI often normal or slightly overweight (vs anorexia). Associated with parotid gland hypertrophy (may see ↑ serum amylase), enamel erosion, Mallory-Weiss syndrome, electrolyte disturbances (eg, ↓ K⁺, ↓ Cl⁻), metabolic alkalosis, dorsal hand calluses from induced vomiting (Russell sign). Treatment: psychotherapy, nutritional rehabilitation, SSRIs (eg, fluoxetine). Bupropion is contraindicated due to seizure risk.
Binge-eating disorder	Recurring episodes of binge eating without purging behaviors at least weekly over the last 3 months. ↑ diabetes risk. Most common eating disorder in adults. Treatment: psychotherapy (first line); SSRIs; lisdexamfetamine.
Pica	Recurring episodes of eating non-food substances (eg, ice, dirt, hair, paint chips) over ≥ 1 month that are not culturally or developmentally recognized as normal. May provide temporary emotional relief. Common in children and during pregnancy. Associated with malnutrition, iron deficiency anemia, developmental disabilities, emotional trauma. Treatment: psychotherapy and nutritional rehabilitation (first line); SSRIs (second line).
Gender dysphoria	Significant incongruence between one's gender identity and one's gender assigned at birth, lasting > 6 months and leading to persistent distress. Individuals experience marked discomfort with their assigned gender, which interferes with social, academic, and other areas of function. Individuals may pursue multiple domains of gender affirmation, including social, legal, and medical. Transgender—any individual who transiently or persistently experiences incongruence between their gender identity and their gender assigned at birth. Some individuals who are transgender will experience gender dysphoria. Nonconformity to one's assigned gender itself is not a mental disorder.
Sexual dysfunction	Includes sexual desire disorders (hypoactive sexual desire or sexual aversion), sexual arousal disorders (erectile dysfunction), orgasmic disorders (anorgasmia, premature ejaculation), sexual pain disorders (genito-pelvic pain/penetration disorder). Differential diagnosis includes (**PENIS**): ▪ Psychological (if nighttime erections still occur) ▪ Endocrine (eg, diabetes, low testosterone) ▪ Neurogenic (eg, postoperative, spinal cord injury) ▪ Insufficient blood flow (eg, atherosclerosis) ▪ Substances (eg, antihypertensives, antidepressants, ethanol)

Sleep terror disorder	Periods of inconsolable terror with screaming in the middle of the night. Most common in children. Occurs during slow-wave/deep (stage N3) non-REM sleep with no memory of the arousal episode, as opposed to nightmares that occur during **REM** sleep (**re**membering a scary dream). Triggers include emotional stress, fever, and lack of sleep. Usually self limited.
Elimination disorders	Inappropriate urination (enuresis) and/or defecation (encopresis) in individuals who should be continent. Typically diagnosed in childhood or adolescence. **Enuresis**—occurs ≥ 2 times/week for ≥ 3 months in individuals ≥ 5 years old, most commonly during sleep (nocturnal enuresis). First-line treatment: behavioral modification (eg, scheduled voids, nighttime fluid restriction) and positive reinforcement. For refractory cases: bedwetting alarm, oral desmopressin (ADH analog; preferred over imipramine due to fewer adverse effects). **Encopresis**—occurs ≥ 1 time/month for ≥ 3 months in individuals ≥ 4 years old. Types include with or without constipation and overflow. Treatment: behavioral therapy, toilet training, and laxatives or enemas (for constipation).
Narcolepsy	Excessive daytime sleepiness (despite awakening well-rested) with recurrent episodes of rapid-onset, overwhelming sleepiness ≥ 3 times/week for the last 3 months. Due to ↓ orexin (hypocretin) production in lateral hypothalamus and dysregulated sleep-wake cycles. Associated with: ▪ Hypna**go**gic (just before **go**ing to sleep) or hypno**pomp**ic (just before awakening; get **pomp**ed up in the morning) hallucinations. ▪ Nocturnal and narcoleptic sleep episodes that start with REM sleep (sleep paralysis). ▪ Cataplexy (loss of all muscle tone following strong emotional stimulus, such as laughter). Treatment: good sleep hygiene (scheduled naps, regular sleep schedule), daytime stimulants (eg, modafinil, solriamfetol, pitolisant, amphetamines) and/or nighttime sodium oxybate (GHB).
Substance use disorder	Maladaptive pattern of substance use involving ≥ 2 of the following in the past year: ▪ Tolerance ▪ Withdrawal ▪ Intense, distracting cravings ▪ Using more, or longer, than intended ▪ Persistent desire but inability to cut down ▪ Time-consuming substance acquisition, use, or recovery ▪ Impaired functioning at work, school, or home ▪ Social or interpersonal conflicts ▪ Reduced recreational activities ▪ > 1 episode of use involving danger (eg, unsafe sex, driving while impaired) ▪ Continued use despite awareness of harm In the case of appropriate medical treatment with prescribed medications (eg, opioid analgesics, sedatives, stimulants), symptoms of tolerance and withdrawal do not indicate a substance use disorder.

Gambling disorder	Persistent, recurrent, problematic gambling that cannot be better explained as a manic episode. Diagnosis made if patient meets ≥ 4 of the following criteria:

- Is preoccupied with gambling
- Requires more gambling to reach desired level of excitement
- Has failed efforts to limit, cut back, or stop gambling
- Becomes restless or irritable when limiting or attempting to stop gambling
- Gambles to escape or relieve feelings of helplessness, guilt, anxiety, or depression
- After losing money gambling, continues gambling in an attempt to recover losses
- Lies to conceal the extent of gambling
- Puts at risk or has lost significant relationship, career, or academic pursuits because of gambling
- Relies on money from others to fix financial collapse due to gambling

Treatment: psychotherapy.

Transtheoretical model of change

STAGE	FEATURES	MOTIVATIONAL STRATEGIES
Precontemplation	Denies problem and its consequences.	Encourage introspection. Use patient's personal priorities in explaining risks. Affirm your availability to the patient.
Contemplation	Acknowledges problem but is ambivalent or unwilling to change.	Discuss pros of changing and cons of maintaining current behavior. Suggest means to support behavior changes.
Preparation/ determination	Committed to and planning for behavior change.	Employ motivational interviewing. Encourage initial changes, promote expectations for positive results, provide resources to assist in planning.
Action/willpower	Executes a plan and demonstrates a change in behavior.	Assist with strategies for self-efficacy, contingency management, and coping with situations that trigger old behaviors.
Maintenance	New behaviors become sustained, integrate into personal identity and lifestyle.	Reinforce developing habits. Evaluate and mitigate relapse risk. Praise progress.
Relapse	Regression to prior behavior (does not always occur).	Varies based on degree of regression. Encourage return to changes. Provide reassurance that change remains possible.

Psychiatric emergencies

	CAUSE	MANIFESTATION	TREATMENT
Serotonin syndrome	Any drug that ↑ 5-HT. Psychiatric drugs: MAO inhibitors, SSRIs, SNRIs, TCAs, vilazodone, vortioxetine, buspirone Nonpsychiatric drugs: tramadol, ondansetron, triptans, linezolid, MDMA, dextromethorphan, meperidine, St. John's wort	3 A's: ↑ activity (neuromuscular; eg, clonus, hyperreflexia, hypertonia, tremor, seizure), autonomic instability (eg, hyperthermia, diaphoresis, diarrhea), altered mental status	Benzodiazepines and supportive care; cyproheptadine (5-HT$_2$ receptor antagonist) if no improvement Prevention: avoid simultaneous serotonergic drugs, and allow a washout period between them
Hypertensive crisis	Eating tyramine-rich foods (eg, aged cheeses, cured meats, wine, chocolate) while taking MAO inhibitors, insufficient washout period when switching antidepressants to or from MAO inhibitors	Hypertensive crisis (tyramine displaces other neurotransmitters [eg, NE] in the synaptic cleft → ↑ sympathetic stimulation)	Phentolamine
Neuroleptic malignant syndrome	Antipsychotics (typical > atypical) + genetic predisposition	Malignant **FEVER**: Myoglobinuria, Fever, Encephalopathy, Vitals unstable, ↑ Enzymes (eg, CK), muscle Rigidity ("lead pipe")	Dantrolene, dopaminergics (eg, bromocriptine, amantadine), benzodiazepines; discontinue causative agent
Delirium tremens	Alcohol withdrawal; occurs 2–4 days after last drink Classically seen in hospital setting when inpatient cannot drink	Altered mental status, hallucinations, autonomic hyperactivity, anxiety, seizures, tremors, psychomotor agitation, insomnia, nausea	Longer-acting benzodiazepines
Acute dystonia	Antipsychotics (typical > atypical), anticonvulsants (eg, carbamazepine), metoclopramide	Sudden onset of muscle spasms, stiffness, and/or oculogyric crisis occurring hours to days after medication use; can lead to laryngospasm requiring intubation	Benztropine or diphenhydramine
Lithium toxicity	↑ lithium dosage, ↓ renal elimination (eg, acute kidney injury), medications affecting clearance (eg, ACE inhibitors, thiazide diuretics, NSAIDs) Narrow therapeutic window	Nausea, vomiting, slurred speech, hyperreflexia, seizures, ataxia, nephrogenic diabetes insipidus	Discontinue lithium, hydrate aggressively with isotonic sodium chloride, consider hemodialysis
Tricyclic antidepressant toxicity	TCA overdose	Sedation, anticholinergic effects, prolonged QT and QRS Tricyclic's: convulsions, coma, cardiotoxicity (arrhythmia due to Na$^+$ channel inhibition)	Supportive treatment, monitor ECG, NaHCO$_3$ (prevents arrhythmia), activated charcoal

Psychoactive drug intoxication and withdrawal

DRUG	MECHANISM	INTOXICATION	WITHDRAWAL
Depressants			
		Nonspecific: mood elevation, ↓ anxiety, sedation, behavioral disinhibition, respiratory depression.	Nonspecific: anxiety, tremor, seizures, insomnia.
Alcohol	GABA-A receptor positive allosteric modulator. Inhibits glutamate-induced excitation of NMDA.	Emotional lability, slurred speech, ataxia, coma, blackouts. **AST** value is 2× **ALT** value ("To**AST** 2 **AL**cohol"). Treatment: supportive (eg, fluids, antiemetics).	Adaptation causes ↑ glutamate receptors; symptoms result from unregulated excess excitation. Treatment: longer-acting benzodiazepines.
Barbiturates	GABA-A receptor positive allosteric modulator.	Low safety margin, marked respiratory depression. Treatment: symptom management (eg, assist respiration, ↑ BP).	Delirium, life-threatening cardiovascular collapse.
Benzodiazepines	GABA-A receptor positive allosteric modulator.	Greater safety margin. Ataxia, minor respiratory depression. Treatment: flumazenil (benzodiazepine receptor antagonist).	Seizures, sleep disturbance, depression.
Opioids	Opioid receptor modulator.	Activation of μ receptors causes the prototypic effect of miosis (pinpoint pupils), ↓ GI motility, respiratory and CNS depression, euphoria, ↓ gag reflex, seizures. Most common cause of drug overdose death. Overdose treatment: naloxone.	Mydriasis, diarrhea, flulike symptoms, rhinorrhea, yawning, nausea, sweating, piloerection ("cold turkey"), lacrimation. Treatment: symptom management, methadone, buprenorphine.
Inhalants	Enhanced GABA signaling.	Disinhibition, euphoria, slurred speech, ataxia, disorientation, drowsiness, periorifical rash. Rapid onset and resolution.	Irritability, dysphoria, sleep disturbance, headache.
Stimulants			
	Nonspecific.	Mood elevation, ↓ appetite, psychomotor agitation, insomnia, cardiac arrhythmias, ↑ HR, anxiety.	Post-use "crash," including depression, lethargy, ↑ appetite, sleep disturbance, vivid nightmares.
Amphetamines	Induces reversal of monoamine transporters (VMAT, DAT, SERT, NET), ↑ neurotransmitter release.	Euphoria, grandiosity, mydriasis, prolonged wakefulness, hyperalertness, hypertension, paranoia, fever. Skin excoriations with **m**ethamphetamine use. Severe: cardiac arrest, seizures. Treatment: benzodiazepines for agitation and seizures.	**M**eth **m**ites (tactile hallucinations)

Psychoactive drug intoxication and withdrawal *(continued)*

DRUG	MECHANISM	INTOXICATION	WITHDRAWAL
Caffeine	Adenosine receptor antagonist.	Palpitation, agitation, tremor, insomnia.	Headache, difficulty concentrating, flulike symptoms.
Cocaine	Blocks reuptake by dopamine (DAT), serotonin (SERT), and norepinephrine (NET) transporters.	Impaired judgment, mydriasis, diaphoresis, hallucinations (including formication), paranoia, angina, sudden cardiac death. Chronic use may lead to perforated nasal septum due to vasoconstriction and resulting ischemic necrosis. Treatment: benzodiazepines.	Restlessness, hunger, severe depression, sleep disturbance.
Nicotine	Stimulates central nicotinic acetylcholine receptors.	Restlessness.	Irritability, anxiety, restlessness, ↓ concentration, ↑ appetite/weight. Treatment: nicotine replacement therapy (eg, patch, gum, lozenge); bupropion/varenicline.
Hallucinogens			
Lysergic acid diethylamide	5-HT$_{2A}$ receptor agonist.	Perceptual distortion (visual, auditory), depersonalization, anxiety, paranoia, psychosis, flashbacks, mydriasis.	
Cannabis/ cannabinoids	CB1 receptor agonist.	Euphoria, anxiety, paranoid delusions, perception of slowed time, impaired judgment, social withdrawal, ↑ appetite, dry mouth, conjunctival injection, hallucinations.	Irritability, anxiety, depression, insomnia, restlessness, ↓ appetite.
MDMA (ecstasy)	Induces reversal of transporters for monoamines (SERT > DAT, NET), → ↑ neurotransmitter release.	Euphoria, hallucinations, disinhibition, hyperactivity, ↑ thirst, bruxism, distorted perceptions, mydriasis. Life-threatening effects include hypertension, tachycardia, hyperthermia, hyponatremia, serotonin syndrome.	Depression, fatigue, change in appetite, difficulty concentrating, anxiety.
Phencyclidine	NMDA receptor antagonist.	Violence, nystagmus, impulsivity, psychomotor agitation, tachycardia, hypertension, analgesia, psychosis, delirium, seizures.	

Alcohol use disorder	Diagnosed using criteria for substance use disorder. Complications: vitamin B_1 (thiamine) deficiency, alcoholic cirrhosis, hepatitis, pancreatitis, peripheral neuropathy, testicular atrophy. Treatment: naltrexone (reduces cravings; avoid in liver failure), acamprosate (contraindicated in renal failure), disulfiram (to condition the patient to abstain from alcohol use). Support groups such as Alcoholics Anonymous are helpful in sustaining abstinence and supporting patient and family.
Wernicke-Korsakoff syndrome	Results from vitamin B_1 deficiency. Symptoms can be precipitated by administering dextrose before vitamin B_1. Triad of confusion, ophthalmoplegia, ataxia (Wernicke encephalopathy). May progress to irreversible memory loss, confabulation, personality change (Korsakoff syndrome). Treatment: IV vitamin B_1 (before dextrose).

▶ PSYCHIATRY—PHARMACOLOGY

Psychotherapy

Behavioral therapy	Teaches patients how to identify and change maladaptive behaviors or reactions to stimuli (eg, systematic desensitization for specific phobia).
Cognitive behavioral therapy	Teaches patients to recognize distortions in their thought processes, develop constructive coping skills, and ↓ maladaptive coping behaviors → greater emotional control and tolerance of distress (eg, recognizing triggers for alcohol consumption).
Dialectical behavioral therapy	Designed for use in borderline personality disorder, but can be used in other psychiatric conditions as well (eg, depression).
Interpersonal therapy	Focused on improving interpersonal relationships and communication skills.
Motivational interviewing	Enhances intrinsic motivation to change by exploring and resolving ambivalence. Used in substance use disorder and weight loss.
Supportive therapy	Utilizes empathy to help individuals during a time of hardship to maintain optimism or hope.

Central nervous system stimulants	Methylphenidate, dextroamphetamine, methamphetamine, lisdexamfetamine.
MECHANISM	↑ catecholamines in the synaptic cleft, especially norepinephrine and dopamine.
CLINICAL USE	ADHD, narcolepsy, binge-eating disorder.
ADVERSE EFFECTS	Nervousness, agitation, anxiety, insomnia, anorexia, tachycardia, hypertension, weight loss, tics, bruxism.

Antipsychotics	Typical (1st-generation) antipsychotics—haloperidol, pimozide, trifluoperazine, fluphenazine, thioridazine, chlorpromazine. Atypical (2nd-generation) antipsychotics—aripiprazole, asenapine, clozapine, olanzapine, quetiapine, iloperidone, paliperidone, risperidone, lurasidone, ziprasidone.
MECHANISM	Block dopamine D_2 receptor (↑ cAMP). Atypical antipsychotics also block serotonin 5-HT_2 receptor. Aripiprazole is a D_2 partial agonist.
CLINICAL USE	Schizophrenia (typical antipsychotics primarily treat positive symptoms; atypical antipsychotics treat both positive and negative symptoms), disorders with concomitant psychosis (eg, bipolar disorder), Tourette syndrome, OCD, Huntington disease. Clozapine is used for treatment-resistant psychotic disorders or those with persistent suicidality (**cloze** to the edge).

ADVERSE EFFECTS	Antihistaminic (sedation), anti-α_1-adrenergic (orthostatic hypotension), antimuscarinic (dry mouth, constipation) (anti-**HAM**). Use with caution in dementia.
	Metabolic: weight gain, hyperglycemia, dyslipidemia. ↑ risk with clozapine and olanzapine (obesity).
	Endocrine: hyperprolactinemia → galactorrhea, oligomenorrhea, gynecomastia (↓ activity in the tuberoinfundibular pathway).
	Cardiac: QT prolongation.
	Neurologic: neuroleptic malignant syndrome.
	Ophthalmologic: chlorpromazine—corneal deposits; thioridazine—retinal deposits.
	Clozapine—agranulocytosis (monitor WBCs **cloze**ly), seizures (dose related), myocarditis, hypersalivation.
	Extrapyramidal symptoms (↓ activity in the nigrostriatal pathway)—**ADAPT**:
	  ▪ Hours to days: **A**cute **D**ystonia (muscle spasm, stiffness, oculogyric crisis). Treatment: benztropine, diphenhydramine.
	  ▪ Days to months:
	    ▪ **A**kathisia (restlessness). Treatment: β-blockers, benztropine, benzodiazepines.
	    ▪ **P**arkinsonism (bradykinesia). Treatment: benztropine, amantadine.
	  ▪ Months to years: **T**ardive dyskinesia (chorea, especially orofacial). Treatment: benzodiazepines, botulinum toxin injections, valbenazine, deutetrabenazine.

NOTES	Lipid soluble → stored in body fat → slow to be removed from body. Typical antipsychotics have greater affinity for D_2 receptor than atypical antipsychotics → ↑ risk for hyperprolactinemia, extrapyramidal symptoms, neuroleptic malignant syndrome. High-potency typical antipsychotics: haloperidol, trifluoperazine, pimozide, fluphenazine (**Hal tries pie to fly high**)—more neurologic adverse effects (eg, extrapyramidal symptoms). Low-potency typical antipsychotics: chlorpromazine, thioridazine (**cheating thieves are low**)—more antihistaminic, anti-α_1-adrenergic, antimuscarinic effects.

Lithium

MECHANISM	Affects neurotransmission (↓ excitatory, ↑ inhibitory) and second messenger systems (eg, G proteins).
CLINICAL USE	Mood stabilizer for bipolar disorder; treats acute manic episodes and prevents relapse.
ADVERSE EFFECTS	Tremor, hypothyroidism, hyperthyroidism, mild hypercalcemia, polyuria (causes nephrogenic diabetes insipidus), teratogenesis (causes Ebstein anomaly). Narrow therapeutic window requires close monitoring of serum levels. Almost exclusively excreted by kidneys; most is reabsorbed at PCT via Na^+ channels. Thiazides, ACE inhibitors, NSAIDs, and other drugs affecting clearance are implicated in lithium toxicity. LiTHIUM: Low Thyroid (hypothyroidism) Heart (Ebstein anomaly) Insipidus (nephrogenic diabetes insipidus) Unwanted Movements (tremor)

Buspirone

MECHANISM	Partial 5-HT_{1A} receptor agonist.
CLINICAL USE	Generalized anxiety disorder. Does not cause sedation, addiction, or tolerance. Begins to take effect after 1–2 weeks. Does not interact with alcohol (vs barbiturates, benzodiazepines). I get anxious if the bus doesn't arrive at one, so I take buspirone.

Antidepressants

It normally takes 4–8 weeks for antidepressants to show appreciable effect.

Selective serotonin reuptake inhibitors	Fluoxetine, fluvoxamine, paroxetine, sertraline, escitalopram, citalopram.
MECHANISM	Inhibit 5-HT reuptake.
CLINICAL USE	Depression, generalized anxiety disorder, panic disorder, OCD, bulimia, binge-eating disorder, social anxiety disorder, PTSD, premature ejaculation, premenstrual dysphoric disorder.
ADVERSE EFFECTS	Fewer than TCAs. Serotonin syndrome, GI distress, SIADH, sexual dysfunction (anorgasmia, erectile dysfunction, ↓ libido), mania precipitation if underlying bipolar disorder.

Serotonin- norepinephrine reuptake inhibitors	Venlafaxine, desvenlafaxine, duloxetine, levomilnacipran, milnacipran.
MECHANISM	Inhibit 5-HT and NE reuptake.
CLINICAL USE	Depression, generalized anxiety disorder, diabetic neuropathy. Venlafaxine is also indicated for social anxiety disorder, panic disorder, PTSD, OCD. Duloxetine and milnacipran are also indicated for fibromyalgia.
ADVERSE EFFECTS	↑ BP, stimulant effects, sedation, sexual dysfunction, nausea.

Tricyclic antidepressants	Amitriptyline, nortriptyline, imipramine, desipramine, clomipramine, doxepin, amoxapine.
MECHANISM	TCAs inhibit 5-HT and NE reuptake.
CLINICAL USE	MDD, peripheral neuropathy, chronic neuropathic pain, migraine prophylaxis, OCD (clomipramine), nocturnal enuresis (imipramine).
ADVERSE EFFECTS	Sedation, α_1-blocking effects including postural hypotension, and atropine-like (anticholinergic) adverse effects (tachycardia, urinary retention, dry mouth). 3° TCAs (amitriptyline) have more anticholinergic effects than 2° TCAs (nortriptyline). Can prolong QT interval. **Tri-CyCliC's**: Convulsions, Coma, Cardiotoxicity (arrhythmia due to Na⁺ channel inhibition); also respiratory depression, hyperpyrexia. Confusion and hallucinations are more common in older adults due to anticholinergic adverse effects (2° amines [eg, nortriptyline] better tolerated). Treatment: NaHCO₃ to prevent arrhythmia.

Monoamine oxidase inhibitors	Tranylcypromine, phenelzine, isocarboxazid, selegiline (selective **MAO-B** inhibitor). (**MAO** takes pride in Shanghai).
MECHANISM	Nonselective MAO inhibition → ↑ levels of amine neurotransmitters (norepinephrine, 5-HT, dopamine).
CLINICAL USE	Atypical depression, anxiety. Parkinson disease (selegiline).
ADVERSE EFFECTS	CNS stimulation; hypertensive crisis, most notably with ingestion of tyramine. Contraindicated with SSRIs, TCAs, St. John's wort, meperidine, dextromethorphan, pseudoephedrine, linezolid (to avoid precipitating serotonin syndrome). Wait 2 weeks after stopping MAO inhibitors before starting serotonergic drugs (risk for serotonin syndrome) or stopping dietary restrictions (risk for tyramine induced hypertensive crisis).

Atypical antidepressants	Atypical Bees Make Tasty Vegan Venison.
Bupropion	Inhibits NE and DA reuptake. Also used for smoking cessation. Adverse effects: stimulant effects (tachycardia, insomnia), headache, seizures in patients with bulimia and anorexia nervosa. ↓ risk of sexual adverse effects and weight gain compared to other antidepressants.
Mirtazapine	α_2-antagonist (↑ release of NE and 5-HT), potent 5-HT$_2$ and 5-HT$_3$ receptor antagonist, and H$_1$ antagonist. Adverse effects: sedation (which may be desirable in depressed patients with insomnia), ↑ appetite, weight gain (which may be desirable in underweight patients), dry mouth. **M**irtazapine makes you **m**unch **m**ore and **m**ove less.
Trazodone	Primarily blocks 5-HT$_2$, α_1-adrenergic, and H$_1$ receptors; also weakly inhibits 5-HT reuptake. Used primarily for insomnia, as high doses are needed for antidepressant effects. Adverse effects: sedation, nausea, priapism, postural hypotension. Think tra**ZZZ**obone due to sedative and male-specific adverse effects.
Vilazodone	Inhibits 5-HT reuptake; 5-HT$_{1A}$ receptor partial agonist. Used for MDD. Adverse effects: headache, diarrhea, nausea, anticholinergic effects. May cause serotonin syndrome if taken with other serotonergic agents.
Vortioxetine	Inhibits 5-HT reuptake; 5-HT$_{1A}$ receptor agonist and 5-HT$_3$ receptor antagonist. Used for MDD. Adverse effects: nausea, sexual dysfunction, sleep disturbances, anticholinergic effects. May cause serotonin syndrome if taken with other serotonergic agents.

Pharmacotherapies for smoking cessation	
Nicotine replacement therapy	Binds to nicotinic ACh receptors. Aim to relieve withdrawal symptoms upon stopping smoking. Long-acting patch and short-acting products (ie, gum, lozenge) can be used in combination. Adverse effects: headache, oral irritation.
Varenicline	Nicotinic ACh receptor partial agonist. Diminishes effect on reward system, but also reduces withdrawal. Adverse effects: GI discomfort, sleep disturbance. Vare**nicline** helps **ni**cotine cravings de**cline**.

Medically supervised opioid withdrawal and relapse prevention	Injection drug use ↑ risk for HBV, HCV, HIV, skin and soft tissue infections, bacteremia, right-sided infective endocarditis.
Methadone	Long-acting oral opioid used for medically supervised opioid (eg, heroin) withdrawal or long-term maintenance therapy.
Buprenorphine	Partial opioid agonist. Sublingual form (film) used to suppress withdrawal and for maintenance therapy. Partial agonists can precipitate withdrawal symptoms in opioid-dependent individuals or when administered shortly after use of a full agonist.
Naloxone	Short-acting opioid antagonist given IM, IV, or as a nasal spray to treat acute opioid overdose, particularly to reverse respiratory and CNS depression.
Naltrexone	Long-acting oral opioid antagonist used after detoxification to prevent relapse. May help alcohol and nicotine cessation, weight loss. Use nal**trex**one for the long **trex** back to sobriety.

Renal

"But I know all about love already. I know precious little still about kidneys."

—Aldous Huxley, *Antic Hay*

"This too shall pass. Just like a kidney stone."

—Hunter Madsen

"Playing dead is difficult with a full bladder."

—Diane Lane

Being able to understand and apply renal physiology will be critical for the exam. Important topics include electrolyte disorders, acid-base derangements, glomerular disorders (including histopathology), acute and chronic kidney disease, urine casts, diuretics, ACE inhibitors, and AT II receptor blockers. Renal anomalies associated with various congenital defects are also high-yield associations to think about when evaluating pediatric vignettes.

▶ RENAL—EMBRYOLOGY

Kidney embryology	Pronephros—week 4 of development; then degenerates.
	
	Mesonephros—week 4 of development; functions as interim kidney for 1st trimester in both sexes. Mesonephric ducts persist in the male genital system as Wolffian duct, forming ductus deferens and epididymis. Mesonephric ducts degenerate in females.
	
	Metanephros—permanent; first appears in week 5 of development; nephrogenesis is normally completed by week 36 of gestation.
	  ▪ Ureteric bud (metanephric diverticulum)—fully canalized by week 10 of development; derived from mesonephric duct to form ureters, pelvises, calyces, and collecting ducts
	  ▪ Metanephric mesenchyme (ie, metanephric blastema)—ureteric bud interacts with this tissue to induce differentiation and formation of glomerulus through distal convoluted tubule (DCT)
	  ▪ Aberrant interaction between these 2 tissues may result in several congenital malformations of the kidney (eg, renal agenesis, multicystic dysplastic kidney)
		Ureteropelvic junction → last part of ureter to canalize; if doesn't fully canalize → congenital obstruction. Can be unilateral or bilateral. Most common pathologic cause of prenatal hydronephrosis. Detected by prenatal ultrasound.
		
		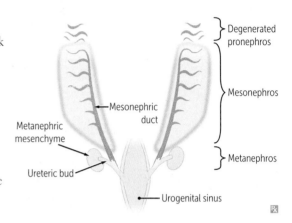

Potter sequence	Oligohydramnios → compression of developing fetus → limb deformities (eg, club feet), facial anomalies (eg, low-set ears and retrognathia, flattened nose), compression of chest and lack of amniotic fluid aspiration into fetal lungs → pulmonary hypoplasia (cause of death).
	
	Caused by chronic placental insufficiency or reduced fetal urine output, including ARPKD, obstructive uropathy (eg, posterior urethral valves), bilateral renal agenesis, preterm premature rupture of membranes, maternal ACE inhibitor use.
		Babies who can't "Pee" in utero develop Potter sequence.
		POTTER sequence associated with:
		  Pulmonary hypoplasia
		  Oligohydramnios (trigger)
		  Twisted face
		  Twisted skin
		  Extremity defects
		  Renal failure (in utero)

Horseshoe kidney

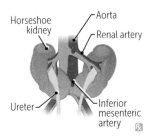

Horseshoe kidney
Aorta
Renal artery
Ureter
Inferior mesenteric artery

Inferior poles of both kidneys fuse abnormally 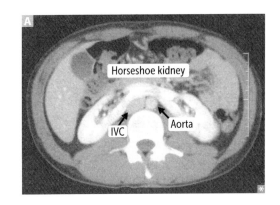. As they ascend from pelvis during fetal development, horseshoe kidneys get trapped under inferior mesenteric artery and remain low in the abdomen. Kidneys can function normally, but associated with hydronephrosis (eg, ureteropelvic junction obstruction), renal stones, infection, ↑ risk of renal cancer.

Higher incidence in chromosomal aneuploidy (eg, Turner syndrome, trisomies 13, 18, 21).

Horseshoe kidney
IVC
Aorta

Congenital solitary functioning kidney

Condition of being born with only one functioning kidney. Majority asymptomatic with compensatory hypertrophy of contralateral kidney, but anomalies in contralateral kidney are common. Often diagnosed prenatally via ultrasound bilateral agenesis or dysplasia leads to Potter sequence.

Unilateral renal agenesis

Ureteric bud fails to develop and induce differentiation of metanephric mesenchyme → complete absence of kidney and ureter.

Multicystic dysplastic kidney

Ureteric bud develops, but fails to induce differentiation of metanephric mesenchyme → nonfunctional kidney consisting of cysts and connective tissue. Nongenetic inheritance, though tends to run in families; usually unilateral.

Duplex collecting system

Bifurcation of ureteric bud before it enters the metanephric blastema creates a Y-shaped bifid ureter. Duplex collecting system can alternatively occur through two ureteric buds reaching and interacting with metanephric blastema. Strongly associated with vesicoureteral reflux and/or ureteral obstruction, ↑ risk for UTIs. Frequently presents with hydronephrosis.

Posterior urethral valves

Membrane remnant in posterior (prostatic) urethra in males; its persistence can lead to urethral obstruction. Diagnosed prenatally by bilateral hydronephrosis and dilated or thick-walled bladder on ultrasound. Severe obstruction in fetus associated with oligohydramnios. Most common cause of bladder outlet obstruction in male infants.

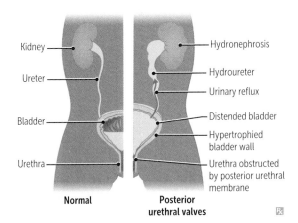

Kidney
Ureter
Bladder
Urethra

Hydronephrosis
Hydroureter
Urinary reflux
Distended bladder
Hypertrophied bladder wall
Urethra obstructed by posterior urethral membrane

Normal

Posterior urethral valves

Vesicoureteral reflux	Retrograde flow of urine from bladder toward upper urinary tract. Can be 1° due to abnormal/insufficient insertion of the ureter within the vesicular wall (ureterovesical junction [UVJ]) or 2° due to abnormally high bladder pressure resulting in retrograde flow via the UVJ. ↑ risk of recurrent UTIs.

▶ RENAL—ANATOMY

Renal blood flow

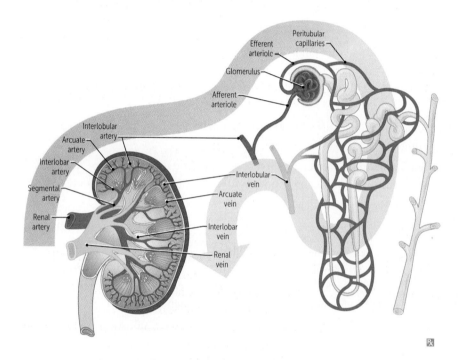

Left renal vein receives two additional veins: left suprarenal and left gonadal veins.

Renal medulla receives significantly less blood flow than the renal cortex. This makes medulla very sensitive to hypoxia and vulnerable to ischemic damage (eg, ATN).

Left kidney is most commonly taken during Living donor transpLantation because it has a Longer renal vein (rule of Ls).

Glomerular anatomy

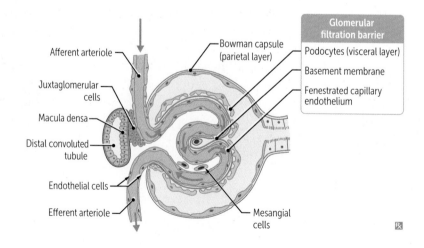

Course of ureters

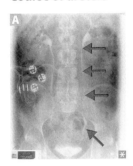

Course of ureter **A**: arises from renal pelvis, travels under gonadal arteries → **over** common iliac artery → **under** uterine artery/vas deferens (retroperitoneal).

Gynecologic procedures (eg, ligation of uterine or ovarian vessels) may damage ureter → ureteral obstruction or leak.

Bladder contraction compresses the intramural ureter, preventing urine reflux.

3 common points of ureteral obstruction: ureteropelvic junction, pelvic inlet, ureterovesical junction.

Water (ureters) flows **over** the iliacs and **under** the bridge (uterine artery or vas deferens).

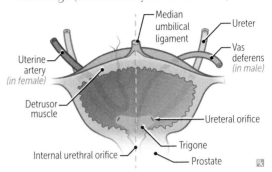

▶ RENAL—PHYSIOLOGY

Fluid compartments

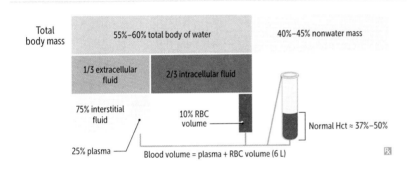

HIKIN': **HI K⁺ IN**tracellularly.

60–40–20 rule (% of body weight for average person):
- 60% total body water
- 40% ICF, mainly composed of K^+, Mg^{2+}, organic phosphates (eg, ATP)
- 20% ECF, mainly composed of Na^+, Cl^-, HCO_3^-, albumin

Plasma volume can be measured by radiolabeling albumin.

Extracellular volume can be measured by inulin or mannitol.

Serum osmolality = 275–295 mOsm/kg H_2O.

Plasma volume = TBV × (1 – Hct).

Glomerular filtration barrier

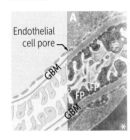

Responsible for filtration of plasma according to size and charge selectivity.

Composed of
- Fenestrated capillary endothelium
- Glomerular basement membrane (GBM) with type IV collagen chains and heparan sulfate
- Visceral epithelial layer consisting of podocyte foot processes (FPs) **A**

Charge barrier—glomerular filtration barrier contains ⊖ charged glycoproteins that prevent entry of ⊖ charged molecules (eg, albumin).

Size barrier—fenestrated capillary endothelium (prevents entry of > 100 nm molecules/blood cells); slit diaphragm (prevents entry of molecules > 40–50 nm).

Podocyte foot processes interpose with GBM—both charge and size barrier.

Renal clearance

$C_x = (U_x V)/P_x$ = volume of plasma from which the substance is completely cleared in the urine per unit time.

If $C_x < GFR$: net tubular reabsorption and/or not freely filtered.

If $C_x > GFR$: net tubular secretion of X.

If $C_x = GFR$: no net secretion or reabsorption.

C_x = clearance of X (mL/min).
U_x = urine concentration of X (eg, mg/mL).
P_x = plasma concentration of X (eg, mg/mL).
V = urine flow rate (mL/min).

Glomerular filtration rate

Inulin clearance can be used to calculate GFR because it is freely filtered and is neither reabsorbed nor secreted.

$$C_{inulin} = GFR = U_{inulin} \times V/P_{inulin}$$
$$= K_f [(P_{GC} - P_{BS}) - (\pi_{GC} - \pi_{BS})]$$

P_{GC} = glomerular capillary hydrostatic pressure; P_{BS} = Bowman space hydrostatic pressure; π_{GC} = glomerular capillary oncotic pressure; π_{BS} = Bowman space oncotic pressure; π_{BS} normally equals zero; K_f = filtration coefficient.

Normal GFR ≈ 100 mL/min.

Creatinine clearance is an approximate measure of GFR. Slightly overestimates GFR because creatinine is moderately secreted by proximal renal tubules.

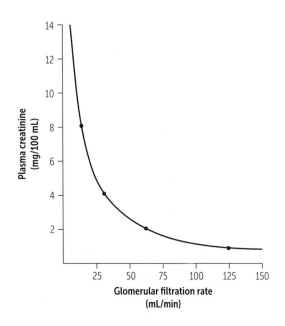

Renal blood flow autoregulation

Autoregulatory mechanisms help maintain a constant RBF and GFR to protect the kidney from rapid fluctuations in renal perfusion pressure that could cause renal injury leading to reduced glomerular filtration. Mechanisms:

Myogenic: ↑ arterial pressure → stretch of afferent arteriole → mechanical activation of vascular smooth muscle → vasoconstriction of afferent arteriole → ↓ RBF.

Tubuloglomerular: ↑ NaCl of the filtrate sensed by macula densa cells → paracrine-driven vasoconstriction of afferent arteriole → ↓ RBF. Can also have the opposite effect on RBF if ↓ NaCl.

Effective renal plasma flow

Effective renal plasma flow (eRPF) can be estimated using *para*-aminohippuric acid (PAH) clearance. Between filtration and secretion, there is nearly complete excretion of all PAH that enters the kidney.

$eRPF = U_{PAH} \times V/P_{PAH} = C_{PAH}$.

Renal blood flow (RBF) = RPF/(1 − Hct). Usually 20–25% of cardiac output.

eRPF underestimates true renal plasma flow (RPF) slightly.

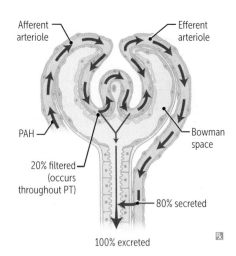

Filtration

Filtration fraction (FF) = GFR/RPF.
Normal FF = 20%.
Filtered load (mg/min) = GFR (mL/min) × plasma concentration (mg/mL).

GFR can be estimated with creatinine clearance.
Prostaglandins **D**ilate **A**fferent arteriole (**PDA**).
Angiotensin II **C**onstricts **E**fferent arteriole (**ACE**). RPF is best estimated with PAH clearance. NSAIDs and ACE inhibitors should not be given together → constriction of afferent and efferent arterioles.

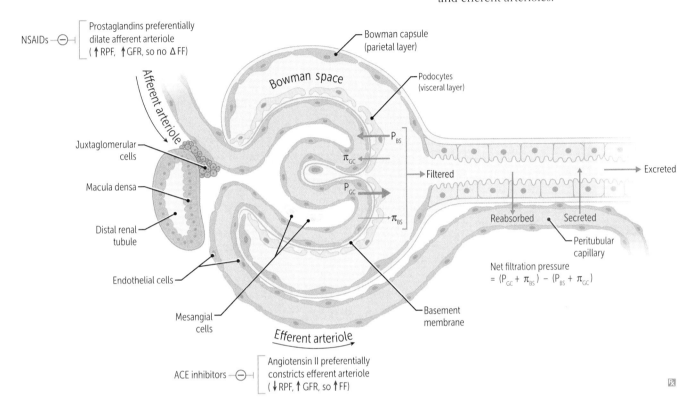

NSAIDs —⊖—| Prostaglandins preferentially dilate afferent arteriole (↑RPF, ↑GFR, so no Δ FF)

ACE inhibitors —⊖—| Angiotensin II preferentially constricts efferent arteriole (↓RPF, ↑GFR, so ↑FF)

Net filtration pressure = $(P_{GC} + \pi_{BS}) - (P_{BS} + \pi_{GC})$

Changes in glomerular dynamics

	GFR	RPF	FF (GFR/RPF)
Afferent arteriole constriction	↓	↓	—
Efferent arteriole constriction	↑	↓	↑
↑ plasma protein concentration	↓	—	↓
↓ plasma protein concentration	↑	—	↑
Constriction of ureter	↓	—	↓
Dehydration	↓	↓↓	↑

Notably for patients undergoing nephrectomy, there is a proportionate decline in renal function (↓ nephron number) → ↓ remaining kidney renal function to ~50% of prenephrectomy value until long-term compensations like hypertrophy develop.

Calculation of reabsorption and secretion rate

Filtered load = GFR × P_x.
Excretion rate = V × U_x.
Reabsorption rate = filtered − excreted.
Secretion rate = excreted − filtered.
FENa = fractional excretion of sodium.

$$FENa = \frac{Na^+ \text{ excreted}}{Na^+ \text{ filtered}} = \frac{V \times U_{Na}}{GFR \times P_{Na}} = \frac{P_{Cr} \times U_{Na}}{U_{Cr} \times P_{Na}} \quad \text{where GFR} = \frac{U_{Cr} \times V}{P_{Cr}}$$

Glucose clearance

Glucose at a normal plasma level (range 60–120 mg/dL) is completely reabsorbed in proximal convoluted tubule (PCT) by Na^+/glucose cotransport.

In adults, at plasma glucose of ~ 200 mg/dL, glucosuria begins (threshold). At rate of ~ 375 mg/min, all transporters are fully saturated (T_m).

Normal pregnancy is associated with ↑ GFR. With ↑ filtration of all substances, including glucose, the glucose threshold occurs at lower plasma glucose concentrations → glucosuria at normal plasma glucose levels.

Sodium-glucose cotransporter 2 (SGLT2) inhibitors (eg, -flozin drugs) lead to glucosuria at plasma concentrations < 200 mg/dL.

Glucosuria is an important clinical clue to diabetes mellitus.

Splay phenomenon—T_m for glucose is reached gradually rather than sharply due to the heterogeneity of nephrons (ie, different T_m points); represented by the portion of the titration curve between threshold and T_m.

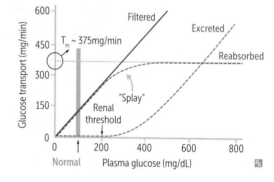

Nephron transport physiology

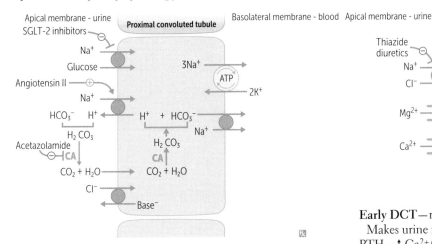

Early PCT—contains brush border. Reabsorbs all glucose
and amino acids and most HCO_3^-, Na^+, Cl^-, PO_4^{3-}, K^+,
H_2O, and uric acid. Isotonic absorption. Generates and
secretes NH_3, which enables the kidney to excrete (via
secretion) more H^+.
PTH—inhibits Na^+/PO_4^{3-} cotransport → ↑ PO_4^{3-} excretion.
AT II—stimulates Na^+/H^+ exchange → ↑ Na^+, H_2O, and
HCO_3^- reabsorption (permitting contraction alkalosis).
65–80% Na^+ and H_2O reabsorbed.

Thin descending loop of Henle—passively reabsorbs H_2O
via medullary hypertonicity (impermeable to Na^+).
Concentrating segment. Makes urine hypertonic.

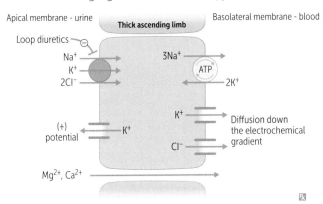

Thick ascending loop of Henle—reabsorbs Na^+, K^+, and
Cl^-. Indirectly induces paracellular reabsorption of Mg^{2+}
and Ca^{2+} through ⊕ lumen potential generated by K^+
backleak. Impermeable to H_2O. Makes urine less
concentrated as it ascends.
10–20% Na^+ reabsorbed.

Early DCT—reabsorbs Na^+, Cl^-. Impermeable to H_2O.
Makes urine fully dilute (hypotonic).
PTH—↑ Ca^{2+}/Na^+ exchange → ↑ Ca^{2+} reabsorption.
5–10% Na^+ reabsorbed.

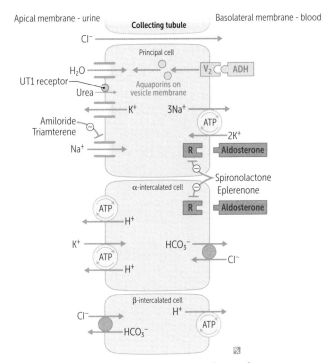

Collecting tubule—reabsorbs Na^+ in exchange for
secreting K^+ and H^+ (regulated by aldosterone).
Aldosterone—acts on mineralocorticoid receptor → mRNA
→ protein synthesis. In principal cells: ↑ apical K^+
conductance, ↑ Na^+/K^+ pump, ↑ epithelial Na^+ channel
(ENaC) activity → lumen negativity → K^+ secretion. In
α-intercalated cells: lumen negativity → ↑ H^+ ATPase
activity → ↑ H^+ secretion → ↑ HCO_3^-/Cl^- exchanger
activity.
ADH—acts at V_2 receptor → insertion of aquaporin H_2O
channels on apical side.
3–5% Na^+ reabsorbed. Urea reabsorption (medullary, not
cortical, duct only).

Renal tubular defects   Order: **Fanconi's BaGeLS**

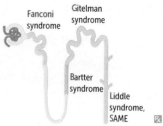

	DEFECTS	EFFECTS	CAUSES	NOTES
Fanconi syndrome	Generalized reabsorption defect in PCT → ↑ excretion of amino acids, glucose, HCO_3^-, and PO_4^{3-}, and all substances reabsorbed by the PCT	Metabolic acidosis (proximal RTA), hypophosphatemia, hypokalemia	Hereditary defects (eg, Wilson disease, tyrosinemia, glycogen storage disease), ischemia, multiple myeloma, drugs (eg, ifosfamide, cisplatin, tenofovir, lead poisoning	Growth restriction and rickets/osteopenia common due to hypophosphatemia Volume depletion also common
Bartter syndrome	Reabsorption defect in thick ascending loop of Henle (affects $Na^+/K^+/2Cl^-$ cotransporter)	Metabolic alkalosis, hypochloremia, hypokalemia, hypercalciuria	Autosomal recessive	Presents similarly to chronic loop diuretic use
Gitelman syndrome	Reabsorption defect of NaCl in DCT	Metabolic alkalosis, hypochloremia, hypomagnesemia, hypokalemia	Autosomal recessive	Presents similarly to chronic thiazide diuretic use Less severe than Bartter syndrome
Liddle syndrome	Gain of function mutation → ↓ Na^+ channel degradation → ↑ Na^+ reabsorption in collecting tubules	Metabolic alkalosis, hypokalemia, hypertension, ↓ serum aldosterone	Autosomal dominant	Presents similarly to hyperaldosteronism, but aldosterone is nearly undetectable Treatment: amiloride
Syndrome of Apparent Mineralocorticoid Excess	Cortisol activates mineralocorticoid receptors; 11β-HSD converts cortisol to cortisone (inactive on these receptors) Hereditary 11β-HSD deficiency → ↑ cortisol → ↑ mineralocorticoid receptor activity	Metabolic alkalosis, hypokalemia, hypertension ↓ serum aldosterone level; cortisol tries to be the **SAME** as aldosterone	Autosomal recessive Can acquire disorder from glycyrrhetinic acid (present in licorice), which blocks activity of 11β-hydroxysteroid dehydrogenase	Treatment: K^+-sparing diuretics (↓ mineralocorticoid effects) or corticosteroids (exogenous corticosteroid ↓ endogenous cortisol production → ↓ mineralocorticoid receptor activation)

Features of renal disorders

CONDITION	BLOOD PRESSURE	PLASMA RENIN	ALDOSTERONE	SERUM Mg²⁺	URINE Ca²⁺
SIADH	—/↑	—/↓	—/↓	—	—
Bartter syndrome	—	↑	↑	—	↑
Gitelman syndrome	—	↑	↑	↓	↓
Renin-secreting tumor	↑	↑	↑	—	—
Primary hyperaldosteronism	↑	↓	↑	—	—
Liddle syndrome, syndrome of apparent mineralocorticoid excess	↑	↓	↓	—	—

↑↓ = important differentiating feature.

Relative concentrations along proximal tubule

[TF/P] > 1 when solute is reabsorbed less quickly than water or when solute is secreted

[TF/P] = 1 when solute and water are reabsorbed at the same rate

[TF/P] < 1 when solute is reabsorbed more quickly than water

$\dfrac{\text{[Tubular fluid]}}{\text{[Plasma]}}$

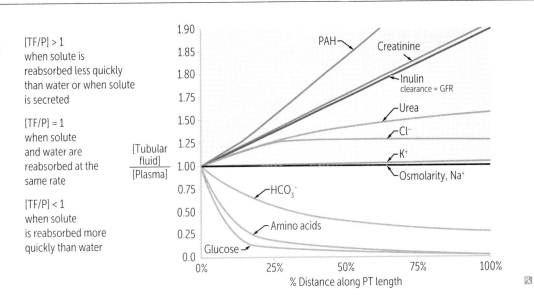

Tubular inulin ↑ in concentration (but not amount) along the PT as a result of water reabsorption. Cl⁻ reabsorption occurs at a slower rate than Na⁺ in early PCT and then matches the rate of Na⁺ reabsorption more distally. Thus, its relative concentration ↑ before it plateaus.

Renin-angiotensin-aldosterone system

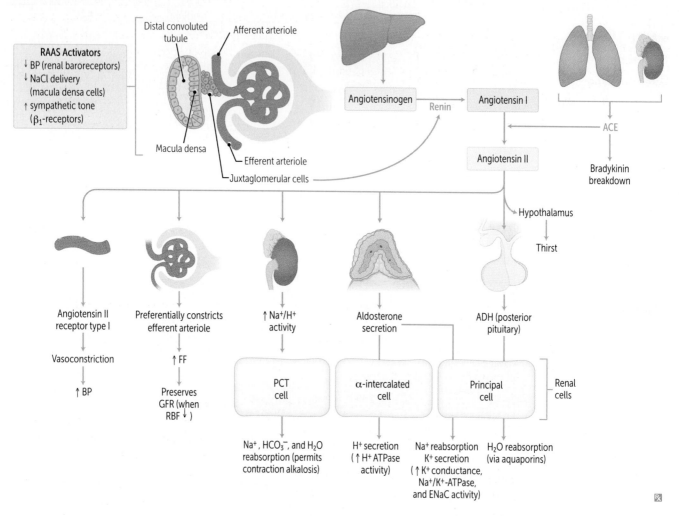

Renin	Secreted by JG cells in response to ↓ renal perfusion pressure (detected in afferent arteriole), ↑ renal sympathetic discharge (β_1 effect), and ↓ NaCl delivery to macula densa cells.
ACE	Catalyzes conversion of angiotensin I to angiotensin II. Located in many tissues but conversion occurs most extensively in the lung. Produced by vascular endothelial cells in the lung.
AT II	Helps maintain blood volume and blood pressure. Affects baroreceptor function; limits reflex bradycardia, which would normally accompany its pressor effects.
ANP, BNP	Released from atria (ANP) and ventricles (BNP) in response to ↑ volume; relaxes vascular smooth muscle via cGMP → ↑ GFR; ↓ renin → angiotensin-aldosterone inhibition. Dilates afferent arteriole, promotes natriuresis.
ADH (vasopressin)	Primarily regulates serum osmolality; also responds to low blood volume states. Stimulates reabsorption of water in collecting ducts. Also stimulates reabsorption of urea in medullary collecting ducts to maximize corticopapillary osmotic gradient.
Aldosterone	Primarily regulates ECF volume and Na^+ content; ↑ release in hypovolemic states. Responds to hyperkalemia by ↑ K^+ excretion.

Juxtaglomerular apparatus	Consists of mesangial cells, JG cells (modified smooth muscle of afferent arteriole), and the macula densa (NaCl sensor located at the DCT). JG cells secrete renin in response to ↓ renal blood pressure and ↑ sympathetic tone (β_1). Macula densa cells sense ↓ NaCl delivery to DCT → ↑ renin release → efferent arteriole vasoconstriction → ↑ GFR. Communication between JG cells and macula densa occurs via gap junctions.	JGA prevents short-term changes in GFR through autoregulation and maintains GFR long-term through regulation of the renin-angiotensin-aldosterone system. β-blockers ↓ BP by ↓ CO and inhibiting β_1-receptors of the JGA → ↓ renin release.

Kidney endocrine/paracrine functions

Erythropoietin	Released by interstitial cells in peritubular capillary bed in response to hypoxia.	Stimulates RBC proliferation in bone marrow. Administered for anemia secondary to chronic kidney disease. Adverse effect: ↑ risk of HTN in some individuals.
Calciferol (vitamin D)	PCT cells convert 25-OH vitamin D_3 to 1,25-$(OH)_2$ vitamin D_3 (calcitriol, active form). Increases calcium absorption in small bowel.	25-OH D_3 (calcidiol) ——[1α-hydroxylase]——→ 1,25-$(OH)_2$ D_3 (calcitriol); 1α-hydroxylase stimulated (⊕) by PTH
Prostaglandins	Paracrine secretion vasodilates afferent arterioles to ↑ RBF.	NSAIDs block renal-protective prostaglandin synthesis → constriction of afferent arteriole and ↓ GFR; this may result in acute kidney injury in low renal blood flow states.
Dopamine	Secreted by PT cells, promotes natriuresis. At low doses; dilates interlobular arteries, afferent arterioles, efferent arterioles → ↑ RBF, little or no change in GFR. At higher doses; acts as vasoconstrictor.	

Hormones acting on kidney

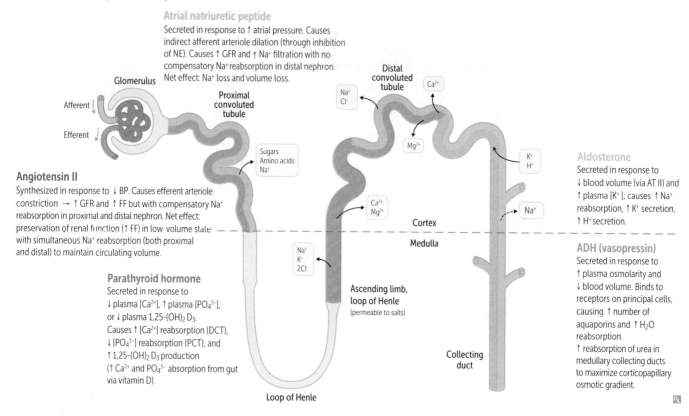

Atrial natriuretic peptide
Secreted in response to ↑ atrial pressure. Causes indirect afferent arteriole dilation (through inhibition of NE). Causes ↑ GFR and ↑ Na⁺ filtration with no compensatory Na⁺ reabsorption in distal nephron. Net effect: Na⁺ loss and volume loss.

Angiotensin II
Synthesized in response to ↓ BP. Causes efferent arteriole constriction → ↑ GFR and ↑ FF but with compensatory Na⁺ reabsorption in proximal and distal nephron. Net effect: preservation of renal function (↑ FF) in low volume state with simultaneous Na⁺ reabsorption (both proximal and distal) to maintain circulating volume.

Parathyroid hormone
Secreted in response to ↓ plasma [Ca²⁺], ↑ plasma [PO₄³⁻], or ↓ plasma 1,25-(OH)₂ D₃. Causes ↑ [Ca²⁺] reabsorption (DCT), ↓ [PO₄³⁻] reabsorption (PCT), and ↑ 1,25-(OH)₂ D₃ production (↑ Ca²⁺ and PO₄³⁻ absorption from gut via vitamin D).

Aldosterone
Secreted in response to ↓ blood volume (via AT II) and ↑ plasma [K⁺]; causes ↑ Na⁺ reabsorption, ↑ K⁺ secretion, ↑ H⁺ secretion.

ADH (vasopressin)
Secreted in response to ↑ plasma osmolarity and ↓ blood volume. Binds to receptors on principal cells, causing ↑ number of aquaporins and ↑ H₂O reabsorption. ↑ reabsorption of urea in medullary collecting ducts to maximize corticopapillary osmotic gradient.

Potassium shifts

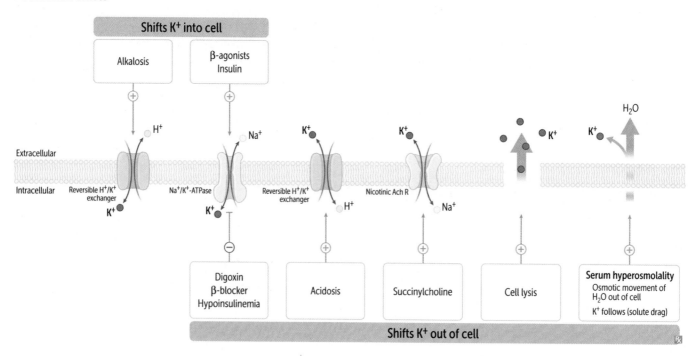

Electrolyte disturbances

ELECTROLYTE	LOW SERUM CONCENTRATION	HIGH SERUM CONCENTRATION
Sodium	Nausea, malaise, stupor, coma, seizures	Irritability, stupor, coma
Potassium	U waves and flattened T waves on ECG, arrhythmias, muscle cramps, spasm, weakness	Wide QRS and peaked T waves on ECG, arrhythmias, muscle weakness
Calcium	Tetany, seizures, QT prolongation, twitching (eg, Chvostek sign), spasm (eg, Trousseau sign)	**Stones** (renal), **bones** (pain), **groans** (abdominal pain), **thrones** (↑ urinary output frequency), **psychiatric overtones** (anxiety, altered mental status)
Magnesium	Tetany, torsades de pointes, hypokalemia, hypocalcemia (when $[Mg^{2+}] < 1.0$ mEq/L)	↓ DTRs, lethargy, bradycardia, hypotension, cardiac arrest, hypocalcemia
Phosphate	Bone loss, osteomalacia (adults), rickets (children)	Renal stones, metastatic calcifications, hypocalcemia

Acid-base physiology

Metabolic acid-base disorders cause HCO_3^- alterations. Respiratory acid-base disorders cause P_{CO_2} alterations.

	pH	P_{CO_2}	$[HCO_3^-]$	COMPENSATORY RESPONSE
Metabolic acidosis	↓	↓	↓	Hyperventilation (immediate)
Metabolic alkalosis	↑	↑	↑	Hypoventilation (immediate)
Respiratory acidosis	↓	↑	↑	↑ renal $[HCO_3^-]$ reabsorption (delayed)
Respiratory alkalosis	↑	↓	↓	↓ renal $[HCO_3^-]$ reabsorption (delayed)

Key: ↓ ↑ = compensatory response.

Henderson-Hasselbalch equation: $pH = 6.1 + \log \dfrac{[HCO_3^-]}{0.03 \, P_{CO_2}}$

Predicted respiratory compensation for a simple metabolic acidosis can be calculated using the Winters formula. If measured P_{CO_2} > predicted P_{CO_2} → concomitant respiratory acidosis; if measured P_{CO_2} < predicted P_{CO_2} → concomitant respiratory alkalosis:

$$P_{CO_2} = 1.5 \, [HCO_3^-] + 8 \pm 2$$

Acidosis and alkalosis

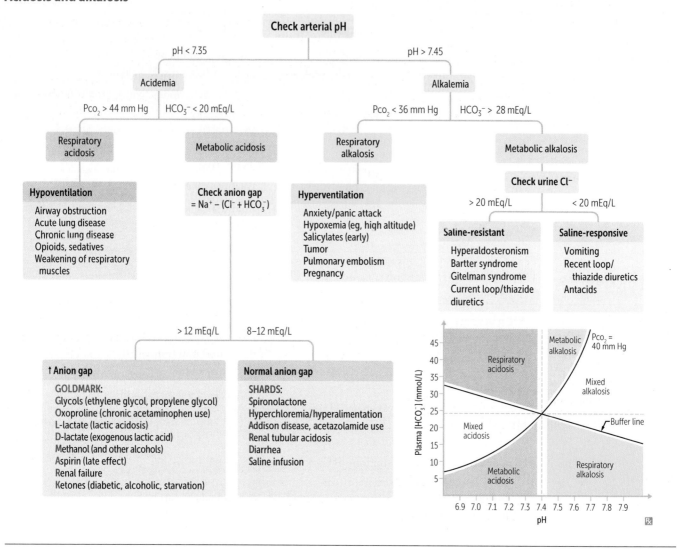

Check arterial pH

pH < 7.35 → **Acidemia**
- Pco_2 > 44 mm Hg → **Respiratory acidosis**
  - **Hypoventilation**
    - Airway obstruction
    - Acute lung disease
    - Chronic lung disease
    - Opioids, sedatives
    - Weakening of respiratory muscles
- HCO_3^- < 20 mEq/L → **Metabolic acidosis**
  - **Check anion gap** = $Na^+ - (Cl^- + HCO_3^-)$
    - > 12 mEq/L → **↑ Anion gap**
      - **GOLDMARK:**
        - Glycols (ethylene glycol, propylene glycol)
        - Oxoproline (chronic acetaminophen use)
        - L-lactate (lactic acidosis)
        - D-lactate (exogenous lactic acid)
        - Methanol (and other alcohols)
        - Aspirin (late effect)
        - Renal failure
        - Ketones (diabetic, alcoholic, starvation)
    - 8–12 mEq/L → **Normal anion gap**
      - **SHARDS:**
        - Spironolactone
        - Hyperchloremia/hyperalimentation
        - Addison disease, acetazolamide use
        - Renal tubular acidosis
        - Diarrhea
        - Saline infusion

pH > 7.45 → **Alkalemia**
- Pco_2 < 36 mm Hg → **Respiratory alkalosis**
  - **Hyperventilation**
    - Anxiety/panic attack
    - Hypoxemia (eg, high altitude)
    - Salicylates (early)
    - Tumor
    - Pulmonary embolism
    - Pregnancy
- HCO_3^- > 28 mEq/L → **Metabolic alkalosis**
  - **Check urine Cl^-**
    - > 20 mEq/L → **Saline-resistant**
      - Hyperaldosteronism
      - Bartter syndrome
      - Gitelman syndrome
      - Current loop/thiazide diuretics
    - < 20 mEq/L → **Saline-responsive**
      - Vomiting
      - Recent loop/thiazide diuretics
      - Antacids

Graph: Plasma $[HCO_3^-]$ (mmol/L) vs pH
- Respiratory acidosis
- Metabolic alkalosis
- Pco_2 = 40 mm Hg
- Mixed alkalosis
- Buffer line
- Mixed acidosis
- Metabolic acidosis
- Respiratory alkalosis

Renal tubular acidosis

	Distal renal tubular acidosis (RTA type 1)	Proximal renal tubular acidosis (RTA type 2)	Hyperkalemic tubular acidosis (RTA type 4)
DEFECT	Inability of α-intercalated cells to secrete $H(1)^+$ → no new HCO_3^- is generated → metabolic acidosis	Defect in PCT bi(2)carbonate (HCO_3^-) reabsorption → ↑ excretion of HCO_3^- in urine → metabolic acidosis. Urine can be acidified by α-intercalated cells in collecting duct, but not enough to overcome ↑ HCO_3^- excretion	Hypoaldosteronism or aldosterone resistance; hyperkalemia → ↓ NH_3 synthesis in PCT → ↓ NH_4^+ excretion
URINE pH	> 5.5	< 5.5 when plasma HCO_3^- below reduced resorption threshold. > 5.5 when filtered HCO_3^- exceeds resorptive threshold	Variable
SERUM K⁺	↓	↓	↑
CAUSES	Amphotericin B toxicity, analgesic nephropathy, congenital anomalies (obstruction) of urinary tract, autoimmune diseases (eg, SLE)	Fanconi syndrome, multiple myeloma, carbonic anhydrase inhibitors	↓ aldosterone production (eg, diabetic hyporeninism, ACE inhibitors, ARB, NSAIDs, heparin, cyclosporine, adrenal insufficiency) or aldosterone resistance (eg, K⁺-sparing diuretics, nephropathy due to obstruction, TMP-SMX)
ASSOCIATIONS	↑ risk for calcium phosphate kidney stones (due to ↑ urine pH and ↑ bone turnover related to buffering)	↑ risk for hypophosphatemic rickets (in Fanconi syndrome)	

▸ RENAL—PATHOLOGY

Casts in urine	Presence of casts indicates that hematuria/pyuria is of glomerular or renal tubular origin. Bladder cancer, kidney stones → hematuria, no casts. Acute cystitis → pyuria, no casts. All casts contain a matrix composed primarily of Tamm-Horsfall mucoprotein (uromodulin), secreted by renal tubular cells to prevent UTIs.
RBC casts A	Glomerulonephritis, hypertensive emergency.
WBC casts	Tubulointerstitial inflammation, acute pyelonephritis, transplant rejection.
Granular casts B	Acute tubular necrosis (ATN). Can be "muddy brown" in appearance.
Fatty casts ("oval fat bodies")	Nephrotic syndrome. Associated with "Maltese cross" sign C.
Waxy casts	End-stage renal disease/chronic kidney disease.
Hyaline casts D	Nonspecific, can be a normal finding with dehydration, exercise, or diuretic therapy.

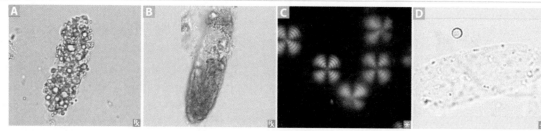

Nomenclature of glomerular disorders

TYPE	CHARACTERISTICS	EXAMPLE
Focal	< 50% of glomeruli are involved	Focal segmental glomerulosclerosis
Diffuse	> 50% of glomeruli are involved	Diffuse proliferative glomerulonephritis
Proliferative	Hypercellular glomeruli	Membranoproliferative glomerulonephritis
Membranous	Thickening of GBM	Membranous nephropathy
Primary glomerular disease	1° disease of the kidney specifically impacting the glomeruli	Minimal change disease
Secondary glomerular disease	Systemic disease or disease of another organ system that also impacts the glomeruli	SLE, diabetic nephropathy

Glomerular diseases

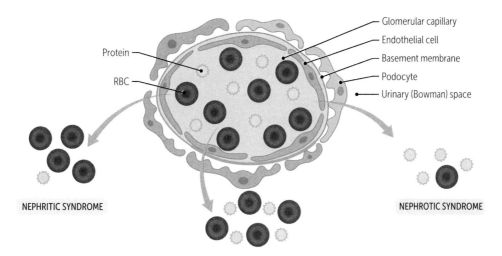

TYPE	ETIOLOGY	CLINICAL PRESENTATION	EXAMPLES
Nephritic syndrome	Glomerular inflammation → GBM damage → loss of RBCs into urine → dysmorphic RBCs, hematuria	Hematuria, RBC casts in urine ↓ GFR → oliguria, azotemia ↑ renin release, HTN Proteinuria often in the subnephrotic range (< 3.5 g/day) but in severe cases may be in nephrotic range	▪ Infection-associated glomerulonephritis ▪ Goodpasture syndrome ▪ IgA nephropathy (Berger disease) ▪ Alport syndrome ▪ Membranoproliferative glomerulonephritis
Nephrotic syndrome	Podocyte damage → impaired charge barrier → proteinuria	Massive proteinuria (> 3.5 g/day) with edema, hypoalbuminemia → ↑ hepatic lipogenesis → hypercholesterolemia Frothy urine with fatty casts Associated with hypercoagulable state (eg, renal vein thrombosis) due to antithrombin loss in urine and ↑ risk of infection (loss of IgGs in urine and soft tissue compromise by edema)	May be 1° (eg, direct podocyte damage) or 2° (podocyte damage from systemic process): ▪ Focal segmental glomerulosclerosis (1° or 2°) ▪ Minimal change disease (1° or 2°) ▪ Membranous nephropathy (1° or 2°) ▪ Amyloidosis (2°) ▪ Diabetic glomerulonephropathy (2°)
Nephritic-nephrotic syndrome	Severe GBM damage → loss of RBCs into urine + impaired charge barrier → hematuria + proteinuria	Nephrotic-range proteinuria (> 3.5 g/day) and concomitant features of nephritic syndrome	Can occur with any form of nephritic syndrome, but is most common with: ▪ Diffuse proliferative glomerulonephritis ▪ Membranoproliferative glomerulonephritis

Nephritic syndrome

	MECHANISM	LIGHT MICROSCOPY	IMMUNOFLUORESCENCE	ELECTRON MICROSCOPY
Infection-related glomerulonephritis	Type III hypersensitivity reaction with consumptive hypocomplementemia Children: seen ~2–4 weeks after group A streptococcal pharyngitis or skin infection Adults: *Staphylococcus* is additional causative agent	Enlarged and hypercellular glomeruli A	Granular ("starry sky") appearance ("lumpy-bumpy") B due to IgG, IgM, and C3 deposition along GBM and mesangium	Subepithelial IC humps
IgA nephropathy (Berger disease)	Occurs concurrently with respiratory or GI tract infections (IgA is secreted by mucosal linings) Renal pathology of IgA vasculitis	Mesangial proliferation	IgA-based IC deposits in mesangium	Mesangial IC deposition
Rapidly progressive (crescentic) glomerulonephritis	Poor prognosis Multiple causes: Type II HSR in Goodpasture syndrome	Crescent moon shape C; crescents consist of fibrin and plasma proteins (eg, C3b) with glomerular parietal cells, monocytes, macrophages	Linear IF due to antibodies to GBM and alveolar basement membrane: Goodpasture syndrome—hematuria/hemoptysis Negative IF/Pauci-immune (no IgC3 deposition): granulomatosis with polyangiitis—PR3-ANCA/c-ANCA, eosinophilic granulomatosis with polyangiitis, or Microscopic polyangiitis—MPO-ANCA/p-ANCA Granular IF—PSGN or DPGN	Goodpasture syndrome: breaks in GBM, necrosis and crescent formation with no deposits Pauci-immune: usually no deposits EM features depend on underlying cause
Diffuse proliferative glomerulonephritis	Often due to SLE (think "wire lupus"); DPGN and MPGN often present as nephritic and nephrotic syndromes concurrently	"Wire looping" of capillaries D	Granular	Subendothelial, sometimes subepithelial or intramembranous IgG-based ICs often with C3 deposition

Nephritic syndrome (continued)

Alport syndrome	Type IV collagen mutation → GBM alterations; mostly X-linked dominant. Eye problems (eg, retinopathy, anterior lenticonus), glomerulonephritis, sensorineural hearing loss (can't see, can't pee, can't hear a bee)	Irregular thinning and thickening and splitting of GBM	Initially negative; nonspecific staining (usually stays negative)	"Basket-weave" appearance due to irregular thickening and longitudinal splitting of GBM
Membrano-proliferative glomerulonephritis	Type I may be 2° to HBV or HCV infection; type II associated with C3 nephritic factor (IgG autoantibody that stabilizes C3 convertase → persistent complement activation → ↓ C3)	Mesangial ingrowth → GBM splitting → "tram-track" on H&E and PAS **E** stains	Granular	Type I—subendothelial IC deposits Type II—intramembranous deposits, also called dense deposit disease

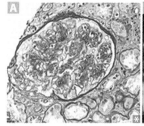 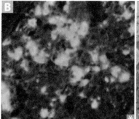 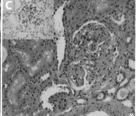 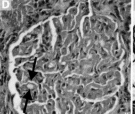 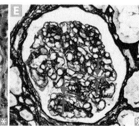

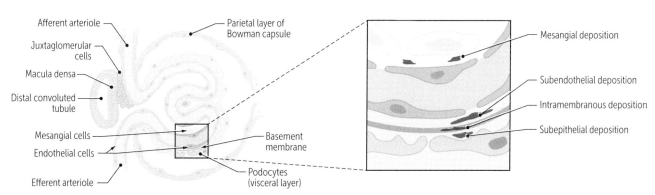

Afferent arteriole — Parietal layer of Bowman capsule
Juxtaglomerular cells
Macula densa
Distal convoluted tubule
Mesangial cells — Basement membrane
Endothelial cells
Efferent arteriole — Podocytes (visceral layer)

Mesangial deposition
Subendothelial deposition
Intramembranous deposition
Subepithelial deposition

Nephrotic syndrome

	MECHANISM	LIGHT MICROSCOPY	IMMUNOFLUORESCENCE	ELECTRON MICROSCOPY
Minimal change disease	Often 1° (idiopathic), triggered by recent infection, immunization, immune stimulus (4 Is); rarely 2° to lymphoma (eg, cytokine-mediated damage). More common in children.	Normal glomeruli (lipid may be seen in PT cells)	⊖	Effacement of podocyte foot processes 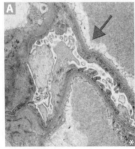
Focal segmental glomerulosclerosis	Can be 1° (idiopathic) or 2° (eg, HIV infection, sickle cell disease, obesity, or congenital malformations); may progress to CKD. More common in Black people.	Segmental sclerosis and hyalinosis 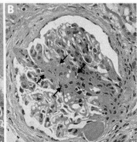	Often ⊖ but may be ⊕ for nonspecific focal deposits of IgM, C3, C1	Effacement of podocyte foot processes
Membranous nephropathy	Also called membranous glomerulo-nephritis. Can be 1° (eg, antibodies to phospholipase A₂ receptor) or 2° to drugs (eg, NSAIDs, penicillamine, gold), infections (eg, HBV, HCV, syphilis), SLE, or solid tumors. ↑ risk of thromboembolism (eg, DVT, renal vein thrombosis).	Diffuse capillary and GBM thickening 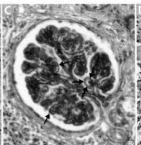	Granular due to immune complex (IC) deposition	"Spike and dome" appearance of subepithelial deposits
Amyloidosis	Kidney most commonly involved organ. Associated with chronic conditions that predispose to amyloid deposition (eg, AL amyloid, AA amyloid, prolonged dialysis).	Congo red stain shows apple-green birefringence (polarized light) due to amyloid deposition in the mesangium	AL amyloidosis: may be positive for lambda and kappa light chains AA amyloidosis: positive for AA protein	Mesangial expansion by amyloid fibrils
Diabetic glomerulo-nephropathy	Most common cause of ESRD in United States. Hyperglycemia → nonenzymatic glycation of tissue proteins → mesangial expansion → GBM thickening and ↑ permeability. Hyperfiltration (glomerular HTN and ↑ GFR) → glomerular hypertrophy and glomerular scarring (glomerulosclerosis) → further progression of nephropathy. Look for albuminuria with ↑ urine albumin-to-creatinine ratio. ACE inhibitors and ARBs are renoprotective.	Mesangial expansion, GBM thickening, eosinophilic nodular glomerulo-sclerosis (Kimmelstiel-Wilson lesions 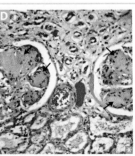)	Non-specific staining. Usually negative.	Prominent thickening of GBM with expanded mesangium, predominantly due to increased mesangial matrix, segmental podocyte effacement

(Image A) (Image B) (Image C) (Image D)

| Kidney stones | Can lead to severe complications such as hydronephrosis, pyelonephritis, and acute kidney injury. Obstructed stone presents with unilateral flank tenderness, colicky pain radiating to groin, hematuria. Treat and prevent by encouraging fluid intake. Radiolucent stones: I can't **c** (see) **u** (you) (**c**ystine and **u**ric acid). |

CONTENT	PRECIPITATES WITH	X-RAY FINDINGS	CT FINDINGS	URINE CRYSTAL	NOTES
Calcium	Calcium oxalate: hypocitraturia	Radiopaque	Hyperdense	Shaped like envelope 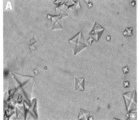 or dumbbell	Calcium stones most common (80%); calcium oxalate more common than calcium phosphate stones. Can result from ethylene glycol (antifreeze) ingestion, vitamin C overuse, hypocitraturia (usually associated with ↓ urine pH), malabsorption (eg, Crohn disease). Treatment: thiazides, citrate, low-sodium diet.
	Calcium phosphate: ↑ pH	Radiopaque	Hyperdense	Wedge-shaped prism	Treatment: low-sodium diet, thiazides.
Ammonium magnesium phosphate (struvite)	↑ pH	Radiopaque	Hyperdense	Coffin lid ("sarcophagus")	Account for 15% of stones. Caused by infection with urease ⊕ bugs (eg, *Proteus mirabilis*, *Staphylococcus saprophyticus*, *Klebsiella*) that hydrolyze urea to ammonia → urine alkalinization. Commonly form staghorn calculi 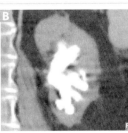. Treatment: eradication of underlying infection, surgical removal of stone.
Uric acid	↓ pH	Radiolucent	Visible	Rhomboid 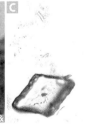 or rosettes	About 5% of all stones. Risk factors: arid climates, acidic pH. Strong association with hyperuricemia (eg, gout). Often seen in diseases with ↑ cell turnover (eg, leukemia). Treatment: alkalinization of urine, allopurinol.
Cystine	↓ pH	Faintly radiopaque	Moderately radiodense	Hexagonal	Hereditary (autosomal recessive) condition in which **C**ystine-reabsorbing PCT transporter loses function, causing cystinuria. Transporter defect also results in poor reabsorption of **O**rnithine, **L**ysine, **A**rginine (**COLA**). Cystine is poorly soluble, thus stones form in urine. Usually begins in childhood. Can form staghorn calculi. Sodium cyanide nitroprusside test ⊕. "**Six**tine" stones have **six** sides. Treatment: low sodium diet, alkalinization of urine, chelating agents (eg, tiopronin, penicillamine) if refractory.

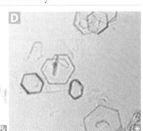

Hydronephrosis

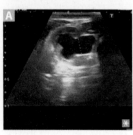

Distention/dilation of renal pelvis and/or calyces A. Mostly caused by urinary tract obstruction (eg, urinary tract stones, severe BPH, congenital obstructions, locally advanced cervical cancer, injury to ureter); other causes include retroperitoneal fibrosis, vesicoureteral reflux. Dilation occurs proximal to site of pathology. Serum creatinine becomes elevated if obstruction is bilateral or if patient has an obstructed solitary kidney. Leads to compression and possible atrophy of renal cortex and medulla.

Urinary incontinence　Mixed incontinence has features of both stress and urgency incontinence.

	Stress incontinence	Urgency incontinence	Overflow incontinence
MECHANISM	Outlet incompetence (urethral hypermobility or intrinsic sphincter deficiency) → leak with ↑ intra-abdominal pressure (eg, sneezing, lifting) ⊕ bladder stress test (directly observed leakage from urethra upon coughing or Valsalva maneuver)	Detrusor overactivity → leak with urge to void immediately	Incomplete emptying (detrusor underactivity or outlet obstruction) → leak with overfilling, ↑ postvoid residual on catheterization or ultrasound
ASSOCIATIONS	Obesity, pregnancy, vaginal delivery, prostate surgery	Bladder irritation from UTI, stones, tumors, pelvic radiation	Urinary retention, polyuria (eg, diabetes), bladder outlet obstruction (eg, BPH), spinal cord injury
TREATMENT	Pelvic floor muscle strengthening (Kegel) exercises, weight loss, pessaries	Pelvic floor physical therapy, bladder training (timed voiding, distraction or relaxation techniques), antimuscarinics (eg, oxybutynin for overactive bladder), mirabegron/vibegron	Catheterization, relieve obstruction (eg, α-blockers for BPH)

Acute cystitis	Inflammation of urinary bladder. Presents as suprapubic pain, dysuria, urinary frequency, urgency. Systemic signs (eg, high fever, chills) are usually absent.
	Risk factors include female sex (short urethra), sexual intercourse, indwelling catheter, diabetes mellitus, impaired bladder emptying.
	Causes:
	▪ *E coli* (most common)
	▪ *Staphylococcus saprophyticus*—seen in sexually active young women (*E coli* is still more common in this group)
	▪ *Klebsiella*
	▪ *Proteus mirabilis*—urine has ammonia scent
	▪ *Enterococcus* spp.
	Labs: ⊕ leukocyte esterase. ⊕ nitrites (indicates presence of Enterobacteriaceae). Sterile pyuria (pyuria with ⊖ urine cultures) could suggest urethritis by *Neisseria gonorrhoeae* or *Chlamydia trachomatis*.
	Treatment: antibiotics (eg, TMP-SMX, nitrofurantoin).

Pyelonephritis

Acute pyelonephritis 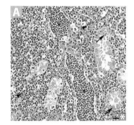	Neutrophils infiltrate renal interstitium 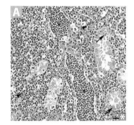. Affects cortex with relative sparing of glomeruli/vessels. Presents with fevers, flank pain (costovertebral angle tenderness), nausea/vomiting, chills.
	Causes include ascending UTI (*E coli* is most common), hematogenous spread to kidney. Presents with WBCs in urine +/− WBC casts. CT would show striated parenchymal enhancement.
	Risk factors include indwelling urinary catheter, urinary tract obstruction, vesicoureteral reflux, diabetes mellitus, pregnancy (progesterone-mediated ↓ in ureter tone and compression by gravid uterus).
	Complications include chronic pyelonephritis, renal papillary necrosis, perinephric abscess (with possible posterior spread to adjacent psoas muscle), urosepsis.
	Treatment: antibiotics.
Chronic pyelonephritis 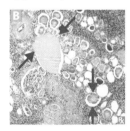	The result of recurrent or inadequately treated episodes of acute pyelonephritis. Typically requires predisposition to infection such as vesicoureteral reflux or chronically obstructing kidney stones.
	Coarse, asymmetric corticomedullary scarring, blunted calyces. Tubules can contain eosinophilic casts resembling thyroid tissue 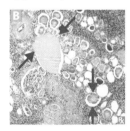 (thyroidization of kidney).

Acute kidney injury

	Prerenal azotemia	Intrinsic renal failure	Postrenal azotemia
ETIOLOGY	Hypovolemia ↓ cardiac output ↓ effective circulating volume (eg, HF, liver failure)	Tubules and interstitium: ■ Acute tubular necrosis (ischemia, nephrotoxins) ■ Acute interstitial nephritis Glomerulus: ■ Acute glomerulonephritis Vascular: ■ Vasculitis ■ Hypertensive emergency ■ TTP-HUS	Stones BPH Neoplasm Congenital anomalies
PATHOPHYSIOLOGY	↓ RBF → ↓ GFR → ↑ reabsorption of Na^+/H_2O and urea	In ATN, patchy necrosis → debris obstructing tubules and fluid backflow → ↓ GFR	Outflow obstruction (bilateral)
URINE OSMOLALITY (mOsm/kg)	>500	<350	Varies
URINE Na^+ (mEq/L)	<20	>40	Varies
FE_{Na}	<1%	>2%	Varies
SERUM BUN/Cr	>20	<15	Varies

Acute interstitial nephritis

Also called tubulointerstitial nephritis. Acute interstitial renal inflammation. Pyuria (classically eosinophils) and azotemia occurring after administration of drugs that act as haptens, inducing hypersensitivity (eg, diuretics, NSAIDs, penicillin derivatives, proton pump inhibitors, rifampin, quinolones, sulfonamides). Less commonly may be 2° to other processes such as systemic infections (eg, *Mycoplasma*) or systemic inflammatory disorders (eg, Sjögren syndrome, SLE, sarcoidosis).

Associated with fever, rash, pyuria, hematuria, and costovertebral angle tenderness, but can be asymptomatic.
Remember the causes of inflammation to your **DRAINS**:
■ **D**iuretics
■ **R**ifampin
■ **A**ntibiotics (penicillins and cephalosporins)
■ **P**roton pump **I**nhibitors
■ **N**SAIDs
■ **S**ulfa drugs

Acute tubular necrosis

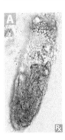

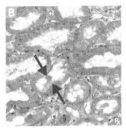

Most common cause of intrinsic acute kidney injury in hospitalized patients. Spontaneously resolves in many cases. Can be fatal, especially during initial oliguric phase. ↑ FE_{Na}.

Key finding: granular casts (often muddy brown in appearance) **A**.

3 stages:
1. Inciting event
2. Maintenance phase—oliguric; lasts 1–3 weeks; risk of hyperkalemia, metabolic acidosis, uremia
3. Recovery phase—polyuric; BUN and serum creatinine fall; risk of hypokalemia and renal wasting of other electrolytes and minerals

Can be caused by ischemic or nephrotoxic injury:
- Ischemic—2° to ↓ renal blood flow (eg, prerenal azotemia). Results in death of tubular cells that may slough into tubular lumen **B** (PT and thick ascending limb are highly susceptible to injury).
- Nephrotoxic—2° to injury resulting from toxic substances (eg, aminoglycosides, radiocontrast agents, lead, cisplatin, ethylene glycol, uric acid in tumor lysis syndrome), myoglobinuria (rhabdomyolysis), hemoglobinuria. PTs are particularly susceptible to injury.

Diffuse cortical necrosis

Acute generalized cortical infarction of both kidneys. Likely due to a combination of vasospasm and DIC.

Associated with obstetric catastrophes (eg, placental abruption), septic shock.

Renal papillary necrosis

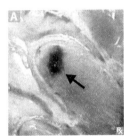

Sloughing of necrotic renal papillae **A** → gross hematuria. May be triggered by recent infection or immune stimulus.

Associated with:
- Sickle cell disease or trait
- Acute pyelonephritis
- Analgesics (eg, NSAIDs)
- Diabetes mellitus

SAAD papa with papillary necrosis.

Consequences of renal failure

Decline in renal filtration can lead to excess retained nitrogenous waste products and electrolyte disturbances.

Consequences (**MAD HUNGER**):
- Metabolic Acidosis
- Dyslipidemia (especially ↑ triglycerides)
- High potassium
- Uremia
- Na^+/H_2O retention (HF, pulmonary edema, hypertension)
- Growth retardation and developmental delay
- Erythropoietin deficiency (anemia)
- Renal osteodystrophy

2 forms of renal failure: acute (eg, ATN) and chronic (eg, hypertension, diabetes mellitus, congenital anomalies).

Incremental reductions in GFR define the stages of chronic kidney disease.

Normal phosphate levels are maintained during early stages of CKD due to ↑ levels of fibroblast growth factor 23 (FGF23), which promotes renal excretion of phosphate. "FGF23 fights f(ph)osphate."

Uremia—syndrome resulting from high serum urea. Can present with Pericarditis, Encephalopathy (seen with asterixis), Anorexia, Nausea (pronounce "Ure-PEAN" [European]).

Renal osteodystrophy	Hypocalcemia, hyperphosphatemia, and failure of vitamin D hydroxylation associated with chronic kidney disease → 2° hyperparathyroidism → 3° hyperparathyroidism (if 2° poorly managed). High serum phosphate can bind with Ca^{2+} → tissue deposits → ↓ serum Ca^{2+}. ↓ $1,25\text{-}(OH)_2D_3$ → ↓ intestinal Ca^{2+} absorption. Causes subperiosteal thinning of bones.

Renal cyst disorders

Autosomal dominant polycystic kidney disease 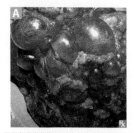	Numerous cysts in cortex and medulla A causing bilateral enlarged kidneys ultimately destroy kidney parenchyma. Presents with combinations of flank pain, hematuria, hypertension, urinary infection; progressive renal failure in ~ 50% of individuals. Mutation in genes encoding polycystin protein: PKD1 (85% of cases, chromosome 16) or PKD2 (15% of cases, chromosome 4). Complications include chronic kidney disease and hypertension (caused by ↑ renin production). Associated with berry aneurysms, mitral valve prolapse, benign hepatic cysts, diverticulosis. Treatment: If hypertension or proteinuria develops, treat with ACE inhibitors or ARBs.
Autosomal recessive polycystic kidney disease 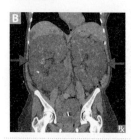	Mutation in *PKHD1* encoding fibrocystin. Cystic dilation of collecting ducts B. Often presents in infancy, and may be seen on prenatal ultrasound. Associated with congenital hepatic fibrosis. Significant oliguric renal failure in utero can lead to Potter sequence. Concerns beyond neonatal period include systemic hypertension, progressive renal insufficiency, and portal hypertension from congenital hepatic fibrosis.
Autosomal dominant tubulointerstitial kidney disease	Also called medullary cystic kidney disease. Causes tubulointerstitial fibrosis and progressive renal insufficiency with inability to concentrate urine. Medullary cysts usually not visualized; smaller kidneys on ultrasound. Poor prognosis.
Simple vs complex renal cysts	Simple cysts are filled with ultrafiltrate (anechoic on ultrasound). Very common and account for majority of all renal masses. Found incidentally and typically asymptomatic. Complex cysts, including those that are septated, enhanced, or have solid components on imaging require follow-up or removal due to possibility of renal cell carcinoma.

Renovascular disease

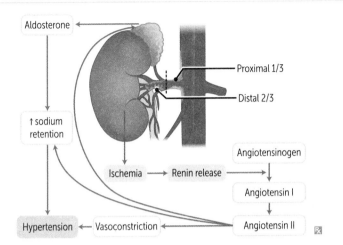

Unilateral or bilateral renal artery stenosis (RAS) → ↓ renal perfusion → ↑ renin → ↑ angiotensin → HTN. Most common cause of 2° HTN in adults.

Main causes of RAS:
- Atherosclerotic plaques: proximal 1/3 of renal artery, usually in older males, smokers.
- Fibromuscular dysplasia: distal 2/3 of renal artery or segmental branches, usually young or middle-aged females

For unilateral RAS, affected kidney can atrophy → asymmetric kidney size. Renal venous sampling will show ↑ renin in affected kidney, ↓ renin in unaffected kidney.

For bilateral RAS, patients can have a sudden rise in creatinine after starting an ACE inhibitor, ARB, or renin inhibitor, due to their interference on RAAS-mediated renal perfusion.

Can present with severe/refractory HTN, flash pulmonary edema, epigastric/flank bruit. Patients with RAS may also have stenosis in other large vessels.

Renal cell carcinoma

Polygonal clear cells 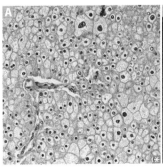 filled with accumulated lipids and carbohydrate. Often golden-yellow 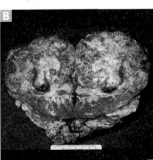 on gross pathology, due to ↑ lipid content.

Originates from PCT → invades renal vein (may develop varicocele if left sided) → IVC → hematogenous spread → metastasis to lung, bone, and liver.

Manifests with flank pain, palpable mass, hematuria (classic triad) as well as anemia, 2° polycythemia (less common), fever, weight loss.

Treatment: surgery/ablation for localized disease. Immunotherapy (eg, ipilimumab) or targeted therapy for metastatic disease, rarely curative. Resistant to radiation and chemotherapy.

Most common 1° renal malignancy 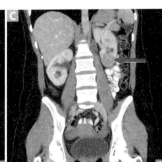.

Most common in males 50–70 years old, ↑ incidence with tobacco smoking and obesity.

Associated with paraneoplastic syndromes, eg, **P**THrP, **E**ctopic EPO, **A**CTH, **R**enin ("**PEAR**"-aneoplastic).

Clear cell (most common subtype) associated with gene deletion on chromosome 3 (sporadic, or inherited as von Hippel-Lindau syndrome).

RCC = **3** letters = chromosome **3** = associated with **VHL** (also 3 letters).

Renal oncocytoma

Benign epithelial cell tumor 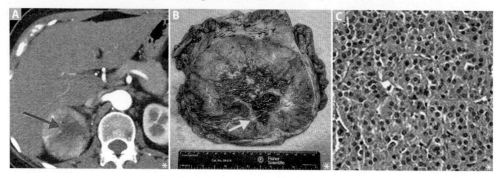 arising from collecting ducts (red arrow in B points to well circumscribed mass; yellow arrow points to central scar). Large eosinophilic cells with abundant mitochondria without perinuclear clearing C (vs chromophobe renal cell carcinoma). Presents with painless hematuria, flank pain, abdominal mass.

Often resected to exclude malignancy (eg, renal cell carcinoma).

Nephroblastoma

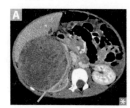

Also called Wilms tumor. Most common renal malignancy of early childhood (ages 2–4). Contains embryonic glomerular structures. Most often present with large, palpable, unilateral flank mass A and/or hematuria and possible HTN.

Can be associated with loss-of-function mutations of tumor suppressor genes *WT1* or *WT2* on chromosome 11 (W11ms tumor).

May be a part of several syndromes:

- **WAGR** complex—**W**ilms tumor, **A**niridia (absence of iris), **G**enitourinary malformations, **R**ange of developmental delays (*WT1* deletion)
- **D**enys-**D**rash syndrome—Wilms tumor, **D**iffuse mesangial sclerosis (early-onset nephrotic syndrome), **D**ysgenesis of gonads (male pseudohermaphroditism), *WT1* mutation
- Beck**with**-**W**iedemann syndrome—**W**ilms tumor, **i**ncrease in organ size (organomegaly), tongue enlargement (macroglossia), **h**emihyperplasia (imprinting defect causing genetic overexpression, associated with *WT2* mutation), omphalocele

Urothelial carcinoma of the bladder

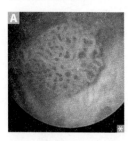

Also called transitional cell carcinoma. Most common tumor of urinary tract system (can occur in renal calyces, renal pelvis, ureters, and bladder) A B. Can be suggested by Painless hematuria (no casts).

Associated with problems in your Pee SAC: Tobacco **S**moking, **A**romatic amines (found in dyes), **C**yclophosphamide.

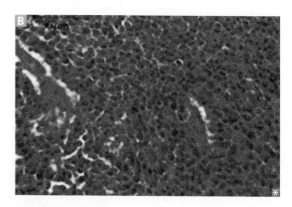

Squamous cell carcinoma of the bladder

Chronic irritation of urinary bladder → squamous metaplasia → dysplasia and squamous cell carcinoma.

Risk factors include 4 S's: *Schistosoma haematobium* infection (Middle East), chronic cystitis ("systitis"), smoking, chronic nephrolithiasis (stones). Presents with painless hematuria (no casts).

▶ **RENAL—PHARMACOLOGY**

Diuretics: site of action

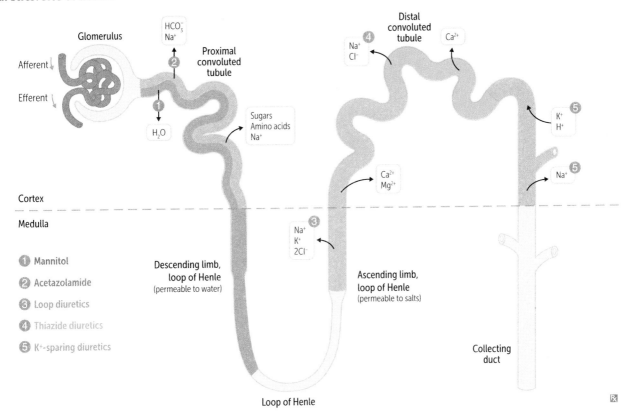

1 Mannitol
2 Acetazolamide
3 Loop diuretics
4 Thiazide diuretics
5 K⁺-sparing diuretics

Diuretics: effects on electrolyte excretion

	Na^+	HCO_3^-	K^+	Cl^-	Ca^{2+}	Mg^{2+}	H^+
Carbonic anhydrase inhibitors	↑	↑↑	↑↑	—/↑	—	—	↓
Loop diuretics	↑↑	↓	↑↑	↑↑	↑↑	↑↑	↑
Thiazide diuretics	↑	↑	↑↑	↑	↓↓	—/↑	↑
K⁺-sparing diuretics	↑	—	↓	↑	↓/—	↓/—	↓

Blood pH	↓ (**acidemia**): carbonic anhydrase inhibitors: ↓ HCO_3^- reabsorption. K⁺ sparing: aldosterone blockade prevents K⁺ secretion and H⁺ secretion. Additionally, hyperkalemia leads to K⁺ entering all cells (via H⁺/K⁺ exchanger) in exchange for H⁺ exiting cells.
	↑ (**alkalemia**): loop diuretics and thiazides cause alkalemia through several mechanisms:
	▪ Volume contraction → ↑ AT II → ↑ Na⁺/H⁺ exchange in PCT → ↑ HCO_3^- reabsorption ("contraction alkalosis")
	▪ K⁺ loss leads to K⁺ exiting all cells (via H⁺/K⁺ exchanger) in exchange for H⁺ entering cells
	▪ In low K⁺ state, H⁺ (rather than K⁺) is exchanged for Na⁺ in cortical collecting tubule → alkalosis and "paradoxical aciduria"

Mannitol

MECHANISM	Osmotic diuretic. ↑ serum osmolality → fluid shift from interstitium to intravascular space → ↑ urine flow, ↓ intracranial/intraocular pressure.
CLINICAL USE	Drug overdose, elevated intracranial/intraocular pressure, augmenting diuresis.
ADVERSE EFFECTS	Dehydration, hypo- or hypernatremia, pulmonary edema. Contraindicated in anuria, HF.

Acetazolamide

MECHANISM	Carbonic anhydrase inhibitor. Causes self-limited $NaHCO_3$ diuresis and ↓ total body HCO_3^- stores. Alkalinizes urine.	
CLINICAL USE	Glaucoma, metabolic alkalosis, altitude sickness (by offsetting respiratory alkalosis), idiopathic intracranial hypertension (pseudotumor cerebri).	
ADVERSE EFFECTS	Proximal renal tubular acidosis (type 2 RTA), paresthesias, NH_3 toxicity, sulfa allergy, hypokalemia. Promotes calcium phosphate stones (insoluble at high urine pH).	"Acid"azolamide causes acidosis.

Loop diuretics

Furosemide, bumetanide, torsemide

MECHANISM	Sulfonamide loop diuretics. Inhibit cotransport system ($Na^+/K^+/2Cl^-$) of thick ascending limb of loop of Henle. Abolish hypertonicity of medulla, preventing concentration of urine. Associated with ↑ PGE (vasodilatory effect on afferent arteriole); inhibited by NSAIDs. ↑ Ca^{2+} excretion. Loops lose Ca^{2+}.	
CLINICAL USE	Edematous states (HF, cirrhosis, nephrotic syndrome, pulmonary edema), hypertension, hypercalcemia.	
ADVERSE EFFECTS	Ototoxicity, Hypokalemia, Hypomagnesemia, Dehydration, Allergy (sulfa), metabolic Alkalosis, Nephritis (interstitial), Gout.	OHH DAANG!

Ethacrynic acid

MECHANISM	Nonsulfonamide inhibitor of cotransport system ($Na^+/K^+/2Cl^-$) of thick ascending limb of **loop** of Henle.	
CLINICAL USE	Diuresis in patients allergic to sulfa drugs.	
ADVERSE EFFECTS	Similar to furosemide, but more ototoxic.	**Loop** earrings hurt your **ears.**

Thiazide diuretics	Hydrochlorothiazide, chlorthalidone, metolazone.	
MECHANISM	Inhibit NaCl reabsorption in early DCT → ↓ diluting capacity of nephron. ↓ Ca^{2+} excretion.	
CLINICAL USE	Hypertension, HF, idiopathic hypercalciuria, nephrogenic diabetes insipidus, osteoporosis. Potentiates loop diuretics in refractory volume overload.	Hypergluc.
ADVERSE EFFECTS	Hypokalemic metabolic alkalosis, hyponatremia, hyperglycemia, hyperlipidemia, hyperuricemia, hypercalcemia. Sulfa allergy.	

Potassium-sparing diuretics	Spironolactone, Eplerenone, Amiloride, Triamterene.	Keep your SEAT.
MECHANISM	Spironolactone and eplerenone are competitive aldosterone receptor antagonists in cortical collecting tubule. Triamterene and amiloride block Na^+ channels at the same part of the tubule.	
CLINICAL USE	Hyperaldosteronism, HF, hepatic ascites (spironolactone), nephrogenic DI (amiloride), antiandrogen (spironolactone).	
ADVERSE EFFECTS	Hyperkalemia (can lead to arrhythmias), endocrine effects with spironolactone (eg, gynecomastia, antiandrogen effects), metabolic acidosis.	

Angiotensin-converting enzyme inhibitors	Captopril, enalapril, lisinopril, ramipril.	
MECHANISM	Inhibit ACE → ↓ AT II → ↓ GFR by preventing constriction of efferent arterioles. ↑ renin due to loss of negative feedback. Inhibition of ACE also prevents inactivation of bradykinin, a potent vasodilator.	
CLINICAL USE	Hypertension, HF (↓ mortality), proteinuria, diabetic nephropathy. Prevent unfavorable heart remodeling as a result of chronic hypertension.	In chronic kidney disease (eg, diabetic nephropathy), ↓ intraglomerular pressure, slowing GBM thickening.
ADVERSE EFFECTS	Cough (dry, nonproductive), Angioedema (both due to ↑ bradykinin; contraindicated in C1 esterase inhibitor deficiency), Teratogen (fetal renal malformations), ↑ Creatinine (↓ GFR), Hyperkalemia, and Hypotension. Used with caution in bilateral renal artery stenosis because ACE inhibitors will further ↓ GFR → renal failure.	Captopril's **CATCHH**.

Angiotensin II receptor blockers	Losartan, candesartan, valsartan.
MECHANISM	Selectively block binding of angiotensin II to AT_1 receptor. Effects similar to ACE inhibitors, but ARBs do not increase bradykinin.
CLINICAL USE	Hypertension, HF, proteinuria, or chronic kidney disease (eg, diabetic nephropathy) with intolerance to ACE inhibitors (eg, cough, angioedema).
ADVERSE EFFECTS	Hyperkalemia, ↓ GFR, hypotension; teratogen.

Aliskiren	
MECHANISM	Direct renin inhibitor, blocks conversion of angiotensinogen to angiotensin I. Ali**skiren kills renin**.
CLINICAL USE	Hypertension.
ADVERSE EFFECTS	Hyperkalemia, ↓ GFR, hypotension, angioedema. Relatively contraindicated in patients already taking ACE inhibitors or ARBs and contraindicated in pregnancy.

Reproductive

"Life is always a rich and steady time when you are waiting for something to happen or to hatch."

—E.B. White, *Charlotte's Web*

"Love is only a dirty trick played on us to achieve continuation of the species."

—W. Somerset Maugham

"I liked that in obstetrics you end up with twice the number of patients you started with."

—Adam Kay

"Life is a sexually transmitted disease and the mortality rate is one hundred percent."

—R.D. Laing

Organizing the reproductive system by key concepts such as embryology, endocrinology, pregnancy, and oncology can help with understanding this complex topic. Study the endocrine and reproductive chapters together, because mastery of the hypothalamic-pituitary-gonadal axis is key to answering questions on ovulation, menstruation, disorders of sexual development, contraception, and many pathologies.

Embryology is a nuanced subject that spans multiple organ systems. Approach it from a clinical perspective. For instance, make the connection between the presentation of DiGeorge syndrome and the 3rd/4th pharyngeal pouch, and between the Müllerian/Wolffian systems and disorders of sexual development.

As for oncology, don't worry about remembering screening or treatment guidelines. It is more important to recognize the clinical presentation (eg, signs and symptoms) of reproductive cancers and their associated labs, histopathology, and risk factors. In addition, some of the testicular and ovarian cancers have distinct patterns of hCG, AFP, LH, or FSH derangements that serve as helpful clues in exam questions.

▶ REPRODUCTIVE—EMBRYOLOGY

Early embryonic development

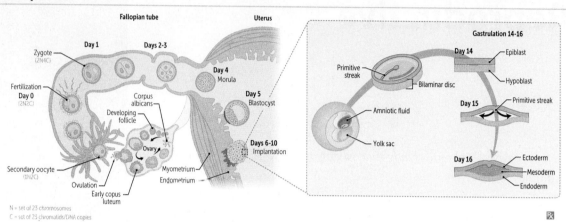

Week 1	hCG secretion begins around the time of blastocyst implantation. Blastocyst "sticks" on day six.
Week 2	Formation of bilaminar embryonic disc; two layers = epiblast, hypoblast.
Week 3	Formation of trilaminar embryonic disc via gastrulation (epiblast cell invagination through primitive streak); three layers = endoderm, mesoderm, ectoderm. Notochord arises from midline mesoderm and induces overlying ectoderm (via SHH) to become neural plate, which gives rise to neural tube via neurulation.
Week 4	Heart begins to beat (four chambers). Cardiac activity visible by transvaginal ultrasound. Upper and lower limb buds begin to form (four limbs).
Week 8	Genitalia have male/female characteristics (pronounce "geneightalia").

Embryologic derivatives

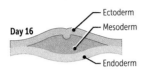 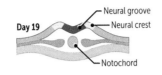 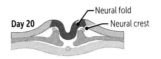 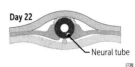

Ectoderm		External/outer layer
Surface ectoderm	Epidermis; adenohypophysis (from Rathke pouch); lens of eye; epithelial linings of oral cavity, sensory organs of ear, and olfactory epithelium; anal canal below the pectinate line; parotid, sweat, mammary glands.	**Craniopharyngioma**—benign Rathke pouch tumor with cholesterol crystals, calcifications.
Neural tube	Brain (neurohypophysis, CNS neurons, oligodendrocytes, astrocytes, ependymal cells, pineal gland), retina, spinal cord.	Neuroectoderm—think CNS.
Neural crest	Enterochromaffin cells, Melanocytes, Odontoblasts, PNS ganglia (cranial, dorsal root, autonomic), Adrenal medulla, Schwann cells, Spiral membrane (aorticopulmonary septum), Endocardial cushions (also derived partially from mesoderm), Skull bones.	**EMO PASSES** Neural crest—think PNS and non-neural structures nearby.
Mesoderm	Muscle, bone, connective tissue, serous linings of body cavities (eg, peritoneum, pericardium, pleura), spleen (develops within foregut mesentery), cardiovascular structures, lymphatics, blood, wall of gut tube, proximal vagina, kidneys, adrenal cortex, dermis, testes, ovaries, microglia, tracheal cartilage. Notochord induces ectoderm to form neuroectoderm (neural plate); its only postnatal derivative is the nucleus pulposus of the intervertebral disc.	Middle/"meat" layer. Mesodermal defects = **VACTERL** association: Vertebral defects Anal atresia Cardiac defects Tracheo-Esophageal fistula Renal defects Limb defects (bone and muscle)
Endoderm	Gut tube epithelium (including anal canal above the pectinate line), most of urethra and distal vagina (derived from urogenital sinus), luminal epithelial derivatives (eg, lungs, liver, gallbladder, pancreas, eustachian tube, thymus, parathyroid, thyroid follicular and parafollicular [C] cells).	"Enternal" layer.

Teratogens   Most susceptible during organogenesis in embryonic period (before week 8 of development). Before implantation, "all-or-none" effect. After week 8 (fetal period), growth and function affected.

TERATOGEN	EFFECT ON FETUS
Medications	
ACE inhibitors	Renal failure, oligohydramnios, hypocalvaria.
Alkylating agents	Multiple anomalies (eg, ear/facial abnormalities, absence of digits).
Aminoglycosides	Ototoxicity. "**A mean guy** hit the baby in the **ear**."
Antiepileptic drugs	Neural tube defects, cardiac defects, cleft palate, skeletal abnormalities (eg, phalanx/nail hypoplasia, facial dysmorphism). Most commonly due to valproate, carbamazepine, phenytoin, phenobarbital; high-dose folate supplementation recommended.
Diethylstilbestrol	Vaginal clear cell adenocarcinoma, congenital Müllerian anomalies.
Fluoroquinolones	Cartilage damage.
Folate antagonists	Neural tube defects. Most commonly due to trimethoprim, methotrexate.
Isotretinoin	Craniofacial (eg, microtia, dysmorphism), CNS, cardiac, and thymic defects. Contraception mandatory. Pronounce "iso**teratin**oin" for its **terato**genicity.
Lithium	Ebstein anomaly.
Methimazole	Aplasia cutis congenita (congenital absence of skin, typically on scalp).
Tetracyclines	Discolored **teeth**, inhibited bone growth. Pronounce "**teeth**racyclines."
Thalidomide	**Limb** defects (eg, phocomelia—flipperlike limbs). Pronounce "tha**limb**domide."
Warfarin	**Bone** and cartilage deformities (stippled epiphyses, nasal and limb hypoplasia), **optic** nerve atrophy, cerebral hemorrhage. Use heparin during pregnancy (does not cross placenta). In **war**, you need strong **bones** to march and **optics** to see the enemy.
Substance use	
Alcohol	Fetal alcohol syndrome.
Cocaine	Preterm birth, low birth weight, fetal growth restriction (FGR). Cocaine → vasoconstriction.
Tobacco smoking	Preterm birth, low birth weight (leading cause in resource-rich countries), FGR, sudden infant death syndrome (SIDS), ADHD. Nicotine → vasoconstriction, CO → impaired O_2 delivery.
Other	
Iodine lack or excess	Congenital hypothyroidism.
Maternal diabetes	Caudal regression syndrome, cardiac defects (eg, transposition of great arteries, VSD), neural tube defects, macrosomia, neonatal hypoglycemia (due to islet cell hyperplasia), polycythemia, respiratory distress syndrome.
Maternal PKU	Fetal growth restriction, microcephaly, intellectual disability, congenital heart defects.
Methylmercury	Neurotoxicity. ↑ concentration in top-predator fish (eg, shark, swordfish, king mackerel, tilefish).
X-rays	Microcephaly, intellectual disability. Effects minimized by use of lead shielding.

Types of errors in morphogenesis

Agenesis	Absent organ due to absent primordial tissue.
Aplasia	Absent organ despite presence of primordial tissue.
Hypoplasia	Incomplete organ development; primordial tissue present.
Disruption	2° breakdown of tissue with normal developmental potential (eg, amniotic band syndrome).
Deformation	Extrinsic mechanical distortion (eg, congenital torticollis); occurs during fetal period.
Malformation	Intrinsic developmental defect (eg, cleft lip/palate); occurs during embryonic period.
Sequence	Abnormalities result from a single 1° embryologic event (eg, oligohydramnios → Potter sequence).
Field defect	Disturbance of tissues that develop in a contiguous physical space (eg, holoprosencephaly).

Fetal alcohol syndrome

One of the leading preventable causes of intellectual disability in the US. 2° to maternal alcohol use during pregnancy. Newborns may present with developmental delay, microcephaly, facial abnormalities (eg, smooth philtrum, thin vermillion border, small palpebral fissures, flat nasal bridge), limb dislocation, heart defects. Holoprosencephaly may occur in more severe presentations. One mechanism is due to impaired migration of neuronal and glial cells.

Treatment: supportive care.

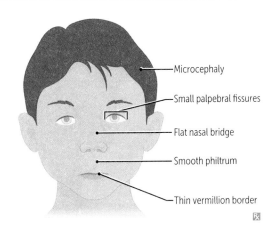

— Microcephaly
— Small palpebral fissures
— Flat nasal bridge
— Smooth philtrum
— Thin vermillion border

Neonatal abstinence syndrome

Complex disorder involving CNS, ANS, and GI systems. 2° to maternal substance use (most commonly opioids) during pregnancy. Newborns may present with uncoordinated sucking reflexes, irritability, high-pitched crying, tremors, tachypnea, sneezing, diarrhea, and possibly seizures.

Treatment (for opioid use): methadone, morphine, buprenorphine.

Universal screening for substance use is recommended in all pregnant patients.

Placenta	1° site of nutrient and gas exchange between mother and fetus.
Fetal component	
Cytotrophoblast	Inner layer of chorionic villi; **c**reates **c**ells.
Syncytiotrophoblast	Outer layer of chorionic villi; **syn**thesizes and secretes hormones, eg, hCG (structurally similar to LH; stimulates corpus luteum to secrete progesterone during first trimester). Lacks MHC I expression → ↓ chance of attack by maternal immune system.
Maternal component	
Decidua basalis	Derived from endometrium. Maternal blood in lacunae.

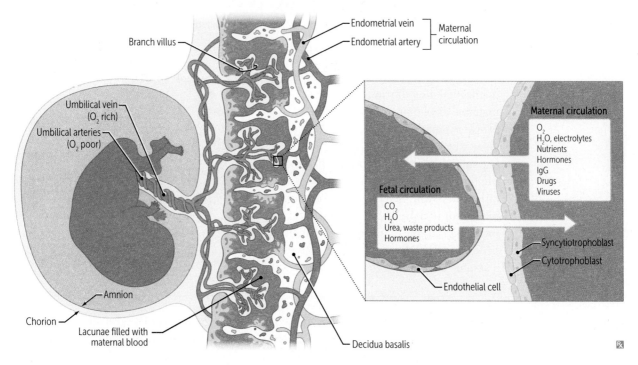

Amniotic fluid

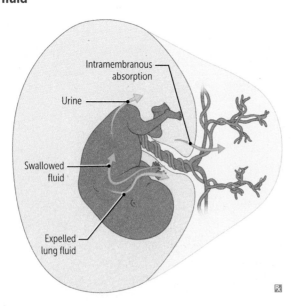

Derived from fetal urine (mainly) and fetal lung liquid.

Cleared by fetal swallowing (mainly) and intramembranous absorption.

Polyhydramnios—too much amniotic fluid. May be idiopathic or associated with fetal malformations (eg, esophageal/duodenal atresia, anencephaly; both result in inability to swallow amniotic fluid), maternal diabetes, fetal anemia, multifetal gestation.

Oligohydramnios—too little amniotic fluid. Associated with placental insufficiency, bilateral renal agenesis, posterior urethral valves (in males); these result in inability to excrete urine. Profound oligohydramnios can cause Potter sequence.

Twinning

Dizygotic ("fraternal") twins arise from 2 eggs that are separately fertilized by 2 different sperm (always 2 zygotes) and will have 2 separate amniotic sacs and 2 separate placentas (chorions).

Monozygotic ("identical") twins arise from 1 fertilized egg (1 egg + 1 sperm) that splits in early pregnancy. The timing of splitting determines chorionicity (number of chorions) and amnionicity (number of amnions) (take **separate** cars or **share** a **CAB**):

- Splitting 0–4 days: **separate** chorion and amnion (di-di)
- Splitting 4–8 days: **shared** Chorion (mo-di)
- Splitting 8–12 days: **shared** chorion and Amnion (mo-mo)
- Splitting 13+ days: **shared** chorion, amnion, and Body (mo-mo; conjoined)

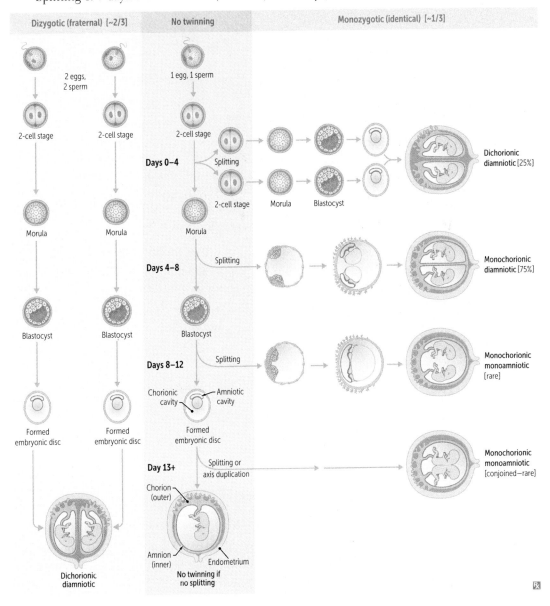

Twin-twin transfusion syndrome

Occurs in monochorionic twin gestations. Unbalanced arteriovenous anastomoses between twins in shared placenta → net blood flow from one twin to the other.

Donor twin → hypovolemia and oligohydramnios ("stuck twin" appearance).

Recipient twin → hypervolemia and polyhydramnios.

Umbilical cord

Two umbilical arteries return deoxygenated blood from fetal internal iliac arteries to placenta.

One umbilical vein supplies oxygenated blood from placenta to fetus; drains into IVC via liver or via ductus venosus.

Single umbilical artery (2-vessel cord) is associated with congenital and chromosomal anomalies.

Umbilical arteries and vein are derived from allantois.

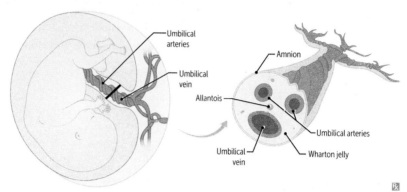

Urachus	Allantois forms from yolk sac and extends into cloaca. Intra-abdominal remnant of allantois is called the urachus, a duct between fetal bladder and umbilicus. Failure of urachus to involute can lead to anomalies that may increase risk of infection and/or malignancy (eg, adenocarcinoma) if not treated. Obliterated urachus is represented by the median umbilical ligament after birth, which is covered by median umbilical fold of the peritoneum.
Patent urachus	Total failure of urachus to obliterate → urine discharge from umbilicus.
Urachal cyst	Partial failure of urachus to obliterate; fluid-filled cavity lined with uroepithelium, between umbilicus and bladder. Cyst can become infected and present as painful mass below umbilicus.
Vesicourachal diverticulum	Slight failure of urachus to obliterate → outpouching of bladder.

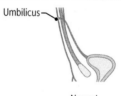   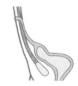

Normal   Patent urachus   Urachal cyst   Vesicourachal diverticulum

Vitelline duct	Also called omphalomesenteric duct. Connects yolk sac to midgut lumen. Obliterates during week 7 of development.
Patent vitelline duct	Total failure of vitelline duct to obliterate → meconium discharge from umbilicus.
Vitelline duct cyst	Partial failure of vitelline duct to obliterate. ↑ risk for volvulus.
Meckel diverticulum	Slight failure of vitelline duct to obliterate → outpouching of ileum (true diverticulum, arrow in A). Usually asymptomatic. May have heterotopic gastric and/or pancreatic tissue → melena, hematochezia, abdominal pain.

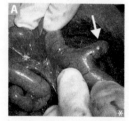

 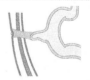

Normal   Patent vitelline duct   Vitelline duct cyst   Meckel diverticulum

Pharyngeal apparatus	Composed of pharyngeal (branchial) clefts, arches, pouches. Pharyngeal clefts—derived from ectoderm. Also called pharyngeal grooves. Pharyngeal arches—derived from mesoderm (muscles, arteries) and neural crest (bones, cartilage). Pharyngeal pouches—derived from endoderm.	**CAP** covers outside to inside: **C**lefts = ectoderm **A**rches = mesoderm + neural crest **P**ouches = endoderm 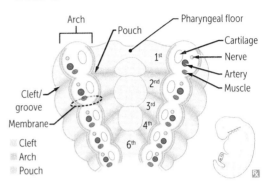

Pharyngeal cleft derivatives	1st cleft develops into external auditory meatus. 2nd through 4th clefts form temporary cervical sinuses, which are obliterated by proliferation of 2nd arch mesenchyme. **Pharyngeal cleft cyst**—persistent cervical sinus; presents as lateral neck mass anterior to sternocleidomastoid muscle that does not move with swallowing (vs thyroglossal duct cyst).

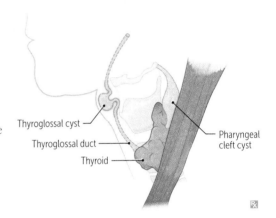

Pharyngeal pouch derivatives

Ear, tonsils, bottom-to-top: 1 (ear), 2 (tonsils), 3 dorsal (bottom = inferior parathyroids), 3 ventral (to = thymus), 4 (top = superior parathyroids).

POUCH	DERIVATIVES	NOTES
1st pharyngeal pouch	Middle ear cavity, eustachian tube, mastoid air cells	1st pouch contributes to endoderm-lined structures of ear
2nd pharyngeal pouch	Epithelial lining of palatine tonsil	
3rd pharyngeal pouch	Dorsal wings → **inferior** parathyroids Ventral wings → thymus	Third pouch contributes to thymus and both inferior parathyroids Structures from 3rd pouch end up **below** those from 4th pouch
4th pharyngeal pouch	Dorsal wings → **superior** parathyroids Ventral wings → ultimopharyngeal body → parafollicular (C) cells of thyroid	4th pharyngeal pouch forms para"4"llicular cells Developmental anomalies in 3rd and 4th pharyngeal pouch are present in DiGeorge syndrome

Pharyngeal arch derivatives	Sensory and motor nerves are not pharyngeal arch derivatives. They grow into the arches and are derived from neural crest (sensory) and neuroectoderm (motor). Arches 3 and 4 form posterior 1/3 of tongue. Arch 5 makes no major developmental contributions.

When at the restaurant of the golden **arches**, children tend to first **chew** (1), then **smile** (2), then **swallow stylishly** (3) or **simply swallow** (4), and then **speak** (6).

ARCH	NERVES	MUSCLES	CARTILAGE
1st pharyngeal arch	CN V$_3$ **chew**	Muscles of mastication (temporalis, masseter, lateral and medial pterygoids), mylohyoid, anterior belly of digastric, tensor tympani, anterior 2/3 of tongue, tensor veli palatini	Maxillary process → maxilla, zygomatic bone Mandibular process → Meckel cartilage → mandible, malleus and incus, sphenomandibular ligament
2nd pharyngeal arch	CN VII (seven) –**smile**	Muscles of facial expression, stapedius, stylohyoid, platysma, posterior belly of digastric	Reichert cartilage → stapes, styloid process, lesser horn of hyoid, stylohyoid ligament
3rd pharyngeal arch	CN IX—**swallow stylishly**	Stylopharyngeus	Greater horn of hyoid
4th and 6th pharyngeal arches	4th arch: CN X (superior laryngeal branch) **simply swallow** 6th arch: CN X (recurrent laryngeal branch) **speak**	4th arch: most pharyngeal constrictors; cricothyroid, levator veli palatini 6th arch: all intrinsic muscles of larynx except cricothyroid	Arytenoids, Cricoid, Corniculate, Cuneiform, Thyroid cartilage (used to sing and **ACCCT**)

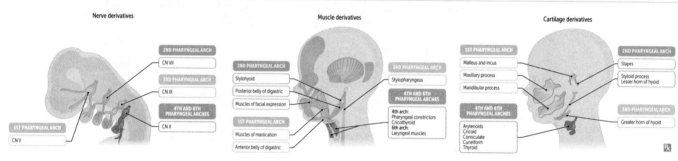

First and second pharyngeal arch syndromes

Pierre Robin sequence	Mandibular hypoplasia (micrognathia) → posteriorly displaced tongue (glossoptosis) → cleft palate, airway compromise. Feeding difficulties are common.
Treacher Collins syndrome	Autosomal dominant neural crest dysfunction → craniofacial abnormalities (eg, zygomatic bone and mandibular hypoplasia), hearing loss, airway compromise.

Orofacial clefts	Cleft lip and cleft palate have distinct, multifactorial etiologies, but often occur together.
Cleft lip	Due to failure of fusion of the intermaxillary segment (merged medial nasal processes) with the maxillary process (formation of 1° palate).
Cleft palate	Due to failure of fusion of the two lateral palatine shelves or failure of fusion of lateral palatine shelf with the nasal septum and/or 1° palate (formation of 2° palate).

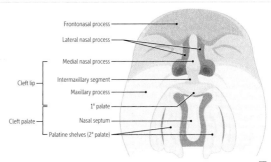

Genital embryology

Female	Default development. Mesonephric duct degenerates and paramesonephric duct develops.
Male	SRY gene on Y chromosome—produces testis-determining factor → testes development. Sertoli cells secrete Müllerian-inhibiting substance (MIS, also called anti-Müllerian hormone) that suppresses development of paramesonephric ducts. Leydig cells secrete androgens that stimulate development of mesonephric ducts.
Paramesonephric (Müllerian) duct	Develops into female internal structures—fallopian tubes, uterus, proximal vagina (distal vagina from urogenital sinus). Male remnant is appendix testis. Müllerian agenesis (Mayer-Rokitansky-Küster-Hauser syndrome)—1° amenorrhea with absent uterus, blind vaginal pouch, normal female external genitalia and 2° sexual characteristics (functional ovaries). Associated with urinary tract anomalies (eg, renal agenesis).
Mesonephric (Wolffian) duct	Develops into male internal structures (except prostate)—Seminal vesicles, Epididymis, Ejaculatory duct, Ductus deferens (**SEED**). Female remnant is Gartner duct.

Sexual differentiation

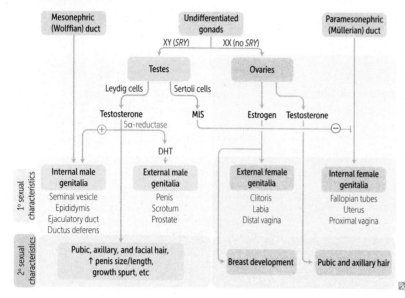

In XY individuals absence of Sertoli cells or lack of Müllerian-inhibiting substance → develop both male and female internal genitalia and male external genitalia (streak gonads)

5α-reductase deficiency—inability to convert testosterone into DHT → male internal genitalia, atypical external genitalia until puberty (when ↑ testosterone levels cause masculinization)

In the testes:

Leydig leads to male (internal and external) sexual differentiation.

Sertoli shuts down female (internal) sexual differentiation.

Uterine (Müllerian duct) anomalies	↓ fertility and ↑ risk of complicated pregnancy (eg, spontaneous abortion, prematurity, FGR, malpresentation). Hysterosalpingogram of normal uterus demonstrates normal uterine cavity and intraperitoneal spill of contrast (indicative of patent fallopian tubes).
Septate uterus	Incomplete resorption of septum A. Common anomaly. Treat with septoplasty.
Bicornuate uterus	Incomplete fusion of Müllerian ducts B.
Uterus didelphys	Complete failure of fusion → double uterus, cervix, vagina.

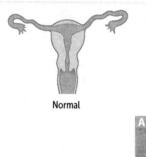
Normal

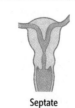
Septate

Bicornuate

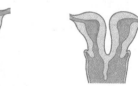
Didelphys

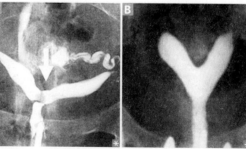

Male/female genital homologs

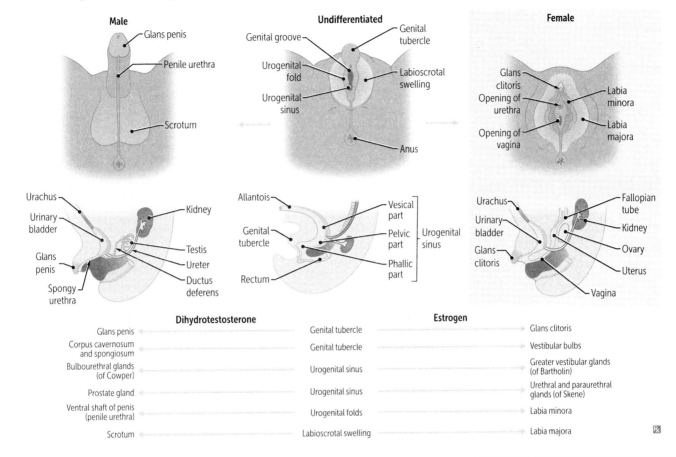

Congenital penile abnormalities

Hypospadias	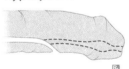	Abnormal opening of penile urethra on ventral (under) surface due to failure of urethral folds to fuse.	Hypospadias is more common than epispadias. Associated with inguinal hernia, cryptorchidism, chordee (downward or upward bending of penis). Can be seen in 5α-reductase deficiency.
Epispadias	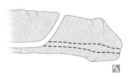	Abnormal opening of penile urethra on dorsal (top) surface due to faulty positioning of genital tubercle.	Exstrophy of the bladder is associated with epispadias.

Descent of testes and ovaries

	DESCRIPTION	MALE REMNANT	FEMALE REMNANT
Gubernaculum	Band of fibrous tissue	Anchors testes within scrotum	Ovarian ligament + round ligament of uterus
Processus vaginalis	Evagination of peritoneum	Forms tunica vaginalis Persistent patent processus vaginalis → hydrocele	Obliterated

▶ REPRODUCTIVE—ANATOMY

Drainage of reproductive organs

Venous drainage

Right ovary/testis → right gonadal vein → IVC.
Left ovary/testis → left gonadal vein → left renal vein → IVC (takes the longer way).
Left testicular vein enters left renal vein at 90° angle → flow is less laminar on the left than on the right → left venous pressure > right venous pressure → varicocele is more common on the left.

Lymphatic drainage

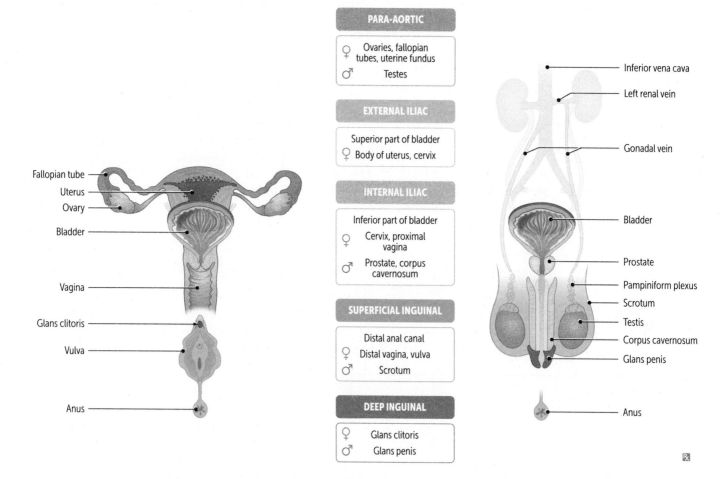

Female reproductive anatomy

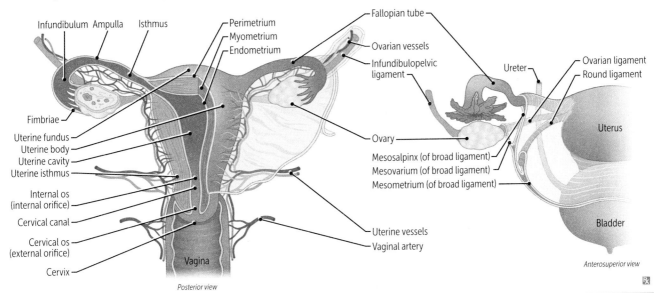

Infundibulum Ampulla Isthmus Perimetrium Myometrium Endometrium Fallopian tube Ovarian vessels Infundibulopelvic ligament Ureter Ovarian ligament Round ligament

Fimbriae Uterine fundus Uterine body Uterine cavity Uterine isthmus Internal os (internal orifice) Cervical canal Cervical os (external orifice) Cervix Vagina Ovary Mesosalpinx (of broad ligament) Mesovarium (of broad ligament) Mesometrium (of broad ligament) Uterine vessels Vaginal artery

Uterus Bladder

Posterior view

Anterosuperior view

LIGAMENT	CONNECTS	STRUCTURES CONTAINED	NOTES
Infundibulopelvic ligament	Ovary to lateral pelvic wall	Ovarian vessels	Also called suspensory ligament of ovary Ovarian vessel ligation during oophorectomy risks damaging the ureter
Utero-ovarian ligament	Ovary to uterine horn		Derivative of gubernaculum
Round ligament	Uterine horn to labia majora		Travels through inguinal canal Derivative of gubernaculum
Broad ligament	Uterus to lateral pelvic wall	Ovary, fallopian tube, round ligament	Fold of peritoneum comprising the mesometrium, mesovarium, and mesosalpinx
Cardinal ligament	Cervix to lateral pelvic wall	Uterine vessels	Condensation at the base of broad ligament Uterine vessel ligation during hysterectomy risks damaging the ureter
Uterosacral ligament	Cervix to sacrum		

Adnexal torsion	Twisting of ovary and fallopian tube around infundibulopelvic ligament and ovarian ligament → compression of ovarian vessels in infundibulopelvic ligament → blockage of lymphatic and venous outflow. Continued arterial perfusion → ovarian edema → complete blockage of arterial inflow → necrosis, local hemorrhage. Associated with ovarian masses/cysts. Presents with acute pelvic pain, adnexal mass, nausea/vomiting. Surgical emergency.

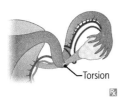

Torsion

Pelvic organ prolapse	Herniation of pelvic organs to or beyond the vaginal walls (anterior, posterior) or apex. Associated with multiparity, ↑ age, obesity. Presents with pelvic pressure, bulging sensation or tissue protrusion from vagina, urinary frequency, constipation, sexual dysfunction. ▪ Anterior compartment prolapse—bladder (cystocele). Most common type. ▪ Posterior compartment prolapse—rectum (rectocele) or small bowel (enterocele). ▪ Apical compartment prolapse—uterus, cervix, or vaginal vault. Uterine procidentia—herniation involving all 3 compartments.

Female reproductive epithelial histology

TISSUE	HISTOLOGY/NOTES
Vulva	Stratified squamous epithelium
Vagina	Stratified squamous epithelium, nonkeratinized
Ectocervix	Stratified squamous epithelium, nonkeratinized
Transformation zone	Squamocolumnar junction (most common area for cervical cancer; sampled in Pap test)
Endocervix	Simple columnar epithelium
Uterus	Simple columnar epithelium with long tubular glands in proliferative phase; coiled glands in secretory phase
Fallopian tube	Simple columnar epithelium, ciliated
Ovary, outer surface	Simple cuboidal epithelium (germinal epithelium covering surface of ovary)

Male reproductive anatomy

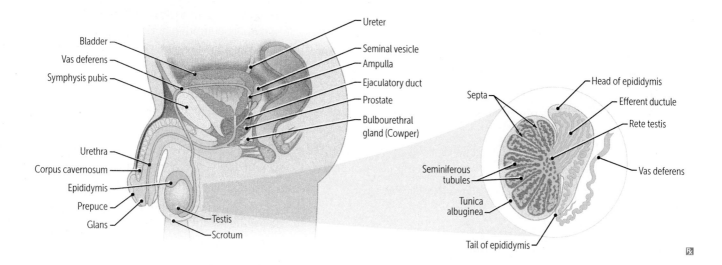

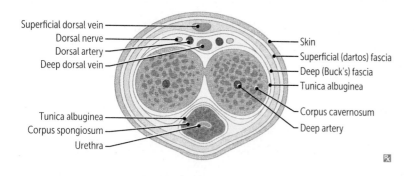

Pathway of sperm during ejaculation—
SEVEN UP:
Seminiferous tubules
Epididymis
Vas deferens
Ejaculatory ducts
(Nothing)
Urethra
Penis

Genitourinary trauma	Most commonly due to blunt trauma (eg, motor vehicle collision).
Renal injury	Presents with bruises, flank pain, hematuria. Caused by direct blows or lower rib fractures.
Bladder injury	Presents with hematuria, suprapubic pain, difficulty voiding. ▪ Superior bladder wall (dome) injury—direct trauma to full bladder (eg, seatbelt) → abrupt ↑ intravesical pressure → dome rupture (weakest part) → intraperitoneal urine accumulation. Peritoneal absorption of urine → ↑ BUN, ↑ creatinine. ▪ Anterior bladder wall or neck injury—pelvic fracture → perforation by bony spicules → extraperitoneal urine accumulation (retropubic space).
Urethral injury	Occurs almost exclusively in males. Presents with blood at urethral meatus, hematuria, difficulty voiding. Urethral catheterization is relatively contraindicated. ▪ Anterior urethral injury—perineal straddle injury → disruption of bulbar (spongy) urethra → scrotal hematoma. If Buck fascia is torn, urine escapes into perineal space. ▪ Posterior urethral injury—pelvic fracture → disruption at bulbomembranous junction (weakest part) → urine leakage into retropubic space and high-riding prostate.

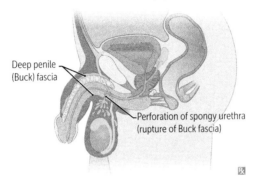

Anterior urethral injury

Deep penile (Buck) fascia

Perforation of spongy urethra (rupture of Buck fascia)

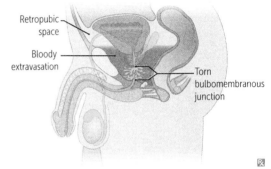

Posterior urethral injury

Retropubic space

Bloody extravasation

Torn bulbomembranous junction

Autonomic innervation of male sexual response	Erection—parasympathetic nervous system (pelvic splanchnic nerves, S2-S4): ▪ NO → ↑ cGMP → smooth muscle relaxation → vasodilation → proerectile. ▪ Norepinephrine → ↑ $[Ca^{2+}]_{in}$ → smooth muscle contraction → vasoconstriction → antierectile. Emission—sympathetic nervous system (hypogastric nerve, T11-L2). Expulsion—visceral and somatic nerves (pudendal nerve).	Point, squeeze, and shoot. S2, 3, 4 keep the penis off the **floor**. PDE-5 inhibitors (eg, sildenafil) → ↓ cGMP breakdown.

Seminiferous tubules

CELL	FUNCTION	LOCATION/NOTES
Spermatogonia	Maintain germ cell pool and produce 1° spermatocytes	Line seminiferous tubules 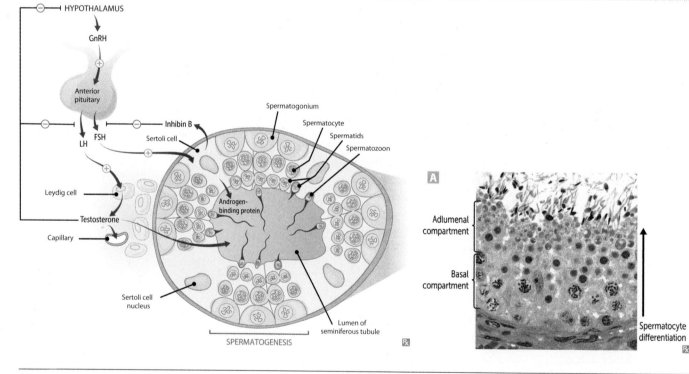A Germ cells
Sertoli cells	Secrete inhibin B → inhibit FSH Secrete androgen-binding protein → maintain local levels of testosterone Produce MIF Tight junctions between adjacent Sertoli cells form blood-testis barrier → isolate gametes from autoimmune attack Support and nourish developing spermatozoa Regulate spermatogenesis Temperature sensitive; ↓ sperm production and ↓ inhibin B with ↑ temperature	Line seminiferous tubules Non–germ cells Convert testosterone and androstenedione to estrogens via aromatase Sertoli cells are temperature sensitive, line seminiferous tubules, support sperm synthesis, and inhibit FSH Homolog of female granulosa cells ↑ temperature seen in varicocele, cryptorchidism
Leydig cells	Secrete testosterone in the presence of LH; testosterone production unaffected by temperature	Interstitium Endocrine cells Homolog of female theca interna cells

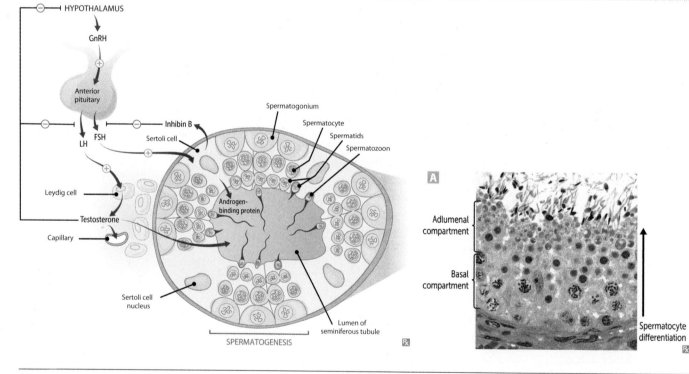

▶ REPRODUCTIVE—PHYSIOLOGY

Spermatogenesis

Begins at puberty with spermatogonia. Full development takes 2 months. Occurs in seminiferous tubules. Produces spermatids that undergo spermiogenesis (loss of cytoplasmic contents, gain of acrosomal cap) to form mature spermatozoa.

"Gonium" is going to be a sperm; "zoon" is "zooming" to egg.

Tail mobility impaired in ciliary dyskinesia/ Kartagener syndrome → infertility.

Tail mobility normal in cystic fibrosis (in CF, absent vas deferens → infertility).

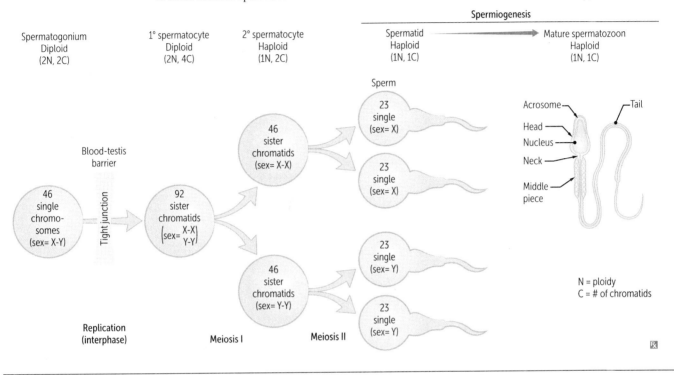

Spermiogenesis

| Spermatogonium Diploid (2N, 2C) | 1° spermatocyte Diploid (2N, 4C) | 2° spermatocyte Haploid (1N, 2C) | Spermatid Haploid (1N, 1C) | Mature spermatozoon Haploid (1N, 1C) |

Blood-testis barrier

Tight junction

46 single chromo-somes (sex= X-Y)

92 sister chromatids (sex= X-X / Y-Y)

46 sister chromatids (sex= X-X)

46 sister chromatids (sex= Y-Y)

Sperm

23 single (sex= X)

23 single (sex= X)

23 single (sex= Y)

23 single (sex= Y)

Replication (interphase)

Meiosis I

Meiosis II

Acrosome — Tail

Head —

Nucleus —

Neck —

Middle piece —

N = ploidy
C = # of chromatids

Estrogen

SOURCE	Ovary (estradiol), placenta (estriol), adipose tissue (estrone via aromatization).	Potency: estradiol > estrone > estriol. Estra**diol** is produced from **2** ovaries.
FUNCTION	Development of internal/external genitalia, breasts, female fat distribution. Growth of follicle, endometrial proliferation, ↑ myometrial excitability. Upregulation of estrogen, LH, and progesterone receptors; feedback inhibition of FSH and LH, then LH surge; stimulation of prolactin secretion, ↓ prolactin action on breasts. ↑ transport proteins, SHBG; ↑ HDL; ↓ LDL.	Pregnancy: ▪ 50-fold ↑ in estradiol and estrone ▪ 1000-fold ↑ in estriol (indicator of fetal well-being) Estrogen receptors expressed in cytoplasm; translocate to nucleus when bound by estrogen.

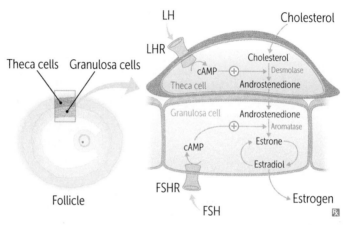

Progesterone

SOURCE	Corpus luteum, placenta, adrenal cortex, testes.	Fall in estrogen and progesterone after delivery disinhibits prolactin → lactation. ↑ progesterone is indicative of ovulation.
FUNCTION	During luteal phase, prepares uterus for implantation of fertilized egg: ▪ Stimulation of endometrial glandular secretions and spiral artery development ▪ Production of thick cervical mucus → inhibits sperm entry into uterus ▪ Prevention of endometrial hyperplasia ▪ ↑ body temperature ▪ ↓ estrogen receptor expression ▪ ↓ gonadotropin (LH, FSH) secretion During pregnancy: ▪ Maintenance of endometrial lining and pregnancy ▪ ↓ myometrial excitability → ↓ contraction frequency and intensity ▪ ↓ prolactin action on breasts	**Progest**erone is **pro-gest**ation. **Prolact**in is **pro-lactat**ion.

Oogenesis

1° oocytes begin meiosis I during fetal life and complete meiosis I just prior to ovulation. Meiosis I is arrested in prophase I (one) for years until ovulation (1° oocytes). Meiosis II is arrested in metaphase II (two) until fertilization (2° oocytes). If fertilization does not occur within 1 day, the 2° oocyte degenerates.

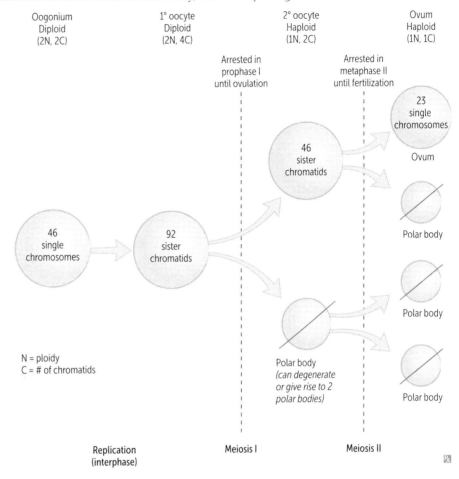

Ovulation

Follicular rupture and 2° oocyte release. Caused by sudden LH release (LH surge) at **mid**cycle. Estrogen normally inhibits LH release, but high estrogen at midcycle transiently stimulates LH release → LH surge → ovulation.

Mittelschmerz ("**middle** hurts")—pain with ovulation. Associated with peritoneal irritation from normal bleeding upon follicular rupture. Typically unilateral and mild, but can mimic acute appendicitis.

Menstrual cycle	Regular cyclic changes periodically preparing the female reproductive system for fertilization and pregnancy. Occurs in phases based on events taking place in ovaries and uterus.	
	1ST DAY OF MENSES TO OVULATION	OVULATION TO 1ST DAY OF NEXT MENSES
Ovarian cycle	Follicular phase—follicular development; late stages are stimulated by FSH; can fluctuate in length.	Luteal phase—corpus luteum formation from follicular remnants; stimulated by LH; lasts a fixed 14 days.
Uterine cycle	Proliferative phase—endometrial development; stimulated by estrogen. Straight, narrow endometrial glands.	Secretory phase—endometrial preparation for implantation; stimulated by progesterone. Tortuous, dilated endometrial glands.

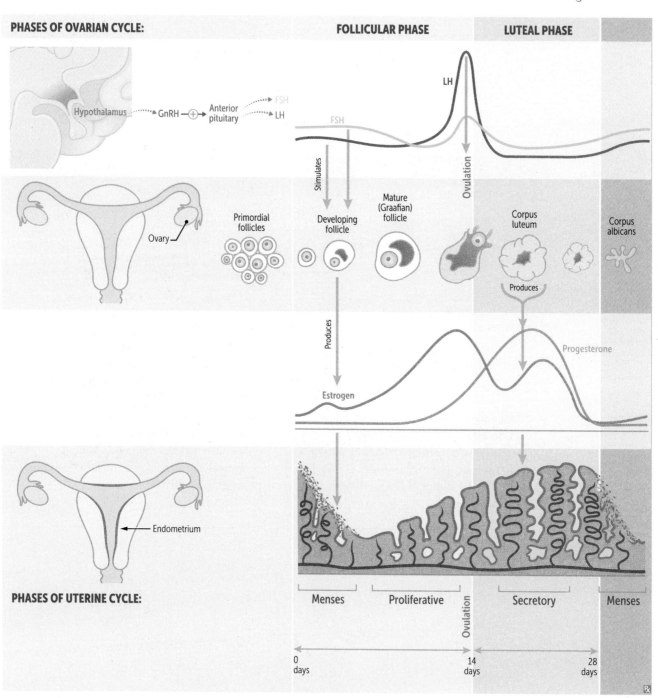

Abnormal uterine bleeding	Deviation from normal menstruation volume, duration, frequency, regularity, or intermenstrual bleeding. Causes (**PALM-COEIN**): ▪ Structural: **P**olyp, **A**denomyosis, **L**eiomyoma, **M**alignancy/hyperplasia ▪ Nonstructural: **C**oagulopathy, **O**vulatory, **E**ndometrial, **I**atrogenic, **N**ot yet classified	Terms such as dysfunctional uterine bleeding, menorrhagia, metrorrhagia, polymenorrhea, and oligomenorrhea are no longer recommended.

Pregnancy	Fertilization (conception) most commonly occurs in upper end of fallopian tube (the ampulla). Occurs within 1 day of ovulation. Implantation in the uterine wall occurs 6 days after fertilization. Syncytiotrophoblasts secrete hCG, which is detectable in blood 1 week after fertilization and on home urine tests 2 weeks after fertilization. Embryonic/developmental age—time since fertilization. Used in embryology. Gestational age—time since first day of last menstrual period. Used clinically. Gravidity ("gravida")—number of pregnancies. Parity ("para")—number of pregnancies that resulted in live births.	Placental hormone secretion generally increases over the course of pregnancy, but hCG peaks at 8–10 weeks of gestation. 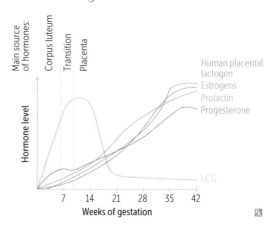

Physiologic changes in pregnancy

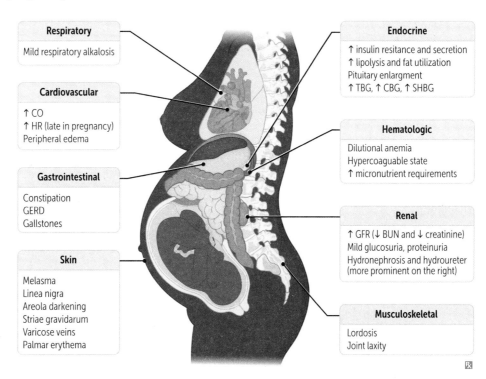

Respiratory

Mild respiratory alkalosis

Cardiovascular

↑ CO
↑ HR (late in pregnancy)
Peripheral edema

Gastrointestinal

Constipation
GERD
Gallstones

Skin

Melasma
Linea nigra
Areola darkening
Striae gravidarum
Varicose veins
Palmar erythema

Endocrine

↑ insulin resitance and secretion
↑ lipolysis and fat utilization
Pituitary enlargment
↑ TBG, ↑ CBG, ↑ SHBG

Hematologic

Dilutional anemia
Hypercoaguable state
↑ micronutrient requirements

Renal

↑ GFR (↓ BUN and ↓ creatinine)
Mild glucosuria, proteinuria
Hydronephrosis and hydroureter
(more prominent on the right)

Musculoskeletal

Lordosis
Joint laxity

Human chorionic gonadotropin

SOURCE	Syncytiotrophoblast of placenta.
FUNCTION	Maintains corpus luteum (and thus progesterone) for first 8–10 weeks of gestation by acting like LH (otherwise no luteal cell stimulation → abortion). Luteal-placental shift is complete after 8–10 weeks; placenta synthesizes its own estriol and progesterone and corpus luteum degenerates. Used to detect pregnancy because it appears early in urine (see above). Has identical α subunit as LH, FSH, TSH. β subunit is unique (detected by pregnancy tests) but structurally similar to that of TSH (states of ↑ hCG can cause hyperthyroidism). hCG is ↑ in multifetal gestation, hydatidiform moles, choriocarcinomas, and Down syndrome; hCG is ↓ in ectopic/failing pregnancy, Edwards syndrome, and Patau syndrome.

Human placental lactogen

	Also called human chorionic somatomammotropin.
SOURCE	Syncytiotrophoblast of placenta.
FUNCTION	Promotes insulin resistance to supply growing fetus with glucose and amino acids. Concurrently stimulates insulin secretion; inability to overcome insulin resistance → gestational diabetes.

Apgar score

	Score 2	Score 1	Score 0
Appearance	Pink	Extremities blue	Pale or blue
Pulse	≥ 100 bpm	< 100 bpm	No pulse
Grimace	Cries and pulls away	Grimaces or weak cry	No response to stimulation
Activity	Active movement	Arms, legs flexed	No movement
Respiration	Strong cry	Slow, irregular	No breathing

Assessment of newborn vital signs following delivery via a 10-point scale evaluated at 1 minute and 5 minutes. **A**pgar score is based on **a**ppearance, **p**ulse, **g**rimace, **a**ctivity, and **r**espiration. Apgar scores < 7 may require further evaluation. If Apgar score remains low at later time points, there is ↑ risk the child will develop long-term neurologic damage.

Neonatal birth weight

	Low birth weight	High birth weight (macrosomia)
DEFINITION	Birth weight < 2500 g	Birth weight > 4000 g
RISK FACTORS	Prematurity, FGR	Fetal: constitutional/genetic Maternal: obesity, diabetes mellitus
COMPLICATIONS	↑ mortality (SIDS), ↑ morbidity	↑ risk of maternal or fetal trauma (eg, shoulder dystocia)

Lactation	After parturition and delivery of placenta, rapid ↓ in estrogen and progesterone disinhibits prolactin → initiation of lactation. Suckling is required to maintain milk production and ejection, since ↑ nerve stimulation → ↑ oxytocin and prolactin. Prolactin—induces and maintains lactation and ↓ reproductive function. Oxytocin—assists in milk letdown; also promotes uterine contractions. Breast milk is the ideal nutrition for infants < 6 months old. Contains immunoglobulins (conferring passive immunity; mostly IgA), macrophages, lymphocytes. Breast milk reduces infant infections and is associated with ↓ risk for child to develop asthma, allergies, diabetes mellitus, and obesity. Exclusively breastfed infants should get vitamin D +/– iron supplementation. Breastfeeding ↓ maternal risk of breast and ovarian cancer and facilitates mother-child bonding.

Menopause	Diagnosed by amenorrhea for 12 months. ↓ estrogen production due to age-linked decline in number of ovarian follicles. Average age at onset is 51 years (earlier in people who smoke tobacco). Usually preceded by 4–5 years of abnormal menstrual cycles. Source of estrogen (estrone) after menopause becomes peripheral conversion of androgens, ↑ androgens → hirsutism. ↑↑ FSH is specific for menopause (loss of negative feedback on FSH due to ↓ estrogen).	Hormonal changes: ↓ estrogen, ↑↑ FSH, ↑ LH (no surge), ↑ GnRH. Causes **HAVOCS**: Hot flashes (most common), Atrophy of the Vagina, Osteoporosis (↑ osteoclast activity), Coronary artery disease, Sleep disturbances. Hormone replacement therapy (HRT) is used to treat menopausal symptoms, but can be associated with ↑ risk of breast and endometrial cancer, CVD, stroke, and thromboembolism. Menopause before age 40 suggests 1° ovarian insufficiency (premature ovarian failure); may occur in females who have received chemotherapy and/or radiation therapy.

Androgens	Testosterone, dihydrotestosterone (DHT), dehydroepiandrosterone (DHEA), androstenedione (adrenal).	
SOURCE	DHT and testosterone (testis), DHEA and androstenedione (adrenal).	Potency: DHT > testosterone > androstenedione > DHEA.
FUNCTION	Testosterone: ▪ Differentiation of epididymis, vas deferens, seminal vesicles (internal genitalia, except prostate) ▪ Growth spurt: penis, seminal vesicles, sperm, muscle, RBCs ▪ Deepening of voice ▪ Closing of epiphyseal plates (via estrogen converted from testosterone) ▪ Libido DHT: ▪ Early—differentiation of penis, scrotum, prostate ▪ Late—prostate growth, androgenetic alopecia, sebaceous gland activity	Testosterone is converted to DHT by 5α-reductase, which is inhibited by finasteride. In the male, androgens are converted to estrogens by aromatase (primarily in adipose tissue and testes). Anabolic-androgenic steroid use—↑ fat-free mass, muscle strength, performance. Suspect in males who present with changes in behavior (eg, aggression), acne, gynecomastia, erythrocytosis (↑ risk of thromboembolism), small testes (exogenous testosterone → hypothalamic-pituitary-gonadal axis inhibition → ↓ intratesticular testosterone → ↓ testicular size, ↓ sperm count, azoospermia). Females may present with virilization (eg, hirsutism, acne, breast atrophy, androgenetic alopecia).

Sexual maturity rating (Tanner stage) of pubertal development

Sexual maturity rating is assigned independently to genitalia, pubic hair, and breast (eg, a person can have stage 2 genitalia, stage 3 pubic hair). Earliest detectable secondary sexual characteristic is breast bud development in females, testicular enlargement in males.

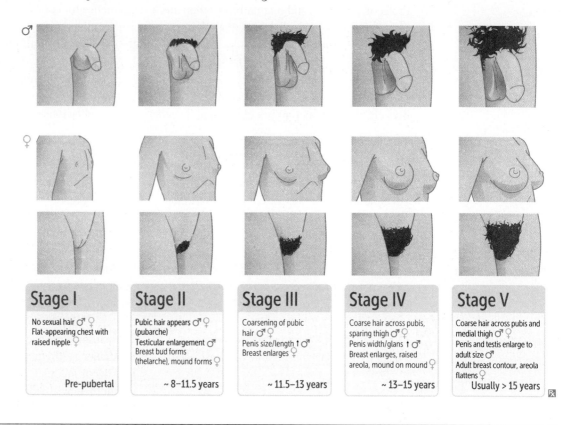

Stage I	Stage II	Stage III	Stage IV	Stage V
No sexual hair ♂ ♀ Flat-appearing chest with raised nipple ♀	Pubic hair appears ♂ ♀ (pubarche) Testicular enlargement ♂ Breast bud forms (thelarche), mound forms ♀	Coarsening of pubic hair ♂ ♀ Penis size/length ↑ ♂ Breast enlarges ♀	Coarse hair across pubis, sparing thigh ♂ ♀ Penis width/glans ↑ ♂ Breast enlarges, raised areola, mound on mound ♀	Coarse hair across pubis and medial thigh ♂ ♀ Penis and testis enlarge to adult size ♂ Adult breast contour, areola flattens ♀
Pre-pubertal	~ 8–11.5 years	~ 11.5–13 years	~ 13–15 years	Usually > 15 years

Precocious puberty

Appearance of 2° sexual characteristics (eg, pubarche, thelarche) before age 8 years in females and 9 years in males. ↑ sex hormone exposure or production → ↑ linear growth, somatic and skeletal maturation (eg, premature closure of epiphyseal plates → short stature). Types include:
- Central precocious puberty (↑ GnRH secretion): idiopathic (most common; early activation of hypothalamic-pituitary gonadal axis), CNS tumors.
- Peripheral precocious puberty (GnRH-independent; ↑ sex hormone production or exposure to exogenous sex steroids): congenital adrenal hyperplasia, estrogen-secreting ovarian tumor (eg, granulosa cell tumor), Leydig cell tumor, McCune-Albright syndrome.

Delayed puberty

Absence of 2° sexual characteristics by age 13 years in females and 14 years in males. Causes:
- Hypergonadotropic (1°) hypogonadism: Klinefelter syndrome, Turner syndrome, gonadal injury (eg, chemotherapy, radiotherapy, infection).
- Hypogonadotropic (2°) hypogonadism: constitutional delay of growth and puberty ("late blooming"), Kallmann syndrome, CNS lesions.

▶ REPRODUCTIVE—PATHOLOGY

Sex chromosome disorders	Aneuploidy most commonly due to meiotic nondisjunction.	
Klinefelter syndrome 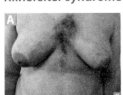	Male, 47,XXY. Small, firm testes; infertility (azoospermia); tall stature with eunuchoid proportions (delayed epiphyseal closure → ↑ long bone length); gynecomastia A; female hair distribution. May present with developmental delay. Presence of inactivated X chromosome (Barr body). Common cause of hypogonadism seen in infertility workup. ↑ risk of breast cancer.	Dysgenesis of seminiferous tubules → ↓ inhibin B → ↑ FSH. Abnormal Leydig cell function → ↓ testosterone → ↑ LH.
Turner syndrome 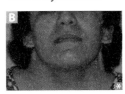	Female, 45,XO. Short stature (preventable with GH therapy), ovarian dysgenesis (streak ovary), broad chest with widely spaced nipples, bicuspid aortic valve, coarctation of the aorta (femoral < brachial pulse), lymphatic defects (result in webbed neck B or cystic hygroma; lymphedema in feet, hands), horseshoe kidney, high-arched palate, shortened 4th metacarpals. Most common cause of 1° amenorrhea. No Barr body.	Menopause before menarche. ↓ estrogen leads to ↑ LH, FSH. Sex chromosome (X, or rarely Y) loss often due to nondisjunction during meiosis or mitosis. Meiosis errors usually occur in paternal gametes → sperm missing the sex chromosome. Mitosis errors occur after zygote formation → loss of sex chromosome in some but not all cells → mosaic karyotype (eg. 45,X/46,XX). (45,X/46,XY) mosaicism associated with ↑ risk for gonadoblastoma. Pregnancy is possible in some cases (IVF, exogenous estradiol-17β and progesterone).
Double Y males	47,XYY. Phenotypically normal (usually undiagnosed), very tall. Normal fertility. May be associated with severe acne, learning disability, autism spectrum disorders.	

Other disorders of sex development	Formerly called intersex states. Discrepancy between phenotypic sex (external genitalia, influenced by hormonal levels) and gonadal sex (testes vs ovaries, corresponds with Y chromosome).
46,XX DSD	Ovaries present, but external genitalia are virilized or atypical. Most commonly due to congenital adrenal hyperplasia (excessive exposure to androgens early in development).
46,XY DSD	Testes present, but external genitalia are feminized or atypical. Most commonly due to androgen insensitivity syndrome (defect in androgen receptor).
Ovotesticular DSD	46,XX > 46,XY. Both ovarian and testicular tissue present (ovotestis); atypical genitalia.

Diagnosing disorders by sex hormones	Testosterone	LH	Diagnosis
	↑	↑	Androgen insensitivity syndrome
	↑	↓	Testosterone-secreting tumor, exogenous androgenic steroids
	↓	↑	Hypergonadotropic (1°) hypogonadism
	↓	↓	Hypogonadotropic (2°) hypogonadism

Diagnosing disorders by physical characteristics	Uterus	Breasts	Diagnosis
	⊕	⊖	Hypergonadotropic (1°) hypogonadism in genotypic female Hypogonadotropic (2°) hypogonadism in genotypic female
	⊖	⊕	Müllerian agenesis in genotypic female Androgen insensitivity syndrome in genotypic male

Aromatase deficiency	Inability to synthesize endogenous estrogens. Autosomal recessive. During fetal life, DHEA produced by fetal adrenal glands cannot be converted to estrogen by the placenta and is converted to testosterone peripherally → virilization of both female infant (atypical genitalia) and mother (acne, hirsutism; fetal androgens can cross placenta).
Androgen insensitivity syndrome	Defect in androgen receptor resulting in female-appearing genetic male (46,XY DSD); breast development and female external genitalia with scant axillary and pubic hair, rudimentary vagina; uterus and fallopian tubes absent due to persistence of anti-Müllerian hormone from testes. Patients develop normal functioning testes (often found in labia majora; surgically removed to prevent malignancy). ↑ testosterone, estrogen, LH (vs sex chromosome disorders).
5α-reductase deficiency	Autosomal recessive; sex limited to genetic males (46,XY DSD). Inability to convert testosterone to DHT. Atypical genitalia until puberty, when ↑ testosterone causes masculinization/↑ growth of external genitalia. Testosterone/estrogen levels are normal; LH is normal or ↑. Internal genitalia are normal.
Kallmann syndrome	Failure to complete puberty; a form of hypogonadotropic hypogonadism. Defective migration of neurons and subsequent failure of olfactory bulbs to develop → ↓ synthesis of GnRH in the hypothalamus; hyposmia/anosmia; ↓ GnRH, FSH, LH, testosterone. Infertility (low sperm count in males; amenorrhea in females).

Placental disorders

Placenta accreta spectrum

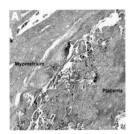

Abnormal invasion of trophoblastic tissue into uterine wall 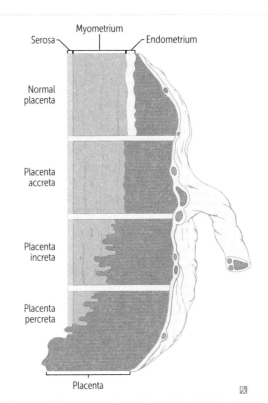. Risk factors: prior C-section or other uterine surgery (areas of uterine scarring impair normal decidualization), placenta previa, ↑ maternal age, multiparity. Three types depending on depth of trophoblast invasion:

- Placenta accreta—attaches to myometrium (instead of overlying decidua basalis) without invading it. Most common type.
- Placenta increta—partially invades into myometrium.
- Placenta percreta—completely invades ("perforates") through myometrium and serosa, sometimes extending into adjacent organs (eg, bladder → hematuria).

Presents with difficulty separating placenta from uterus after fetal delivery and severe postpartum hemorrhage upon attempted manual removal of placenta (often extracted in pieces). Treatment: hysterectomy.

Placenta previa

Attachment of placenta over internal cervical os (a "**preview**" of the placenta is visible through cervix). Risk factors: prior C-section, multiparity.

Presents with painless vaginal bleeding in third trimester.

Low-lying placenta—located < 2 cm from, but not covering, the internal cervical os.

Vasa previa

Fetal vessels run over, or < 2 cm from, the internal cervical os. Risk factors: velamentous insertion of umbilical cord (inserts in chorioamniotic membrane rather than placenta → fetal vessels travel to placenta unprotected by Wharton jelly), bilobed or succenturiate placenta.

Presents with painless vaginal bleeding (fetal blood from injured vessels) upon rupture of membranes accompanied by fetal heart rate abnormalities (eg, bradycardia). May lead to fetal death from exsanguination.

Placental abruption

Also called abruptio placentae. Premature separation of placenta from uterus prior to fetal delivery. Risk factors: maternal hypertension, preeclampsia, smoking, cocaine use, abdominal trauma.

Presents with **abrupt**, painful vaginal bleeding in third trimester; can lead to maternal hypovolemic shock (due to hemorrhage) and DIC (due to release of tissue factor from injured placenta), fetal distress (eg, hypoxia). May be life threatening for both mother and fetus.

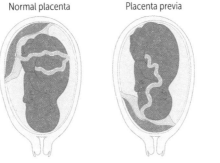
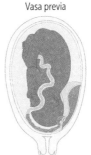
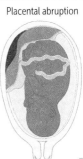

Normal placenta   Placenta previa   Vasa previa   Placental abruption

Uterine rupture

Full-thickness disruption of uterine wall. Risk factors: prior C-section (usually occurs during labor in a subsequent pregnancy), abdominal trauma.

Presents with painful vaginal bleeding, fetal heart rate abnormalities (eg, bradycardia), easily palpable fetal parts, loss of fetal station. May be life threatening for both mother and fetus.

Postpartum hemorrhage

Greater-than-expected blood loss after delivery. Leading cause of maternal mortality worldwide.

Etiology (4 T's): Tone (uterine atony → soft, boggy uterus; most common), Trauma (eg, lacerations, incisions, uterine rupture), Tissue (retained products of conception), Thrombin (coagulopathy).

Treatment: uterine massage, oxytocin. If refractory, surgical ligation of uterine or internal iliac arteries (fertility is preserved since ovarian arteries provide collateral circulation).

Ectopic pregnancy

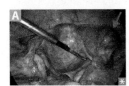

Implantation of fertilized ovum in a site other than the uterus, most often in ampulla of fallopian tube A. Risk factors: tubal pathologies (eg, scarring from salpingitis [PID] or surgery), previous ectopic pregnancy, IUD, IVF.

Presents with first-trimester bleeding and/or lower abdominal pain. Often clinically mistaken for appendicitis. Suspect in patients with history of amenorrhea, lower-than-expected rise in hCG based on dates. Confirm with ultrasound, which may show extraovarian adnexal mass.

Treatment: methotrexate, surgery.

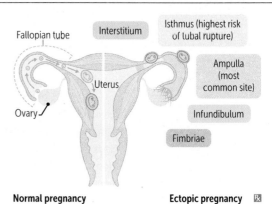

Fallopian tube — Interstitium — Isthmus (highest risk of tubal rupture)

Ampulla (most common site)

Uterus

Infundibulum

Ovary

Fimbriae

Normal pregnancy   **Ectopic pregnancy** ℞

Hydatidiform mole

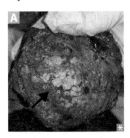
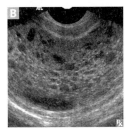

Cystic swelling of chorionic villi and proliferation of chorionic epithelium (only trophoblast).
Presents with vaginal bleeding, emesis, uterine enlargement more than expected, pelvic pressure/
pain. Associated with hCG-mediated sequelae: hyperthyroidism, theca lutein cysts, hyperemesis
gravidarum, early preeclampsia (before 20 weeks of gestation).
Treatment: dilation and curettage +/− methotrexate. Monitor hCG.

	Complete mole	Partial mole
KARYOTYPE	46,XX (most common); 46,XY	69,XXX; 69,XXY; 69,XYY
COMPONENTS	Most commonly enucleated egg + single sperm (subsequently duplicates paternal DNA)	2 sperm + 1 egg
HISTOLOGY	Hydropic villi, circumferential and diffuse trophoblastic proliferation	Only some villi are hydropic, focal/minimal trophoblastic proliferation
FETAL PARTS	No	Yes (**partial** = fetal **parts**)
STAINING FOR P57 PROTEIN	⊖ (paternally imprinted) Complete mole is complete male	⊕ (maternally expressed) Partial mole is P57 positive
UTERINE SIZE	↑	—
hCG	↑↑↑↑	↑
IMAGING	"Honeycombed" uterus or "clusters of grapes" A, "snowstorm" B on ultrasound	Fetal parts
RISK OF INVASIVE MOLE	15–20%	< 5%
RISK OF CHORIOCARCINOMA	2%	Rare

Choriocarcinoma

Rare malignancy of trophoblastic tissue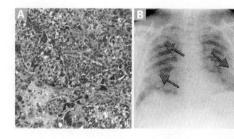
(cytotrophoblasts, syncytiotrophoblasts),
without chorionic villi present. Most
commonly occurs after an abnormal
pregnancy (eg, hydatidiform mole, abortion);
can occur nongestationally in gonads.
Presents with abnormal uterine bleeding,
hCG-mediated sequelae, dyspnea,
hemoptysis. Hematogenous spread to lungs
→ "cannonball" metastases B.
Treatment: methotrexate.

Hypertension in pregnancy

Gestational hypertension	BP > 140/90 mm Hg after 20 weeks of gestation. No preexisting hypertension. No proteinuria or end-organ damage. Hypertension prior to 20 weeks of gestation suggests chronic hypertension. Treatment: antihypertensives (Hydralazine, α-methyldopa, labetalol, nifedipine), deliver at 37–39 weeks. Hypertensive moms love nifedipine.
Preeclampsia	New-onset hypertension with either proteinuria or end-organ dysfunction after 20 weeks of gestation (onset of preeclampsia < 20 weeks of gestation may suggest molar pregnancy). Caused by abnormal placental spiral arteries → endothelial dysfunction, vasoconstriction, ischemia. Risk factors: history of preeclampsia, multifetal gestation, nulliparity, chronic hypertension, diabetes, chronic kidney disease, autoimmune disorders (eg, antiphospholipid syndrome), obesity. Complications: placental abruption, coagulopathy, renal failure, pulmonary edema, uteroplacental insufficiency; may lead to eclampsia and/or HELLP syndrome. Treatment: antihypertensives, IV magnesium sulfate (to prevent seizure); definitive is delivery. Prophylaxis: aspirin.
Eclampsia	Preeclampsia with seizures. Death due to stroke, intracranial hemorrhage, ARDS. Treatment: IV magnesium sulfate, antihypertensives, immediate delivery.
HELLP syndrome	Preeclampsia with thrombotic microangiopathy of the liver. Hemolysis, Elevated Liver enzymes, Low Platelets. May occur in the absence of hypertension and proteinuria. Blood smear shows schistocytes. Can lead to hepatic subcapsular hematomas (rupture → severe hypotension) and DIC (due to release of tissue factor from injured placenta). Treatment: immediate delivery.

Supine hypotensive syndrome	Also called aortocaval compression syndrome. Seen at > 20 weeks of gestation. Supine position → compression of abdominal aorta and IVC by gravid uterus → ↓ placental perfusion (can lead to pregnancy loss) and ↓ venous return (hypotension). Relieved by left lateral decubitus position.

Gynecologic tumor epidemiology	Incidence (US)—endometrial > ovarian > cervical; cervical cancer is more common worldwide due to lack of screening or HPV vaccination. Prognosis: Cervical (**best** prognosis, diagnosed < 45 years old) > Endometrial (middle-aged, about 55 years old) > Ovarian (**worst** prognosis, > 65 years).	**CEO**s often go from **best** to **worst** as they get older.

Vulvar pathology

Non-neoplastic

Bartholin cyst and abscess	Due to blockage of Bartholin gland duct causing accumulation of gland fluid. May lead to abscess 2° to obstruction and inflammation 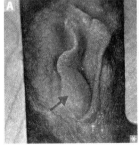. Usually in reproductive-age females.
Lichen sclerosus	Chronic, progressive inflammatory disease characterized by porcelain-white plaques 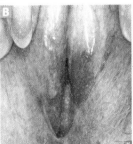 that can be hemorrhagic, eroded, or ulcerated. May extend to anus producing figure-eight appearance. ↑ incidence in prepubertal and peri-/postmenopausal females. Presents with intense pruritus, dyspareunia, dysuria, dyschezia. Benign, but slightly ↑ risk for SCC.
Lichen simplex chronicus	Hyperplasia of vulvar squamous epithelium. Presents with leathery, thick vulvar skin with enhanced skin markings due to chronic rubbing or scratching. Benign, no risk of SCC.

Neoplastic

Vulvar carcinoma	Carcinoma from squamous epithelial lining of vulva 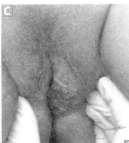. Usually seen in postmenopausal females. Presents with leukoplakia, biopsy often required to distinguish carcinoma from other causes. HPV-related vulvar carcinoma—associated with high-risk HPV types 16, 18. Non-HPV vulvar carcinoma—usually from long-standing lichen sclerosus.
Extramammary Paget disease	Intraepithelial adenocarcinoma. Carcinoma in situ, low risk of underlying carcinoma (vs Paget disease of the breast, which is always associated with underlying carcinoma). Presents with pruritus, erythema, crusting, ulcers 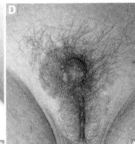.

Imperforate hymen	Incomplete degeneration of the central portion of the hymen. Accumulation of vaginal mucus at birth → self-resolving bulge in introitus. If untreated, leads to 1° amenorrhea, cyclic abdominal pain, hematocolpos (accumulation of menstrual blood in vagina → bulging and bluish hymenal membrane).

Vaginal tumors

Squamous cell carcinoma	Usually 2° to cervical SCC; 1° vaginal carcinoma rare.
Clear cell adenocarcinoma	Arises from vaginal adenosis (persistence of glandular columnar epithelium in proximal vagina), found in females who had exposure to diethylstilbestrol in utero.
Sarcoma botryoides	Embryonal rhabdomyosarcoma variant. Affects females < 4 years old; spindle-shaped cells; desmin ⊕. Presents with clear, grapelike, polypoid mass emerging from vagina.

Anovulatory infertility	Infertility 2° to lack of ovulation. Causes: 　▪ PCOS (most common) 　▪ Primary ovarian insufficiency 　▪ Hypogonadotropic hypogonadism 　▪ Hyperprolactinemia	Anovulation is normal during pregnancy, breastfeeding, and near menarche or menopause.

Polycystic ovary syndrome 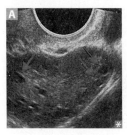	Unknown cause; associated with dysregulation of ovarian steroidogenesis. ↑ LH:FSH, ↑ androgens (eg, testosterone) from theca interna cells, ↓ rate of follicular maturation → unruptured follicles (cysts) + anovulation. Common cause of ↓ fertility in females. Diagnosed based on ≥ 2 of the following: cystic/enlarged ovaries on ultrasound (arrows in A), oligo-/anovulation, hyperandrogenism (eg, hirsutism, acne). Associated with obesity, insulin resistance, acanthosis nigricans. ↑ risk of endometrial cancer 2° to unopposed estrogen from repeated anovulatory cycles. Treatment: cycle regulation via weight reduction (↓ peripheral estrone formation), OCPs (prevent endometrial hyperplasia due to unopposed estrogen); ovulation induction for infertility; spironolactone, finasteride, flutamide to treat hirsutism.

Primary ovarian insufficiency	Also called premature ovarian failure. Premature atresia of ovarian follicles in females of reproductive age. Most often idiopathic; associated with chromosomal abnormalities (eg, Turner syndrome, fragile X syndrome premutation), autoimmunity. Need karyotype screening. Patients present with signs of menopause after puberty but before age 40. ↓ estrogen, ↑ LH, ↑ FSH.

Functional hypothalamic amenorrhea	Also called exercise-induced amenorrhea. Severe caloric restriction, ↑ energy expenditure, and/or stress → functional disruption of pulsatile GnRH secretion → ↓ LH, FSH, estrogen. Pathogenesis includes ↓ leptin (due to ↓ fat) and ↑ cortisol (stress, excessive exercise). Associated with eating disorders and "female athlete triad" (↓ calorie availability/excessive exercise, ↓ bone mineral density, menstrual dysfunction).

Cervical pathology

Dysplasia and carcinoma in situ 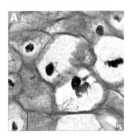	Disordered squamous epithelial growth; begins at basal layer of squamocolumnar junction (transformation zone) and extends outward. Classified as CIN 1, CIN 2, or CIN 3 (severe dysplasia or carcinoma in situ is unlikely to return to normal), depending on extent of dysplasia. Associated with HPV-16 and HPV-18, which produce both the E6 gene product (inhibits *TP53*) and E7 gene product (inhibits *pRb*) (**6** before **7**; **P** before **R**). Koilocytes (cells with wrinkled "raisinoid" nucleus and perinuclear halo **A**) are pathognomonic of HPV infection. May progress slowly to invasive carcinoma if left untreated. Typically asymptomatic (detected with Pap smear) or presents as abnormal vaginal bleeding (often postcoital). Risk factors: multiple sexual partners, HPV, smoking, early coitarche, DES exposure, immunocompromise (eg, HIV, transplant).
Invasive carcinoma	Often squamous cell carcinoma. Pap smear can detect cervical dysplasia before it progresses to invasive carcinoma. Diagnose via colposcopy and biopsy. Lateral invasion can block ureters → hydronephrosis → renal failure.

Primary dysmenorrhea	Painful menses, caused by uterine contractions to ↓ blood loss → ischemic pain. Mediated by prostaglandins. Treatment: NSAIDs, acetaminophen, hormonal contraceptives.

Ovarian cysts

Ovarian cysts	Usually asymptomatic, but may rupture, become hemorrhagic, or lead to adnexal torsion.
Follicular cyst	Functional (physiologic) cyst. Most common ovarian mass in young females. Caused by failure of mature follicle to rupture and ovulate. May produce excess estrogen. Usually resolves spontaneously.
Corpus luteal cyst	Functional cyst. Caused by failure of corpus luteum to involute after ovulation. May produce excess progesterone. Usually resolves spontaneously.
Theca lutein cyst	Also called hyperreactio luteinalis. Caused by hCG overstimulation. Often bilateral/multiple. Associated with gestational trophoblastic disease (eg, hydatidiform mole, choriocarcinoma).

Ovarian tumors

Most common adnexal mass in females > 55 years old. Present with abdominal distention, bowel obstruction, pleural effusion.

Risk ↑ with advanced age, ↑ number of lifetime ovulations (early menarche, late menopause, nulliparity), endometriosis, genetic predisposition (eg, *BRCA1/BRCA2* mutations, Lynch syndrome).

Risk ↓ with previous pregnancy, history of breastfeeding, OCPs, tubal ligation.

Epithelial tumors are typically serous (lined by serous epithelium natively found in fallopian tubes, and often bilateral) or mucinous (lined by mucinous epithelium natively found in cervix). Monitor response to therapy/relapse by measuring CA 125 levels (not good for screening).

Germ cell tumors can differentiate into somatic structures (eg, teratomas), or extra-embryonic structures (eg, yolk sac tumors), or can remain undifferentiated (eg, dysgerminoma).

Sex cord stromal tumors develop from embryonic sex cord (develops into theca and granulosa cells of follicle, Sertoli and Leydig cells of seminiferous tubules) and stromal (ovarian cortex) derivatives.

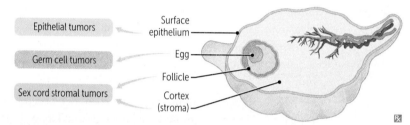

TYPE	CHARACTERISTICS
Epithelial tumors	
Serous cystadenoma	Benign. Most common ovarian neoplasm. Lined by fallopian tube–like epithelium.
Mucinous cystadenoma	Benign. Multiloculated, large. Lined by mucus-secreting epithelium .
Brenner tumor	Usually benign. Nests of urothelial-like (bladderlike) epithelium with "coffee bean" nuclei.
Serous carcinoma	Most common malignant ovarian neoplasm. Psammoma bodies.
Mucinous carcinoma	Malignant. Rare. May be metastatic from appendiceal or other GI tumors. Can result in pseudomyxoma peritonei (intraperitoneal accumulation of mucinous material, also knows as omental caking).
Germ cell tumors	
Mature cystic teratoma	Also called dermoid cyst. Benign. Most common ovarian tumor in young females. Cystic mass with elements from all 3 germ layers (eg, teeth, hair, sebum) . May be painful 2° to ovarian enlargement or torsion. Monodermal form with thyroid tissue (struma ovarii) may present with hyperthyroidism. Malignant transformation rare (usually to squamous cell carcinoma).
Immature teratoma	Malignant, aggressive. Contains fetal tissue, neuroectoderm. Commonly diagnosed before age 20. Typically represented by immature/embryoniclike neural tissue.
Dysgerminoma	Malignant. Most common in adolescents. Equivalent to male seminoma but rarer. Sheets of uniform "fried egg" cells . Tumor markers: ↑ hCG, ↑ LDH.
Yolk sac tumor	Also called endodermal sinus tumor. Malignant, aggressive. Yellow, friable (hemorrhagic) mass. 50% have Schiller-Duval bodies (resemble glomeruli). Tumor marker: ↑ AFP. Occurs in children and young adult females.

Ovarian tumors (continued)

TYPE	CHARACTERISTICS
Sex cord stromal tumors	
Fibroma	Benign. Bundle of spindle-shaped fibroblasts. Meigs syndrome—triad of ovarian fibroma, ascites, pleural effusion. "Pulling" sensation in groin.
Thecoma	Mostly benign; may produce estrogen. Usually presents as abnormal uterine bleeding in a postmenopausal female.
Sertoli-Leydig cell tumor	Benign. Gray to yellow-brown mass. Resembles testicular histology with seminiferous tubules lined by Sertoli cells and surrounded by interstitial Leydig cells. May produce androgens → virilization (eg, hirsutism, androgenetic alopecia, clitoral enlargement).
Granulosa cell tumor	Most common malignant sex cord stromal tumor. Predominantly occurs in females in their 50s. Often produces estrogen and/or progesterone. Presents with postmenopausal bleeding, endometrial hyperplasia, sexual precocity (in preadolescents), breast tenderness. Histology shows **Call**-Exner bodies (granulosa cells arranged haphazardly around collections of eosinophilic fluid, resembling primordial follicles; arrow in **F**). Tumor marker: ↑ inhibin. "Give **Gran**ny a **Call**."

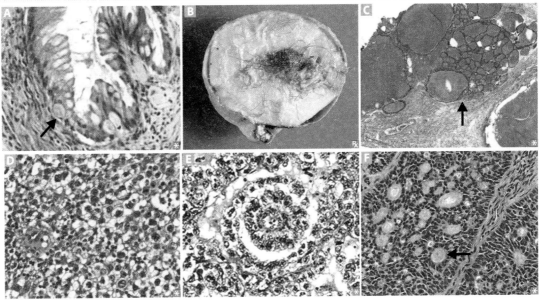

Uterine conditions

TYPE	CHARACTERISTICS
Non-neoplastic	
Adenomyosis	Presence of endometrial tissue (glands and stroma) in myometrium. May be due to invagination of basal layer of endometrium or metaplasia of remnant progenitor cells. Presents with abnormal uterine bleeding, dysmenorrhea. Diffusely enlarged ("globular"), soft ("boggy") uterus on exam.
Endometriosis	Presence of endometrial tissue outside of the uterus. May be due to ectopic implantation (via retrograde menses, lymphatics, or blood vessels) or metaplasia of remnant progenitor cells. Presents with dysmenorrhea, dyspareunia, infertility, abnormal uterine bleeding. Physical exam is usually normal. However, findings may include immobile uterus, adnexal mass, uterosacral tenderness, and/or nodularity, but are non-diagnostic. Typically involves pelvic sites, such as superficial peritoneum (yellow-brown "powder burn" lesions 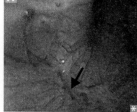) and ovaries (forms blood-filled "chocolate" cysts called endometrioma).
Endometrial hyperplasia	Abnormal endometrial gland proliferation. Usually caused by excess estrogen unopposed by progesterone. Associated with obesity, chronic anovulation (eg, PCOS), nulliparity, HRT, tamoxifen. Presents with abnormal uterine bleeding. ↑ risk for endometrial carcinoma (especially with nuclear atypia).
Endometritis	Inflammation of endometrium 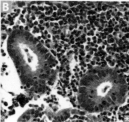. Usually occurs after delivery due to inoculation of uterine cavity by vaginal microbiota. C-section is the most important risk factor (sutures and necrotic tissue act as nidus for polymicrobial infection). Presents with fever, uterine tenderness, purulent lochia.
Intrauterine adhesions	Fibrous bands/tissue within endometrial cavity. Caused by damage to basal layer of endometrium, usually after dilation and curettage. Presents with abnormal uterine bleeding (↓ menses), infertility, recurrent pregnancy loss, dysmenorrhea. Also called Asherman syndrome when symptomatic.
Neoplastic	
Leiomyoma	Benign tumor of myometrium (also called fibroid). Most common gynecological tumor. Arises in reproductive-age females. ↑ incidence in Black population. Typically multiple; subtypes based on location: submucosal, intramural, or subserosal. Usually asymptomatic, but may present with abnormal uterine bleeding, pelvic pressure/pain, reproductive dysfunction. Estrogen sensitive; tumor size ↑ with pregnancy and ↓ with menopause. Enlarged uterus with nodular contour on exam 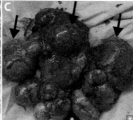. Histology: whorled pattern of smooth muscle bundles 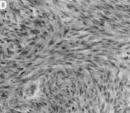 and well-demarcated borders.
Endometrial carcinoma	Malignant tumor of endometrium. Most common gynecological cancer in resource-rich countries. Usually arises in postmenopausal females. Presents with abnormal uterine bleeding. **Endometrioid carcinoma**—most common subtype of endometrial carcinoma. Associated with long-term exposure to unopposed estrogen. Histology: confluent endometrial glands without intervening stroma 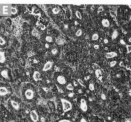.

Breast pathology

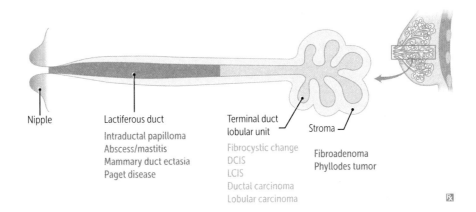

Nipple

Lactiferous duct
Intraductal papilloma
Abscess/mastitis
Mammary duct ectasia
Paget disease

Terminal duct
lobular unit
Fibrocystic change
DCIS
LCIS
Ductal carcinoma
Lobular carcinoma

Stroma

Fibroadenoma
Phyllodes tumor

Benign breast diseases

Fibrocystic changes	Most common in premenopausal females 20–50 years old. Present with premenstrual breast pain or lumps; often bilateral and multifocal. Nonproliferative lesions include simple cysts (fluid-filled duct dilation, blue dome), papillary apocrine change/metaplasia, stromal fibrosis. Risk of cancer is usually not increased. Proliferative lesions include ▪ Sclerosing adenosis—acini and stromal fibrosis, associated with calcifications. Slight ↑ risk for cancer. ▪ Epithelial hyperplasia—cells in terminal ductal or lobular epithelium. ↑ risk of carcinoma with atypical cells.
Inflammatory processes	Fat necrosis—benign, usually painless, lump due to injury to breast tissue. Calcified oil cyst on mammography; necrotic fat and giant cells on biopsy. Up to 50% of patients may not report trauma. Lactational mastitis—occurs during breastfeeding, ↑ risk of bacterial infection through cracks in nipple. *S aureus* is most common pathogen. Treat with antibiotics and continue breastfeeding. Mammary duct ectasia—dilation of subareolar ducts with inflammation and fibrosis. Associated with smoking. Presents with areolar pain, multicolored discharge, inverted nipple, periareolar mass.
Benign tumors	Fibroadenoma—most common in females < 35 years old. Small, well-defined, mobile mass. Tumor composed of fibrous tissue and glands. ↑ size and tenderness with ↑ estrogen (eg, pregnancy, prior to menstruation). Risk of cancer is usually not increased. Intraductal papilloma—small fibroepithelial tumor within lactiferous ducts, typically beneath areola. Most common cause of nipple discharge (often unilateral, serous or bloody). Slight ↑ risk for cancer. Phyllodes tumor—large mass of connective tissue and cysts with "leaflike" lobulations A. Most common in 5th decade. Some may become malignant.
Gynecomastia	Breast enlargement in males due to ↑ estrogen compared with androgen activity. Physiologic in newborn, pubertal, and older males, but may persist after puberty. Other causes include cirrhosis, hypogonadism (eg, Klinefelter syndrome), testicular tumors, drugs (eg, spironolactone).

Breast cancer

Commonly postmenopausal. Often presents as a palpable hard mass A most often in upper outer quadrant. Invasive cancer can become fixed to pectoral muscles, deep fascia, Cooper ligaments, and overlying skin → nipple retraction/skin dimpling.

Usually arises from terminal duct lobular unit. Amplification/overexpression of estrogen/progesterone receptors or HER2 (an EGF receptor) is common; triple negative (ER ⊖, PR ⊖, and HER2 ⊖) form more aggressive.

Risk factors in females: ↑ age; history of atypical hyperplasia; family history of breast cancer; race (White patients at highest risk, Black patients at ↑ risk for triple ⊖ breast cancer); *BRCA1/BRCA2* mutations; ↑ estrogen exposure (eg, nulliparity); postmenopausal obesity (adipose tissue converts androstenedione to estrone); ↑ total number of menstrual cycles; absence of breastfeeding; later age of first pregnancy; alcohol intake. In males: *BRCA2* mutation, Klinefelter syndrome.

Axillary lymph node metastasis most important prognostic factor in early-stage disease.

TYPE	CHARACTERISTICS	NOTES
Noninvasive carcinomas		
Ductal carcinoma in situ	Fills ductal lumen (black arrow in B indicates neoplastic cells in duct; blue arrow shows engorged blood vessel). Arises from ductal atypia. Often seen early as microcalcifications on mammography.	Early malignancy without basement membrane penetration. Usually does not produce a mass.
Paget disease	Extension of underlying DCIS/invasive breast cancer up the lactiferous ducts and into the contiguous skin of nipple → eczematous patches over nipple and areolar skin C.	Paget cells = intraepithelial adenocarcinoma cells.
Lobular carcinoma in situ	↓ E-cadherin expression. No mass or calcifications → incidental biopsy finding.	↑ risk of cancer in either breast (vs DCIS, same breast and quadrant).
Invasive carcinomas		
Invasive ductal	Firm, fibrous, "rock-hard" mass with sharp margins and small, glandular, ductlike cells in desmoplastic stroma.	Most common type of invasive breast cancer.
Invasive lobular	↓ E-cadherin expression → orderly row of cells ("single file" D) and no duct formation. Often lacks desmoplastic response.	Often bilateral with multiple lesions in the same location. Lobular carcinoma lacks cadherin and forms lines of cells.
Inflammatory	Dermal lymphatic space invasion → breast pain with warm, swollen, erythematous skin around exaggerated hair follicles (peau d'orange) E.	Poor prognosis (50% survival at 5 years). Often mistaken for mastitis or Paget disease. Usually lacks a palpable mass.

Penile pathology

Peyronie disease

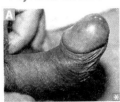

Abnormal curvature of penis 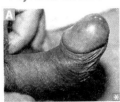 due to fibrous plaque within tunica albuginea. Associated with repeated minor trauma during intercourse. Can cause pain, anxiety, erectile dysfunction. Consider surgical repair or treatment with collagenase injections once curvature stabilizes. Distinct from penile fracture (rupture of tunica albuginea due to forced bending).

Ischemic priapism

Painful sustained erection lasting > 4 hours. Associated with sickle cell disease (sickled RBCs block venous drainage of corpus cavernosum vascular channels), medications (eg, sildenafil, trazodone). Treat immediately with corporal aspiration, intracavernosal phenylephrine, or surgical decompression to prevent ischemia.

Squamous cell carcinoma

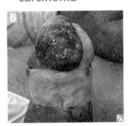

Seen in the US, but more common in Asia, Africa, South America. Most common type of penile cancer B. Precursor in situ lesions: Bowen disease (in penile shaft, presents as leukoplakia "white plaque"), erythroplasia of Queyrat (carcinoma in situ of the glans, presents as erythroplakia "red plaque"), Bowenoid papulosis (carcinoma in situ of unclear malignant potential, presenting as reddish papules). Associated with uncircumcised males and HPV-16.

Cryptorchidism

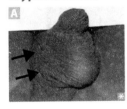

Descent failure of one A or both testes. Impaired spermatogenesis (since sperm develop best at temperatures < 37°C) → subfertility. Can have normal testosterone levels (Leydig cells are mostly unaffected by temperature). Associated with ↑ risk of germ cell tumors. Prematurity ↑ risk of cryptorchidism. ↓ inhibin B, ↑ FSH, ↑ LH; testosterone ↓ in bilateral cryptorchidism, normal in unilateral. Most cases resolve spontaneously; otherwise, orchiopexy performed before 2 years of age.

Testicular torsion

Rotation of testicle around spermatic cord and vascular pedicle. Commonly presents in males 12–18 years old. Associated with congenital inadequate fixation of testis to tunica vaginalis → horizontal positioning of testes ("bell clapper" deformity). May occur after an inciting event (eg, trauma) or spontaneously. Characterized by acute, severe pain, high-riding testis, and absent cremasteric reflex. ⊖ Prehn sign.

Treatment: surgical correction (orchiopexy) within 6 hours, manual detorsion if surgical option unavailable in timeframe. If testis is not viable, orchiectomy. Orchiopexy, when performed, should be bilateral because the contralateral testis is at risk for subsequent torsion.

Varicocele

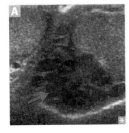

Dilated veins in pampiniform plexus due to ↑ venous pressure; most common cause of scrotal enlargement in adult males. Most often on left side because of ↑ resistance to flow from left gonadal vein drainage into left renal vein. Right-sided varicocele may indicate IVC obstruction (eg, from RCC invading right renal vein). Can cause infertility because of ↑ temperature. Diagnosed by standing clinical exam/Valsalva maneuver (distension on inspection and "bag of worms" on palpation; augmented by Valsalva) or ultrasound A. Does not transilluminate. Treatment: consider surgical ligation or embolization if associated with pain or infertility.

Extragonadal germ cell tumors	Arise in midline locations. In adults, most commonly in retroperitoneum, mediastinum, pineal, and suprasellar regions. In infants and young children, sacrococcygeal teratomas are most common.

Benign scrotal lesions	Testicular masses that can be transilluminated 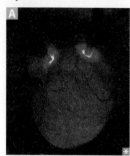 (vs solid testicular tumors).
Hydrocele	Accumulation of serous fluid within tunica vaginalis. Types: ▪ Congenital (communicating)—due to incomplete obliteration of processus vaginalis. Common cause of scrotal swelling in infants. Most resolve spontaneously within 1 year. ▪ Acquired (noncommunicating)—due to infection, trauma, tumor. Termed hematocele if bloody.
Spermatocele	Cyst due to dilated epididymal duct or rete testis. Paratesticular fluctuant nodule on palpation.

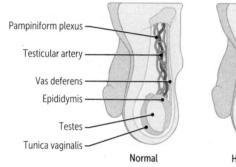
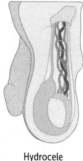
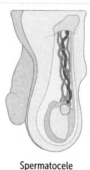
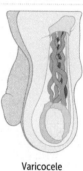
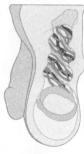

Pampiniform plexus · Testicular artery · Vas deferens · Epididymis · Testes · Tunica vaginalis

Normal　　Hydrocele　　Spermatocele　　Varicocele　　Testicular torsion

Testicular tumors	Germ cell tumors account for ~ 95% of all testicular tumors. Arise from germ cells that produce sperm. Most often occur in young males. Risk factors: cryptorchidism, Klinefelter syndrome. Can present as mixed germ cell tumors. Do not transilluminate. Usually not biopsied (risk of seeding scrotum), removed via radical orchiectomy. Sex cord stromal tumors develop from embryonic sex cord (develops into Sertoli and Leydig cells of seminiferous tubules, theca and granulosa cells of follicle) derivatives. 5% of all testicular tumors. Mostly benign.

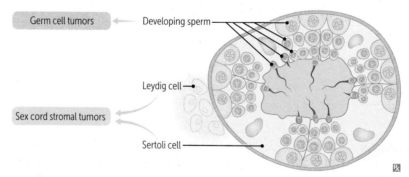

Germ cell tumors ← Developing sperm

Leydig cell

Sex cord stromal tumors

Sertoli cell

Testicular tumors *(continued)*

TYPE	CHARACTERISTICS
Germ cell tumors	
Seminoma	Malignant. Painless, homogenous testicular enlargement. Most common testicular tumor. Analogous to ovarian dysgerminoma. Does not occur in infancy. Large cells in lobules with watery cytoplasm and "fried egg" appearance on histology A, ↑ placental alkaline phosphatase (PLAP). Highly radiosensitive. Late metastasis, excellent prognosis.
Embryonal carcinoma	Malignant. Painful, hemorrhagic mass with necrosis. "Pure" embryonal carcinoma is rare; most commonly mixed with other tumor types. May present with metastases. May be associated with ↑ hCG and normal AFP levels when pure (↑ AFP when mixed). Worse prognosis than seminoma.
Teratoma	Mature teratoma may be malignant in adult males. Benign in children and females.
Yolk sac tumor	Also called endodermal sinus tumor. Malignant, aggressive. Yellow, mucinous. Analogous to ovarian yolk sac tumor. Schiller-Duval bodies resemble primitive glomeruli. ↑ AFP is highly characteristic. Most common testicular tumor in children < 3 years old.
Choriocarcinoma	Malignant. Disordered syncytiotrophoblastic and cytotrophoblastic elements. Hematogenous metastases to lungs and brain. ↑ hCG. May produce gynecomastia, symptoms of hyperthyroidism (hCG and TSH share an identical α subunit and a similar β subunit, which determines their hormonal function).
Non–germ cell tumors	
Leydig cell tumor	Mostly benign. Golden brown color; contains Reinke crystals (eosinophilic cytoplasmic inclusions). Produces androgens or estrogens → precocious puberty, gynecomastia.
Sertoli cell tumor	Also called androblastoma (arises from sex cord **stroma**). Mostly benign.
Primary testicular lymphoma	Malignant, aggressive. Typically diffuse large B-cell lymphoma. Often bilateral. Most common testicular cancer in males > 60 years old.

Hormone levels in germ cell tumors

	SEMINOMA	YOLK SAC TUMOR	CHORIOCARCINOMA	TERATOMA	EMBRYONAL CARCINOMA
PLAP	↑	–	–	–	–
AFP	–	↑↑	–	–/↑	–/↑ (when mixed)
β-hCG	–/↑	–/↑	↑↑	–	↑

Epididymitis and orchitis

Most common causes:
- *C trachomatis* and *N gonorrhoeae* (young males)
- *E coli* and *Pseudomonas* (older males, associated with UTI and BPH)
- Autoimmune (eg, granulomas involving seminiferous tubules)

Epididymitis	Inflammation of epididymis. Presents with localized pain and tenderness over posterior testis. ⊕ Prehn sign (pain relief with scrotal elevation). May progress to involve testis.
Orchitis	Inflammation of testis. Presents with testicular pain and swelling. Mumps orchitis ↑ infertility risk. Rare in males < 10 years old.

Benign prostatic hyperplasia

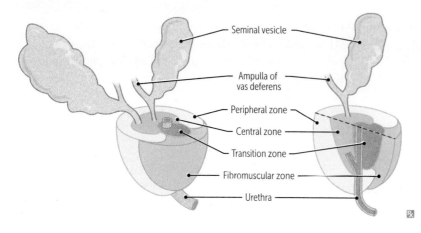

Seminal vesicle

Ampulla of vas deferens

Peripheral zone

Central zone

Transition zone

Fibromuscular zone

Urethra

Common in males > 50 years old. Characterized by smooth, elastic, firm nodular enlargement (hyperplasia not hypertrophy) of transition zone, which compress the urethra into a vertical slit. Not premalignant.

Often presents with ↑ frequency of urination, nocturia, difficulty starting and stopping urine stream, dysuria. May lead to distention and hypertrophy of bladder, hydronephrosis, UTIs. ↑ total PSA, with ↑ fraction of free PSA. PSA is made by prostatic epithelium stimulated by androgens.

Treatment: α_1-antagonists (terazosin, tamsulosin), which cause relaxation of smooth muscle; 5α-reductase inhibitors (eg, finasteride); PDE-5 inhibitors (eg, tadalafil); surgical resection (eg, TURP, ablation).

Prostatitis

Characterized by dysuria, frequency, urgency, low back pain. Warm, tender, enlarged prostate.

Acute bacterial prostatitis—in older males most common bacterium is *E coli*; in young males consider *C trachomatis*, *N gonorrhoeae*.

Chronic prostatitis—either bacterial or nonbacterial (eg, 2° to previous infection, nerve problems, chemical irritation).

Prostatic adenocarcinoma

Common in males > 50 years old. Arises most often from posterior lobe (peripheral zone) of prostate gland and is most frequently diagnosed by ↑ PSA and subsequent needle core biopsies (transrectal, ultrasound-guided). Histologically graded using **Gl**eason grade, which is based on **gl**andular architecture and correlates closely with metastatic potential. Prostatic acid phosphatase (PAP) and PSA are useful tumor markers (↑ total PSA, with ↓ fraction of free PSA). Osteoblastic metastases in bone may develop in late stages, as indicated by lower back pain and ↑ serum ALP and PSA. Metastasis to the spine often occurs via Batson (vertebral) venous plexus.

Control of reproductive hormones

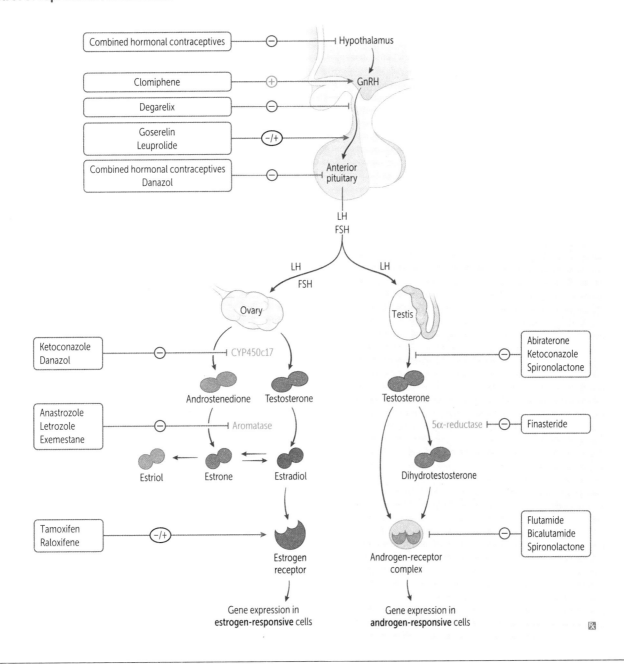

Gonadotropin-releasing hormone analogs	Leuprolide, goserelin, nafarelin, histrelin.
MECHANISM	Act as GnRH agonists when used in pulsatile fashion. When used in continuous fashion, first transiently act as GnRH agonists (tumor flare), but subsequently act as GnRH antagonists (downregulate GnRH receptor in pituitary → ↓ FSH and ↓ LH → ↓ estrogen in females and ↓ testosterone in males). Can be used in lieu of GnRH.
CLINICAL USE	Uterine fibroids, endometriosis, precocious puberty, prostate cancer, infertility. Pulsatile for pregnancy, continuous for cancer.
ADVERSE EFFECTS	Hypogonadism, ↓ libido, erectile dysfunction, nausea, vomiting.

Degarelix	
MECHANISM	GnRH antagonist. No start-up flare.
CLINICAL USE	Prostate cancer.
ADVERSE EFFECTS	Hot flashes, liver toxicity.

Ethinyl estradiol	
MECHANISM	Binds estrogen receptors.
CLINICAL USE	Hypogonadism or ovarian failure, contraception (combined with progestins), HRT in postmenopausal females (use for < 5 years to lower risk of adverse effects).
ADVERSE EFFECTS	↑ risk of endometrial cancer (when given without progesterone), bleeding in postmenopausal patients, hepatic adenoma, breast tenderness, ↑ risk of thrombi. Contraindications—people > 35 years old who smoke tobacco (↑ risk of cardiovascular events), patients with ↑ risk of cardiovascular disease (including history of venous thromboembolism, coronary artery disease, stroke), migraine (especially with aura), breast cancer, liver disease.

Selective estrogen receptor modulators	
Clomiphene	Antagonist at estrogen receptors in hypothalamus. Prevents normal feedback inhibition and ↑ release of LH and FSH from pituitary, which stimulates ovulation. Used to treat infertility due to anovulation (eg, PCOS). May cause hot flashes, ovarian enlargement, multiple simultaneous pregnancies, visual disturbances.
Tamoxifen	Antagonist at breast, partial agonist at uterus, bone. Hot flashes, ↑ risk of thromboembolic events (especially with tobacco smoking), and endometrial hyperplasia and/or cancer. Used to treat and prevent recurrence of ER/PR ⊕ breast cancer and to prevent gynecomastia in patients undergoing prostate cancer therapy.
Raloxifene	Antagonist at breast, uterus; agonist at bone; hot flashes, ↑ risk of thromboembolic events (especially with tobacco smoking), but no increased risk of endometrial cancer (vs tamoxifen, so you can "**relax**"); used primarily to treat postmenopausal osteoporosis.

Aromatase inhibitors	Anastrozole, letrozole, exemestane.
MECHANISM	Inhibit peripheral conversion of androgens to estrogen.
CLINICAL USE	ER ⊕ breast cancer in postmenopausal females. Letrozole can be used to treat infertility from anovulation (eg, PCOS).

Progestins	Levonorgestrel, medroxyprogesterone, etonogestrel, norethindrone, megestrol.
MECHANISM	Bind progesterone receptors, ↓ growth and ↑ vascularization of endometrium, thicken cervical mucus.
CLINICAL USE	Contraception (forms include pill, intrauterine device, implant, depot injection), endometrial cancer, abnormal uterine bleeding. Progestin challenge: presence of bleeding upon withdrawal of progestins excludes anatomic defects (eg, Asherman syndrome) and chronic anovulation without estrogen.

Antiprogestins	Mifepristone, ulipristal.
MECHANISM	Competitive inhibitors of progestins at progesterone receptors.
CLINICAL USE	Termination of pregnancy (mifepristone with misoprostol); emergency contraception (ulipristal).

Contraception	Birth control.		
	METHOD	MECHANISM	NOTES
Hormonal	Estrogen combined with progestins Progestin-only	Prevent ovulation by ↓ GnRH → ↓ LH/FSH → no estrogen surge → no LH surge Progestins also thicken cervical mucus (↓ sperm entry) and thin endometrium (less suitable for implantation)	Forms include pill (OCPs), transdermal patch, vaginal ring
Intrauterine device	Copper IUD (hormone free)	Copper IUD causes local inflammation that is toxic to sperm and ova preventing fertilization and implantation	IUDs ↑ risk for abnormal uterine bleeding; insertion contraindicated in patients with active STI and heavy menstrual bleeding
	Progesterone IUD	Same as progestins	
Surgical	Males—vasectomy Females—tubal ligation	No sperm in ejaculate Sperm cannot reach ova	Irreversible

Tocolytics	Medications that relax the uterus; include Terbutaline (β_2-agonist action), Indomethacin (NSAID), Nifedipine (Ca^{2+} channel blocker). Used to ↓ contraction frequency in preterm labor and allow time for administration of glucocorticoids (to promote fetal lung maturity) or transfer to appropriate medical center with obstetrical care. Keep baby in the **TIN**.

Danazol

MECHANISM	Synthetic androgen that acts as partial agonist at androgen receptors.
CLINICAL USE	Endometriosis, hereditary angioedema.
ADVERSE EFFECTS	Weight gain, edema, acne, hirsutism, masculinization, ↓ HDL levels, hepatotoxicity, idiopathic-intracranial hypertension.

Testosterone, methyltestosterone

MECHANISM	Agonists at androgen receptors.
CLINICAL USE	Treat hypogonadism and promote development of 2° sex characteristics.
ADVERSE EFFECTS	Virilization in females; testicular atrophy in males. Premature closure of epiphyseal plates. Risk of acne, ↑ erythrocytosis, ↑ LDL, ↑ HDL.

Antiandrogens

DRUG	MECHANISM	CLINICAL USE	ADVERSE EFFECTS
Abiraterone	17α-hydroxylase/17,20-lyase inhibitor (↓ steroid synthesis)	Prostate cancer	Hypertension, hypokalemia (↑ mineralocorticoids)
Finasteride	5α-reductase inhibitor (↓ conversion of testosterone to DHT)	BPH, androgenetic alopecia	Gynecomastia, sexual dysfunction
Flutamide, bicalutamide	Nonsteroidal competitive inhibitors at androgen receptor (↓ steroid binding)	Prostate cancer	Gynecomastia, sexual dysfunction
Ketoconazole	17α-hydroxylase/17,20-lyase inhibitor	Prostate cancer	Gynecomastia
Spironolactone	Androgen receptor and 17α-hydroxylase/17,20-lyase inhibitor	PCOS	Amenorrhea

Tamsulosin

MECHANISM	α_1-antagonist selective for $\alpha_{1A/D}$ receptors in prostate (vs vascular α_{1B} receptors) → ↓ smooth muscle tone → ↑ urine flow.
CLINICAL USE	BPH.

Minoxidil

MECHANISM	Direct arteriolar vasodilator.
CLINICAL USE	Androgenetic alopecia, severe refractory hypertension.

Respiratory

"Whenever I feel blue, I start breathing again."

—L. Frank Baum

"Until I feared I would lose it, I never loved to read. One does not love breathing."

—Scout, *To Kill a Mockingbird*

"Love is anterior to life, posterior to death, initial of creation, and the exponent of breath."

—Emily Dickinson

"Love and a cough cannot be concealed."

—Anne Sexton

Group key respiratory, cardiovascular, and renal concepts together for study whenever possible. Respiratory physiology is challenging but high yield, especially as it relates to the pathophysiology of respiratory diseases. Develop a thorough understanding of normal respiratory function. Get familiar with obstructive vs restrictive lung disorders, ventilation/perfusion mismatch, lung volumes, mechanics of respiration, and hemoglobin physiology. Lung cancers and other causes of lung masses are also high yield. Be comfortable reading basic chest x-rays, CT scans, and PFTs.

▶ RESPIRATORY—EMBRYOLOGY

Lung development	Occurs in five stages. Begins with the formation of lung bud from distal end of respiratory diverticulum during week 4 of development. Every pulmonologist can see alveoli.	
STAGE	STRUCTURAL DEVELOPMENT	NOTES
Embryonic (weeks 4–7)	Lung bud → trachea → bronchial buds → mainstem bronchi → secondary (lobar) bronchi → tertiary (segmental) bronchi.	Errors at this stage can lead to tracheoesophageal fistula, tracheal atresia/stenosis and pulmonary agenesis.
Pseudoglandular (weeks 5–17)	Endodermal tubules → terminal bronchioles. Surrounded by modest capillary network.	Respiration impossible, incompatible with life.
Canalicular (weeks 16–25)	Terminal bronchioles → respiratory bronchioles → alveolar ducts. Surrounded by prominent capillary network.	Airways increase in diameter. Pneumocytes develop starting at week 20 (surfactant synthesis). Respiration capable at week 25.
Saccular (week 24–birth)	Alveolar ducts → terminal sacs. Terminal sacs separated by 1° septae.	
Alveolar (week 36–8 years)	Terminal sacs → adult alveoli (due to 2° septation).	In utero, "breathing" occurs via aspiration and expulsion of amniotic fluid → ↑ pulmonary vascular resistance through gestation. At birth, air replaces fluid → ↓ pulmonary vascular resistance.

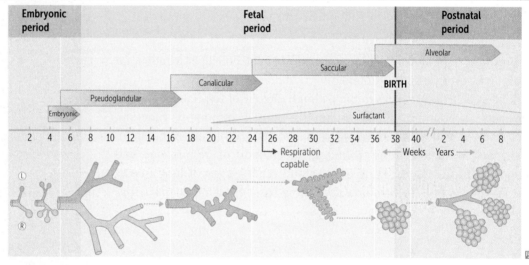

| Choanal atresia | Blockage of posterior nasal opening. Often associated with bony abnormalities of the midface. Most often unilateral. When bilateral, is an emergency and presents with upper airway obstruction, noisy breathing, and/or cyanosis that worsens during feeding and improves with crying. Diagnosed by failure to pass nasogastric tube (beyond the pharynx) and confirmed with CT scan. | Often part of multiple malformation syndromes, such as **CHARGE** syndrome:
 ▪ **C**oloboma of eye
 ▪ **H**eart defects
 ▪ **A**tresia of choanae
 ▪ **R**estricted growth and development
 ▪ **G**enitourinary defects
 ▪ **E**ar defects |

Lung malformations

Pulmonary hypoplasia	Poorly developed bronchial tree with abnormal histology. Associated with congenital diaphragmatic hernia (usually left-sided), bilateral renal agenesis (Potter sequence).
Bronchogenic cysts	Caused by abnormal budding of the foregut and dilation of terminal or large bronchi. Discrete, round, sharply defined, fluid-filled densities on CXR (air-filled if infected). Generally asymptomatic but can drain poorly → airway compression, recurrent respiratory infections.

Club cells

Microciliated; low columnar/cuboidal with secretory granules. Located in bronchioles. Degrade toxins (P-450); secrete surfactant-like component; progenitor for club and ciliated cells.

Alveolar cell types

Type I pneumocytes	Squamous. 97% of alveolar surfaces. Thinly line the alveoli A for optimal gas exchange.	Pores of Kohn—anatomical communications between alveoli that allow for passing of air, fluid, phagocytes, and bacteria (in pneumonia).
Type II pneumocytes	Cuboidal and clustered B. 2 functions: 1. Serve as stem cell precursors for 2 cell types (type I and type II pneumocytes); proliferate during lung damage. 2. Secrete surfactant from lamellar bodies (arrowheads in B). Application of Law of Laplace in alveoli–alveoli have ↑ tendency to collapse on expiration as radius ↓.	Surfactant—↓ alveolar surface tension, ↓ alveolar collapse, ↓ lung recoil, and ↑ compliance. Composed of multiple lecithins, mainly dipalmitoylphosphatidylcholine (DPPC). Synthesis begins ~20 weeks of gestation and achieves mature levels ~35 weeks of gestation. Glucocorticoids are important for fetal surfactant synthesis and lung development. Collapsing pressure = 2 (surface tension)/radius
Alveolar macrophages (dust cells)	Phagocytose foreign materials; release cytokines and alveolar proteases.	Hemosiderin-laden macrophages may be found (eg, pulmonary edema, alveolar hemorrhage).

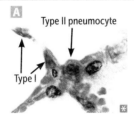
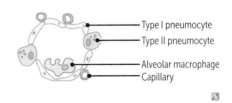
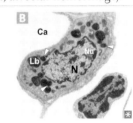

Neonatal respiratory distress syndrome

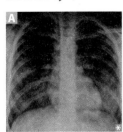

Surfactant deficiency → ↑ surface tension → alveolar collapse ("ground-glass" appearance of lung fields) A.

Risk factors: prematurity, diabetes during pregnancy (due to ↑ fetal insulin), C-section delivery (↓ release of fetal glucocorticoids; less stressful than vaginal delivery).

Treatment: maternal glucocorticoids before birth; exogenous surfactant for infant.

Therapeutic supplemental O_2 → **R**etinopathy of prematurity, **I**ntraventricular hemorrhage, **B**ronchopulmonary dysplasia (**RIB**).

Persistently low O_2 tension → risk of PDA.

Screening tests for fetal lung maturity: lamellar body count and lecithin-sphingomyelin (L/S) ratio in amniotic fluid (≥ 2 is healthy; < 1.5 predictive of NRDS), foam stability index, surfactant-albumin ratio.

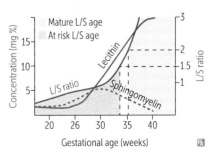

▶ RESPIRATORY—ANATOMY

Respiratory tree

Conducting zone	Large airways consist of nose, pharynx, larynx, trachea, and bronchi. Airway resistance highest in the large- to medium-sized bronchi. Small airways consist of bronchioles that further divide into terminal bronchioles (large numbers in parallel → least airway resistance). Warms, humidifies, and filters air but does not participate in gas exchange → "anatomic dead space." Cartilage and goblet cells extend to the end of bronchi. Pseudostratified ciliated columnar cells primarily make up epithelium of bronchus and extend to beginning of terminal bronchioles, then transition to cuboidal cells. Clear mucus and debris from lungs (mucociliary escalator). Airway smooth muscle cells extend to end of terminal bronchioles (sparse beyond this point).
Respiratory zone	Lung parenchyma; consists of respiratory bronchioles, alveolar ducts, and alveoli. Participates in gas exchange. Mostly cuboidal cells in respiratory bronchioles, then simple squamous cells up to alveoli. Cilia terminate in respiratory bronchioles. Alveolar macrophages clear debris and participate in immune response.

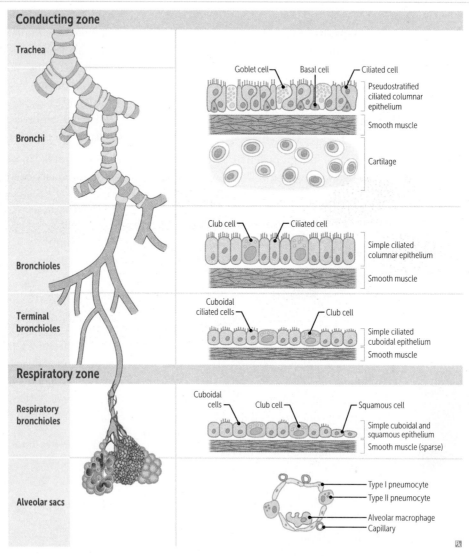

Lung anatomy

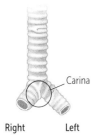

Trachea

Carina

Right bronchus   Left bronchus

Right lung has 3 lobes; Left has less lobes (2) and lingula (homolog of right middle lobe). Instead of a middle lobe, left lung has a space occupied by the heart **A**.

Relation of the pulmonary artery to the bronchus at each lung hilum is described by **RALS**—**R**ight **A**nterior; **L**eft **S**uperior. Carina is posterior to ascending aorta and anteromedial to descending aorta **B**.

Right lung is a more common site for inhaled foreign bodies because right main stem bronchus is wider, more vertical, and shorter than the left. If you aspirate a peanut:

- While supine—usually enters superior segment of right lower lobe or sometimes enters posterior segment of right upper lobe.
- While lying on right side or prone—usually enters right upper lobe.
- While upright—usually enters right lower lobe.

Thoracentesis—pleural space between visceral and parietal pleura. Thoracentesis → remove liquid or air from this space. Needle above the rib → avoid neurovascular bundle below each rib. Avoid below 9th rib → risk of injuring abdominal structures (ie, right hepatic lobe, spleen).

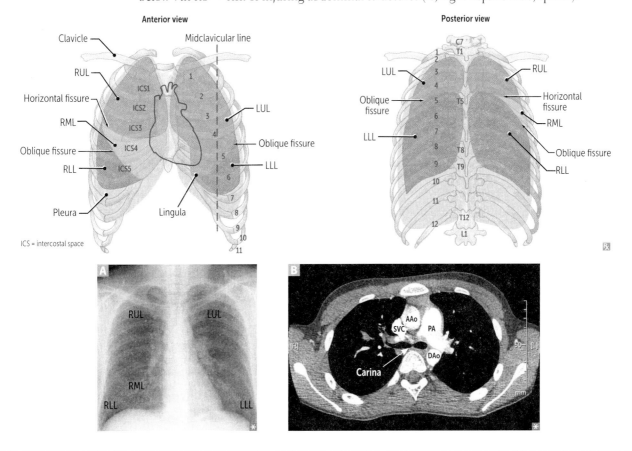

Anterior view

Clavicle
Midclavicular line
RUL
Horizontal fissure
ICS1
ICS2
RML
ICS3
Oblique fissure
ICS4
RLL
ICS5
Pleura
Lingula
LUL
Oblique fissure
LLL

ICS = intercostal space

Posterior view

C7
T1
LUL
RUL
Oblique fissure
T5
Horizontal fissure
RML
LLL
T8
Oblique fissure
T9
RLL
T12
L1

A — RUL LUL RML RLL LLL

B — AAo SVC PA DAo Carina

Diaphragm structures

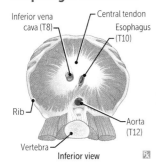

Inferior vena cava (T8)
Central tendon
Esophagus (T10)
Rib
Aorta (T12)
Vertebra
Inferior view

Structures perforating diaphragm:
- At T8: IVC, right phrenic nerve
- At T10: esophagus, vagus (CN 10; 2 trunks)
- At T12: aorta (red), thoracic duct (white), azygos vein (blue) ("At T-1-2 it's the **red, white,** and **blue**")

Diaphragm innervated by C3-5 (phrenic). Pain from diaphragm irritation can be referred to shoulder (C5) and trapezius ridge (C3, 4). Phrenic nerve injury causes elevation of the ipsilateral hemidiaphragm on x-ray.

Number of letters = T level:
  T8: vena cava (**IVC**)
  T10: (**O**)esophagus
  T12: aortic hiatus

I ate (8) **ten eggs at twelve.**

C3, 4, 5 keeps the diaphragm **alive.**

Other bifurcations:
- The Common Carotid bi**four**cates at C4.
- The Trachea bi**four**cates at T4.
- The abdominal aorta bi**four**cates at L4.

▶ RESPIRATORY—PHYSIOLOGY

Lung volumes and capacities	There are 4 volumes and 4 capacities. Note: a capacity is a sum of ≥ 2 physiologic volumes.
Tidal volume	Air that moves into lung with each quiet inspiration, 6–8 mL/kg, typically ~500 mL.
Inspiratory reserve volume	Air that can still be breathed in after normal inspiration
Expiratory reserve volume	Air that can still be breathed out after normal expiration
Residual volume	Air in lung after maximal expiration; RV and any lung capacity that includes RV cannot be measured by spirometry
Inspiratory capacity	IRV + V_T Air that can be breathed in after normal exhalation
Functional residual capacity	RV + ERV Volume of gas in lungs after normal expiration; outward pulling force of chest wall is balanced with inward collapsing force of lungs
Vital capacity	IRV + V_T + ERV Maximum volume of gas that can be expired after a maximal inspiration
Total lung capacity	IRV + V_T + ERV + RV = VC + RV Volume of gas present in lungs after a maximal inspiration

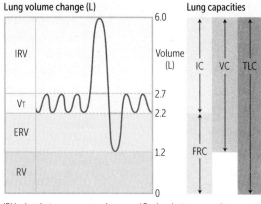

IRV = inspiratory reserve volume
V_T = tidal volume
ERV = expiratory reserve volume
RV = residual volume

IC = inspiratory capacity
FRC = functional residual capacity
VC = vital capacity
TLC = total lung capacity

Work of breathing	Refers to the energy expended or O_2 consumed by respiratory muscles to produce the ventilation needed to meet the body's metabolic demand. Combination of flow-resistive and elastic work (ie, work = force × distance = pressure × volume)—needed to overcome both elastic recoil and airway resistance. Minimized by optimizing respiratory rate (RR) and V_T. ↑ in restrictive diseases (↑ work to overcome elastic recoil resistance achieved with ↑ RR and ↓ V_T) and obstructive diseases (↑ work to overcome airway resistance achieved with ↓ RR and ↑ V_T).

Determination of physiologic dead space	$V_D = V_T \times \dfrac{Pa_{CO_2} - Pe_{CO_2}}{Pa_{CO_2}}$ V_D = physiologic dead space = anatomic dead space of conducting airways plus alveolar dead space; apex of healthy lung is largest contributor of alveolar dead space. V_D = volume of inspired air that does not take part in gas exchange. Pa_{CO_2} = arterial P_{CO_2}. Pe_{CO_2} = expired air P_{CO_2}.	Physiologic dead space—approximately equivalent to anatomic dead space in normal lungs. May be greater than anatomic dead space in lung diseases with ventilation/perfusion mismatch.

Ventilation

Minute ventilation	Abbreviated as V$_E$. Total volume of gas entering and exiting the lungs per minute. V$_E$ = V$_T$ × RR	Normal values: ▪ RR = 12–20 breaths/min ▪ V$_T$ = 500 mL/breath ▪ V$_D$ = 150 mL/breath
Alveolar ventilation	Abbreviated as V$_A$. Total volume of gas that reaches alveoli each minute. V$_A$ = (V$_T$ − V$_D$) × RR	

Lung and chest wall properties	Lung inflation follows a different pressure-volume curve than lung deflation due to the need to overcome surface tension forces during inflation. **Hysteresis**—difference between pressure of inhalation (volume increasing) and pressure of exhalation (volume decreasing). Because of historical reasons and small pressures, pulmonary pressures are always presented in cm H$_2$O.	
Elastic recoil	Tendency for lungs to collapse inward and chest wall to spring outward. At FRC, airway and alveolar pressures equal atmospheric pressure (P$_B$; called zero), and intrapleural pressure is negative (preventing atelectasis). The inward pull of the lung is balanced by the outward pull of the chest wall. System pressure is atmospheric. Pulmonary vascular resistance (PVR) is at a minimum.	
Compliance	Change in lung volume for a change in pressure (ΔV/ΔP). Inversely proportional to wall stiffness and increased by surfactant. ▪ ↑ compliance = lung easier to fill (eg, emphysema, older adults) ▪ ↓ compliance = lung more difficult to fill (eg, pulmonary fibrosis, pneumonia, ARDS, pulmonary edema)	

Pulmonary circulation

Normally a low-resistance, high-compliance system. A ↓ in P_{AO_2} causes hypoxic vasoconstriction that shifts blood away from poorly ventilated regions of lung to well-ventilated regions of lung.

Perfusion limited—O_2 (normal health), CO_2, N_2O. Gas equilibrates early along the length of the capillary. Exchange can be ↑ only if blood flow ↑.

Diffusion limited—O_2 (emphysema, fibrosis), CO. Gas does not equilibrate by the time blood reaches the end of the capillary.

O_2 diffuses slowly, while CO_2 diffuses very rapidly across the alveolar membrane. Disease states that lead to diffusion limitation (eg, pulmonary fibrosis) are more likely to cause early hypoxia than hypercapnia.

Chronic hypoxic vasoconstriction may lead to pulmonary hypertension +/– cor pulmonale.

$$\text{Diffusion } (J) = A \times D_k \times \frac{P_1 - P_2}{\Delta_x} \text{ where}$$

A = area, Δ_x = alveolar wall thickness,
D_k = diffusion coefficient of gas,
$P_1 - P_2$ = difference in partial pressures.
- A ↓ in emphysema.
- Δ_x ↑ in pulmonary fibrosis.

DLCO is the extent to which CO passes from air sacs of lungs into blood.

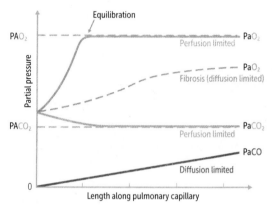

Pa = partial pressure of gas in pulmonary capillary blood
PA = partial pressure of gas in alveolar air

Pulmonary vascular resistance

$$PVR = \frac{P_{pulm\ artery} - P_{L\ atrium}}{\dot{Q}}$$

Remember: $\Delta P = \dot{Q} \times R$, so $R = \Delta P / \dot{Q}$

$$R = \frac{8\eta l}{\pi r^4}$$

$P_{pulm\ artery}$ = pressure in pulmonary artery
$P_{L\ atrium}$ ≈ pulmonary artery occlusion pressure (also called pulmonary capillary wedge pressure)
$\dot{Q}$ = cardiac output (mL/min)
R = resistance
η = viscosity of blood ("stickiness")
l = vessel length
r = vessel radius

Ventilation/perfusion mismatch

Ideally, ventilation (V) is matched to perfusion (Q) per minute (ie, $\dot{V}/\dot{Q}$ ratio = 1) for adequate gas exchange.

Lung zones:
- $\dot{V}/\dot{Q}$ at apex of lung = 3 (wasted ventilation)
- $\dot{V}/\dot{Q}$ at base of lung = 0.6 (wasted perfusion)

Both ventilation and perfusion are greater at the base of the lung than at the apex of the lung.

With exercise (↑ cardiac output), there is vasodilation of apical capillaries → $\dot{V}/\dot{Q}$ ratio approaches 1.

Certain organisms that thrive in high O_2 (eg, TB) flourish in the apex.

$\dot{V}/\dot{Q}$ = 0 = "oirway" obstruction (shunt). In shunt, 100% O_2 does not improve Pao_2 (eg, foreign body aspiration).

$\dot{V}/\dot{Q}$ = ∞ = blood flow obstruction (physiologic dead space). Assuming < 100% dead space, 100% O_2 improves Pao_2 (eg, pulmonary embolus).

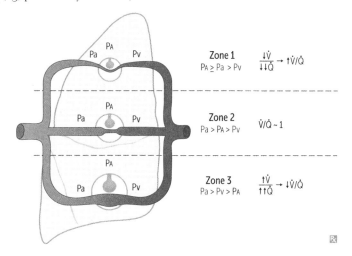

Alveolar gas equation

$$PAO_2 = PIO_2 - \frac{Paco_2}{RQ}$$

$$\approx 150 \text{ mm Hg}^a - \frac{Paco_2}{0.8}$$

[a]At sea level breathing room air

PAO_2 = alveolar Po_2 (mm Hg)
PIO_2 = Po_2 in inspired air (mm Hg)
$Paco_2$ = arterial Pco_2 (mm Hg)
RQ = respiratory quotient = CO_2 produced/ O_2 consumed
A-a gradient = $PAO_2 - Pao_2$. Normal A-a gradient estimated as (age/4) + 4 (eg, for a person < 40 years old, gradient should be < 14).

Carbon dioxide transport

Majority of CO_2 (90%) must be converted to HCO_3^- in RBCs ❶ → carried in the plasma to the lungs (and released via the carbonic anhydrase reaction). CO_2 (5%) also binds to various plasma proteins (carbamino compounds) including the N-terminus of globin in deoxygenated hemoglobin in RBCs → carbaminohemoglobin or $HbCO_2$ ❷. Small percentage of CO_2 (5%) can be dissolved into plasma itself ❸.

In the lungs, Hb oxygenation promotes dissociation of H^+ → equilibrium shifts towards CO_2 production → CO_2 is released from RBCs (Haldane effect).

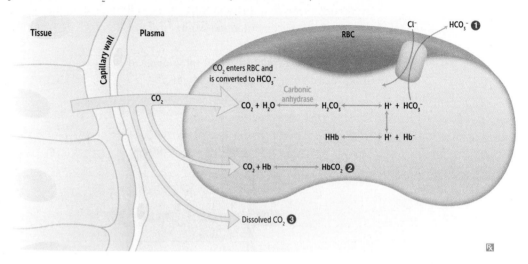

Hypoxia and hypoxemia

Hypoxia	↓ O_2 delivery to tissues. Commonly due to ↓ cardiac output, hypoxemia (insufficient oxygenation of blood with ↓ PaO_2), ischemia, anemia, CO/ cyanide poisoning.

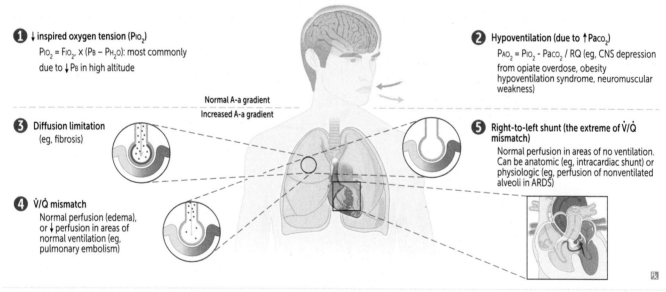

❶ ↓ inspired oxygen tension (PIO_2)
$PIO_2 = FIO_2$ x ($PB – PH_2O$): most commonly due to ↓PB in high altitude

❷ Hypoventilation (due to ↑$PaCO_2$)
$PAO_2 = PIO_2 – PaCO_2 / RQ$ (eg, CNS depression from opiate overdose, obesity hypoventilation syndrome, neuromuscular weakness)

Normal A-a gradient
Increased A-a gradient

❸ Diffusion limitation (eg, fibrosis)

❺ Right-to-left shunt (the extreme of V̇/Q̇ mismatch)
Normal perfusion in areas of no ventilation. Can be anatomic (eg, intracardiac shunt) or physiologic (eg, perfusion of nonventilated alveoli in ARDS)

❹ V̇/Q̇ mismatch
Normal perfusion (edema), or ↓ perfusion in areas of normal ventilation (eg, pulmonary embolism)

Hypoxemia	Insufficient oxygenation of blood (↓ PaO_2).

Hemoglobin 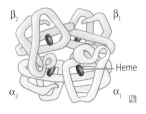	Normal adult hemoglobin (Hb) is composed of 4 polypeptide subunits (2 α and 2 β) that each bind one O_2 molecule. Hb is an allosteric protein that exhibits positive cooperativity when binding to O_2, such that: ▪ Oxygenated Hb has high affinity for O_2 (300×). ▪ Deoxygenated Hb has low affinity for O_2 → promotes release/unloading of O_2.	The protein component of hemoglobin acts as buffer for H^+ ions and CO_2. Myoglobin is composed of a single polypeptide chain associated with one heme moiety. Higher affinity for oxygen than Hb. Essential for full oxygenation of aerobically active muscle.

Oxygen content of blood

O_2 content = (O_2 bound to hemoglobin) + (O_2 solubilized in plasma) = ($1.34 \times Hb \times Sao_2$) + ($0.003 \times Pao_2$).

Sao_2 = percent saturation of arterial blood with O_2.

0.003 = solubility constant of O_2; Pao_2 = partial pressure of O_2 in arterial blood.

Normally 1 g Hb can bind 1.34 mL O_2; normal Hb amount in blood is 15 g/dL.
O_2 binding (carrying) capacity ≈ 20 mL O_2/dL of blood.
With ↓ Hb there is ↓ O_2 content of arterial blood, but no change in O_2 saturation and Pao_2.
O_2 delivery to tissues = cardiac output × O_2 content of blood.

	Hb CONCENTRATION	Sao_2	Pao_2	TOTAL O_2 CONTENT
CO poisoning	Normal	↓ (CO competes with O_2)	Normal	↓
Anemia	↓	Normal	Normal	↓
Polycythemia	↑	Normal	Normal	↑
Methemoglobinemia	Normal	↓ (Fe^{3+} poor at binding O_2)	Normal	↓
Cyanide toxicity	Normal	Normal	Normal	Normal

Oxyhemoglobin dissociation curve

Shifts in oxyhemoglobin dissociation curve (ODC) reflect local tissue oxygen needs. Can be helpful (meets metabolic needs) or harmful (in toxicities, pathophysiologic situations).

Right shift in ODC reflects ↓ Hb affinity for O_2 → ↑ O_2 unloading at tissue. Physiologically occurs with ↑ O_2 needs: exercise, ↓ pH, ↑ temperature/fever, hypoxia (↑ 2,3-BPG); at the cellular level, caused by ↑ H^+ and ↑ CO_2 created by tissue metabolism (Bohr effect).

Left shift in ODC reflects ↑ Hb affinity for O_2 → ↓ O_2 unloading at tissue. Physiologically occurs with ↓ O_2 needs (↓ temperature) and pregnancy (fetal Hb has higher O_2 affinity than adult Hb, and ↑ O_2 binding due to ↓ affinity for 2,3-BPG → left shift, driving O_2 across placenta to fetus). Pathologically occurs with ↑ CO, ↑ MetHb, genetic mutation (↓ 2,3-BPG). **Left is lower.**

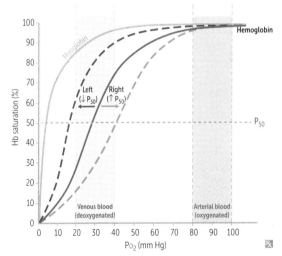

ODC has sigmoidal shape due to positive cooperativity (ie, tetrameric Hb molecule can bind 4 O_2 molecules and has higher affinity for each subsequent O_2 molecule bound). Myoglobin is monomeric and thus does not show positive cooperativity; curve lacks sigmoidal appearance.

Response to high altitude	Constant F_{IO_2} but ↓ P_B → ↓ atmospheric oxygen (P_{IO_2}) → ↓ Pa_{O_2} → ↑ ventilation → ↓ Pa_{CO_2} → respiratory alkalosis → altitude sickness (headaches, nausea, fatigue, lightheadedness, sleep disturbance). Chronic ↑ in ventilation. ↑ erythropoietin (primarily from kidneys) → ↑ Hct and Hb (due to chronic hypoxemia). ↑ 2,3-BPG (binds to Hb → rightward shift of oxyhemoglobin dissociation curve → ↑ O_2 release) due to increased glycolysis and isomerization by BPG mutase. Cellular changes (↑ mitochondria). ↑ renal excretion of HCO_3^- to compensate for respiratory alkalosis (can augment with acetazolamide). Chronic hypoxic pulmonary vasoconstriction → ↑ pulmonary vascular resistance → pulmonary hypertension, right ventricular hypertrophy (RVH).

Response to exercise	↑ HR and ↑ SV → ↑ $\dot{Q}$ → ↑ pulmonary blood flow → ↑ $\dot{V}/\dot{Q}$ ratio from base to apex (becoming more uniform). ↑ cellular respiration → ↑ CO_2 production and ↓ pH at tissues → right shift of ODC → tissue offloading of more O_2 → ↑ O_2 consumption (↑ O_2 difference in arteries and veins). ↑ RR to meet ↑ O_2 demand and remove excess CO_2 → ↑ pulmonary blood flow. Pa_{O_2} and Pa_{CO_2} are maintained by homeostatic mechanisms. ↓ $P\bar{v}_{O_2}$ due to ↑ O_2 consumption. ↑ $P\bar{v}_{CO_2}$ due to ↑ CO_2 production.

Methemoglobin	Iron in Hb is normally in a reduced state (ferrous Fe^{2+}; "just the 2 of **us**"). Oxidized form of Hb (ferric, Fe^{3+}) has reduced O_2 affinity → tissue hypoxia from ↓ O_2 saturation and ↓ O_2 content. Fe^{3+} also has ↑ affinity for cyanide. This oxidized form is called methemoglobinemia. While typical concentrations are 1–2%, methemoglobinemia will occur at higher levels and may present with cyanosis (does not improve with supplemental O_2) and with chocolate-colored blood.	Dapsone, local anesthetics (eg, benzocaine), and nitrites (eg, from dietary intake or polluted water sources) cause poisoning by oxidizing Fe^{2+} to Fe^{3+}. **Meth**emoglobinemia can be treated with **meth**ylene blue and vitamin C.

	Cyanide	Carbon monoxide
Cyanide vs carbon monoxide poisoning	Both inhibit aerobic metabolism via inhibition of complex IV of ETC (cytochrome c oxidase) → hypoxia that does not fully correct with supplemental O_2 and ↑ anaerobic metabolism.	
EXPOSURE	Synthetic product combustion, amygdalin ingestion (found in apricot seeds), cyanide ingestion (eg, in suicide attempts), fire victims. Risk of cyanide toxicity with use of nitroprusside in hypertensive emergencies.	From tobacco smoke, furnaces, space heaters, fires, motor exhaust (incomplete combustion of carbon-containing compounds). Odorless, tasteless, colorless, non-irritating. Leading worldwide cause of death by poisoning.
PRESENTATION	Headache, dyspnea, drowsiness, seizure, coma. Skin may appear flushed ("cherry red") due to bright red venous blood. Venules in retina appear bright red. Breath may have bitter almond odor.	Headache, vomiting, confusion, visual disturbances, coma. May have cherry-red skin with bullous skin lesions. Multiple victims may be involved (eg, family due to faulty furnace).
LABS	Normal PaO_2. ↑ lactate → anion gap metabolic acidosis.	Normal PaO_2. ↑ carboxyhemoglobin on co-oximetry (cannot be distinguished with pulse oximetry). Classically associated with bilateral globus pallidus lesions on MRI 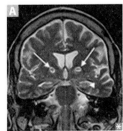, although can rarely be seen with cyanide toxicity.
EFFECT ON OXYGEN-HEMOGLOBIN CURVE	Cyanide binds cytochrome a3 in complex IV → ample O_2 but cannot be used due to ineffective oxidative phosphorylation. Curve normal. O_2 saturation may appear normal initially.	Left shift in ODC → ↑ affinity for O_2 → ↓ O_2 unloading in tissues. Binds competitively to Hb with > 200× greater affinity than O_2 to form carboxyhemoglobin → ↓ %O_2 saturation of Hb.
TREATMENT	Decontamination (eg, remove clothing). 100% O_2 is ineffective; instead give treatments to remove and excrete the cyanide: ▪ Hydroxocobalamin (binds cyanide → cyanocobalamin → renal excretion) ▪ Nitrites (oxidize Hb → methemoglobin → binds cyanide → cyanomethemoglobin → ↓ toxicity) ▪ Sodium thiosulfate (↑ cyanide conversion to thiocyanate → renal excretion)	Give 100% O_2 to overcome the increased affinity for CO. Hyperbaric oxygen if severe. CO-Hb half-life is ~300 mins → ↓ to ~80 mins on 100% O_2 → ↓ to ~20 mins in a hyperbaric O_2 chamber. If concurrent CO and cyanide poisoning are suspected (eg, in victims of a fire), give hydroxocobalamin, rather than nitrites or sodium thiosulfate, to avoid increasing methylglobin.

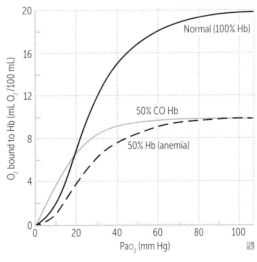

Rhinosinusitis

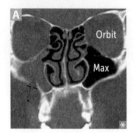

Obstruction of sinus drainage into nasal cavity → inflammation and pain over affected area. Typically affects maxillary sinuses, which drain against gravity due to ostia located superomedially (red arrow points to fluid-filled right maxillary sinus in A).

Superior meatus—drains posterior ethmoid; middle meatus—drains frontal, maxillary, and anterior ethmoid; inferior meatus—drains nasolacrimal duct.

Acute rhinosinusitis is most commonly caused by viruses (eg, rhinovirus); may lead to superimposed bacterial infection, most commonly nontypeable *H influenzae*, *S pneumoniae*, *M catarrhalis*.

Paranasal sinus infections may extend to the orbits, cavernous sinus, and brain, causing complications (eg, orbital cellulitis, cavernous sinus syndrome, meningitis).

Epistaxis

Nose bleed. Most commonly occurs in anterior segment of nostril (**Kiesselbach plexus** at caudal septum). Life-threatening hemorrhages occur in posterior segment (sphenopalatine artery, a branch of maxillary artery). Common causes include foreign body, trauma, allergic rhinitis, and nasal angiofibromas (common in adolescent males).

Kiesselbach drives his **Lexus** with his **LEGS**: superior **L**abial artery, anterior and posterior **E**thmoidal arteries, **G**reater palatine artery, **S**phenopalatine artery.

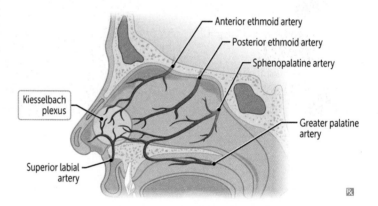

Head and neck cancer

Mostly squamous cell carcinoma. Risk factors include tobacco, alcohol, HPV-16 (oropharyngeal), EBV (nasopharyngeal). Field cancerization: carcinogen damages wide mucosal area → multiple tumors develop independently after exposure.

Nasopharyngeal carcinoma may present with unilateral nasal obstruction, discharge, epistaxis. Eustachian tube obstruction may lead to otitis media +/– effusion, hearing loss.

Laryngeal papillomatosis—also called recurrent respiratory papillomatosis. Benign laryngeal tumor, commonly affecting areas of stratified squamous epithelium such as the true vocal cords, especially in children (possibly from HPV transmitted from mother to baby during labor). Associated with HPV-6 and HPV-11. Symptoms may guide location of pathology (supraglottic → dysphagia, infraglottic/glottic → hoarseness).

Pulmonary emboli	Obstruction of the pulmonary artery or its branches by foreign material (usually thrombus) that originated elsewhere. Affected alveoli are ventilated but not perfused ($\dot{V}/\dot{Q}$ mismatch). May present with sudden-onset dyspnea, pleuritic chest pain, tachypnea, tachycardia, hypoxemia, respiratory alkalosis. Large emboli or saddle embolus (red arrows show filling defects in 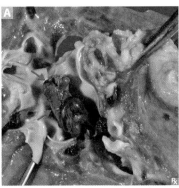) may cause sudden death due to clot preventing blood from filling LV and increased RV size further compromising LV filling (obstructive shock). CT pulmonary angiography is imaging test of choice for PE (look for filling defects 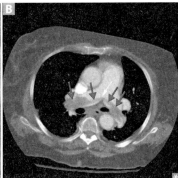). ECG may show sinus tachycardia or, less commonly, S1Q3T3 abnormality.

Lines of Zahn 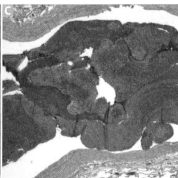 are interdigitating areas of pink (platelets, fibrin) and red (RBCs) found only in thrombi formed before death; help distinguish pre- and postmortem thrombi.

Treatment: anticoagulation (eg, heparin, direct thrombin/factor Xa inhibitors), IVC filter (if anticoagulation is contraindicated).

Types: Fat, Air, Thrombus, Bacteria, Amniotic fluid, Tumor. An embolus moves like a **FAT BAT**.

Fat emboli—associated with long bone fractures and liposuction; classic triad of hypoxemia, neurologic abnormalities, petechial rash.

Air emboli—nitrogen bubbles precipitate in ascending divers (caisson disease/decompression sickness); treat with hyperbaric O_2; or, can be iatrogenic 2° to invasive procedures (eg, central line placement).

Amniotic fluid emboli—typically occurs during labor or postpartum, but can be due to uterine trauma. Can lead to DIC. Rare, but high mortality.

Mediastinal pathology	Normal mediastinum contains heart, thymus, lymph nodes, esophagus, and aorta.
Mediastinal masses	Some pathologies (eg, lymphoma, lung cancer, abscess) can occur in any compartment, but there are common associations: ▪ Anterior—4 T's: thyroid (substernal goiter), thymic neoplasm, teratoma, "terrible" lymphoma. ▪ Middle—metastases, hiatal hernia, bronchogenic cysts. ▪ Posterior—esophageal cancer (may present as mass in, or spread to, middle mediastinum), neurogenic tumor (eg, neurofibroma), multiple myeloma.
Mediastinitis	Inflammation of mediastinal tissues. Commonly due to postoperative complications of cardiothoracic procedures (≤ 14 days), esophageal perforation (common with repetitive vomiting), or contiguous spread of odontogenic/retropharyngeal infection. Chronic mediastinitis—also called fibrosing mediastinitis; due to ↑ proliferation of connective tissue in mediastinum. *Histoplasma capsulatum* is common cause. Clinical features: fever, tachycardia, leukocytosis, chest pain, and sternal wound drainage.
Pneumomediastinum	Presence of gas (usually air) in the mediastinum. Can either be spontaneous (due to rupture of pulmonary bleb) or 2° (eg, trauma, iatrogenic, Boerhaave syndrome). Ruptured alveoli allow tracking of air into the mediastinum via peribronchial and perivascular sheaths. Clinical features: chest pain, dyspnea, voice change, subcutaneous emphysema, ⊕ Hamman sign (crepitus on cardiac auscultation).

Flow-volume loops

FLOW-VOLUME PARAMETER	Normal	Obstructive lung disease	Restrictive lung disease
RV		↑	↓
FRC		↑	↓
TLC		↑	↓
FEV$_1$	>80% predicted	↓↓	↓
FVC	>80% predicted	Normal or ↓	↓
FEV$_1$/FVC	>70%	↓ FEV$_1$ decreased more than FVC	Normal or ↑ FEV$_1$ decreased proportionately to FVC

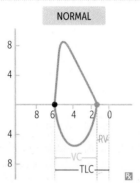

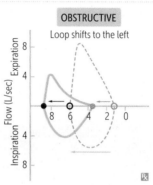

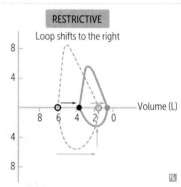

Obstructive lung diseases	Obstruction of air flow (↓↓ FEV$_1$, ↓ FVC ↓ FEV$_1$/FVC ratio) → air trapping in lungs (↑ RV, →↑ FRC and ↑ TLC) due to premature airway closure at high lung volumes. Includes COPD (chronic bronchitis and emphysema), asthma, and bronchiectasis.
Chronic obstructive pulmonary disease	Often due to tobacco use (most important risk factor), pollutants, or allergens. Includes chronic bronchitis and emphysema, which often co-exist. Exacerbation: acute worsening of symptoms, often associated with viral or bacterial upper respiratory tract infection.
Chronic bronchitis	
DIAGNOSIS	Clinical diagnosis. Criteria: productive cough for ≥ 3 months in ≥ 2 consecutive years. May also have dyspnea, wheezes, crackles (due to mucus), cyanosis (hypoxemia due to shunting), 2° polycythemia. Leads to metaplasia of pseudostratified ciliated columnar epithelium into stratified squamous epithelium.
MECHANISMS	Hypertrophy and hyperplasia of mucus-secreting glands in bronchi.
NOTES	↑ Reid index (thickness of mucosal gland layer to thickness of wall between epithelium and cartilage) > 50%.
Emphysema	
DIAGNOSIS	Radiologic or biopsy diagnosis. CXR: barrel chest, ↑ AP diameter (best seen in lateral **A**), flattened diaphragm, ↑ lung field lucency.
MECHANISMS	Alveolar wall destruction **B** → ↑ compliance of lung, ↓ recoil, and damage to alveolar capillary membrane → ↓ DLCO; results in ↑ air space. Centriacinar—spares distal alveoli, frequently in upper lobes. Associated with tobacco smoking **C D**. Panacinar—affects respiratory bronchioles and alveoli, frequently in lower lobes. Associated with α$_1$-antitrypsin deficiency.

Obstructive lung diseases *(continued)*

NOTES	Mediated by oxidative stress, chronic inflammation (CD8+ T cells, neutrophils, and macrophages), and imbalance of proteases and antiproteases ($\uparrow$ elastase activity → $\uparrow$ loss of elastic fibers → alveolar destruction). Defect/deficiency/absence of α_1-antitrypsin (antiprotease that inhibits neutrophil elastase) leads to unopposed elastase activity.

Asthma

Intermittent obstructive lung disease often triggered by allergens, viral URIs, stress. Associated with atopy.

NSAID- or aspirin-exacerbated respiratory disease—asthma, nasal polyps, and COX-inhibitor sensitivity (leukotriene overproduction → airway constriction) (Samter's triad).

DIAGNOSIS	Clinical diagnosis. Intermittent episodes of dyspnea, coughing, wheezing, tachypnea. Diagnosis supported by spirometry (obstructive pattern with bronchodilator response, but may be normal when not in exacerbation) +/– methacholine challenge.
MECHANISMS	Type I hypersensitivity reaction → smooth muscle hypertrophy and hyperplasia. Hyperresponsive bronchi → reversible bronchoconstriction. Mucus plugging E.
OTHER	Curschmann spirals F—shed epithelium forms whorled mucus plugs. Charcot-Leyden crystals G—eosinophilic, hexagonal, double-pointed crystals formed from breakdown of eosinophils in sputum.

Bronchiectasis

Obstructive lung disease. Most commonly associated with cystic fibrosis.

DIAGNOSIS	Characterized by chronic cough and daily purulent sputum production. Often have recurrent pulmonary infections. Confirmed by imaging demonstrating airway dilation and bronchial thickening. Supported by obstructive PFT pattern.
PATHOPHYSIOLOGY	Initial insult of pulmonary infection combined with obstruction or impaired clearance → dysregulated host response → bronchial inflammation → permanently dilated airways.
NOTES	Many etiologies, including airway obstruction (eg, foreign body aspiration, mass), poor ciliary motility (eg, tobacco smoking, Kartagener syndrome), cystic fibrosis (H shows a coughed up inspissated mucus plug), allergic bronchopulmonary aspergillosis, pulmonary infections (eg, *Mycobacterium avium*).

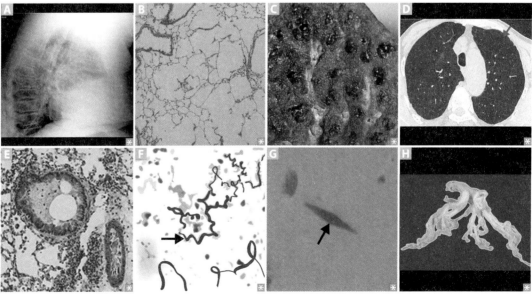

Restrictive lung diseases

May lead to ↓ lung volumes (↓ FVC and TLC). PFTs: normal or ↑ FEV_1/FVC ratio. Patient presents with short, shallow breaths, crackles (velcro-type).

Types:
- Altered respiratory mechanics (extrapulmonary, normal D_{LCO}, normal A-a gradient):
  - Respiratory muscle weakness—polio, myasthenia gravis, Guillain-Barré syndrome, ALS
  - Chest wall abnormalities—scoliosis, severe obesity
- Diffuse parenchymal lung diseases, also called interstitial lung diseases (pulmonary, ↓ D_{LCO}, ↑ A-a gradient):
  - Pneumoconioses (eg, coal workers' pneumoconiosis, silicosis, asbestosis)
  - Sarcoidosis: bilateral hilar lymphadenopathy, noncaseating granulomas; ↑ ACE and Ca^{2+}
  - Idiopathic pulmonary fibrosis
  - Granulomatosis with polyangiitis
  - Pulmonary Langerhans cell histiocytosis (eosinophilic granuloma)
  - Hypersensitivity pneumonitis
  - Drug toxicity (eg, bleomycin, busulfan, amiodarone, methotrexate)
  - Acute respiratory distress syndrome
  - **Radiation-induced lung injury**—associated with proinflammatory cytokine release (eg, TNF-α, IL-1, IL-6). May be asymptomatic but most common symptoms are dry cough and dyspnea +/– low-grade fever. Acute radiation pneumonitis develops within 3–12 weeks (exudative phase); radiation fibrosis may develop after 6–12 months.

Idiopathic pulmonary fibrosis

Progressive fibrotic lung disease of unknown etiology. May involve multiple cycles of lung injury, inflammation, and fibrosis. Associated with tobacco smoking, environmental pollutants, genetic defects.

Findings: progressive dyspnea, fatigue, nonproductive cough, crackles, clubbing. Imaging shows peripheral reticular opacities with traction bronchiectasis +/– "honeycomb" appearance of lung (advanced disease). Histologic pattern: usual interstitial pneumonia. ↓ type 1 pneumocytes, ↑ type 2 pneumocytes, ↑ fibroblasts.

Complications: pulmonary hypertension, right heart failure, arrhythmias, coronary artery disease, respiratory failure, lung cancer.

Hypersensitivity pneumonitis

Mixed type III/IV hypersensitivity reaction to environmental antigens such as thermophilic *Actinomyces* and *Aspergillus*. Often seen in farmers and bird-fanciers. Acutely, causes dyspnea, cough, chest tightness, fever, headache. Often self-limiting if stimulus is removed. Chronically, leads to irreversible fibrosis with noncaseating granuloma, alveolar septal thickening, traction bronchiectasis.

Sarcoidosis

Characterized by immune-mediated, widespread noncaseating granulomas **A**, elevated serum ACE levels, and elevated CD4/CD8 ratio in bronchoalveolar lavage fluid. More common in Black females. Often asymptomatic except for enlarged lymph nodes. CXR shows bilateral adenopathy and coarse reticular opacities **B**, including ground glass opacities; CT of the chest better demonstrates the extensive hilar and mediastinal adenopathy **C**.

Associated with **B**ell palsy, parotid enlargement, granulomas (noncaseating epithelioid, containing microscopic **S**chaumann and **A**steroid bodies), **R**heumatoid arthritis–like arthropathy, ↑ **C**alcium, **O**cular uveitis, **I**nterstitial fibrosis, vitamin **D** activation (due to ↑ 1α-hydroxylase in macrophages), **S**kin changes (eg, lupus pernio, erythema nodosum) (**SARCOIDS**).

Treatment: glucocorticoids (if symptomatic).

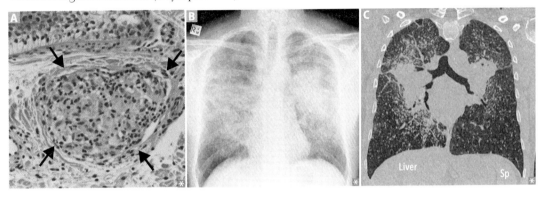

Mesothelioma

Malignancy of the pleura associated with asbestosis. May result in hemorrhagic pleural effusion (exudative), pleural thickening.

Histology may show psammoma bodies. EM may show polygonal tumor cells with microvilli, desmosomes, tonofilaments. Calretinin and cytokeratin 5/6 ⊕ in almost all mesotheliomas, ⊖ in most carcinomas. Tobacco smoking is not a risk factor.

Pneumoconioses	**Asbestos** is from the **roof** (was common in insulation), but affects the **base** (lower lobes). **Silica**, **coal**, and **berries** are from the **base** (earth), but affect the **roof** (upper lobes).	
Asbestos-related disease	Asbestos causes asbestosis (pulmonary fibrosis), pleural disease, malignancies. Associated with shipbuilding, roofing, plumbing. "Ivory white," calcified, supradiaphragmatic and pleural **A** plaques are pathognomonic. Risk of bronchogenic carcinoma > risk of mesothelioma. ↑ risk of Caplan syndrome (rheumatoid arthritis and pneumoconioses with intrapulmonary nodules).	Affects lower lobes. Asbestos (ferruginous) bodies are golden-brown fusiform rods resembling dumbbells, found in alveolar sputum sample, visualized using Prussian blue stain **B**, often obtained by bronchoalveolar lavage. ↑ risk of pleural effusions.
Berylliosis	Associated with exposure to beryllium in aerospace and manufacturing industries. Granulomatous (noncaseating) **C** on histology and therefore occasionally responsive to glucocorticoids. ↑ risk of cancer and cor pulmonale.	Affects upper lobes.
Coal workers' pneumoconiosis	Prolonged coal dust exposure → macrophages laden with carbon → inflammation and fibrosis. Also called black lung disease. ↑ risk of Caplan syndrome.	Affects upper lobes. Small, rounded nodular opacities seen on imaging. Anthracosis—asymptomatic condition found in many urban dwellers exposed to sooty air.
Silicosis	Associated with **sand**blasting, **found**ries, **mines**. Macrophages respond to silica and release fibrogenic factors, leading to fibrosis. It is thought that silica may disrupt phagolysosomes and impair macrophages, increasing susceptibility to TB. ↑ risk of lung cancer, cor pulmonale, and Caplan syndrome.	Affects upper lobes. "Eggshell" calcification of hilar lymph nodes on CXR. The **silly egg sand**wich **I found** is **mine**!

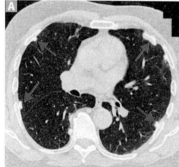
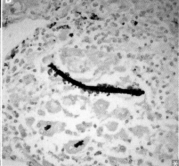
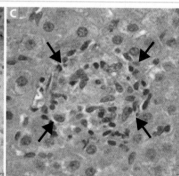

Acute respiratory distress syndrome

PATHOPHYSIOLOGY	Alveolar insult → release of pro-inflammatory cytokines → neutrophil recruitment, activation, and release of toxic mediators (eg, reactive oxygen species, proteases, etc) → capillary endothelial damage and ↑ vessel permeability → leakage of protein-rich fluid into alveoli → formation of intra-alveolar hyaline membranes (arrows in 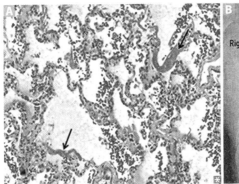) and noncardiogenic pulmonary edema (normal PCWP) → ↓ compliance and $\dot{V}/\dot{Q}$ mismatch → hypoxic vasoconstriction → ↑ pulmonary vascular resistance. Loss of surfactant also contributes to alveolar collapse (eg, preterm infants, drowning).
CAUSES	Sepsis (most common), aspiration pneumonia, burns, trauma, pancreatitis, drowning injuries.
DIAGNOSIS	Diagnosis of exclusion with the following criteria (**ARDS**): ▪ **A**bnormal chest X-ray (bilateral lung opacities) 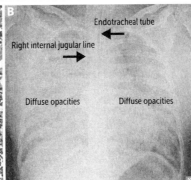 ▪ **R**espiratory failure within 1 week of alveolar insult ▪ **D**ecreased Pa_{O_2}/F_{IO_2} (ratio < 300, hypoxemia due to ↑ intrapulmonary shunting and diffusion abnormalities) ▪ **S**ymptoms of respiratory failure are not due to HF/fluid overload
CONSEQUENCES	Impaired gas exchange, ↓ lung compliance; pulmonary hypertension.
MANAGEMENT	Treat the underlying cause. Mechanical ventilation: ↓ tidal volume, ↑ PEEP (keeps alveoli open during expiration).

Labels for image B: Endotracheal tube; Right internal jugular line; Diffuse opacities; Diffuse opacities

Sleep apnea	Repeated cessation of breathing > 10 seconds during sleep → disrupted sleep → daytime somnolence. Diagnosis confirmed by sleep study (polysomnography). Nocturnal hypoxia → systemic and pulmonary hypertension, arrhythmias (atrial fibrillation/flutter), sudden death. Hypoxia → ↑ EPO release → ↑ erythropoiesis.
Obstructive sleep apnea	Respiratory effort against airway obstruction. Pa_{O_2} is usually normal during the day. Associated with obesity, loud snoring, daytime sleepiness. Usually caused by excess parapharyngeal/oropharyngeal tissue in adults, adenotonsillar hypertrophy in children. Treatment: weight loss, CPAP, dental devices, hypoglossal nerve stimulation, upper airway surgery.
Central sleep apnea	Impaired respiratory effort due to CNS injury/toxicity, Congestive HF, opioids. May be associated with Cheyne-Stokes respirations (oscillations between apnea and hyperpnea). Treatment: positive airway pressure.
Obesity hypoventilation syndrome	Also called Pickwickian syndrome. Obesity (BMI ≥ 30 kg/m²) → hypoventilation → ↑ Pa_{CO_2} during waking hours (retention); ↓ Pa_{O_2} and ↑ Pa_{CO_2} during sleep. Treatment: weight loss, positive airway pressure.

Pulmonary hypertension	Elevated mean pulmonary artery pressure (> 20 mm Hg) at rest. Results in arteriosclerosis, medial hypertrophy, intimal fibrosis of pulmonary arteries, plexiform lesions. ↑ pulmonary vascular resistance → ↑ RV pressure → RVH (parasternal heave on examination), RV failure.

ETIOLOGIES

Pulmonary arterial hypertension (group 1)	Often idiopathic. Females > males. Heritable PAH can be due to an inactivating mutation in *BMPR2* gene (normally inhibits vascular smooth muscle proliferation); poor prognosis. Pulmonary vasculature endothelial dysfunction results in ↑ vasoconstrictors (eg, endothelin) and ↓ vasodilators (eg, NO and prostacyclins). Other causes include drugs (eg, amphetamines, cocaine), connective tissue disease, HIV infection, portal hypertension, congenital heart disease, schistosomiasis.
Left heart disease (group 2)	Causes include systolic/diastolic dysfunction and valvular disease.
Lung diseases or hypoxia (group 3)	Destruction of lung parenchyma (eg, COPD), lung inflammation/fibrosis (eg, interstitial lung diseases), hypoxemic vasoconstriction (eg, obstructive sleep apnea, living in high altitude).
Chronic thromboembolic (group 4)	Recurrent microthrombi → ↓ cross-sectional area of pulmonary vascular bed.
Multifactorial (group 5)	Causes include hematologic, systemic, and metabolic disorders, along with compression of the pulmonary vasculature by a tumor.

Physical findings in select lung diseases

ABNORMALITY	BREATH SOUNDS	PERCUSSION	FREMITUS	TRACHEAL DEVIATION
Pleural effusion	↓	Dull	↓	None if small Away from side of lesion if large
Atelectasis	↓	Dull	↓	Toward side of lesion
Simple pneumothorax	↓	Hyperresonant	↓	None
Tension pneumothorax	↓	Hyperresonant	↓	Away from side of lesion
Consolidation (lobar pneumonia, pulmonary edema)	Bronchial breath sounds; late inspiratory crackles, egophony, whispered pectoriloquy	Dull	↑	None

Digital clubbing	Increased angle between nail bed and nail plate (> 180°) 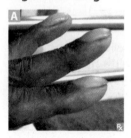. Pathophysiology not well understood; in patients with intrapulmonary shunt, platelets and megakaryocytes become lodged in digital vasculature → local release of PDGF and VEGF. Can be hereditary or acquired. Causes include respiratory diseases (eg, idiopathic pulmonary fibrosis, cystic fibrosis, bronchiectasis, lung cancer), cardiovascular diseases (eg, cyanotic congenital heart disease), infections (eg, lung abscess, TB), and others (eg, IBD). Not typically associated with COPD or asthma.

Atelectasis

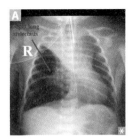

Alveolar collapse (right upper lobe collapse against mediastinum in 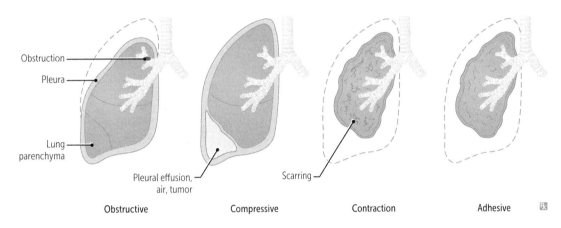). Multiple causes:
- Obstructive—airway obstruction prevents new air from reaching distal airways, old air is resorbed (eg, foreign body, mucous plug, tumor)
- Compressive—external compression on lung decreases lung volumes (eg, space-occupying lesion, pleural effusion)
- Contraction (cicatrization)—scarring of lung parenchyma that distorts alveoli (eg, sarcoidosis)
- Adhesive—due to lack of surfactant (eg, NRDS in premature infants)

Decreased via incentive spirometry or ↑ PEEP during mechanical ventilation.

Obstructive	Compressive	Contraction	Adhesive

Pleural effusions

Excess accumulation of fluid A between pleural layers → restricted lung expansion during inspiration. Can be treated with thoracentesis to remove/reduce fluid B. Based on the Light's criteria, fluid is consistent with an exudate if pleural fluid protein/serum protein > 0.5, pleural fluid LDH/serum LDH > 0.6, or pleural fluid LDH > 2/3 upper limit of normal serum LDH.

Exudate

Cloudy fluid (cellular). Due to infection (eg, pneumonia, tuberculosis), malignancy, connective tissue disease, lymphatic (chylothorax), trauma. Often requires drainage due to ↑ risk of infection.

Transudate

Clear fluid (hypocellular). Due to ↑ hydrostatic pressure (eg, HF, Na⁺ retention) and/or ↓ oncotic pressure (eg, nephrotic syndrome, cirrhosis).

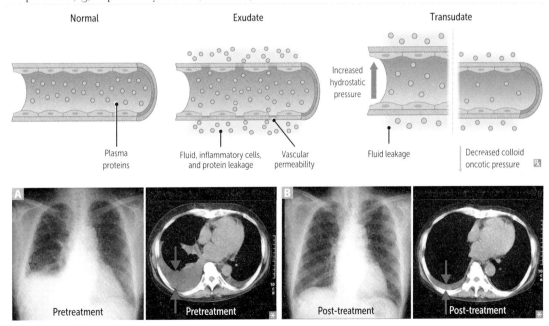

Normal	Exudate	Transudate

Pneumothorax	Accumulation of air in pleural space 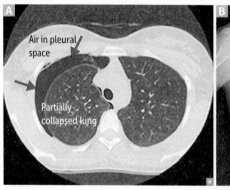. Dyspnea, uneven chest expansion. Chest pain, ↓ tactile fremitus, hyperresonance, and diminished breath sounds, all on the affected side.
Primary spontaneous pneumothorax	Due to rupture of apical subpleural bleb or cysts. Occurs most frequently in tall, thin, young males. Associated with tobacco smoking and vaping.
Secondary spontaneous pneumothorax	Due to diseased lung (eg, bullae in emphysema, Marfan syndrome, infections), mechanical ventilation with use of high pressures → barotrauma.
Traumatic pneumothorax	Caused by blunt (eg, rib fracture), penetrating (eg, gunshot), or iatrogenic (eg, central line placement, lung biopsy, barotrauma due to mechanical ventilation) trauma.
Tension pneumothorax	Can be from any of the above. Air enters pleural space but cannot exit. Increasing trapped air → tension pneumothorax. Trachea deviates away from affected lung 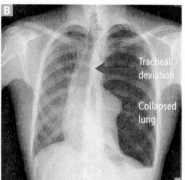. May lead to increased intrathoracic pressure → mediastinal displacement → kinking of IVC → ↓ venous return → ↓ cardiac output, obstructive shock (hypotension, tachycardia), jugular venous distention. Needs immediate needle decompression and chest tube placement.

Pneumonia

TYPE	TYPICAL ORGANISMS	CHARACTERISTICS
Lobar pneumonia	*S pneumoniae* (most common), *Legionella*, *Klebsiella*.	Intra-alveolar exudate → consolidation A; may involve entire lobe or the whole lung.
Bronchopneumonia	*S pneumoniae, S aureus, H influenzae, Klebsiella*.	Acute inflammatory infiltrates from bronchioles into adjacent alveoli; patchy distribution involving ≥ 1 lobe.
Interstitial (atypical) pneumonia	*Mycoplasma, Chlamydophila pneumoniae, Chlamydophila psittaci, Legionella, Coxiella burnetii*, viruses (RSV, CMV, influenza, adenovirus).	Diffuse patchy inflammation localized to interstitial areas at alveolar walls; CXR shows bilateral multifocal opacities B. Generally follows a more indolent course ("walking" pneumonia).
Cryptogenic organizing pneumonia	Etiology unknown. ⊖ sputum and blood cultures, often responds to glucocorticoids but not to antibiotics.	Formerly called bronchiolitis obliterans organizing pneumonia (BOOP). Noninfectious pneumonia characterized by inflammation of bronchioles and surrounding structure.
Aspiration pneumonia	Aspiration of oropharyngeal or gastric contents → pulmonary infection. Risk factors: altered mental status (↓ cough reflex or glottic closure), dysphagia, neurologic disorders (eg, stroke), invasive tubes (eg, nasogastric tube).	Presents days after aspiration event in dependent lung segment. More common in RLL if sitting up and RUL if lying down (recumbent) due to bronchial anatomy. Can progress to abscess. Aspiration (chemical) pneumonitis—presents hours after aspiration event. Due to gastric acid–mediated inflammation. Presents with infiltrates in lower lobe(s) and resolves with supportive treatment.

Natural history of lobar pneumonia

	Congestion	Red hepatization	Gray hepatization	Resolution
DAYS	1–2	3–4	5–7	8+
FINDINGS	Red-purple, partial consolidation of parenchyma Exudate with mostly bacteria	Red-brown consolidation Exudate with fibrin, bacteria, RBCs, WBCs Reversible	Uniformly gray Exudate full of WBCs, lysed RBCs, and fibrin	Enzymatic digestion of exudate by macrophages

Healthy alveolus
Macrophage
Capillary
WBC

Normal

Bacteria
Exudate

Congestion

RBC   Fibrin

Red hepatization

Lysed RBC   Exudate

Gray hepatization

Resolution

Lung abscess

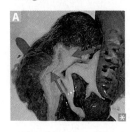

Localized collection of pus within parenchyma. Caused by aspiration of oropharyngeal contents (especially in patients predisposed to loss of consciousness [eg, alcohol overuse, epilepsy]) or bronchial obstruction (eg, cancer).
Air-fluid levels often seen on CXR; presence suggests cavitation. Due to anaerobes (eg, *Bacteroides*, *Fusobacterium*, *Peptostreptococcus*) or *S aureus*.
Treatment: antibiotics, drainage, or surgery.

Lung abscess A 2° to aspiration is most often found in right lung. Location depends on patient's position during aspiration: RLL if upright, RUL or RML if recumbent.

Lung cancer	Leading cause of cancer death. Presentation: cough, hemoptysis, bronchial obstruction, wheezing, pneumonic "coin" lesion on CXR or noncalcified nodule on CT. Sites of metastases from lung cancer: **liver** (jaundice, hepatomegaly), adrenals, **bone** (pathologic fracture), **brain**; "Lung 'mets' Love affective **bone**heads and **brain**iacs." In the lung, metastases (usually multiple lesions) are more common than 1° neoplasms. Most often from breast, colon, prostate, and bladder cancer.	**SPHERE** of complications: **S**uperior vena cava/thoracic outlet syndromes, **P**ancoast tumor, **H**orner syndrome, **E**ndocrine (paraneoplastic), **R**ecurrent laryngeal nerve compression (hoarseness), **E**ffusions (pleural or pericardial). Risk factors include tobacco smoking, secondhand smoke, radiation, environmental exposures (eg, radon, asbestos), pulmonary fibrosis, family history. Squamous and small cell carcinomas are **s**entral (central) and often caused by tobacco smoking. Hamartomas are found incidentally on imaging, appearing as well-circumscribed mass.

TYPE	LOCATION	CHARACTERISTICS	HISTOLOGY
Small cell			
Small cell (oat cell) carcinoma	Central	Undifferentiated → very aggressive. May cause **neurologic** paraneoplastic syndromes (eg, Lambert-Eaton myasthenic syndrome, paraneoplastic myelitis, encephalitis, subacute cerebellar degeneration) and **endocrine** paraneoplastic syndromes (Cushing syndrome, SIADH). Amplification of *myc* oncogenes common. Managed with chemotherapy +/− radiation.	Neoplasm of **neuroendocrine** Kulchitsky cells → small dark blue cells 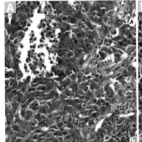. Chromogranin A ⊕, neuron-specific enolase ⊕, synaptophysin ⊕.
Non–small cell			
Adenocarcinoma	Peripheral	Most common 1° lung cancer. Most common subtype in people who do not smoke. More common in females than males. Activating mutations include *KRAS*, *EGFR*, and *ALK*. Associated with hypertrophic osteoarthropathy (clubbing). Bronchioloalveolar subtype (adenocarcinoma in situ): CXR often shows hazy infiltrates similar to pneumonia; better prognosis.	Glandular pattern, often stains mucin ⊕ 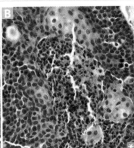. Bronchioloalveolar subtype: grows along alveolar septa → apparent "thickening" of alveolar walls. Tall, columnar cells containing mucus.
Squamous cell carcinoma	Central	Hilar mass 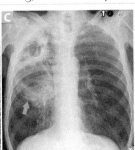 arising from bronchus; **c**avitation; **c**igarettes; hyper**c**alcemia (produces PTHrP).	Keratin pearls 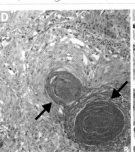 and intercellular bridges (desmosomes).
Large cell carcinoma	Peripheral	Highly anaplastic undifferentiated tumor. Strong association with tobacco smoking. May produce hCG → gynecomastia (en**larged** breasts). Less responsive to chemotherapy; removed surgically. Poor prognosis.	Pleomorphic **giant** cells 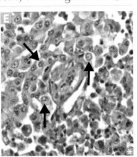.
Bronchial carcinoid tumor	Central or peripheral	Excellent prognosis; metastasis rare. Symptoms due to mass effect (wheezing) or carcinoid syndrome (flushing, diarrhea).	Nests of neuroendocrine cells; chromogranin A ⊕.

Pancoast tumor 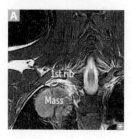	Also called superior sulcus tumor. Carcinoma (most commonly NSCLC) that occurs in the apex of lung 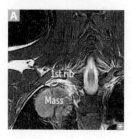 may cause Pancoast syndrome by invading/compressing local structures. Compression of locoregional structures may cause array of findings: • Recurrent laryngeal nerve → hoarseness • Stellate ganglion → Horner syndrome (ipsilateral ptosis, miosis, anhidrosis) • Superior vena cava → SVC syndrome • Brachiocephalic vein → brachiocephalic syndrome (unilateral symptoms) • Brachial plexus → shoulder pain, sensorimotor deficits (eg, atrophy of intrinsic muscles of the hand) • Phrenic nerve → hemidiaphragm paralysis (hemidiaphragm elevation on CXR)
Superior vena cava syndrome 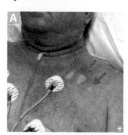	Obstruction of the SVC (eg, thrombus, tumor) impairs blood drainage from the head ("facial plethora"; note blanching after fingertip pressure in A), neck (jugular venous distension, laryngeal/pharyngeal edema), and upper extremities (edema). Commonly caused by malignancy (eg, mediastinal mass, Pancoast tumor) and thrombosis from indwelling catheters. Medical emergency. Can raise intracranial pressure (if obstruction is severe) → headaches, dizziness, ↑ risk of aneurysm/ rupture of intracranial arteries. 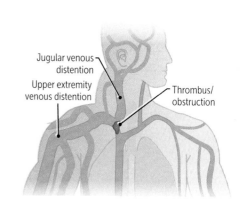

▶ RESPIRATORY—PHARMACOLOGY

Asthma drugs	Bronchoconstriction is mediated by (1) inflammatory processes and (2) parasympathetic tone; therapy is directed at these 2 pathways.
Inhaled β₂-agonists	**Albuterol (short-acting), salmeterol, formoterol**—relax bronchial smooth muscle. Can cause tremor, arrhythmia. Albuterol is for acute symptoms.
Inhaled or oral glucocorticoids	**Fluticasone, budesonide**—inhibit the synthesis of virtually all cytokines. Inactivate NF-κB, the transcription factor that induces production of TNF-α and other inflammatory agents. 1st-line therapy for chronic asthma. Use a spacer or rinse mouth after use to prevent oral thrush.
Muscarinic antagonists	**Tiotropium, ipratropium**—competitively block muscarinic receptors, preventing bronchoconstriction. Also used for COPD. Tiotropium is long acting.
Antileukotrienes	**Montelukast, zafirlukast**—block leukotriene receptors (CysLT1). Especially good for aspirin-induced and exercise-induced asthma. **Zileuton**—5-lipoxygenase inhibitor. ↓ conversion of arachidonic acid to leukotrienes. Hepatotoxic.
Anti-IgE monoclonal therapy	**Omalizumab**—binds mostly unbound serum IgE and blocks binding to FcεRI. Used in allergic asthma with ↑ IgE levels resistant to inhaled glucocorticoids and long-acting β₂-agonists.
Methylxanthines	**Theophylline**—likely causes bronchodilation by inhibiting phosphodiesterase → ↑ cAMP levels due to ↓ cAMP hydrolysis. Limited use due to narrow therapeutic index (cardiotoxicity, neurotoxicity); metabolized by cytochrome P-450. Blocks actions of adenosine.
PDE-4 Inhibitors	**Roflumilast**—inhibits phosphodiesterase → ↑ cAMP → bronchodilation, ↓ airway inflammation. Used in COPD to reduce exacerbations.
Chromones	**Cromolyn**—prevents mast cell degranulation. Prevents acute asthma symptoms. Rarely used.

Asthma drugs *(continued)*

Biologics	**Mepolizumab, reslizumab**—against IL-5. **Benralizumab**—against IL-5 receptor α. Prevent eosinophil differentiation, maturation, activation, and survival mediated by IL-5 stimulation. For maintenance therapy in severe eosinophilic asthma. **Dupilumab**—against IL-4 and IL-13.

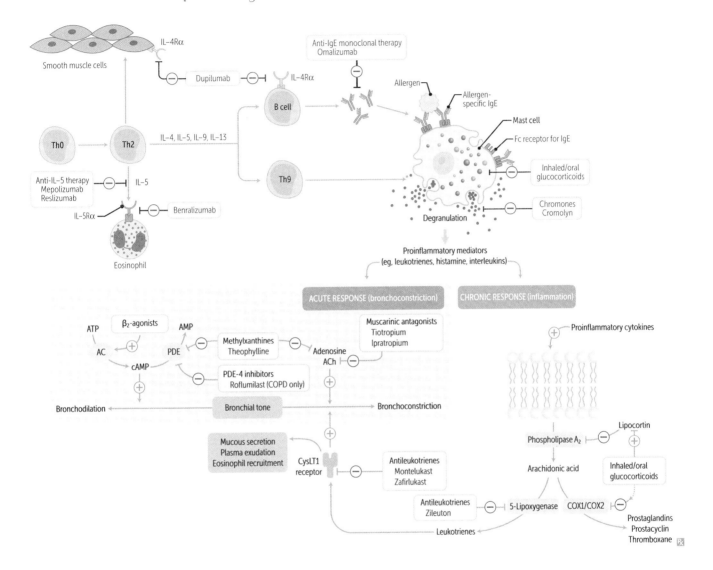

H_1-blockers	Also called antihistamines. Reversible inhibitors of H_1 histamine receptors (inverse agonists).
First generation	Diphenhydramine, dimenhydrinate, chlorpheniramine, doxylamine. Names usually contain "-en/-ine" or "-en/-ate."
CLINICAL USE	Allergy, motion sickness, vomiting in pregnancy, sleep aid.
ADVERSE EFFECTS	Sedation, antimuscarinic, anti-α-adrenergic.
Second generation	Loratadine, fexofenadine, desloratadine, cetirizine. Names usually end in "-adine." **Se**tirizine (cetirizine) is **se**cond-generation agent.
CLINICAL USE	Allergy.
ADVERSE EFFECTS	Far less sedating than 1st generation because of ↓ entry into CNS.

Dextromethorphan

Antitussive (antagonizes NMDA glutamate receptors can act as a hallucinogenic dissociative agent similar to ketamine at high doses (and may be combined with bupropion as a fast acting antidepressant). Synthetic codeine analog. Has mild opioid effect when used in excess. Naloxone can be given for overdose. Mild abuse potential. May cause serotonin syndrome if combined with other serotonergic agents.

Pseudoephedrine, phenylephrine

MECHANISM	Activation of α-adrenergic receptors in nasal mucosa → local vasoconstriction.
CLINICAL USE	Reduce hyperemia, edema (used as nasal decongestants); open obstructed eustachian tubes.
ADVERSE EFFECTS	Hypertension. Rebound congestion (rhinitis medicamentosa) if used more than 4–6 days. Associated with tachyphylaxis. Can also cause CNS stimulation/anxiety (pseudoephedrine).

Pulmonary hypertension drugs

DRUG	MECHANISM	CLINICAL NOTES
Endothelin receptor antagonists	Competitively antagonizes endothelin-1 receptors → ↓ pulmonary vascular resistance.	Hepatotoxic (monitor LFTs). Example: bosentan.
PDE-5 inhibitors	Inhibits PDE-5 → ↑ cGMP → prolonged vasodilatory effect of NO.	Also used to treat erectile dysfunction. Contraindicated when taking nitroglycerin or other nitrates (due to risk of severe hypotension). Example: sildenafil.
Prostacyclin analogs	PGI$_2$ (prostacyclin) with direct vasodilatory effects on pulmonary and systemic arterial vascular beds. Inhibits platelet aggregation.	Adverse effects: flushing, jaw pain. Examples: epoprostenol, iloprost.

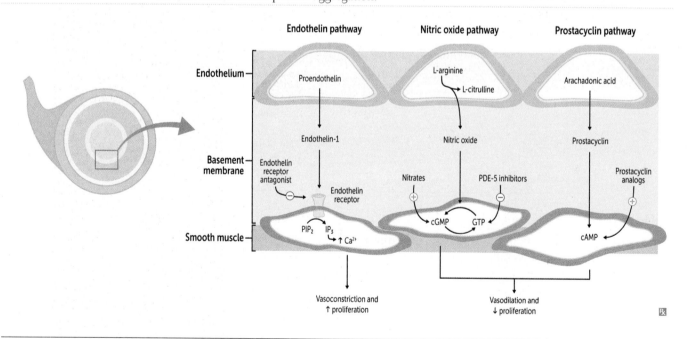

Rapid Review

"Study without thought is vain: thought without study is dangerous."
—Confucius

"It is better, of course, to know useless things than to know nothing."
—Lucius Annaeus Seneca

"For every complex problem there is an answer that is clear, simple, and wrong."
—H. L. Mencken

The following tables represent a collection of high-yield information about diseases and their pathophysiological mechanisms, clinical findings, and key associations.

We have added a high-yield Pathophysiology of Important Diseases section for review of disease mechanisms and removed the Classic/Relevant Treatments section to accommodate the change in focus of the USMLE from pharmacology to pathophysiology.

▶ PATHOPHYSIOLOGY OF IMPORTANT DISEASES

CONDITION	MECHANISM	PAGE
Lesch-Nyhan syndrome	Defective HGPRT → ↑ de novo purine synthesis → ↑ uric acid production	35
Lynch syndrome (HNPCC)	Mutation of MMR genes (*MLH1*, *MSH2*) → Failure of mismatch repair during the S phase → microsatellite instability → CRC (80%)	37, 395
β-thalassemia	Mutation at splice site or promoter sequences on chromosome 11 → ↓ or absent β-globin synthesis	38, 425
Osteogenesis imperfecta	Mutation in *COL1A1* and *COL1A2* genes → Type 1 collagen defect → inability to form triple helices	49
Ehlers-Danlos syndrome	Faulty collagen synthesis → hyperextensible skin, hypermobile joints, easy bruising	49
Menkes disease	Defective ATP7A protein → impaired copper absorption and transport → ↓ lysyl oxidase activity → ↓ collagen cross-linking	49
Marfan syndrome	*FBN1* mutation on chromosome 15 → defective fibrillin-1 glycoprotein (normally forms sheath around elastin)	50
Prader-Willi syndrome	Imprinting or maternal uniparental disomy (25%) → deletion or mutated expression of paternal allele on chromosome 15	56
Angelman syndrome	Imprinting or paternal uniparental disomy (5%) → deletion or mutated expression of *UBE3A* on maternal chromosome 15	56
Cystic fibrosis	ΔF508 deletion in *CFTR* gene on chromosome 7 → impaired ATP-gated Cl⁻ channel → impaired secretion of Cl⁻ in lungs/GI tract and reabsorption of Cl⁻ in sweat glands	58
Duchenne muscular dystrophy	Dystrophin gene frameshift or nonsense mutations → loss of anchoring protein to ECM (dystrophin) → myonecrosis	59
Becker muscular dystrophy	Non-frameshift deletion of dystrophin gene; less severe than Duchenne	59
Myotonic dystrophy	CTG trinucleotide repeat expansion in *DMPK* gene → abnormal expression of myotonin protein kinase → myotonia	59
Fragile X syndrome	CGG trinucleotide repeat in *FMR1* gene → hypermethylation of cytosine residues → ↓ expression	60
Bitot spots in vitamin A deficiency	↓ differentiation of epithelial cells into specialized tissue → conjunctival squamous metaplasia → keratin buildup	64
Wernicke encephalopathy in patient with alcohol use disorder given glucose	Thiamine deficiency → impaired glucose breakdown → ATP depletion worsened by glucose infusion	64
Pellagra in malignant carcinoid syndrome	Tryptophan is diverted towards serotonin synthesis by tumor → B₃ deficiency (B₃ is derived from tryptophan)	65
Kwashiorkor	Protein malnutrition → ↓ plasma oncotic pressure (→ edema), ↓ apolipoprotein synthesis (→ fatty changes in the liver)	69
Lactic acidosis, fasting hypoglycemia, hepatic steatosis in patient with alcohol use disorder	↑ NADH/NAD⁺ ratio due to ethanol metabolism	70
Aspirin-induced hyperthermia	↑ permeability of inner mitochondrial membrane → ↓ proton gradient and ↑ O₂ consumption (uncoupling) → heat production	76
Hereditary fructose intolerance	Aldolase B deficiency → Fructose-1-phosphate accumulation → ↓ available phosphate → inhibition of glycogenolysis and gluconeogenesis	78

CONDITION	MECHANISM	PAGE
Essential fructosuria	Fructokinase deficiency → ↑ fructose; hexokinase pathway converts fructose to fructose-6-phosphate	78
Classic galactosemia	Galactose-1-phosphate uridyltransferase deficiency → accumulation of toxic substances (eg, galactitol in eye lens → cataracts)	78
Galactokinase deficiency	Galactokinase deficiency → ↑ galactose; aldose reductase converts galactose to galactitol	78
Cataracts, retinopathy, nephropathy, peripheral neuropathy in DM	Excess glucose → sorbitol (via aldose reductase) and sorbitol → fructose (via sorbitol dehydrogenase); lens, retina, kidney, and Schwann cells lack sorbitol dehydrogenase → intracellular sorbitol accumulation → osmotic damage	79
Recurrent *Neisseria* bacteremia	Terminal complement deficiencies (C5–C9) → failure of MAC formation	105
Hereditary angioedema	C1 inhibitor deficiency → unregulated activation of kallikrein → ↑ bradykinin	105
Paroxysmal nocturnal hemoglobinuria	*PIGA* gene mutation → ↓ GPI anchors for complement inhibitors (DAF/CD55, MIRL/CD59) → complement-mediated intravascular hemolysis → ↓ haptoglobin	105
Type I hypersensitivity	Immediate (minutes): antigen crosslinks IgE on mast cells → degranulation → release of histamine, tryptase, leukotrienes Late (hours): mast cells secrete chemokines (attract inflammatory cells and other mediators) → inflammation, tissue damage	110
Type II hypersensitivity	Antibodies bind to cell-surface antigens or ECM → inflammation, cellular destruction, and dysfunction	110
Type III hypersensitivity	Antigen-antibody complexes activate complement → attract neutrophils → release of lysosomal enzymes	111
Type IV hypersensitivity	T cell–mediated (no antibodies involved); APCs activate CD4+ T cells (→ release of cytokines) or CD8+ T cells (→ direct cell cytotoxicity)	111
Acute hemolytic transfusion reaction	Type II hypersensitivity reaction against donor RBCs (usually ABO antigens)	112
X-linked (Bruton) agammaglobulinemia	Defect in *BTK* gene → no B-cell maturation → absent B cells in peripheral blood, ↓ Ig of all classes	114
DiGeorge syndrome	22q11 microdeletion → failure to develop 3rd and 4th branchial (pharyngeal) pouches → absent thymus and parathyroid	114
Hyper-IgM syndrome	Defective CD40L on Th cells → class switching defect	115
Leukocyte adhesion deficiency (type 1)	LFA-1 integrin (CD18) defect → impaired phagocyte migration and chemotaxis	115
Chédiak-Higashi syndrome	*LYST* mutation → microtubule dysfunction → phagosome-lysosome fusion defect	115
Chronic granulomatous disease	NADPH oxidase defect → ↓ ROS, ↓ respiratory burst in neutrophils → ↑ susceptibility to catalase ⊕ organisms	115
Candida infection in immunodeficiency	↓ granulocytes (systemic), ↓ T cells (local)	114, 116
Graft-versus-host disease	Type IV hypersensitivity reaction; HLA mismatch → donor T cells attack host cells	117
Recurrent S aureus, Serratia, B cepacia infections in CGD	Catalase ⊕ organisms degrade H_2O_2 before it can be converted to microbicidal products by the myeloperoxidase system	126

CONDITION	MECHANISM	PAGE
Hemolytic-uremic syndrome	Shiga/Shiga-like toxins inactivate 60S ribosome → ↑ cytokine release	130, 432
Tetanus	Tetanospasmin cleaves SNARE → inhibition of release of inhibitory neurotransmitters (GABA and glycine) from Renshaw cells	130
Botulism	Toxin (protease) cleaves SNARE → ↓ neurotransmitter (ACh) release at NMJ	130
Gas gangrene	Alpha toxin (a phospholipase/lecithinase) degrades phospholipids → myonecrosis, crepitus	131, 136
Toxic shock syndrome, scarlet fever	TSST-1 and erythrogenic exotoxin A cross-link β region of TCR to MHC class II on APCs outside of antigen binding site → ↑↑ IL-1, IL-2, IFN-γ, TNF-α	131
Shock and DIC caused by gram ⊖ bacteria	Lipid A of LPS macrophage activation (TLR4/CD14), complement activation, tissue factor activation	131
Prosthetic device infection by S epidermidis	Biofilm production	126, 133
Endocarditis 2° to S sanguinis	Dextrans (biofilm) production → fibrin-platelet aggregates bind to damaged heart valves	126, 134
Pseudomembranous colitis 2° to C difficile	Toxins A and B damage enterocytes → watery diarrhea	136
Diphtheria	Exotoxin inhibits protein synthesis via ADP-ribosylation of EF-2 → possible necrosis	137
Virulence of M tuberculosis	Cord factor activates macrophages (promoting granuloma formation), induces release of TNF-α; sulfatides (surface glycolipids) inhibit phagolysosomal fusion	138
Tuberculoid leprosy	Th1 immune response, mild symptoms	139
Lepromatous leprosy	Predominantly Th2 response, can be lethal	139
Lack of effective vaccine for N gonorrhoeae	Antigenic variation of pilus proteins	140
Cystitis and pyelonephritis 2° to E coli	Fimbriae (P pili)	143
Pneumonia, neonatal meningitis 2° to E coli	K capsule	143
Chlamydiae resistance to β-lactam antibiotics	Lack of classic peptidoglycan due to reduced muramic acid	146
Influenza pandemics	RNA segment reassortment → antigenic shift	166
Influenza epidemics	Mutations in hemagglutinin, neuraminidase → antigenic drift	166
CNS invasion by rabies	Binds to ACh receptors → retrograde transport (dynein)	169
HIV infection	Binds CD4 along with CCR5 on macrophages (early), or CXCR4 on T cells (late)	172
Granuloma	Macrophages present antigens to CD4+ and secrete IL-12 → CD4+ differentiation into Th1 → IFN-γ secretion → macrophage activation	213
Limitless replicative potential of cancer cells	Reactivation of telomerase → maintains and lengthens telomeres → prevention of chromosome shortening and aging	217
Tissue invasion by cancer	↓ E-cadherin function → ↓ intercellular junctions → basement membrane and ECM degradation by metalloproteinases → cell attachment to ECM proteins (laminin, fibronectin) → locomotion → vascular dissemination	217

CONDITION	MECHANISM	PAGE
Persistent truncus arteriosus	Failure of aorticopulmonary septum formation	285, 302
D-transposition of great arteries	Failure of the aorticopulmonary septum to spiral	285, 302
"Tet spells" in tetralogy of Fallot	Crying, fever, exercise → ↑ RV outflow obstruction → ↑ right-to-left flow across VSD	302
Eisenmenger syndrome	Uncorrected left-to-right shunt → ↑ pulmonary blood flow → remodeling of vasculature → pulmonary hypertension → RVH → right-to-left shunting	303
Atherosclerosis	Endothelial cell dysfunction → macrophage and LDL accumulation → foam cell formation → fatty streaks → smooth muscle cell migration, ECM deposition → fibrous plaque → complex atheromas	305
Thoracic aortic aneurysm	Cystic medial degeneration; associated with 3° syphilis	306
Myocardial infarction	Rupture of coronary artery atherosclerotic plaque → acute thrombosis	308
NSTEMI	Subendocardial infarcts	308
STEMI	Transmural infarcts	308
Death within 0-24 hours post-MI	Ventricular arrhythmia	309, 314
Death or shock within 3–14 days post-MI	Macrophage-mediated ruptures: papillary muscle (2–7 days), interventricular septum (3–5 days), free wall (5–14 days)	309, 314
Wolff-Parkinson-White	Abnormal accessory pathway from atria to ventricle bypasses the AV node → ventricles begin to partially depolarize earlier → delta wave; reentrant circuit → supraventricular tachycardia	311
Hypertrophic obstructive cardiomyopathy (HOCM)	Sarcomere protein gene mutation → concentric hypertrophy (sarcomeres added in parallel); death due to arrhythmia	315
Syncope, dyspnea in HOCM	Asymmetric septal hypertrophy, systolic anterior motion of mitral valve → outflow obstruction	315
Hypovolemic shock	↓ preload → ↓ SV → ↓ CO	317
Cardiogenic shock	↓ CO due to left heart dysfunction	317
Obstructive shock	↓ CO due to blockage of vessels/structures outside the heart	317
Distributive shock	↓ SVR (afterload)	317
Rheumatic fever	Antibodies to M protein cross-react with self-antigens; type II hypersensitivity reaction	319
Deep venous thrombosis	Stasis, hypercoagulability, endothelial damage (Virchow triad) → blood clot within deep vein	321
Most common congenital adrenal hyperplasia	21-hydroxylase deficiency → ↓ mineralocorticoids, ↓ cortisol, ↑ sex hormones, ↑ 17-hydroxyprogesterone	339
Euvolemic hyponatremia in SIADH	↑ ADH → water retention → ↓ aldosterone, ↑ ANP, ↑ BNP → ↑ urinary Na$^+$ secretion	342
Heat intolerance, weight loss in hyperthyroidism	↑ Na$^+$/K$^+$-ATPase → ↑ basal metabolic rate → ↑ calorigenesis	344
Myxedema in hypothyroidism	↑ GAGs in interstitial space → ↑ osmotic pressure → ↑ water retention	344
Graves ophthalmopathy	Lymphocytic infiltration, fibroblast secretion of GAGs → ↑ osmotic muscle swelling, inflammation	346

CONDITION	MECHANISM	PAGE
1° hyperparathyroidism	Parathyroid adenoma or hyperplasia → ↑ PTH	349
2° hyperparathyroidism	↓ Ca^{2+} and/or ↑ PO_4^{3-} → parathyroid hyperplasia → ↑ PTH, ↑ ALP	349
Vascular disease in DM	Nonenzymatic glycation of proteins; small vessel hyaline arteriosclerosis; large vessel atherosclerosis	350
Diabetic ketoacidosis	↓ insulin or ↑ insulin requirement → ↑ lipolysis → ↑ free fatty acid oxidation → ↑ ketogenesis	351
Hyperosmolar hyperglycemic state	Hyperglycemia → ↑ serum osmolality, excessive osmotic diuresis	351
Zollinger-Ellison syndrome	Gastrinoma in pancreas or duodenum → recurrent ulcers in duodenum/jejunum, malabsorption	357
Duodenal atresia	Recanalization failure	366
Jejunal/ileal atresia	Disruption of mesenteric vessels (most commonly SMA) → ischemic necrosis of fetal intestine	366
Superior mesenteric artery syndrome	Diminished mesenteric fat → compression of transverse (3rd) portion of duodenum by SMA and aorta	370
Achalasia	Degeneration of inhibitory neurons in myenteric plexus of esophageal wall → failure of LES relaxation	383
Barrett esophagus	Chronic GERD → metaplasia of nonkeratinized stratified squamous epithelium to intestinal epithelium (nonciliated columnar with goblet cells)	385
Acute gastritis 2° to NSAIDs	↓ PGE_2 → ↓ gastric mucosa protection	386
Celiac disease	Autoimmune-mediated intolerance of gliadin (found in wheat) → malabsorption (distal duodenum, proximal jejunum), steatorrhea	388
Fistula formation in Crohn disease	Transmural inflammation	389
Meckel diverticulum	Persistence of the vitelline (omphalomesenteric) duct	391
Hirschsprung disease	Loss of function mutation in *RET* → failure of neural crest migration → lack of ganglion cells/enteric nervous plexuses in distal colon	391
Adenoma-carcinoma sequence in colorectal cancer	Loss of APC (↓ intercellular adhesion, ↑ proliferation) → *KRAS* mutation (unregulated intracellular signaling) → loss of tumor suppressor genes (*TP53*, *DCC*)	395
Fibrosis in cirrhosis	Occurs via stellate cell production of ECM	374, 396
Reye syndrome	Aspirin ↓ β-oxidation via reversible inhibition of mitochondrial enzymes	398
Hepatic encephalopathy	Cirrhosis → portosystemic shunts → ↓ NH_3 metabolism	399
$α_1$-antitrypsin deficiency	Liver: misfolded proteins aggregate in hepatocellular ER → cirrhosis; lungs: ↓ $α_1$-antitrypsin → uninhibited elastase in alveoli → panacinar emphysema	400
Wilson disease	Mutated hepatocyte copper-transporting ATPase (*ATP7B* on chromosome 13) → copper incorporation into apoceruloplasmin, excretion into bile → ↑ serum ceruloplasmin, copper in tissues and urine	402
Hemochromatosis	*HFE* mutation on chromosome 6 → ↓ hepcidin production, ↑ intestinal absorption → iron overload (↑ ferritin, ↑ iron, ↓ TIBC → ↑ transferrin saturation)	402
Gallstone ileus	Fistula between gallbladder and GI tract → stone enters GI lumen → obstruction of ileocecal valve (narrowest point)	403
Acute cholangitis	Biliary tree obstruction → stasis/bacterial overgrowth	403

CONDITION	MECHANISM	PAGE
Acute pancreatitis	Autodigestion of pancreas by pancreatic enzymes	404
Rh hemolytic disease of the newborn	Rh ⊖ mother forms antibodies (maternal anti-D IgG) against RBCs of Rh ⊕ fetus	411
Anemia in lead poisoning	Lead inhibits ferrochelatase and ALA dehydratase →↓ heme synthesis, ↑ RBC protoporphyrin	425
Anemia of chronic disease	Inflammation → ↑ hepcidin → ↓ release of iron from macrophages, ↓ iron absorption from gut	427
G6PD deficiency	G6PD defect → ↓ NADPH → ↓ reduced glutathione → ↑ RBC susceptibility to oxidant stress	428
Sickle cell anemia	Point mutation → substitution of glutamic acid with valine in β chain → low O_2, high altitude, acidosis precipitate sickling (polymerization of deoxygenated HbS) → anemia, vaso-occlusive disease	428
Bernard-Soulier syndrome	↓ GpIb → ↓ platelet-to-vWF adhesion	432
Glanzmann thrombasthenia	↓ GpIIb/IIIa → ↓ platelet-to-platelet aggregation, defective platelet plug formation	432
Thrombotic thrombocytopenic purpura	↓ ADAMTS13 (vWF metalloprotease) → ↓ degradation of vWF multimers → ↑ platelet adhesion and aggregation (microthrombi formation)	432
von Willebrand disease	↓ vWF → ↓ platelet-to-vWF adhesion, possibly ↑ PTT (vWF protects factor VIII)	433
Factor V Leiden	Arg506Gln mutation in factor V → resistance to degradation by protein C → hypercoagulable state	433
Heparin-induced thrombocytopenia	Type 1: Heparin administration (within 2 days) → mild, transient drop in platelets; not clinically significant Type 2: Heparin administration (5–10 days) → IgG antibodies against heparin-bound platelet factor 4 complex → complex binds and activates platelets → thrombosis, removal by splenic macrophages → ↓↓ platelet count (significant thrombocytopenia)	440
Warfarin-induced skin/tissue necrosis	Warfarin administration → rapid ↓ in protein C levels due to its shorter half-life → procoagulant state due to delay in depletion of other existing clotting factors with longer half-lives → hypercoagulation and microthrombosis → skin/tissue necrosis	433, 441
Axillary nerve injury	Fractured surgical neck or anterior dislocation of humerus → flattened deltoid, arm at side, ↓ shoulder sensation	450
Radial nerve injury ("Saturday night palsy")	Axilla compression (use of crutches), midshaft humerus fracture, repetitive pronation/supination of forearm → wrist drop, ↓ grip strength	450
Median nerve injury (hand of benediction)	Proximal lesion: supracondylar fracture → loss of wrist flexion and function of LOAF muscles; loss of sensation over thenar eminence, dorsal and palmar aspect of lateral 3½ fingers Distal lesion: carpal tunnel syndrome	450
Ulnar nerve injury	Proximal lesion: fractured medial epicondyle → radial deviation of wrist on flexion Distal lesion: fractured hook of hamate (fall on outstretched hand) → ulnar claw on digital extension, loss of sensation over ulnar digits	450
Erb palsy (waiter's tip)	Traction/tear of C5-C6 roots on infant's neck during delivery, or due to trauma in adults	452

CONDITION	MECHANISM	PAGE
Klumpke palsy (claw hand)	Traction/tear of C8-T1 roots on infant's arm during delivery, or on trying to grab a branch in adults	452
Winged scapula	Injury to long thoracic nerve (C5-C7); seen after mastectomy, stab wounds	452
Common peroneal nerve injury	Trauma to lateral leg, fibular neck fracture → foot drop with "steppage gait"	457
Superior gluteal nerve injury	Iatrogenic injury during IM injection in gluteal region → Trendelenburg sign: lesion contralateral to side of hip that drops due to abductor weakness	457
Pudendal nerve injury	Injury during horseback riding or prolonged cycling; can be blocked during delivery at the ischial spine → ↓ sensation in perineal and genital area +/– fecal/urinary incontinence	457
Radial head subluxation (nursemaid's elbow)	Due to sudden pull on arm (in children; radial head slips out of immature annular ligament)	466
Slipped capital femoral epiphysis	Obese young adolescent with hip/knee pain; ↑ axial force on femoral head → epiphysis displaces relative to femoral neck	466
Achondroplasia	Constitutive activation of $FGFR3$ → ↓ chondrocyte proliferation → failure of endochondral ossification → short limbs	467
Osteoporosis	↑ osteoclast activity → ↓ bone mass 2° to ↓ estrogen levels, old age, and long-term use of medications like steroids	467
Osteopetrosis	Carbonic anhydrase II mutations → ↓ ability of osteoclasts to generate acidic environment → ↓ bone resorption → dense bones prone to fracture, pancytopenia (↓ marrow space)	468
Osteitis deformans (Paget disease of bone)	↑ osteoclast activity followed by ↑ osteoblast activity → formation of poor quality, fracture-prone bone	468
Osteoarthritis	Mechanical degeneration of articular cartilage → inflammation with inadequate repair, osteophyte formation	472
Rheumatoid arthritis	Autoimmune inflammation → pannus formation, erosion of articular cartilage and bone	472
Sjögren syndrome	Autoimmune reaction → lymphocyte-mediated damage of exocrine glands	474
Systemic lupus erythematosus	Predominantly a type III hypersensitivity reaction with ↓ clearance of immune complexes; hematologic manifestations are a type II hypersensitivity reaction	476
Blindness in giant cell (temporal) arteritis	Ophthalmic artery occlusion	478
Myasthenia gravis	Autoantibodies to postsynaptic nicotinic (ACh) receptors	480
Lambert-Eaton myasthenic syndrome	Autoantibodies to presynaptic calcium channels → ↓ ACh release	480
Albinism	Normal melanocyte number but ↓ melanin production	484
Vitiligo	Autoimmune destruction of melanocytes	484
Atopic dermatitis	Epidermal barrier dysfunction, genetic factors (ie, loss-of-function mutations in the filaggrin [FLG] gene), immune dysregulation, altered skin microbiome, environmental triggers of inflammation	485
Allergic contact dermatitis	Type IV hypersensitivity reaction; during the sensitization phase, allergen activates Th1 cells → memory CD4+ and CD8+ cell formation; upon re-exposure → CD4+ cells release cytokines and CD8+ cells kill targeted cells	485

CONDITION	MECHANISM	PAGE
Pemphigus vulgaris	Type II hypersensitivity reaction; IgG autoantibodies form against desmoglein 1 and 3 in desmosomes → separation of keratinocytes in stratum spinosum from stratum basale; Nikolsky sign ⊕	489
Bullous pemphigoid	Type II hypersensitivity reaction; IgG autoantibodies against hemidesmosomes → separation of epidermis from dermis; Nikolsky sign ⊖	489
Spina bifida occulta, meningocele, myelomeningocele, myeloschisis	Failure of caudal neuropore to fuse by 4th week of development	501
Anencephaly	Failure of rostral neuropore to close → no forebrain, open calvarium	501
Holoprosencephaly	Failure of the forebrain (prosencephalon) to divide into 2 cerebral hemispheres; developmental field defect typically occurring at weeks 3–4 of development; associated with *SHH* mutations	501
Lissencephaly	Failure of neuronal migration → smooth brain surface lacking sulci and gyri	501
Chiari I malformation	Downward displacement of cerebellar tonsils through foramen magnum	502
Chiari II malformation	Herniation of cerebellum (vermis and tonsils) and medulla through foramen magnum	502
Dandy-Walker malformation	Agenesis of cerebellar vermis → cystic enlargement of 4th ventricle, which fills the enlarged posterior fossa	502
Syringomyelia	Fluid-filled, gliosis-lined cavity within spinal cord; damages crossing spinothalamic tract fibers → cape-like loss of pain and temperature	502
Gerstmann syndrome	Lesion in the dominant parietal cortex → agraphia, acalculia, finger agnosia, left-right disorientation	524
Hemispatial neglect syndrome	Lesion in the nondominant parietal cortex → agnosia of contralateral side	524
Klüver-Bucy syndrome	Bilateral lesions in the amygdala; seen in HSV-1 encephalitis → disinhibition, including hyperphagia, hypersexuality, hyperorality	524
Parinaud syndrome	Compression of dorsal midbrain (often due to pineal gland tumors) → upward gaze palsy, convergence-retraction nystagmus, light-near dissociation	524, 542
Cerebral edema	Fluid accumulation in the brain parenchyma → ↑ ICP; may be cytotoxic or vasogenic	525
Aphasia	Stroke in dominant (usually left) hemisphere, in either the superior temporal gyrus of temporal lobe (Wernicke; receptive aphasia) or inferior frontal gyrus of frontal lobe (Broca; expressive aphasia)	526, 529
Locked-in syndrome	Stroke of the basilar artery; loss of horizontal, but not vertical, eye movements	526
Lateral pontine syndrome	Stroke of the anterior inferior cerebellar artery	526
Lateral medullary (Wallenberg) syndrome	Stroke of the posterior inferior cerebellar artery	527
Medial medullary syndrome	Stroke of the anterior spinal artery	527
Neonatal intraventricular hemorrhage	Reduced glial fiber support and impaired autoregulation of BP in premature infants → bleeding into the ventricles, originating in the germinal matrix (a highly vascularized layer within the subventricular zone)	527
Epidural hematoma	Rupture of middle meningeal artery, often 2° to skull fracture involving the pterion	528
Subdural hematoma	Rupture of bridging veins; acute (traumatic, high-energy impact, sudden deceleration injury) or chronic (mild trauma, cerebral atrophy, ↑ age, chronic alcohol overuse, shaken baby syndrome)	528

CONDITION	MECHANISM	PAGE
Subarachnoid hemorrhage	Trauma, rupture of aneurysm (such as a saccular aneurysm), or AVM → bleeding	528
Intraparenchymal hemorrhage	Systemic hypertension (most often occurs in the putamen of basal ganglia, thalamus, pons, and cerebellum), amyloid angiopathy, AVM, vasculitis, neoplasm, or secondary to reperfusion injury in ischemic stroke → bleeding	528
Phantom limb pain	Most commonly following amputation → reorganization of 1° somatosensory cortex → sensation of pain in a limb that is no longer present	529
Diffuse axonal injury	Traumatic shearing of white matter tracts during rapid acceleration and/or deceleration of the brain (eg, motor vehicle accident) → multiple punctate hemorrhages involving white matter tracts → neurologic injury, often causing coma or persistent vegetative state	529
Conduction aphasia	Damage to the arcuate fasciculus	529
Global aphasia	Damage to both Broca and Wernicke areas	529
Heat stroke	Inability of body to dissipate heat (eg, exertion) → CNS dysfunction (eg, confusion), rhabdomyolysis, acute kidney injury, ARDS, DIC	530
Migraine	Irritation of CN V, meninges, or blood vessels (release of vasoactive neuropeptides such as substance P, calcitonin gene-related peptide)	532
Parkinson disease	Loss of dopaminergic neurons of substantia nigra pars compacta	534
Huntington disease	Trinucleotide (CAG) repeat expansion in huntingtin (*HTT*) gene on chromosome 4 → toxic gain of function → atrophy of caudate and putamen with ex vacuo ventriculomegaly; ↑ dopamine, ↓ GABA, ↓ ACh → neuronal death via glutamate excitotoxicity and NMDA receptor binding	534
Alzheimer disease	Widespread cortical atrophy, narrowing of gyri, and widening of sulci; senile plaques in gray matter composed of beta-amyloid core; neurofibrillary tangles composed of intracellular, hyperphosphorylated tau protein; Hirano bodies	534
Frontotemporal dementia (Pick disease)	Frontotemporal lobe degeneration → ↓ executive function and behavioral inhibition	535
Vascular dementia	Multiple arterial infarcts and/or chronic ischemia	535
HIV-associated dementia	Secondary to diffuse gray matter and subcortical atrophy in advanced HIV infection	535
Idiopathic intracranial hypertension	↑ ICP, associated with dural venous sinus stenosis; impaired optic nerve axoplasmic flow → papilledema	536
Communicating hydrocephalus	↓ CSF absorption by arachnoid granulations → ↑ ICP, papilledema, herniation	536
Normal pressure hydrocephalus	Idiopathic, CSF pressure elevated only episodically, no ↑ subarachnoid space volume; expansion of ventricles distorts the fibers of the corona radiata → "wobbly, wacky, wet" triad	536
Noncommunicating hydrocephalus	Structural blockage of CSF circulation within ventricular system (eg, stenosis of aqueduct of Sylvius, colloid cyst blocking foramen of Monro, tumor)	536
Ex vacuo ventriculomegaly	↓ brain tissue and neuronal atrophy → appearance of ↑ CSF on imaging	536
Multiple sclerosis	Autoimmune inflammation and demyelination of CNS (brain and spinal cord) → axonal damage	537

CONDITION	MECHANISM	PAGE
Osmotic demyelination syndrome	Rapid osmotic changes, most commonly iatrogenic correction of hyponatremia but also rapid shifts of other osmolytes (eg, glucose) → massive axonal demyelination in pontine white matter	538
Acute inflammatory demyelinating polyneuropathy (subtype of Guillain-Barré syndrome)	Autoimmune destruction of Schwann cells via inflammation and demyelination of motor and sensory fibers and peripheral nerves; likely facilitated by molecular mimicry and triggered by inoculations or stress	538
Charcot-Marie-Tooth disease	Defective production of proteins involved in the structure and function of peripheral nerves or the myelin sheath	538
Progressive multifocal leukoencephalopathy	Destruction of oligodendrocytes 2° to reactivation of latent JC virus infection → demyelination of CNS	538
Sturge-Weber syndrome	Somatic mosaicism of an activating mutation in one copy of the *GNAQ* gene → congenital anomaly of neural crest derivatives → capillary vascular malformation, ipsilateral leptomeningeal angioma with calcifications, episcleral hemangioma	539
Pituitary adenoma	Hyperplasia of only one type of endocrine cells found in pituitary (most commonly from prolactin-producing lactotrophs)	540
Spinal muscular atrophy	Congenital degeneration of anterior horns due to *SMN1* mutation → defective snRNP assembly → LMN apoptosis	544
Amyotrophic lateral sclerosis	Combined UMN and LMN degeneration; familial form associated with *SOD1* mutation	544
Tabes dorsalis	Degeneration/demyelination of dorsal columns and roots (in 3° syphilis) → progressive sensory ataxia (impaired proprioception → poor coordination)	544
Poliomyelitis	Poliovirus infection spreads from lymphoid tissue of oropharynx to small intestine then to CNS via bloodstream → cell destruction in anterior horn of spinal cord (LMN death)	544
Friedreich ataxia	Trinucleotide repeat (GAA) on chromosome 9 in frataxin gene (iron-binding protein) → impaired mitochondrial function → degeneration of lateral corticospinal tract, spinocerebellar tract, dorsal columns, and dorsal root ganglia	545
Noise-induced hearing loss	Damage to stereociliated cells in organ of Corti → loss of high-frequency hearing first	548
Presbycusis	Aging-related progressive bilateral/symmetric sensorineural hearing loss (often of higher frequencies) due to destruction of hair cells at the cochlear base	548
Cholesteatoma	Abnormal growth of keratinized squamous epithelium in middle ear; 1° from tympanic membrane retraction pocket; 2° from tympanic membrane perforation	548
Ménière disease	↑ endolymph in inner ear → vertigo, sensorineural hearing loss, tinnitus, ear fullness	548
Hyperopia	Eye too short for refractive power of cornea and lens → light focused behind retina	549
Myopia	Eye too long for refractive power of cornea and lens → light focused in front of retina	549
Astigmatism	Irregular or asymmetric curvature of the cornea or lens → different refractive power at different axes	549

CONDITION	MECHANISM	PAGE
Presbyopia	Age-related impaired accommodation, likely primarily due to ↓ lens elasticity	550
Glaucoma	Optic neuropathy → progressive vision loss (peripheral → central), usually with ↑ intraocular pressure	551
Open-angle glaucoma	Associated with ↑ resistance to aqueous humor drainage through trabecular meshwork	551
Angle-closure glaucoma	Anterior chamber angle narrowed or closed; associated anatomic abnormalities (eg, anteriorly displaced lens resting against central iris) → ↓ aqueous flow through pupil → ↑ pressure in posterior chamber → peripheral iris pushes against cornea → drainage pathways obstructed by iris	551
Diabetic retinopathy	Chronic hyperglycemia → ↑ permeability and occlusion of retinal vessels → microaneurysms, hemorrhages (nonproliferative); retinal neovascularization due to chronic hypoxia (proliferative)	552
Hypertensive retinopathy	Chronic hypertension → spasm, sclerosis, and fibrinoid necrosis of retinal vessels	552
Retinal artery occlusion	Central or branch retinal artery blockage usually due to embolism (carotid artery atherosclerosis > cardiogenic); less commonly due to giant cell arteritis	552
Retinal vein occlusion	Central occlusion due to 1° thrombosis; branch occlusion due to 2° thrombosis at arteriovenous crossings	552
Retinal detachment	Neurosensory retina separates from underlying retinal pigment epithelium → choroidal blood supply loss → hypoxia and degeneration of photoreceptors; due to retinal tears (rhegmatogenous) or tractional or exudative (fluid accumulation) (nonrhegmatogenous)	552
Retinitis pigmentosa	Progressive degeneration of photoreceptors and retinal pigment epithelium	552
Papilledema	↑ ICP (eg, 2° to mass effect) → impaired axoplasmic flow in optic nerve → optic disc swelling (usually bilateral)	553
Relative afferent pupillary defect (Marcus Gunn pupil)	Unilateral or asymmetric lesions of afferent limb of pupillary reflex (eg, retina, optic nerve)	554
Horner syndrome	Lesions along sympathetic chain: 1st neuron (pontine hemorrhage, lateral medullary syndrome, spinal cord lesion above T1 like Brown-Sequard syndrome or late-stage syringomyelia); 2nd neuron (stellate ganglion compression by Pancoast tumor); 3rd neuron (carotid dissection)	555
Cavernous sinus syndrome	2° to pituitary tumor mass effect, carotid-cavernous fistula, or cavernous sinus thrombosis related to infection (spreads due to lack of valves in dural venous sinuses)	557
Delirium	Usually 2° to illness (eg, CNS disease, infection, trauma, substance use, metabolic/electrolyte imbalance, hemorrhage, urinary/fecal retention) or medication (eg, anticholinergics)	575
Schizophrenia	Altered dopaminergic activity, ↑ serotonergic activity, ↓ dendritic branching	577
Distal renal tubular acidosis (RTA type 1)	Inability of α-intercalated cells to secrete H^+ → no new HCO_3^- generated → metabolic acidosis	611
Proximal RTA (type 2)	Defective PCT HCO_3^- reabsorption → ↑ urinary excretion of HCO_3^- → metabolic acidosis	611
Hyperkalemic RTA (type 4)	Hypoaldosteronism/aldosterone resistance → ↑ K^+ → ↓ NH_3 synthesis in PCT → ↓ NH_4^+ excretion → metabolic acidosis	611

CONDITION	MECHANISM	PAGE
Nephritic syndrome	Glomerular inflammation → GBM damage → dysmorphic RBCs in urine, hematuria; ↓ GFR → oliguria, azotemia, ↑ renin release	613
Nephrotic syndrome	Podocyte damage → impaired charge barrier → proteinuria; hypoalbuminemia → ↑ hepatic lipogenesis → hypercholesterolemia; antithrombin loss → hypercoagulability; IgG loss → infections	613
Nephritic-nephrotic syndrome	Severe GBM damage → RBCs lost in urine + impaired charge barrier → hematuria + proteinuria	613
Infection-related glomerulonephritis	Type III hypersensitivity reaction with consumptive hypocomplementemia	614
Alport syndrome	Type IV collagen mutation (X-linked dominant) → irregular thinning, thickening, and splitting of GBM → nephritic syndrome	615
Stress incontinence	Outlet incompetence (urethral hypermobility/intrinsic sphincter deficiency) → leak with ↑ intraabdominal pressure (eg, sneezing, lifting)	618
Urge incontinence	Detrusor overactivity → leak with urge to void immediately	618
Overflow incontinence	Incomplete emptying (detrusor underactivity or outlet obstruction) → leak with overfilling	618
Prerenal azotemia	↓ RBF → ↓ GFR → ↑ reabsorption of Na^+/H_2O and urea	620
Intrinsic renal failure	Patchy necrosis → debris obstructing tubules and fluid backflow → ↓ GFR	620
Postrenal azotemia	Outflow obstruction (bilateral)	620
Adnexal torsion	Twisting of ovary/fallopian tube around infundibulopelvic ligament and ovarian ligament → venous/lymphatic blockage; arterial inflow continues → edema → blockade of arterial inflow → necrosis/hemorrhage	643
Preeclampsia	Abnormal placental spiral arteries → endothelial dysfunction, vasoconstriction, ischemia → new-onset HTN with proteinuria	660
Supine hypotensive syndrome	Supine position → gravid uterus compresses abdominal aorta and IVC → ↓ placental perfusion, ↓ venous return	661
Polycystic ovary syndrome	Hyperinsulinemia and/or insulin resistance → altered hypothalamic feedback response → ↑ LH:FSH, ↑ androgens, ↑ rate of follicular maturation → unruptured follicles (cysts), anovulation	662
Functional hypothalamic amenorrhea	Severe caloric restriction, ↑ energy expenditure, and/or stress → altered pulsatile GnRH secretion → ↓ LH, FSH, estrogen	663
Varicocele	↑ venous pressure → dilated veins in pampiniform plexus → enlarged scrotum ("bag of worms")	669
Methemoglobin	↑ oxidized Hb (Fe^{3+}) 2° to dapsone, local anesthetics, nitrites → ↓ O_2 binding but ↑ cyanide affinity → tissue hypoxia	688
Sarcoidosis-associated hypercalcemia	Noncaseating granulomas → ↑ macrophage activity → ↑ 1α-hydroxylase activity in macrophages → vitamin D activation → ↑ Ca^{2+}	695
ARDS	Alveolar injury → inflammation → capillary endothelial damage and ↑ vessel permeability → leakage of protein-rich fluid into alveoli → intra-alveolar hyaline membranes and noncardiogenic pulmonary edema → ↓ compliance and V/Q mismatch → hypoxic vasoconstriction → ↑ pulmonary vascular resistance	697
Sleep apnea	Respiratory effort against airway obstruction (obstructive); impaired respiratory effort due to CNS injury/toxicity, CHF, opioids (central); obesity → hypoventilation → ↑ $PaCO_2$ during waking hours	697

▶ CLASSIC PRESENTATIONS

CLINICAL PRESENTATION	DIAGNOSIS/DISEASE	PAGE
Gout, intellectual disability, self-mutilating behavior in a boy	Lesch-Nyhan syndrome (HGPRT deficiency, X-linked recessive)	35
Situs inversus, chronic ear infections, sinusitis, bronchiectasis, infertility	Primary ciliary dyskinesia (Kartagener syndrome)	47
Blue sclera, multiple fractures, dental problems, conductive/mixed hearing loss	Osteogenesis imperfecta (type I collagen defect)	49
Elastic skin, joint hypermobility, bleeding tendency	Ehlers-Danlos syndrome (type V collagen defect, type III collagen defect seen in vascular subtype)	49
Arachnodactyly, lens dislocation (upward and temporal), aortic dissection, hyperflexible joints	Marfan syndrome (defective fibrillin-1)	50
Arachnodactyly, pectus deformity, lens dislocation (downward and nasal)	Homocystinuria (autosomal recessive cystathionine synthase deficiency)	50
Café-au-lait spots (unilateral), polyostotic fibrous dysplasia, precocious puberty, multiple endocrine abnormalities	McCune-Albright syndrome (G_s-protein activating mutation)	55
Meconium ileus in neonate, recurrent pulmonary infections, nasal polyps, pancreatic insufficiency, infertility/subfertility, malabsorption/vitamin deficiencies	Cystic fibrosis (*CFTR* gene defect, chromosome 7, ΔF508)	58
Calf pseudohypertrophy	Muscular dystrophy (most commonly Duchenne, due to X-linked recessive frameshift mutation of dystrophin gene)	59
Child uses arms to stand up from squat	Duchenne muscular dystrophy (Gowers sign)	59
Slow, progressive muscle weakness in boys	Becker muscular dystrophy (X-linked non-frameshift deletions in dystrophin; less severe than Duchenne)	59
Infant with cleft lip/palate, microcephaly or holoprosencephaly, polydactyly, cutis aplasia	Patau syndrome (trisomy 13)	61
Infant with microcephaly, rocker-bottom feet, clenched hands, structural heart defect	Edwards syndrome (trisomy 18)	61
Single palmar crease, flat facies, prominent epicanthal folds, congenital heart disease, intellectual disability	Down syndrome (trisomy 21)	61
Microcephaly, high-pitched cry, intellectual disability	Cri-du-chat (cry of the cat) syndrome; congenital deletion on short arm of chromosome 5	62
Confusion, ophthalmoplegia/nystagmus, ataxia	Wernicke encephalopathy (add confabulation/memory loss and personality changes for Korsakoff syndrome)	64
Dilated cardiomyopathy/high-output heart failure, edema, alcoholism or malnutrition	Wet beriberi (thiamine [vitamin B_1] deficiency)	64
Dermatitis, dementia, diarrhea	Pellagra (niacin [vitamin B_3] deficiency)	65
"Burning feet syndrome," dermatitis, enteritis, alopecia	Pantothenic acid (vitamin B_5) deficiency	65
Megaloblastic anemia, subacute combined degeneration, paresthesias, cognitive changes	Cobalamin (vitamin B_{12}) deficiency; malabsorption, decreased intrinsic factor, absent terminal ileum	67
Swollen gums, mucosal bleeding, poor wound healing, petechiae, corkscrew hairs, perifollicular hemorrhages	Scurvy (vitamin C deficiency: inability to hydroxylate proline/lysine for collagen synthesis); tea and toast diet	67

CLINICAL PRESENTATION	DIAGNOSIS/DISEASE	PAGE
Bowlegs (children), bone pain, and muscle weakness	Vitamin D deficiency: rickets (children), osteomalacia (adults); ↓ sun exposure, chronic kidney disease	68
Hemorrhagic disease of newborn with ↑ aPTT, normal bleeding time	Vitamin K deficiency	69
Intellectual disability, musty body odor, hypopigmented skin, eczema	Phenylketonuria (tetrahydrobiopterin [BH_4] deficiency)	82
Bluish-black connective tissue, ear cartilage, sclerae; severe arthralgias; urine turns black on prolonged exposure to air	Alkaptonuria (homogentisate oxidase deficiency; ochronosis)	82
Infant with hypoglycemia, hepatomegaly, cardiomyopathy	Cori disease (debranching enzyme deficiency) or von Gierke disease (glucose-6-phosphatase deficiency, more severe)	85
Chronic exercise intolerance with myalgia, fatigue, painful cramps, myoglobinuria	McArdle disease (skeletal muscle glycogen phosphorylase deficiency)	85
"Cherry-red spot" on macula	Tay-Sachs (ganglioside accumulation; no hepatosplenomegaly); Niemann-Pick disease (sphingomyelin accumulation; hepatosplenomegaly); central retinal artery occlusion	86, 552
Hepatosplenomegaly, pancytopenia, osteoporosis, avascular necrosis of femoral head, bone crises	Gaucher disease (glucocerebrosidase [β-glucosidase] deficiency)	86
Achilles tendon xanthoma, corneal arcus	Familial hypercholesterolemia (↓ LDL receptor signaling)	92
Male child, recurrent infections, no mature B cells	Bruton disease (X-linked agammaglobulinemia [*BTK* gene defect])	114
Anaphylaxis following blood transfusion, atopy, airway/GI infections, autoimmune disease	Selective IgA deficiency	114
Recurrent cold (noninflamed) abscesses, eczema, ↑ serum IgE, eosinophils	Hyper-IgE syndrome (Job syndrome: neutrophil chemotaxis abnormality; *STAT3* mutation)	114
Late separation (> 30 days) of umbilical cord, no pus, recurrent skin and mucosal bacterial infections	Leukocyte adhesion deficiency (type 1; defective LFA-1 [CD18] integrin)	115
Recurrent infections and granulomas with catalase ⊕ organisms	Chronic granulomatous disease (defective NADPH oxidase)	115
Fever, vomiting, diarrhea, desquamating rash after prolonged use of nasal pack or tampon	Staphylococcal toxic shock syndrome	133
"Strawberry tongue"	Scarlet fever (sandpaper rash); Kawasaki disease (lymphadenopathy, high fever for 5 days)	134, 478
Colon cancer associated with infective endocarditis	*Streptococcus gallolyticus* (formerly S *bovis*)	135
Descending flaccid paralysis in newborn after honey ingestion	*Clostridium botulinum* infection (floppy baby syndrome)	136
Abdominal pain, diarrhea, leukocytosis, recent antibiotic use	*Clostridioides difficile* infection	136
Grayish-white pseudomembranous pharyngitis with "bull's neck" appearance	*Corynebacterium diphtheriae* infection	137
Back pain, fever, night sweats	Pott disease (vertebral TB)	138
Acute adrenal insufficiency, fever, bilateral adrenal hemorrhage	Waterhouse-Friderichsen syndrome (meningococcemia)	140, 353

CLINICAL PRESENTATION	DIAGNOSIS/DISEASE	PAGE
Red "currant jelly" sputum in patients with alcohol overuse or diabetes	*Klebsiella pneumoniae*	143
Fever, chills, headache, myalgia following antibiotic treatment for syphilis	Jarisch-Herxheimer reaction (host response to sudden release of bacterial antigens)	144
Large rash with bull's-eye appearance, flu-like symptoms	Erythema migrans from *Ixodes* tick bite (Lyme disease: *Borrelia* bacteria)	144
Ulcerated genital lesion	Nonpainful, indurated: chancre (1° syphilis, *Treponema pallidum*) Painful, with exudate: chancroid (*Haemophilus ducreyi*)	145, 180
Smooth, moist, painless, wartlike white lesions on genitals	Condylomata lata (2° syphilis)	145
Pupil accommodates but doesn't react to light	Argyll Robertson pupil (3° syphilis/neurosyphilis)	145
Dog or cat bite resulting in infection (cellulitis, osteomyelitis)	*Pasteurella multocida* (cellulitis at inoculation site)	147
Atypical "walking pneumonia" with x-ray looking worse than the patient	*Mycoplasma pneumoniae* infection	148
Rash on palms and soles	Coxsackie A infection, Rocky Mountain spotted fever, 2° syphilis	148
Black eschar on face of patient with diabetic ketoacidosis and/or neutropenia	*Mucor* or *Rhizopus* fungal infection	150
Chorioretinitis, hydrocephalus, intracranial calcifications, +/– blueberry muffin rash	Congenital toxoplasmosis	153, 180
Pruritus, serpiginous rash after walking barefoot, microcytic anemia	Hookworm (*Ancylostoma spp*, *Necator americanus*)	156
Febrile child later develops red facial rash with subsequent spread to body	Erythema infectiosum/fifth disease ("slapped cheeks" appearance, caused by parvovirus B19)	161
Fever, cough, conjunctivitis, coryza, diffuse rash, Koplik spots (small, irregular red spots on buccal/lingual mucosa with blue-white centers)	Measles (rubeola) virus	167
Systolic ejection murmur (crescendo-decrescendo), "pulsus parvus et tardus," syncope, angina, dyspnea on exertion	Aortic stenosis	296
Hyperdynamic pulses, wide pulse pressure, early diastolic murmur (decrescendo), head bobbing	Aortic regurgitation	296
Continuous "machinelike" murmur	PDA (close with indomethacin; keep open with PGE1 and PGE2 analogs)	296
Chest pain on exertion	Angina (stable: with moderate exertion; unstable: with minimal exertion or at rest)	308
Chest pain with ST depressions on ECG	Angina (⊖ troponins) or NSTEMI (⊕ troponins)	308
Chest pain, pericardial effusion/friction rub, persistent fever following MI	Postcardiac injury syndrome (autoimmune-mediated post-MI pericarditis, weeks to several months after acute episode)	314
Distant heart sounds, distended neck veins, hypotension	Beck triad of cardiac tamponade	317
Painful, raised red/purple lesions on pads of fingers/toes	Osler nodes (immune complex deposition in infective endocarditis)	318

CLINICAL PRESENTATION	DIAGNOSIS/DISEASE	PAGE
Painless erythematous lesions on palms and soles	Janeway lesions (septic emboli/microabscesses in infective endocarditis)	318
Splinter hemorrhages in fingernails	Infective endocarditis	318
Retinal hemorrhages with pale centers	Roth spots (infective endocarditis)	318
Telangiectasias, recurrent epistaxis, skin discoloration, arteriovenous malformations, GI bleeding, hematuria	Hereditary hemorrhagic telangiectasia (Osler-Weber-Rendu syndrome)	320
Polyuria, polydipsia	Primary polydipsia, diabetes mellitus (type 1 or 2), diabetes insipidus (central, nephrogenic)	342, 350
No lactation postpartum, absent menstruation, cold intolerance	Sheehan syndrome (severe postpartum hemorrhage → pituitary infarction)	343
Heat intolerance, weight loss, palpitations, fine tremor, hyperreflexia	Hyperthyroidism	344
Cold intolerance, weight gain, brittle hair, depressed mood, hyporeflexia	Hypothyroidism	344
Cutaneous/dermal edema due to deposition of mucopolysaccharides in connective tissue	Myxedema (caused by hypothyroidism or hyperthyroidism [Graves disease])	344
Facial muscle spasm upon tapping	Chvostek sign (hypocalcemia)	348
Carpal spasm upon BP cuff inflation	Trousseau sign (hypocalcemia)	348
Rapid, deep, labored breathing/hyperventilation	Diabetic ketoacidosis (Kussmaul respirations)	351
Skin hyperpigmentation, orthostatic hypotension, fatigue, weakness, muscle aches, weight loss, GI disturbances	Chronic 1° adrenal insufficiency (Addison disease) → ↑ ACTH, ↑ MSH	353
Shock, altered mental status, vomiting, abdominal pain, weakness, fatigue in patient on glucocorticoid therapy	Acute adrenal insufficiency (adrenal crisis)	353
Pancreatic, pituitary, parathyroid tumors	MEN1 (autosomal dominant *MEN1* mutation)	356
Medullary thyroid carcinoma, parathyroid hyperplasia, pheochromocytoma	MEN2A (autosomal dominant *RET* mutation)	356
Medullary thyroid carcinoma, pheochromocytoma, mucosal neuromas, marfanoid habitus	MEN2B (autosomal dominant *RET* mutation)	356
Cutaneous flushing, diarrhea, bronchospasm, right-sided heart murmur	Carcinoid syndrome (urinary 5-HIAA); indicates systemic dissemination (eg, post–liver metastases)	357
Jaundice, palpable distended nontender gallbladder	Courvoisier sign (distal obstruction of common bile duct by pancreatic head malignancy)	375, 405
Hematemesis +/– abdominal/back pain	Mallory-Weiss syndrome (partial thickness esophageal lacerations in a patient with alcohol use disorder, bulimia nervosa)	384
Dysphagia (esophageal webs), glossitis, iron deficiency anemia	Plummer-Vinson syndrome (may progress to esophageal squamous cell carcinoma)	384
Enlarged, firm left supraclavicular node	Virchow node (metastasis from stomach malignancy)	386
Hematemesis, melena	Upper GI bleed (eg, peptic ulcer disease)	387
Hematochezia	Lower GI bleed (eg, colonic diverticulosis)	387
Arthralgias, cardiac and neurological symptoms, diarrhea	Whipple disease (*Tropheryma whipplei*)	388
Severe RLQ pain with palpation of LLQ	Rovsing sign (acute appendicitis)	390
Severe RLQ pain with deep palpation	McBurney sign (acute appendicitis)	390

CLINICAL PRESENTATION	DIAGNOSIS/DISEASE	PAGE
Hamartomatous GI polyps, hyperpigmented macules on mouth, lips, hands, genitalia	Peutz-Jeghers syndrome (autosomal dominant, benign polyposis can cause bowel obstruction; ↑ breast/GI cancer risk)	394
Thousands of colon polyps, osteomas/soft tissue tumors, impacted/supernumerary teeth	Gardner syndrome (subtype of familial adenomatous polyposis)	394
Severe jaundice, kernicterus (neurological changes) in neonate	Crigler-Najjar syndrome, type I (congenital unconjugated hyperbilirubinemia)	401
Golden brown rings around peripheral cornea	Wilson disease (Kayser-Fleischer rings due to copper accumulation)	402
Female, fat (obese), fertile (multiparity), forty, fair, feeds (TPN), fasting (rapid weight loss)	Cholelithiasis (gallstones)	403
Bluish line on gingiva	Burton line (lead poisoning)	425
Short stature, café-au-lait spots, thumb/radial defects, ↑ incidence of tumors/leukemia, aplastic anemia (pancytopenia)	Fanconi anemia (genetic defect in DNA crosslink repair; often progresses to AML)	427
Red/pink urine in the morning, pancytopenia, venous thrombosis	Paroxysmal nocturnal hemoglobinuria	428
Painful blue fingers/toes, hemolytic anemia	Cold autoimmune hemolytic anemia (caused by *Mycoplasma pneumoniae*, infectious mononucleosis, CLL)	429
Petechiae, mucosal bleeding, ↑ bleeding time	Platelet disorders (eg, Glanzmann thrombasthenia, Bernard Soulier, HUS, TTP, ITP, uremic platelet dysfunction)	432
Low-grade fever, night sweats, weight loss	"B" symptoms of malignancy	434
Erythematous patches → plaques → tumors	Mycosis fungoides (cutaneous T-cell lymphoma) or	435
Neonate with arm in "waiter's tip" position following difficult birth	Erb palsy (superior trunk [C5-C6] brachial plexus injury)	452
Anterior drawer sign ⊕ (tibia glides anteriorly with respect to femur when knee is at 90° angle)	Anterior cruciate ligament (ACL) injury	454
Mosaic pattern of bone, long bone chalk-stick fractures, skull thickening, hearing loss	Osteitis deformans (Paget disease of bone, ↑ osteoblastic and osteoclastic activity)	468
Swollen, hard, painful finger joints in an elderly individual, pain worse with activity	Osteoarthritis (osteophytes on PIP [Bouchard nodes], DIP [Heberden nodes])	472
Sudden swollen/painful big toe joint, tophi	Gout/podagra (hyperuricemia)	473
Dry eyes and mouth, arthritis, parotid enlargement	Sjögren syndrome (autoimmune destruction of exocrine glands)	474
Urethritis, conjunctivitis, arthritis	Reactive arthritis associated with HLA-B27	475
"Butterfly" facial rash, arthritis, cytopenia, and fever in a female of reproductive age	Systemic lupus erythematosus	476
Cervical lymphadenopathy, desquamating rash, coronary aneurysms, red conjunctivae and tongue, hand-foot changes (edema, erythema), fever ≥ 5 days	Kawasaki disease (mucocutaneous lymph node syndrome, treat with IVIG and aspirin)	478
Palpable purpura on buttocks/legs, joint pain, abdominal pain, hematuria in a child	IgA vasculitis (Henoch-Schönlein purpura, affects skin and kidneys)	479

CLINICAL PRESENTATION	DIAGNOSIS/DISEASE	PAGE
Painful fingers/toes changing color from white to blue to red with cold or stress	Raynaud phenomenon (vasospasm in extremities)	480
Dark purple skin/mouth nodules in a patient with AIDS	Kaposi sarcoma, associated with HHV-8	486
Pruritic, purple, polygonal planar papules and plaques (6 Ps)	Lichen planus	492
Dorsiflexion of large toe with fanning of other toes upon plantar scrape	Babinski sign (UMN lesion)	523, 543
Intention tremor, limb ataxia, loss of balance (fall toward injured side)	Cerebellar lesion (hemispheric affects voluntary movement of extremities; vermis affects axial and proximal movement)	524
Hyperphagia, hypersexuality, hyperorality	Klüver-Bucy syndrome (bilateral amygdala lesion; HSV-1 encephalitis)	524
Resting tremor, athetosis, chorea	Basal ganglia lesion (eg, Huntington disease, Parkinson disease)	524
Dysphagia, hoarseness, ↓ gag reflex, nystagmus, ipsilateral Horner syndrome	Lateral medullary (Wallenberg) syndrome (posterior inferior cerebellar artery lesion)	527
Lucid interval after traumatic brain injury	Epidural hematoma (middle meningeal artery rupture; branch of maxillary artery; lentiform collection not crossing suture lines)	528
"Worst headache of my life"	Subarachnoid hemorrhage	528
Resting tremor, rigidity, akinesia (shuffling gait, micrographia), postural instability	Parkinson disease (loss of dopaminergic neurons in substantia nigra pars compacta)	534
Chorea, dementia, caudate degeneration	Huntington disease (loss of GABAergic neurons in striatum; autosomal dominant CAG repeat expansion)	534
Urinary incontinence, gait apraxia, cognitive dysfunction	Normal pressure hydrocephalus (ventricle expansion → distortion of corona radiata fibers)	536
Relapsing and remitting nystagmus, intention tremor, optic neuritis, scanning speech, bilateral internuclear ophthalmoplegia	Multiple sclerosis	537
Progressive, ascending symmetric limb weakness and hyporeflexia after GI/upper respiratory infection	Guillain-Barré syndrome (acute inflammatory demyelinating polyneuropathy)	538
Café-au-lait spots, Lisch nodules (iris hamartomas), cutaneous neurofibromas, pheochromocytomas, optic gliomas	Neurofibromatosis type I	539
Bilateral vestibular schwannomas	Neurofibromatosis type II	539
Vascular birthmark (port-wine stain) on face	Nevus flammeus (benign, associated with Sturge-Weber syndrome)	539
Bilateral renal cell carcinomas, hemangioblastomas, angiomatosis, pheochromocytomas	von Hippel-Lindau disease (VHL deletion on chromosome 3p)	539
Hyperreflexia, hypertonia, ⊕ Babinski sign	UMN damage	543
Hyporeflexia, hypotonia, atrophy, fasciculations	LMN damage	543
Staggering gait, frequent falls, nystagmus, hammer toes, diabetes mellitus, hypertrophic cardiomyopathy	Friedreich ataxia	545
Unilateral facial drooping involving forehead	LMN facial nerve (CN VII) palsy; UMN lesions spare forehead due to bilateral innervation	546

CLINICAL PRESENTATION	DIAGNOSIS/DISEASE	PAGE
Episodic vertigo, tinnitus, sensorineural hearing loss	Ménière disease (↑ endolymph in inner ear)	548
Ptosis, miosis, anhidrosis	Horner syndrome (sympathetic chain lesion)	555
Conjugate horizontal gaze palsy, horizontal diplopia	Internuclear ophthalmoplegia (MLF lesion; unilateral or bilateral)	558
Acute onset, reversible "waxing and waning" level of consciousness (acute onset), ↓ attention span, ↓ arousal	Delirium (usually 2° to other cause)	575
Polyuria, renal tubular acidosis type II, growth retardation, electrolyte imbalances, hypophosphatemic rickets	Fanconi syndrome (generalized reabsorption defect of proximal convoluted tubule)	604, 611
Periorbital and/or peripheral edema, proteinuria (> 3.5 g/day; frothy urine), hypoalbuminemia, hypercholesterolemia	Nephrotic syndrome (podocyte damage)	613
Hereditary nephritis, sensorineural hearing loss, retinopathy, anterior lenticonus	Alport syndrome (type IV collagen mutation)	615
Wilms tumor, macroglossia, organomegaly, hemihyperplasia, omphalocele	Beckwith-Wiedemann syndrome (*WT2* mutation)	624
Streak ovaries, congenital heart disease, horseshoe kidney, cystic hygroma, short stature, webbed neck, lymphedema	Turner syndrome (45,XO)	655
Ovarian fibroma, ascites, pleural effusion	Meigs syndrome	665
Red, itchy, swollen rash of nipple/areola	Paget disease of the breast (sign of underlying neoplasm)	668
Fibrous plaques in tunica albuginea of penis with abnormal curvature	Peyronie disease (associated with repeated minor trauma during intercourse)	669
Hypoxemia, polycythemia, hypercapnia	Chronic bronchitis (hypertrophy and hyperplasia of mucus-secreting glands)	692
Pink complexion, dyspnea, hyperventilation	Emphysema (centriacinar [tobacco smoking] or panacinar [α_1-antitrypsin deficiency])	692
Bilateral hilar adenopathy, uveitis, arthropathy, skin changes	Sarcoidosis (immune-mediated noncaseating granulomas)	695

▶ CLASSIC LABS/FINDINGS

LAB/DIAGNOSTIC FINDING	DIAGNOSIS/DISEASE	PAGE
Colonies of *Pseudomonas* in lungs, ↑ Cl⁻ on sweat test, ↑ immunoreactive trypsinogen	Cystic fibrosis (autosomal recessive mutation in *CFTR* gene → fat-soluble vitamin deficiency and mucous plugs)	58
↓ AFP on second trimester screening	Down syndrome, Edwards syndrome	61
↑ β-hCG, ↓ PAPP-A on first trimester screening	Down syndrome	61
Homocysteine, methylmalonic acid, folate	Vitamin B_{12} deficiency	67
Anti-histone antibodies	Drug-induced lupus	113
↓ T cells, ↓ PTH, ↓ Ca^{2+}, absent thymic shadow on CXR	Thymic aplasia (22q11 microdeletion: DiGeorge syndrome, velocardiofacial syndrome)	114
Recurrent infections, eczema, thrombocytopenia, ↑ IgE and IgA, ↓/normal IgG and IgM	Wiskott-Aldrich syndrome (*WAS* gene mutation)	115

LAB/DIAGNOSTIC FINDING	DIAGNOSIS/DISEASE	PAGE
Giant granules in phagocytes, pancytopenia (immunodeficiency)	Chédiak-Higashi disease (*LYST* gene mutation: congenital failure of phagolysosome formation)	115
Optochin sensitivity	Sensitive: *S pneumoniae*; resistant: viridans streptococci (*S mutans, S sanguis, S mitis*)	132
Novobiocin response	Sensitive: *S epidermidis*; resistant: *S saprophyticus*	132
Bacitracin response	Sensitive: *S pyogenes* (group A); resistant: *S agalactiae* (group B)	132
Branching gram ⊕ rods with "sulfur granules"	*Actinomyces israelii*	137
Hilar lymphadenopathy, peripheral granulomatous lesion in middle or lower lung lobes (can calcify)	Ghon complex (1° TB: *Mycobacterium bacilli*)	138
"Thumb sign" on lateral neck x-ray	Epiglottitis (*Haemophilus influenzae*)	140
Bacteria-covered vaginal epithelial cells, ⊕ whiff test	"Clue cells" (*Gardnerella vaginalis*)	147
Ring-enhancing brain lesion on CT/MRI in AIDS	*Toxoplasma gondii* (multiple), CNS lymphoma (may be solitary)	153, 173
Dilated cardiomyopathy with apical atrophy, megacolon, megaesophagus	Chagas disease (*Trypanosoma cruzi*)	155
Atypical lymphocytes, heterophile antibodies	Infectious mononucleosis (EBV infection)	162
Narrowing of upper trachea and subglottis (Steeple sign) on x-ray	Croup (parainfluenza virus)	167
Cytoplasmic inclusions in Purkinje cells of cerebellum and in hippocampal neurons	Negri bodies of rabies	169
Concentrically laminated calcified spherules (psammoma bodies)	Papillary thyroid carcinoma, somatostatinoma, meningioma, mesothelioma, ovarian serous papillary cystadenocarcinoma, prolactinoma	207
Boot-shaped heart on x-ray	Tetralogy of Fallot (due to RVH)	302
Rib notching (inferior surface, on x-ray)	Coarctation of the aorta	304
Delta wave and shortened PR interval on ECG; may lead to supraventricular tachycardia	Wolff-Parkinson-White syndrome (bundle of Kent bypasses AV node)	311
Electrical alternans (alternating amplitude of R waves on ECG)	Cardiac tamponade	317
Granuloma with giant cells after pharyngeal infection	Aschoff bodies (rheumatic fever)	319
↑ level of fibrin degradation products (D-dimer)	DVT, DIC	321, 433
Empty-appearing nuclei with central clearing in thyroid cells	"Orphan Annie" eyes (papillary thyroid carcinoma)	347
"Brown" tumor of bone	Hyperparathyroidism or osteitis fibrosa cystica (deposited hemosiderin from hemorrhages causes brown color)	349, 469
Hypertension, hypokalemia, metabolic alkalosis, ↑ aldosterone, ↓ renin	1° hyperaldosteronism (eg, Conn syndrome)	354
Mucin-filled cell with peripheral nucleus	"Signet ring" cells (diffuse gastric carcinoma)	386
Anti-transglutaminase/anti-deamidated gliadin/anti-endomysial antibodies	Celiac disease (diarrhea, weight loss)	388
Narrowing of bowel lumen on small bowel follow-through	"String sign" (Crohn disease)	389

LAB/DIAGNOSTIC FINDING	DIAGNOSIS/DISEASE	PAGE
"Lead pipe" appearance of colon on imaging	Ulcerative colitis (loss of haustra)	389
Thousands of polyps on colonoscopy after puberty	Familial adenomatous polyposis (autosomal dominant *APC* gene mutation)	394
"Apple core" lesion on barium enema x-ray	Colorectal cancer (usually left-sided)	395
"Nutmeg" (mottled) appearance of liver	Chronic passive congestion of liver due to right heart failure, Budd-Chiari syndrome	397
Eosinophilic cytoplasmic inclusion of damaged keratin within hepatocyte	Mallory body (alcoholic hepatitis)	398
Fatty infiltration of hepatocytes → cellular "ballooning", eventual necrosis	Fatty liver disease (associated with alcohol use or metabolic syndrome)	398
Anti-smooth muscle antibodies (ASMAs), anti-liver/kidney microsomal-1 (anti-LKM1) antibodies	Autoimmune hepatitis	399
Antimitochondrial antibodies (AMAs)	1° biliary cholangitis (female, cholestasis, portal hypertension)	402
↓ serum ceruloplasmin	Wilson disease	402
Migratory thrombophlebitis (leading to migrating DVTs and vasculitis)	Trousseau syndrome (pancreatic adenocarcinoma)	405
Basophilic stippling of RBCs (basophilic ribosomal precipitates)	Sideroblastic anemia, thalassemias	421
Basophilic nuclear remnants in RBCs	Howell-Jolly bodies (due to splenectomy or nonfunctional spleen)	421
Hypochromic, microcytic anemia	Iron deficiency anemia, lead poisoning, thalassemia (fetal hemoglobin sometimes present), sideroblastic anemia	424, 425
"Hair on end" ("crew cut") appearance on skull x-ray	β-thalassemia, sickle cell anemia (marrow expansion)	425, 428
Hypersegmented neutrophils	Megaloblastic anemia (vitamin B_{12} deficiency: neurologic symptoms; folate deficiency: no neurologic symptoms)	426
Anti-GpIIb/IIIa antibodies	Immune thrombocytopenia	432
Giant B cells featuring bilobed nuclei with prominent inclusions ("owl's eye")	Reed-Sternberg cells (Hodgkin lymphoma)	434
Sheets of lymphocytes with interspersed "tingible body" macrophages ("starry sky" histology)	Burkitt lymphoma [t(8:14) c-*myc* activation, associated with EBV; "starry sky" made up of malignant cells]	435
Lytic ("punched-out") bone lesions on x-ray	Multiple myeloma	436
Monoclonal spike on serum protein electrophoresis	Multiple myeloma (usually IgG or IgA); Waldenström macroglobulinemia (IgM); monoclonal gammopathy of undetermined significance	436
Stacks of RBCs	Rouleaux formation (↑ ESR, multiple myeloma)	436
Myeloperoxidase ⊕ cytoplasmic inclusions in myeloblasts, ↑↑↑ circulating myeloblasts	Auer rods (APL)	437
WBCs that look "smudged"	CLL	437
"Tennis racket"-shaped cytoplasmic organelles (on EM) in Langerhans cells	Birbeck granules (Langerhans cell histiocytosis)	439

LAB/DIAGNOSTIC FINDING	DIAGNOSIS/DISEASE	PAGE
"Soap bubble" in femur or tibia on x-ray	Giant cell tumor of bone (generally benign)	470
Elevated periosteum (creating a "Codman triangle") or sunburst pattern on x-ray	Osteosarcoma (osteogenic sarcoma)	471
"Onion skin" periosteal reaction	Ewing sarcoma (malignant small blue cell tumor)	471
IgM antibodies that target IgG Fc region, anti-cyclic citrullinated peptide antibodies	Rheumatoid arthritis (systemic inflammation, joint pannus, boutonniere and swan neck deformities)	472
Needle-shaped, ⊖ birefringent crystals	Gout (monosodium urate crystals)	473
↑ uric acid levels	Gout, Lesch-Nyhan syndrome, tumor lysis syndrome, loop and thiazide diuretics	473
Rhomboid, ⊕ birefringent crystals	Pseudogout (calcium pyrophosphate dihydrate crystals)	473
"Bamboo spine" (vertebral fusion) on x-ray	Ankylosing spondylitis (chronic inflammatory arthritis, associated with HLA-B27)	475
Antinuclear, anti-Smith, anti-dsDNA, antiphospholipid antibodies	SLE (type III, and to a lesser degree, type II hypersensitivity)	476
Antineutrophil cytoplasmic antibodies (ANCAs)	Microscopic polyangiitis, eosinophilic granulomatosis with polyangiitis, and primary sclerosing cholangitis (MPO-ANCA/p-ANCA); granulomatosis with polyangiitis (PR3-ANCA/c-ANCA)	402, 478
Anti-Scl-70 (anti-DNA topoisomerase-I) and anti-RNA polymerase III antibodies	Diffuse scleroderma	481
Anti-centromere antibodies	Limited scleroderma (CREST syndrome)	481
Anti-desmoglein 3 +/− 1 (anti-desmosome) antibodies	Pemphigus vulgaris	489
Anti-hemidesmosome antibodies	Bullous pemphigoid	489
Keratin pearls on skin biopsy	Squamous cell carcinoma	494
↑ AFP in maternal serum	Dating error, open neural tube defects	501
Bloody or yellow CSF on lumbar puncture	Xanthochromia (due to subarachnoid hemorrhage)	528
Loss of dopaminergic (pigmented) neurons in substantia nigra	Parkinson disease	534
Intracellular eosinophilic inclusion in neuron	Lewy body, composed of α-synuclein (Parkinson disease and Lewy body dementia)	534, 535
Extracellular amyloid deposition in gray matter of brain	Senile plaques (Alzheimer disease)	534
Hyperphosphorylated tau protein aggregates in neurons	Neurofibrillary tangles (Alzheimer disease) and Pick bodies (frontotemporal dementia)	534, 535
"Pseudopalisading" pleomorphic tumor cells on brain biopsy	Glioblastoma	540
Small blue cells surrounding central area of neuropil	Homer-Wright rosettes (neuroblastoma, medulloblastoma)	354, 542
RBC casts in urine	Glomerulonephritis, hypertensive emergency	612
WBC casts in urine	Acute pyelonephritis, transplant rejection, tubulointerstitial inflammation	612
Granular, "muddy-brown" casts in urine	Acute tubular necrosis (eg, ischemia or toxic injury)	612
Waxy casts with very low urine flow	End-stage renal disease/chronic kidney disease	612

LAB/DIAGNOSTIC FINDING	DIAGNOSIS/DISEASE	PAGE
"Lumpy-bumpy" appearance of glomeruli on immunofluorescence	Infection-related glomerulonephritis (due to IgG, IgM, and C3 deposition)	614
Anti–glomerular basement membrane antibodies, linear appearance of IgG deposition on glomerular and alveolar basement membranes	Goodpasture syndrome (hematuria, hemoptysis)	614
		614
Necrotizing vasculitis (lungs) and necrotizing glomerulonephritis	Granulomatosis with polyangiitis (PR3-ANCA/c-ANCA) and Goodpasture syndrome (anti–basement membrane antibodies)	614, 479
Cellular crescents in Bowman's space on light microscopy	Rapidly progressive (crescentic) glomerulonephritis	614
"Wire loop" glomerular capillary on light microscopy	Diffuse proliferative glomerulonephritis (usually seen with lupus)	614
"Tram-track" appearance of capillary loops of glomerular basement membranes on light microscopy	Membranoproliferative glomerulonephritis	615
Effacement of podocyte foot processes on EM	Minimal change disease (child with nephrotic syndrome), focal segmental glomerulosclerosis (nephrotic syndrome more common in Black individuals)	616
"Spike and dome" appearance of subepithelial deposits	Membranous nephropathy (nephrotic syndrome)	616
Eosinophilic nodular glomerulosclerosis	Kimmelstiel-Wilson lesions (diabetic glomerulonephropathy)	616
Thyroid-like appearance of kidney	Chronic pyelonephritis	619
↑ hCG	Multifetal gestation, hydatidiform mole, choriocarcinoma, dysgerminoma, Down syndrome	652
Dysplastic squamous cervical cells with "raisinoid" nuclei and perinuclear halo	Koilocytes (HPV infection; predisposes to cervical cancer)	663
Sheets of uniform "fried egg" cells, ↑ hCG, ↑ LDH	Dysgerminoma	664
Schiller-Duval bodies (resemble glomeruli), ↑ AFP	Yolk sac tumor	664
Disarrayed granulosa cells arranged around collections of eosinophilic fluid	Call-Exner bodies (granulosa cell tumor of the ovary)	665
"Chocolate cyst" in ovary	Endometriosis	666
Mammary gland ("blue domed") simple cyst	Fibrocystic change of the breast	667
Eosinophilic cytoplasmic inclusions in Leydig cells	Reinke crystals (Leydig cell tumor)	671
Interdigitating layers of pink and red in arterial thrombi	Lines of Zahn (layers of platelets and RBCs seen only in thrombi formed before death)	691
Eosinophilic, hexagonal, double-pointed crystals in bronchial secretions	Charcot-Leyden crystals (asthma)	693
Whorled mucus plugs formed from shed bronchial epithelium	Curschmann spirals (asthma)	693
"Honeycomb" appearance of the lung on CXR or CT	Idiopathic pulmonary fibrosis	694
Golden-brown fusiform rods resembling dumbbells in alveolar sputum, visualized with Prussian blue stain	Asbestos (ferruginous) bodies	696
Bronchogenic apical lung tumor on imaging	Pancoast (superior sulcus) tumor (can compress cervical sympathetic chain → Horner syndrome)	704

▶ KEY ASSOCIATIONS

DISEASE/FINDING	MOST COMMON/IMPORTANT ASSOCIATIONS	PAGE
Mitochondrial inheritance	Disease occurs in all offspring of affected females (maternal inheritance pattern), heteroplasmy	55, 57
Intellectual disability	Down syndrome (sporadic), fragile X syndrome (inherited)	60, 61
Vitamin deficiency (USA)	Folate (pregnant women are at ↑ risk; body stores only a 3–4 month supply)	66
Lysosomal storage disease	Gaucher disease	86
HLA-DR3	Type I DM, SLE, Graves disease, Hashimoto thyroiditis, Addison disease	98
HLA-DR4	Rheumatoid arthritis, type I DM, Addison disease	98
Bacteria associated with gastritis, peptic ulcer disease, and gastric malignancies (eg, adenocarcinoma, MALToma)	*H pylori*	144
Opportunistic respiratory infection in AIDS	*Pneumocystis jirovecii*	151
Viral encephalitis affecting temporal lobe	HSV-1	162
Viral infection 2° to blood transfusion	Hepatitis C	171
Food poisoning (exotoxin-mediated)	*S aureus, B cereus*	174
Healthcare-associated pneumonia	*S aureus, Pseudomonas*, other enteric gram ⊖ rods	175
Bacterial meningitis (0–6 months old)	Group B streptococcus, *E coli, Listeria*	176
Bacterial meningitis (> 6 months old)	*S pneumoniae*	176
Osteomyelitis	*S aureus* (most common overall)	176
Osteomyelitis in sickle cell disease	*Salmonella, S aureus*	176
Osteomyelitis with injection drug use	*S aureus, Pseudomonas, Candida*	176
UTI	*E coli, Staphylococcus saprophyticus*	178
Bacterial STI	*C trachomatis* (D–K)	179
Pelvic inflammatory disease (PID)	*C trachomatis* (subacute), *N gonorrhoeae* (acute)	181
Metastases to bone	Prostate, breast >> lung > kidney, colon	219
Metastases to liver	Colon > breast >> pancreas, lung, prostate	219
Metastases to brain	Lung > breast >> melanoma > colon, prostate	219
S3 heart sound	↑ ventricular filling pressure (eg, MR, AR, HF, thyrotoxicosis), common in dilated ventricles	292
S4 heart sound	Stiff/hypertrophic ventricle (aortic stenosis, restrictive cardiomyopathy)	292
Holosystolic murmur	VSD, tricuspid regurgitation, mitral regurgitation	296
Ejection click	Aortic stenosis	296
Mitral stenosis	Rheumatic heart disease (late and highly specific sequelae of rheumatic fever)	296
Opening snap	Mitral stenosis	296
Heart murmur, congenital	Mitral valve prolapse	296

DISEASE/FINDING	MOST COMMON/IMPORTANT ASSOCIATIONS	PAGE
Cyanotic heart disease (early)	Tetralogy of Fallot (most common), D-transposition of great arteries, persistent truncus arteriosus, total anomalous pulmonary venous return, tricuspid atresia (right-to-left shunts)	302
Congenital heart disease (left-to-right shunts)	VSD > ASD > PDA	303
Late cyanotic shunt (uncorrected left-to-right shunt becomes right-to-left)	Eisenmenger syndrome (caused by VSD, ASD, PDA)	303
2° hypertension	Renal/renovascular diseases (eg, fibromuscular dysplasia, atherosclerotic renal artery stenosis), 1° hyperaldosteronism, OSA	304
Sites of atherosclerosis	Abdominal aorta > coronary artery > popliteal artery > carotid artery > circle of Willis	305
Aortic aneurysm, thoracic	Marfan syndrome (cystic medial degeneration), 3° syphilis (obliterative endarteritis of vasa vasorum)	306
Aortic aneurysm, abdominal	Atherosclerosis, tobacco use	306
Aortic dissection	Hypertension (most important risk factor)	307
Irregularly irregular rhythm on ECG with no discrete P waves	Atrial fibrillation (associated with ↑ risk of emboli)	311
Right heart failure due to a pulmonary cause	Cor pulmonale	316
Heart valve in infective endocarditis	Mitral > aortic, tricuspid (injection drug use)	318
Infective endocarditis presentation associated with bacteria	S aureus (acute, injection drug use, tricuspid valve), viridans streptococci (subacute, dental procedure), S gallolyticus (colon cancer), gram ⊖ (HACEK), culture ⊖ (Coxiella, Bartonella)	318
Cardiac tumor (adults)	Metastasis, myxoma (75%–80% in left atrium; "ball valve")	320
Cardiac 1° tumor (children)	Rhabdomyoma (associated with tuberous sclerosis)	320
Hypercoagulability, endothelial damage, blood stasis	Virchow triad (↑ risk of thrombosis)	321
Congenital adrenal hyperplasia	21-hydroxylase deficiency	339
Hypopituitarism	Pituitary adenoma (under-secretion due to mass effect)	343
Congenital hypothyroidism	Thyroid dysgenesis/dyshormonogenesis, iodine deficiency	345
Thyroid cancer	Papillary carcinoma (RET/PTC rearrangements, BRAF mutations, childhood irradiation)	347
Hypoparathyroidism	Accidental excision during thyroidectomy	348
1° hyperparathyroidism	Adenomas, hyperplasia	349
2° hyperparathyroidism	Hypocalcemia of chronic kidney disease	349
Cushing syndrome (↑ cortisol)	Exogenous glucocorticoids; adrenocortical adenoma (secretes excess cortisol); ACTH-secreting pituitary adenoma (Cushing disease); paraneoplastic (due to ACTH secretion by tumors)	352
Cushing disease	↓ ACTH and ↓ cortisol in high-dose dexamethasone suppression test, ↑ ACTH and ↑ cortisol in CRH stimulation test	352
1° hyperaldosteronism	Bilateral adrenal hyperplasia or adenoma (Conn syndrome)	354
Tumor of the adrenal medulla (children)	Neuroblastoma (malignant)	354
Tumor of the adrenal medulla (adults)	Pheochromocytoma (usually benign)	355

DISEASE/FINDING	MOST COMMON/IMPORTANT ASSOCIATIONS	PAGE
Refractory peptic ulcers and ↑ gastrin levels (even after the secretin test)	Zollinger-Ellison syndrome (due to gastrin-secreting tumor of the duodenum or pancreas), associated with MEN1	357
Esophageal cancer	Squamous cell carcinoma (worldwide); adenocarcinoma (US)	385
Acute gastric ulcer associated with CNS injury	Cushing ulcer (↑ vagal stimulation → ↑ ACh → ↑ H⁺ production)	386
Acute gastric ulcer associated with severe burns	Curling ulcer (hypovolemia → mucosal ischemia)	386
Chronic atrophic gastritis	↑ risk of gastric cancers, pernicious anemia (if autoimmune)	386
Bilateral ovarian metastases from gastric carcinoma	Krukenberg tumor (mucin-secreting signet ring cells)	386
Alternating areas of transmural inflammation and normal colon	Skip lesions (Crohn disease)	389
Site of diverticulosis	Sigmoid colon	390
False pharyngoesophageal diverticulum	Zenker diverticulum	391
Hepatocellular carcinoma	HBV (+/– cirrhosis), other causes of cirrhosis (HCV, alcoholic liver disease), specific carcinogens (eg, aflatoxins)	399
Inherited conjugated hyperbilirubinemia 2° to hepatocyte inability to secrete conjugated bilirubin in bile	Dubin-Johnson syndrome (black liver), Rotor syndrome (uncolored liver)	401
Inherited benign unconjugated hyperbilirubinemia	Gilbert syndrome	401
Inherited *ATP7B* mutation (copper buildup in liver, brain, cornea [Kayser-Fleischer rings], kidneys)	Wilson disease	402
Multiple blood transfusions or hereditary *HFE* mutation (can result in heart failure, "bronze diabetes," and ↑ risk of hepatocellular carcinoma)	Hemochromatosis	402
Pancreatitis (acute)	Gallstones, alcohol	404
Pancreatitis (chronic)	Alcohol (adults), cystic fibrosis (children)	404
Microcytic anemia	Iron deficiency, thalassemia, lead poisoning, sideroblastic anemia	424, 425
Autosplenectomy (fibrosis and shrinkage), Howell-Jolly bodies	Sickle cell anemia (hemoglobin S)	428
Inherited platelet disorder with GpIb deficiency	Bernard-Soulier syndrome (↓ platelet-to-vWF adhesion)	432
Inherited platelet disorder with GpIIb/IIIa deficiency	Glanzmann thrombasthenia (↓ platelet-to-platelet aggregation, defective platelet plug formation)	432
Hereditary thrombophilia commonly associated with recurrent pregnancy loss	Factor V Leiden (mutant factor V resistant to degradation)	433
Disseminated Intravascular Coagulopathy (DIC)	Heat stroke, snake bite, sepsis, trauma, obstetric complications, acute pancreatitis, malignancy, nephrotic syndrome, transfusion	433
Common malignancy associated with noninfectious fever and bimodal age distribution	Hodgkin lymphoma	434
Type of Hodgkin lymphoma (most common)	Nodular sclerosis	434
t(14;18)	Follicular lymphoma (*BCL-2* activation, anti-apoptotic oncogene)	435, 439

DISEASE/FINDING	MOST COMMON/IMPORTANT ASSOCIATIONS	PAGE
t(8;14)	Burkitt lymphoma (c-*myc* fusion, transcription factor oncogene)	435, 439
Type of non-Hodgkin lymphoma (most common in adults)	Diffuse large B-cell lymphoma	435
Age ranges for patient with ALL/CLL/AML/CML	ALL: child, CLL: adult > 60, AML: adult ~ 65, CML: adult 45–85	437
t(9;22)	Philadelphia chromosome, CML (*BCR-ABL* oncogene, tyrosine kinase activation), more rarely associated with ALL	437, 439
Vertebral compression fracture	Osteoporosis	467
HLA-B27	Psoriatic arthritis, ankylosing spondylitis, IBD-associated arthritis, reactive arthritis	475
Death in SLE	Renal disease (most common), infections, cardiovascular disease (accelerated CAD)	476
Giant cell arteritis	Risk of ipsilateral blindness due to occlusion of ophthalmic artery; associated with polymyalgia rheumatica	478
Recurrent inflammation/thrombosis of medium-sized vessels in extremities	Buerger disease (strongly associated with tobacco smoking, Raynaud phenomenon)	478
Benign vascular tumor of infancy	Infantile hemangioma (grows rapidly then involutes starting at age 1)	486
Herald patch (followed by scaly erythematous plaques in a "Christmas tree" distribution)	Pityriasis rosea	492
Actinic keratosis	Precursor to squamous cell carcinoma	494
Cerebellar tonsillar herniation	Chiari I malformation (associated with spinal cord cavitations [eg, syringomyelia])	502
Bilateral mamillary body lesions with thiamine deficiency	Wernicke-Korsakoff syndrome	524
Epidural hematoma	Rupture of middle meningeal artery (trauma; biconvex/lentiform-shaped)	528
Subdural hematoma	Rupture of bridging veins (trauma, cerebral atrophy; crescent-shaped)	528
Dementia	Alzheimer disease, vascular dementia (multiple infarcts, stepwise decline)	534, 535
Demyelinating disease in young women	Multiple sclerosis	537
Brain tumor (adults)	Metastasis, glioblastoma (malignant), meningioma, hemangioblastoma	540
Galactorrhea, amenorrhea	Prolactinoma	540
Brain tumor (children)	Overall: pilocytic astrocytoma (benign) Infratentorial: medulloblastoma (most common malignant) Supratentorial: craniopharyngioma (malignant)	542
Combined UMN and LMN degeneration	Amyotrophic lateral sclerosis	544
Degeneration of dorsal column fibers	Tabes dorsalis (3° syphilis), subacute combined degeneration (Vitamin B_{12} deficiency; dorsal columns, lateral corticospinal, spinocerebellar tracts affected)	544
Nephrotic syndrome (children)	Minimal change disease	616

DISEASE/FINDING	MOST COMMON/IMPORTANT ASSOCIATIONS	PAGE
Kidney stones (radiolucent)	Uric acid	617
Kidney stones (radiopaque)	Calcium (most common), struvite (ammonium), cystine (faintly radiopaque)	617
Renal malignancy (in males)	Renal cell carcinoma: associated with tobacco smoking and VHL (clear cell subtype); may present with paraneoplastic syndromes (EPO, renin, PTHrP, ACTH)	623
1° amenorrhea	Turner syndrome (45,XO or 45,XO/46,XX mosaic)	655
Hypogonadotropic hypogonadism with anosmia	Kallmann syndrome (neuron migration failure)	656
Clear cell adenocarcinoma of the vagina	DES exposure in utero	662
Ovarian tumor (benign, bilateral)	Serous cystadenoma	664
Ovarian tumor (malignant)	Serous carcinoma	664
Benign tumor of myometrium	Leiomyoma (estrogen sensitive, not precancerous)	666
Gynecologic malignancy (most common)	Endometrial carcinoma (most common in resource-rich countries); cervical cancer (most common worldwide)	663–666
Breast mass	Fibrocystic change (in premenopausal females); carcinoma (in postmenopausal females)	667, 668
Breast tumor (benign, young woman)	Fibroadenoma	667
Breast cancer	Invasive ductal carcinoma	668
Bloody nipple discharge	Intraductal papilloma (no palpable mass); invasive ductal carcinoma (hard palpable mass)	
Testicular tumor	Seminoma (malignant, radiosensitive, ↑ placental alkaline phosphatase [PLAP])	670, 671
Bladder outlet obstruction in men	BPH	672
Pulmonary hypertension	Idiopathic, left heart disease, lung disease/hypoxia, chronic thromboembolism, multifactorial	698
SIADH	Small cell carcinoma of the lung	703

▶ EQUATION REVIEW

TOPIC	EQUATION	PAGE
Volume of distribution	$V_d = \dfrac{\text{amount of drug in the body}}{\text{plasma drug concentration}}$	229
Half-life	$t_{1/2} = \dfrac{0.7 \times V_d}{CL}$	229
Drug clearance	$CL = \dfrac{\text{rate of elimination of drug}}{\text{plasma drug concentration}} = V_d \times K_e$ (elimination constant)	229
Loading dose	$LD = \dfrac{C_p \times V_d}{F}$	229
Maintenance dose	$\text{Maintenance dose} = \dfrac{C_p \times CL \times \tau}{F}$	229
Therapeutic index	$TI = \text{median toxic dose/median effective dose} = TD_{50}/ED_{50}$	233

TOPIC	EQUATION	PAGE
Odds ratio (for case-control studies)	$OR = \dfrac{a/c}{b/d} = \dfrac{ad}{bc}$	258
Relative risk	$RR = \dfrac{a/(a+b)}{c/(c+d)}$	258
Attributable risk	$AR = \dfrac{a}{a+b} - \dfrac{c}{c+d}$	258
Relative risk reduction	$RRR = (ARC - ART)/ARC$	258
Absolute risk reduction	$ARR = \dfrac{c}{c+d} - \dfrac{a}{a+b}$	258
Number needed to treat	$NNT = 1/ARR$	258
Number needed to harm	$NNH = 1/AR$	258
Likelihood ratio +	$LR+ = sensitivity/(1 - specificity) = TP\ rate/FP\ rate$	259
Likelihood ratio −	$LR- = (1 - sensitivity)/specificity = FN\ rate/TN\ rate$	259
Sensitivity	$Sensitivity = TP / (TP + FN)$	260
Specificity	$Specificity = TN / (TN + FP)$	260
Positive predictive value	$PPV = TP / (TP + FP)$	260
Negative predictive value	$NPV = TN / (TN + FN)$	260
Cardiac output	$CO = \dfrac{\text{rate of } O_2 \text{ consumption}}{(\text{arterial } O_2 \text{ content} - \text{venous } O_2 \text{ content})}$ $CO = \text{stroke volume} \times \text{heart rate}$	290
Mean arterial pressure	$MAP = CO \times \text{total peripheral resistance (TPR)}$ $MAP \text{ (at resting HR)} = \tfrac{2}{3} DBP + \tfrac{1}{3} SBP = DBP + \tfrac{1}{3} PP$	290
Stroke volume	$SV = EDV - ESV$	290
Ejection fraction	$EF = \dfrac{SV}{EDV} = \dfrac{EDV - ESV}{EDV}$	290
Resistance	$Resistance = \dfrac{\text{driving pressure } (\Delta P)}{\text{flow } (Q)} = \dfrac{8\eta \ (\text{viscosity}) \times \text{length}}{\pi r^4}$	291
Capillary fluid exchange	$J_v = \text{net fluid flow} = K_f[(P_c - P_i) - \sigma(\pi_c - \pi_i)]$	301
Reticulocyte production index	$RPI = \% \text{ reticulocytes} \times \left(\dfrac{\text{actual Hct}}{\text{normal Hct}}\right) / \text{maturation time}$	423
Renal clearance	$C_x = (U_x V)/P_x$	600
Glomerular filtration rate	$C_{inulin} = GFR = U_{inulin} \times V/P_{inulin}$ $= K_f [(P_{GC} - P_{BS}) - (\pi_{GC} - \pi_{BS})]$	600
Effective renal plasma flow	$eRPF = U_{PAH} \times \dfrac{V}{P_{PAH}} = C_{PAH}$	600
Filtration fraction	$FF = \dfrac{GFR}{RPF}$	601

TOPIC	EQUATION	PAGE
Fractional excretion of sodium	$Fe_{Na^+} = V \times U_{Na} \,/\, GFR \times P_{Na} = P_{Cr} \times U_{Na} \,/\, U_{Cr} \times P_{Na}$	602
Henderson-Hasselbalch equation (for extracellular pH)	$pH = 6.1 + \log \dfrac{[HCO_3^-]}{0.03\ Pco_2}$	609
Winters formula (for predicted respiratory compensation for simple metabolic acidosis)	$Pco_2 = 1.5\,[HCO_3^-] + 8 \pm 2$	609
Anion gap	$Na^+ - (Cl^- + HCO_3^-)$	610
Physiologic dead space	$V_D = V_T \times \dfrac{Paco_2 - Peco_2}{Paco_2}$	682
Pulmonary vascular resistance	$PVR = \dfrac{P_{pulm\ artery} - P_{L\ atrium}}{Cardiac\ output}$	684
Alveolar gas equation	$Pao_2 = Pio_2 - \dfrac{Paco_2}{RQ} = 150\ mm\ Hg^a - Paco_2 \,/\, 0.8$	685

▶ EASILY CONFUSED MEDICATIONS

DRUG	CLINICAL USE/MECHANISM OF ACTION
Amiloride	HTN, K^+-sparing diuretic (blocks epithelial Na^+ channels in the late distal convoluted tubule and collecting duct)
Amiodarone	Ventricular arrhythmia, atrial fibrillation, supraventricular tachycardia (K^+ channel blocker; class III antiarrhythmic)
Amlodipine	HTN, angina (dihydropyridine Ca^{2+} channel blocker)
Benztropine	Parkinson disease, extrapyramidal symptoms (cholinergic antagonist)
Bromocriptine	Parkinson disease, hyperprolactinemia (dopamine agonist; rarely used)
Buspirone	Generalized anxiety disorder (partial $5\text{-}HT_{1A}$-receptor agonist)
Bupropion	Depression, smoking cessation (norepinephrine-dopamine reuptake inhibitor)
Cimetidine	Gastritis, peptic ulcer (H_2-receptor antagonist)
Cetirizine	Allergy (2nd-generation H_1-receptor antagonist)
Chloramphenicol	Antibiotic (blocks 50S subunit)
Chlordiazepoxide	EtOH withdrawal (↑ frequency of Cl^- channel opening in GABAergic neuron membranes; long-acting benzodiazepine)
Chlorpromazine	Schizophrenia (typical antipsychotic, D2-receptor blockade)
Chlorpropamide	Diabetes (1st-generation sulfonylurea)
Chlorpheniramine	Allergy (1st-generation H_1-receptor antagonist)
Chlorthalidone	HTN, edema (inhibits Na^+ and Cl^- reabsorption in the distal convoluted tubule; thiazide diuretic
Clozapine	Schizophrenia (atypical antipsychotic, D2-receptor partial agonist)
Clomipramine	Depression, anxiety, chronic pain (tricyclic antidepressant)

DRUG	CLINICAL USE/MECHANISM OF ACTION
Clomiphene	Infertility due to anovulation (selective estrogen receptor modulator in hypothalamus)
Clonidine	Hypertensive urgency, ADHD (α_2-receptor agonist)
Doxepin	Depression, anxiety, bipolar disorder (tricyclic antidepressant)
Doxazosin	BPH, HTN (α_1-receptor antagonist)
Eplerenone	HTN, K^+-sparing diuretic (selective mineralocorticoid receptor antagonist)
Propafenone	Ventricular arrhythmia, paroxysmal atrial fibrillation/flutter or supraventricular tachycardia (Na^+ channel blocker; class Ic antiarrhythmic)
Fluoxetine	Depression (selective serotonin reuptake inhibitor)
Fluphenazine	Schizophrenia (typical antipsychotic, D_2-receptor antagonist)
Mifepristone	Pregnancy termination (progesterone receptor antagonist)
Misoprostol	Used with mifepristone for pregnancy termination (synthetic PGE_1 analog)
Naloxone	Opioid overdose (opioid receptor antagonist)
Naltrexone	Alcohol and opioid use disorder (opioid receptor antagonist)
Nitroprusside	Hypertensive emergency (↑ cGMP/NO)
Nitroglycerin	Angina (↑ cGMP/NO)
Omeprazole	GERD (inhibits H^+/K^+-ATPase in parietal cells)
Ketoconazole	Antifungal (inhibits fungal sterol synthesis)
Aripiprazole	Schizophrenia (atypical antipsychotic, D_2 partial agonist)
Anastrozole	ER ⊕ breast cancer in postmenopausal women (aromatase inhibitor)
Rifaximin	Hepatic encephalopathy (inhibits DNA-dependent RNA polymerase → ↓ ammoniagenic bacteria)
Rifampin	Antituberculous drug/antimicrobial (inhibits DNA-dependent RNA polymerase)
Sertraline	Depression, PTSD (selective serotonin reuptake inhibitor)
Selegiline	Parkinson disease (MAO-B inhibitor)
Trazodone	Insomnia (blocks 5-HT_2, α_1-adrenergic, and H_1 receptors; also weakly inhibits 5-HT reuptake)
Tramadol	Chronic pain (weak opioid agonist)
Varenicline	Smoking cessation (nicotinic ACh receptor partial agonist)
Venlafaxine	Depression, diabetic neuropathy (serotonin-norepinephrine reuptake inhibitor)

SECTION IV

Top-Rated Review Resources

"Some books are to be tasted, others to be swallowed, and some few to be chewed and digested."

—Sir Francis Bacon

"Always read something that will make you look good if you die in the middle of it."

—P.J. O'Rourke

"So many books, so little time."

—Frank Zappa

"If one cannot enjoy reading a book over and over again, there is no use in reading it at all."

—Oscar Wilde

"Start where you are. Use what you have. Do what you can."

—Arthur Ashe

▶ HOW TO USE THE DATABASE

This section is a database of top-rated basic science review books, sample examination books, websites, apps, and commercial review courses that have been marketed to medical students studying for the USMLE Step 1. For each recommended resource, we list (where applicable) the **Title**, the **First Author** (or editor), the **Series Name**, the **Current Publisher**, the **Copyright Year**, the **Number of Pages**, the **ISBN**, the **Approximate List Price**, the **Format** of the resource, and the **Number of Test Questions**. We also include **Summary Comments** that describe their style and overall utility for studying. Finally, each recommended resource receives a **Rating**. Within each section, resources are arranged first by Rating and then alphabetically by the first author within each Rating group.

A letter rating scale with six different grades reflects the detailed student evaluations for **Rated Resources**. Each rated resource receives a rating as follows:

A+	Excellent for boards review.
A A–	Very good for boards review; choose among the group.
B+ B	Good, but use only after exhausting better resources.
B–	Fair, but there are many better resources in the discipline; or low-yield subject material.

The rating is meant to reflect the overall usefulness of the resource in helping medical students prepare for the USMLE Step 1. This is based on a number of factors, including:

- The importance of the discipline for the USMLE Step 1
- The appropriateness and accuracy of the material
- The readability of the text, where applicable
- The quality and number of sample questions
- The quality of written answers to sample questions
- The cost
- The quality of the user interface and learning experience, for web and mobile apps
- The quality and appropriateness of the images and illustrations
- The length of the text (longer is not necessarily better)
- The quality and number of other resources available in the same discipline

Please note that ratings do not reflect the quality of the resources for purposes other than reviewing for the USMLE Step 1. Many books with lower ratings are well written and informative but are not ideal for boards preparation. We have not listed or commented on general textbooks available for the basic sciences.

Evaluations are based on the cumulative results of formal and informal surveys of thousands of medical students at many medical schools across the country. The summary comments and overall ratings represent a consensus opinion, but there may have been a broad range of opinion or limited student feedback on any particular resource.

Please note that the data listed are subject to change in that:

- Publisher and app store prices change frequently.
- Retail and online bookstores may set their own prices.
- New editions and app versions come out frequently, and the quality of updating varies.
- The same book may be reissued through another publisher.

We actively encourage medical students and faculty to submit their opinions and ratings of these basic science review materials so that we may update our database. In addition, we ask that publishers and authors submit for evaluation review copies of basic science review books, including new editions and books not included in our database. We also solicit reviews of new books, mobile apps, websites, flash cards, and commercial review courses.

Disclaimer/Conflict of Interest Statement

None of the ratings reflects the opinion or influence of the publisher. All errors and omissions will gladly be corrected if brought to the attention of the authors through our blog at firstaidteam.com. Please note that USMLE-Rx, ScholarRx, and the entire *First Aid for the USMLE* series are publications by certain authors of *First Aid for the USMLE Step 1*; the following ratings are based solely on recommendations from the student authors of *First Aid for the USMLE Step 1* as well as data from the student survey and feedback forms.

▶ TOP-RATED REVIEW RESOURCES

Question Banks

		AUTHOR	PUBLISHER	TYPE	PRICE
A⁺	*NBME Practice Exams*	National Board of Medical Examiners	nbme.org/examinees/self-assessments	Test/200 q	$62
A⁺	*UWorld Qbank*	UWorld	uworld.com	Test/3600+ q	$319–$719
A⁻	*AMBOSS*	Amboss	amboss.com	Test/2700+ q	$149–$299
A⁻	*USMLE-Rx Qmax*	USMLE-Rx	usmle-rx.com/products/step-1-qmax/	Test/2600+ q	$129–$399
B⁺	*Kaplan Qbank*	Kaplan	kaptest.com	Test/3200+ q	$159–$499

Web and Mobile Apps

		AUTHOR	PUBLISHER	TYPE	PRICE
A	*Anki*		ankiweb.net	Flash cards	Free
A	*Armando Hasudungan*		youtube.com/user/armandohasudungan	Review	Free
A	*Boards and Beyond*		boardsbeyond.com/step-1-p	Review/Test/2300+ q	$24–$399
A	*Free 120*		orientation.nbme.org/launch/usmle/stpf1	Test/120 q	Free
A	*Mehlman Medical*		mehlmanmedical.com	Review/Test/1050+ q	Free–$70
A	*Pixorize*		pixorize.com	Review	$185–$249
A	*Rx Bricks*		usmle-rx.com/products/rx-bricks	Review/Study plan	$29–$129
A	*SketchyMedical*		sketchy.com	Review	$300–$600
A⁻	*AMBOSS Library*		amboss.com	Review	$15–$129
A⁻	*Blueprint*		blueprintprep.com/medical/med-school	Study plan	Free
A⁻	*Dirty Medicine*		youtube.com/DirtyMedicine	Review	Free
A⁻	*Divine Intervention Podcast*		divineinterventionpodcasts.com	Review	Free
A⁻	*USMLE-Rx Step 1 Express*		usmle-rx.com/products/step-1-express-videos	Review/Test	49–$179
A⁻	*USMLE-Rx Step 1 Flash Facts*		usmle-rx.com/products/step-1-flash-facts	Flash cards	$29–$99
B⁺	*Lecturio*		lecturio.com/medical/usmle-step-1	Review/Test/4700+ q	$300–$720
B⁺	*Medbullets*		step1.medbullets.com	Review/Test/3400+ q	Free–$250

Web and Mobile Apps (continued)

B+	*Ninja Nerd Medicine*	youtube.com/ninjanerdscience	Review	Free
B+	*OnlineMedEd*	onlinemeded.org	Review	$79–$429
B+	*Osmosis*	osmosis.org	Test	$318–$618
B+	*Physeo*	physeo.com	Review	Free–$450
B+	*Picmonic*	picmonic.com	Review	$25–$288
B	*Kaplan USMLE® Step 1 Prep*	kaptest.com/usmle-step-1	Review/ Test/3200+ q	$1999–$3999
B	*Radiopaedia.org*	radiopaedia.org	Cases/Test	Free

Comprehensive

		AUTHOR	PUBLISHER	TYPE	PRICE
A	*First Aid Cases for the USMLE Step 1*	Le	McGraw-Hill, 2018, 4th ed., 496 pages, ISBN 9781260143133	Cases	$61
A	*First Aid for the Basic Sciences: General Principles*	Le	McGraw-Hill, 2017, 3rd ed., 528 pages, ISBN 9781259587016	Review	$92
A	*First Aid for the Basic Sciences: Organ Systems*	Le	McGraw-Hill, 2017, 3rd ed., 912 pages, ISBN 9781259587030	Review	$80
A	*Crush Step 1: The Ultimate USMLE Step 1 Review*	O'Connell	Elsevier, 2023, 3rd ed., 736 pages, ISBN 9780323878869	Review	$53
A	*USMLE Step 1 Secrets in Color*	O'Connell	Elsevier, 2022, 5th ed., 736 pages, ISBN 9780323810609	Review	$48
B+	*USMLE Step 1 Made Ridiculously Simple*	Carl	MedMaster, 2023, 8th ed., 424 pages, ISBN 9781935660729	Review	$40
B+	*medEssentials for the USMLE Step 1*	Kaplan	Kaplan Medical, 2022, 6th ed., 536 pages, ISBN 9781506254609	Review	$60
B+	*USMLE Step 1 Lecture Notes 2024–2025*	Kaplan	Kaplan Test Prep, 2024, 2576 pages, ISBN 9781506285597	Review	$350
B	*Kaplan USMLE Step 1 Qbook*	Kaplan	Kaplan Test Prep, 2022, 10th ed., 456 pages, ISBN 9781506276410	Test/850 q	$55

Anatomy, Embryology, and Neuroscience

		AUTHOR	PUBLISHER	TYPE	PRICE
B+	*High-Yield Neuroanatomy*	Gould	Lippincott Williams & Wilkins, 2014, 5th ed., 208 pages, ISBN 9781451193435	Review/ Test/50 q	$57
B+	*Crash Course: Anatomy and Physiology*	Hall	Elsevier, 2019, 5th ed., 350 pages, ISBN 9780702073755	Review	$42
B+	*Netter's Anatomy Flash Cards*	Hansen	Elsevier, 2022, 6th ed., 680 pages, ISBN 9789323834179	Flash cards	$43
B+	*Netter's Essential Systems-Based Anatomy (Netter Basic Science)*	Lyons	Elsevier, 2021, 1st ed., 416 pages, ISBN 9780323694971	Text/Review	$53

Anatomy, Embryology, and Neuroscience (continued)

		AUTHOR	PUBLISHER	TYPE	PRICE
B	*BRS Embryology*	Dudek	Lippincott Williams & Wilkins, 2014, 6th ed., 336 pages, ISBN 9781451190380	Review/Test/220 q	$62
B	*Anatomy—An Essential Textbook*	Gilroy	Thieme, 2021, 3rd ed., 634 pages, ISBN 9781684202591	Text/Test	$60
B⁻	*Complete Anatomy*		3d4medical.com	Review	$75

Behavioral Science

		AUTHOR	PUBLISHER	TYPE	PRICE
A	*Randy Neil Biostatistics*		youtube.com/@RandyNeilMD	Review	Free
A⁻	*BRS Behavioral Science*	Fadem	Lippincott Williams & Wilkins, 2021, 8th ed., 384 pages, ISBN 9781975188856	Review/Test/600 q	$69
B⁺	*Kahn's Cases: Medical Ethics*	Kahn	CreateSpace Independent Publishing Platform, 2020, 253 pages, ISBN 9781481959483	Review	$10
B	*Biostatistics and Epidemiology: A Primer for Health and Biomedical Professionals*	Wassertheil-Smoller	Springer, 2024, 5th ed., 251 pages, ISBN 9783031530425	Review	$97

Biochemistry

		AUTHOR	PUBLISHER	TYPE	PRICE
B⁺	*Lippincott Illustrated Reviews: Biochemistry*	Abali	Lippincott Williams & Wilkins, 2021, 8th ed., 640 pages, ISBN 9781975155063	Review/Test/200 q	$88
B⁺	*BRS Biochemistry, Molecular Biology, and Genetics*	Lieberman	Lippincott Williams & Wilkins, 2019, 7th ed., 448 pages, ISBN 9781496399236	Review/Test/500 q	$64
B	*Lange Flashcards: Biochemistry and Genetics*	Baron	McGraw-Hill, 2017, 3rd ed., 184 flash cards, ISBN 9781259837210	Flash cards	$34

Cell Biology and Histology

		AUTHOR	PUBLISHER	TYPE	PRICE
B⁺	*Thieme Test Prep for the USMLE®: Medical Histology and Embryology Q&A*	Das	Thieme, 2017, 1st ed., 266 pages, ISBN 9781626233348	Test/600 q	$50
B⁺	*Crash Course: Cell Biology and Genetics*	Stubbs	Mosby, 2015, 4th ed., 216 pages, ISBN 9780723438762	Review/Print + online	$47
B	*BRS Cell Biology and Histology*	Gartner	Lippincott Williams & Wilkins, 2024, 9th ed., 464 pages, ISBN 9781975219741	Review/Test/400 q	$63

Microbiology and Immunology

		AUTHOR	PUBLISHER	TYPE	PRICE
A⁻	*Medical Microbiology and Immunology Flash Cards*	Rosenthal	Elsevier, 2016, 2nd ed., 192 flash cards, ISBN 9780323462242	Flash cards	$43
B⁺	*Basic Immunology*	Abbas	Elsevier, 2023, 7th ed., 352 pages, ISBN 9780443105197	Review	$78

Microbiology and Immunology *(continued)*

B+	*Clinical Microbiology Made Ridiculously Simple*	Gladwin	MedMaster, 2022, 9th ed., 448 pages, ISBN 9781935660491	Review	$50
B+	*Crash Course: Haematology and Immunology*	Redhouse White	Elsevier, 2019, 5th ed., 223 pages, ISBN 9780702073632	Review	$43
B+	*Lange Microbiology and Infectious Diseases Flash Cards*	Somers	McGraw-Hill, 2018, 3rd ed., ISBN 9781259859823	Flash cards	$55
B	*Levinson's Review of Medical Microbiology and Immunology*	Chin-Hong	McGraw-Hill, 2024, 18th ed., 856 pages, ISBN 9781265126001	Review/Test/650 q	$69
B	*Lippincott Illustrated Reviews: Microbiology*	Cornelissen	Lippincott Williams & Wilkins, 2019, 4th ed., 448 pages, ISBN 9781496395856	Review/Test/Few q	$85
B	*How the Immune System Works*	Sompayrac	Wiley-Blackwell, 2022, 7th ed., 176 pages, ISBN 9781119890683	Review	$46

Pathology

		AUTHOR	PUBLISHER	TYPE	PRICE
A+	*Pathoma: Fundamentals of Pathology*	Sattar	Pathoma, 2021, 218 pages, ISBN 9780983224631	Review/Lecture	$85–$120
A	*Goljan Rapid Review: Pathology*	Alfrey	Elsevier, 2023, 6th ed., 416 pages, ISBN 9780323870573	Review/Test/500 q	$67
A-	*Robbins and Cotran Review of Pathology*	Klatt	Elsevier, 2021, 5th ed., 488 pages, ISBN 9780323640220	Test/1500 q	$59
A-	*Crash Course: Pathology*	McKinney	Elsevier, 2023, 5th ed., 438 pages, ISBN 9780702073540	Review	$42
B	*BRS Pathology*	Gupta	Lippincott Williams & Wilkins, 2020, 6th ed., 496 pages, ISBN 9781975136628	Review/Test/450 q	$64
B	*Pocket Companion to Robbins and Cotran Pathologic Basis of Disease*	Mitchell	Elsevier, 2023, 10th ed., 1028 pages, ISBN 9780323653909	Review	$46

Pharmacology

		AUTHOR	PUBLISHER	TYPE	PRICE
B+	*Crash Course: Pharmacology*	Page	Elsevier, 2019, 5th ed., 336 pages, ISBN 9780702073441	Review	$42
B	*Lange Pharmacology Flash Cards*	Baron	McGraw-Hill, 2023, 5th ed., 266 flash cards, ISBN 9781264779963	Flash cards	$42
B	*BRS Pharmacology*	Lerchenfeldt	Lippincott Williams & Wilkins, 2019, 5th ed., 384 pages, ISBN 9781975105495	Review/Test/200 q	$68
B-	*Katzung & Trevor's Pharmacology: Examination and Board Review*	Trevor	McGraw-Hill, 2024, 14th ed., 624 pages, ISBN 9781265084905	Review/Test/1000 q	$62
B-	*Lippincott Illustrated Reviews: Pharmacology*	Whalen	Lippincott Williams & Wilkins, 2022, 8th ed., 704 pages, ISBN 9781975170554	Review/Test/380 q	$81

Physiology

		AUTHOR	PUBLISHER	TYPE	PRICE
A⁻	*Physiology*	Costanzo	Elsevier, 2021, 7th ed., 528 pages, ISBN 9780323793339	Text	$69
A⁻	*West's Pulmonary Pathophysiology: The Essentials*	West	Lippincott Williams & Wilkins, 2021, 10th ed., 272 pages, ISBN 9781975152819	Review/ Test/75 q	$62
B⁺	*BRS Physiology*	Costanzo	Lippincott Williams & Wilkins, 2022, 8th ed., 336 pages, ISBN 9781975153601	Review/ Test/350 q	$60
B⁺	*Pathophysiology of Heart Disease*	Lilly	Lippincott Williams & Williams, 2020, 7th ed., 480 pages, ISBN 9781975120597	Review	$64
B⁺	*Lippincott Illustrated Reviews: Physiology*	Preston	Lippincott Williams & Wilkins, 2024, 3rd ed., 590 pages, ISBN 9781975196332	Review	$82
B	*Vander's Renal Physiology*	Eaton	McGraw-Hill, 2023, 10th ed., 240 pages, ISBN 9781264278527	Text	$49
B	*Endocrine Physiology*	Molina	McGraw-Hill, 2023, 6th ed., 320 pages, ISBN 9781264278459	Review	$59
B	*Netter's Physiology Flash Cards*	Mulroney	Elsevier, 2024, 3rd ed., 458 pages, ISBN 9780443113444	Flash cards	$46

SECTION IV

Abbreviations and Symbols

ABBREVIATION	MEANING
1st MC*	1st metacarpal
A-a	alveolar-arterial [gradient]
AA	Alcoholics Anonymous, amyloid A
AAA	abdominal aortic aneurysm
AAMC	Association of American Medical Colleges
AAo*	ascending aorta
Ab	antibody
ABPA	allergic bronchopulmonary aspergillosis
AC	adenylyl cyclase
ACA	anterior cerebral artery
Acetyl-CoA	acetyl coenzyme A
ACD	anemia of chronic disease
ACE	angiotensin-converting enzyme
ACh	acetylcholine
AChE	acetylcholinesterase
ACL	anterior cruciate ligament
ACom	anterior communicating [artery]
ACS	acute coronary syndrome
ACTH	adrenocorticotropic hormone
AD	Alzheimer disease, autosomal dominant
ADA	adenosine deaminase, Americans with Disabilities Act
ADH	antidiuretic hormone
ADHD	attention-deficit hyperactivity disorder
ADP	adenosine diphosphate
ADPKD	autosomal-dominant polycystic kidney disease
AFP	α-fetoprotein
Ag	antigen, silver
AICA	anterior inferior cerebellar artery
AIDS	acquired immunodeficiency syndrome
AIHA	autoimmune hemolytic anemia
AKI	acute kidney injury
AKT	protein kinase B
AL	amyloid light [chain]
ALA	aminolevulinate
ALI	acute lung injury
ALK	anaplastic lymphoma kinase
ALL	acute lymphoblastic (lymphocytic) leukemia
ALP	alkaline phosphatase
ALS	amyotrophic lateral sclerosis
ALT	alanine transaminase
AMA	American Medical Association, antimitochondrial antibody
AML	acute myelogenous (myeloid) leukemia
AMP	adenosine monophosphate

ABBREVIATION	MEANING
ANA	antinuclear antibody
ANCA	antineutrophil cytoplasmic antibody
ANOVA	analysis of variance
ANP	atrial natriuretic peptide
ANS	autonomic nervous system
Ant*	anterior
Ao*	aorta
AOA	American Osteopathic Association
AP	action potential, A & P [ribosomal binding sites]
APC	antigen-presenting cell, activated protein C
APL	Acute promyelocytic leukemia
Apo	apolipoprotein
APP	amyloid precursor protein
APRT	adenine phosphoribosyltransferase
aPTT	activated partial thromboplastin time
APUD	amine precursor uptake decarboxylase
AR	attributable risk, autosomal recessive, aortic regurgitation
ARB	angiotensin receptor blocker
ARC	absolute risk of events in a control group
ARDS	acute respiratory distress syndrome
Arg	arginine
ARPKD	autosomal-recessive polycystic kidney disease
ART	antiretroviral therapy, absolute risk of events in an exposed or treatment group
AS	aortic stenosis
ASA	anterior spinal artery
Asc*	ascending
Asc Ao*	ascending aorta
ASD	atrial septal defect
ASO	anti–streptolysin O
AST	aspartate transaminase
AT	angiotensin, antithrombin
ATN	acute tubular necrosis
ATP	adenosine triphosphate
ATPase	adenosine triphosphatase
ATTR	transthyretin-mediated amyloidosis
AV	atrioventricular
AZT	azidothymidine
BAL	British anti-Lewisite [dimercaprol]
BBB	blood-brain barrier
BCG	bacille Calmette-Guérin
bd*	bile duct
BH$_4$	tetrahydrobiopterin
BM	basement membrane

*Image abbreviation only

ABBREVIATION	MEANING
BOOP	bronchiolitis obliterans organizing pneumonia
BP	bisphosphate, blood pressure
BPG	bisphosphoglycerate
BPH	benign prostatic hyperplasia
BT	bleeding time
BUN	blood urea nitrogen
C*	caudate
Ca*	capillary
Ca^{2+}	calcium ion
CAD	coronary artery disease
CAF	common application form
cAMP	cyclic adenosine monophosphate
CBG	corticosteroid-binding globulin
CBSE	Comprehensive Basic Science Examination
CBSSA	Comprehensive Basic Science Self-Assessment
CBT	computer-based test, cognitive behavioral therapy
CCK	cholecystokinin
CCS	computer-based case simulation
CD	cluster of differentiation
CDK	cyclin-dependent kinase
cDNA	complementary deoxyribonucleic acid
CEA	carcinoembryonic antigen
CETP	cholesteryl-ester transfer protein
CF	cystic fibrosis
CFTR	cystic fibrosis transmembrane conductance regulator
CGD	chronic granulomatous disease
cGMP	cyclic guanosine monophosphate
CGRP	calcitonin gene–related peptide
$C_H1–C_H3$	constant regions, heavy chain [antibody]
ChAT	choline acetyltransferase
CHD*	common hepatic duct
χ^2	chi-squared
CI	confidence interval
CIN	candidate identification number, carcinoma in situ, cervical intraepithelial neoplasia
CIS	Communication and Interpersonal Skills
CK	clinical knowledge, creatine kinase
CKD	chronic kidney disease
CK-MB	creatine kinase, MB fraction
C_L	constant region, light chain [antibody]
CL	clearance
Cl^-	chloride ion
CLL	chronic lymphocytic leukemia
CMC	carpometacarpal (joint)
CML	chronic myelogenous (myeloid) leukemia
CMV	cytomegalovirus
CN	cranial nerve
CN^-	cyanide ion
CNS	central nervous system
CNV	copy number variation
CO	carbon monoxide, cardiac output
CO_2	carbon dioxide
CoA	coenzyme A
Coarct*	coarctation

ABBREVIATION	MEANING
COL1A1	collagen, type I, alpha 1
COL1A2	collagen, type I, alpha 2
COMT	catechol-O-methyltransferase
COP	coat protein
COPD	chronic obstructive pulmonary disease
CoQ	coenzyme Q
COVID-19	Coronavirus disease 2019
COX	cyclooxygenase
C_p	plasma concentration
CPAP	continuous positive airway pressure
CPR	cardiopulmonary resuscitation
Cr	creatinine
CRC	colorectal cancer
CREST	calcinosis, Raynaud phenomenon, esophageal dysfunction, sclerosis, and telangiectasias [syndrome]
CRH	corticotropin-releasing hormone
CRP	C-reactive protein
CS	clinical skills
C-section	cesarean section
CSF	cerebrospinal fluid
CT	computed tomography
CTP	cytidine triphosphate
CXR	chest x-ray
CysLT1	cysteinyl leukotriene-1
DA	dopamine
DAF	decay-accelerating factor
DAG	diacylglycerol
DAo*	descending aorta
DAT	dopamine transporter
dATP	deoxyadenosine triphosphate
DCIS	ductal carcinoma in situ
DCT	distal convoluted tubule
ddI	didanosine
DES	diethylstilbestrol
Desc Ao*	descending aorta
DEXA	dual-energy x-ray absorptiometry
DHAP	dihydroxyacetone phosphate
DHEA	dehydroepiandrosterone
DHF	dihydrofolic acid
DHT	dihydrotestosterone
DI	diabetes insipidus
DIC	disseminated intravascular coagulation
DIP	distal interphalangeal [joint]
DKA	diabetic ketoacidosis
DLCO	diffusing capacity for carbon monoxide
DM	diabetes mellitus
DNA	deoxyribonucleic acid
DNR	do not resuscitate
dNTP	deoxynucleotide triphosphate
DO	doctor of osteopathy
DOPAC	3,4-dihydroxyphenylacetic acid
DPGN	diffuse proliferative glomerulonephritis
DPM	doctor of podiatric medicine
DPP-4	dipeptidyl peptidase-4
DPPC	dipalmitoylphosphatidylcholine

*Image abbreviation only

ABBREVIATION	MEANING
DRESS	Drug reaction with eosinophilia and systemic symptoms
DS	double stranded
dsDNA	double-stranded deoxyribonucleic acid
dsRNA	double-stranded ribonucleic acid
DRG	dorsal root ganglion
d4T	didehydrodeoxythymidine [stavudine]
dTMP	deoxythymidine monophosphate
DTR	deep tendon reflex
DTs	delirium tremens
dUDP	deoxyuridine diphosphate
dUMP	deoxyuridine monophosphate
DVT	deep venous thrombosis
E*	euthromatin, esophagus
EBV	Epstein-Barr virus
ECA*	external carotid artery
ECF	extracellular fluid
ECFMG	Educational Commission for Foreign Medical Graduates
ECG	electrocardiogram
ECL	enterochromaffin-like [cell]
ECM	extracellular matrix
ECT	electroconvulsive therapy
ED_{50}	median effective dose
EDRF	endothelium-derived relaxing factor
EDTA	ethylenediamine tetra-acetic acid
EDV	end-diastolic volume
EEG	electroencephalogram
EF	ejection fraction
EGF	epidermal growth factor
EHEC	enterohemorrhagic E coli
EIEC	enteroinvasive E coli
ELISA	enzyme-linked immunosorbent assay
EM	electron micrograph/microscopy
EMB	eosin–methylene blue
EPEC	eneteropathogenic E coli
Epi	epinephrine
EPO	erythropoietin
EPS	extrapyramidal system
ER	endoplasmic reticulum, estrogen receptor
ERAS	Electronic Residency Application Service
ERCP	endoscopic retrograde cholangiopancreatography
ERP	effective refractory period
eRPF	effective renal plasma flow
ERT	estrogen replacement therapy
ERV	expiratory reserve volume
ESR	erythrocyte sedimentation rate
ESRD	end-stage renal disease
ESV	end-systolic volume
ETEC	enterotoxigenic E coli
EtOH	ethyl alcohol
EV	esophageal vein
F	bioavailability
FA	fatty acid
Fab	fragment, antigen-binding
FAD	flavin adenine dinucleotide

ABBREVIATION	MEANING
$FADH_2$	reduced flavin adenine dinucleotide
FAP	familial adenomatous polyposis
F1,6BP	fructose-1,6-bisphosphate
F2,6BP	fructose-2,6-bisphosphate
FBPase	fructose bisphosphatase
FBPase-2	fructose bisphosphatase-2
Fc	fragment, crystallizable
FcR	Fc receptor
5f-dUMP	5-fluorodeoxyuridine monophosphate
Fe^{2+}	ferrous ion
Fe^{3+}	ferric ion
Fem*	femur
FENa	excreted fraction of filtered sodium
FEV_1	forced expiratory volume in 1 second
FF	filtration fraction
FFA	free fatty acid
FGF	fibroblast growth factor
FGFR	fibroblast growth factor receptor
FGR	fetal growth restriction
FISH	fluorescence in situ hybridization
FIO_2	fraction of inspired oxygen
FIT	fecal immunochemical testing
FKBP	FK506 binding protein
fMet	formylmethionine
FMG	foreign medical graduate
FMN	flavin mononucleotide
FN	false negative
FOXP3	forkhead box P3
FP, FP*	false positive, foot process
FRC	functional residual capacity
FSH	follicle-stimulating hormone
FSMB	Federation of State Medical Boards
FTA-ABS	fluorescent treponemal antibody—absorbed
FTD*	frontotemporal dementia
5-FU	5-fluorouracil
FVC	forced vital capacity
GABA	γ-aminobutyric acid
GAG	glycosaminoglycan
Gal	galactose
GBM	glomerular basement membrane
GC	glomerular capillary
G-CSF	granulocyte colony-stimulating factor
GERD	gastroesophageal reflux disease
GFAP	glial fibrillary acid protein
GFR	glomerular filtration rate
GGT	γ-glutamyl transpeptidase
GH	growth hormone
GHB	γ-hydroxybutyrate
GHRH	growth hormone–releasing hormone
G_I	G protein, I polypeptide
GI	gastrointestinal
GIP	gastric inhibitory peptide
GIST	gastrointestinal stromal tumor
GLP-1	glucagon-like peptide-1

*Image abbreviation only

ABBREVIATION	MEANING
GLUT	glucose transporter
GM	granulocyte macrophage
GM-CSF	granulocyte-macrophage colony stimulating factor
GMP	guanosine monophosphate
GnRH	gonadotropin-releasing hormone
Gp	glycoprotein
G6P	glucose-6-phosphate
G6PD	glucose-6-phosphate dehydrogenase
GPe	globus pallidus externa
GPi	globus pallidus interna
GPI	glycosyl phosphatidylinositol
GRP	gastrin-releasing peptide
G_S	G protein, S polypeptide
GSH	reduced glutathione
GSSG	oxidized glutathione
GTP	guanosine triphosphate
GTPase	guanosine triphosphatase
GU	genitourinary
H*	heterochromatin
H^+	hydrogen ion
H_1, H_2	histamine receptors
H_2S	hydrogen sulfide
ha*	hepatic artery
HAV	hepatitis A virus
HAVAb	hepatitis A antibody
Hb	hemoglobin
HBcAb/HBcAg	hepatitis B core antibody/antigen
HBeAb/HBeAg	hepatitis B early antibody/antigen
HBsAb/HBsAg	hepatitis B surface antibody/antigen
$HbCO_2$	carbaminohemoglobin
HBV	hepatitis B virus
HCC	hepatocellular carcinoma
hCG	human chorionic gonadotropin
HCO_3^-	bicarbonate
Hct	hematocrit
HCTZ	hydrochlorothiazide
HCV	hepatitis C virus
HDL	high-density lipoprotein
HDN	hemolytic disease of the newborn
HDV	hepatitis D virus
H&E	hematoxylin and eosin
5-HETE	5-Hydroxyeicosatetraenoic acid
HEV	hepatitis E virus
HF	heart failure
Hfr	high-frequency recombination [cell]
HFpEF	heart failure with preserved ejection fraction
HFrEF	heart failure with reduced ejection fraction
HGPRT	hypoxanthine-guanine phosphoribosyltransferase
HHb	deoxygenated hemoglobin
HHS	hyperosmolar hyperglycemic state
HHV	human herpesvirus
5-HIAA	5-hydroxyindoleacetic acid
Hib	*Haemophilus influenzae* type b
HIT	heparin-induced thrombocytopenia

ABBREVIATION	MEANING
HIV	human immunodeficiency virus
HL	hepatic lipase
HLA	human leukocyte antigen
HMG-CoA	hydroxymethylglutaryl-coenzyme A
HMP	hexose monophosphate
HMWK	high-molecular-weight kininogen
HNPCC	hereditary nonpolyposis colorectal cancer
hnRNA	heterogeneous nuclear ribonucleic acid
H_2O_2	hydrogen peroxide
HOCM	hypertrophic obstructive cardiomyopathy
HPA	hypothalamic-pituitary-adrenal [axis]
HPO	hypothalamic-pituitary-ovarian [axis]
HPV	human papillomavirus
HR	heart rate
HSL	hormone-sensitive lipase
HSP	Henoch-Schönlein purpura
HSV	herpes simplex virus
5-HT	5-hydroxytryptamine (serotonin)
HTLV	human T-cell leukemia virus
HTN	hypertension
HUS	hemolytic-uremic syndrome
HVA	homovanillic acid
IBD	inflammatory bowel disease
IBS	irritable bowel syndrome
IC	inspiratory capacity, immune complex
I_{Ca}	calcium current [heart]
I_f	funny current [heart]
ICA	internal carotid artery
ICAM	intercellular adhesion molecule
ICD	implantable cardioverter-defibrillator
ICE	Integrated Clinical Encounter
ICF	intracellular fluid
ICP	intracranial pressure
ID	identification
ID_{50}	median infective dose
IDL	intermediate-density lipoprotein
IF	immunofluorescence, initiation factor
IFN	interferon
Ig	immunoglobulin
IGF	insulinlike growth factor
I_K	potassium current [heart]
IL	interleukin
IM	intramuscular
IMA	inferior mesenteric artery
IMG	international medical graduate
IMP	inosine monophosphate
IMV	inferior mesenteric vein
I_{Na}	sodium current [heart]
INH	isoniazid
INO	internuclear ophthalmoplegia
INR	International Normalized Ratio
IO	inferior oblique [muscle]
IOP	intraocular pressure
IP_3	inositol triphosphate

*Image abbreviation only

ABBREVIATION	MEANING
IPV	inactivated polio vaccine
IR	current × resistance [Ohm's law], inferior rectus [muscle]
IRV	inspiratory reserve volume
ITP	idiopathic thrombocytopenic purpura
IUD	intrauterine device
IV	intravenous
IVC	inferior vena cava
IVIG	intravenous immunoglobulin
JAK/STAT	Janus kinase/signal transducer and activator of transcription [pathway]
JGA	juxtaglomerular apparatus
JVD	jugular venous distention
JVP	jugular venous pulse
K^+	potassium ion
KatG	catalase-peroxidase produced by *M tuberculosis*
K_e	elimination constant
K_f	filtration constant
KG	ketoglutarate
Kid*	kidney
K_m	Michaelis-Menten constant
KOH	potassium hydroxide
L	left, lentiform, liver
LA	left atrial, left atrium
LAD	left anterior descending coronary artery
LAP	leukocyte alkaline phosphatase
Lat cond*	lateral condyle
Lb*	lamellar body
LCA	left coronary artery
LCAT	lecithin-cholesterol acyltransferase
LCC*	left common carotid artery
LCFA	long-chain fatty acid
LCL	lateral collateral ligament
LCME	Liaison Committee on Medical Education
LCMV	lymphocytic choriomeningitis virus
LCX	left circumflex coronary artery
LD	loading dose
LD_{50}	median lethal dose
LDH	lactate dehydrogenase
LDL	low-density lipoprotein
LES	lower esophageal sphincter
LFA	leukocyte function–associated antigen
LFT	liver function test
LH	luteinizing hormone
Liv*	liver
LLL*	left lower lobe (of lung)
LLQ	left lower quadrant
LM	lateral meniscus, left main coronary artery, light microscopy
LMN	lower motor neuron
LOS	lipooligosaccharide
LP	lumbar puncture
LPA*	left pulmonary artery
LPL	lipoprotein lipase
LPS	lipopolysaccharide
LR	lateral rectus [muscle]

ABBREVIATION	MEANING
LT	labile toxin, leukotriene
LUL*	left upper lobe (of lung)
LV	left ventricle, left ventricular
M_1-M_5	muscarinic (parasympathetic) ACh receptors
MAC	membrane attack complex, minimum alveolar concentration
MALT	mucosa-associated lymphoid tissue
MAO	monoamine oxidase
MAP	mean arterial pressure, mitogen-activated protein
MASLD	metabolic dysfunction–associated steatotic liver disease
Max*	maxillary sinus
MBL-MASP	mannose-binding lectin–associated serine protease
MC	midsystolic click, metacarpal
MCA	middle cerebral artery
MCAD	medium-chain acyl-coA dehydrogenase
MCAT	Medical College Admissions Test
MCHC	mean corpuscular hemoglobin concentration
MCL	medial collateral ligament
MCP	metacarpophalangeal [joint]
MCV	mean corpuscular volume
MD	maintenance dose
MDD	major depressive disorder
MDMA	3,4-methylenedioxymethamphetamine, ecstasy
Med cond*	medial condyle
MELAS syndrome	mitochondrial encephalopathy, lactic acidosis, and stroke-like episodes
MEN	multiple endocrine neoplasia
MERS	Middle East respiratory syndrome
Mg^{2+}	magnesium ion
$MgSO_4$	magnesium sulfate
MHC	major histocompatibility complex
MI	myocardial infarction
MIF	müllerian inhibiting factor
MIRL	membrane inhibitor of reactive lysis
MLCK	myosin light-chain kinase
MLF	medial longitudinal fasciculus
MMC	migrating motor complex
MMR	measles, mumps, rubella [vaccine]
MODY	maturity-onset diabetes of the young
6-MP	6-mercaptopurine
MPGN	membranoproliferative glomerulonephritis
MPO	myeloperoxidase
MPO-ANCA/ p-ANCA	myeloperoxidase/perinuclear antineutrophil cytoplasmic antibody
MR	medial rectus [muscle], mitral regurgitation
MRI	magnetic resonance imaging
miRNA	microribonucleic acid
mRNA	messenger ribonucleic acid
MRSA	methicillin-resistant *S aureus*
MS	mitral stenosis, multiple sclerosis
MSH	melanocyte-stimulating hormone
mtDNA	mitochondrial DNA
mTOR	mammalian target of rapamycin
MTP	metatarsophalangeal [joint]
MTX	methotrexate

*Image abbreviation only

ABBREVIATION	MEANING
MVO_2	myocardial volume oxygen consumption
MVP	mitral valve prolapse
N*	nucleus
Na^+	sodium ion
NAAT	nucleic acid amplification test
NAD	nicotinamide adenine dinucleotide
NAD^+	oxidized nicotinamide adenine dinucleotide
NADH	reduced nicotinamide adenine dinucleotide
$NADP^+$	oxidized nicotinamide adenine dinucleotide phosphate
NADPH	reduced nicotinamide adenine dinucleotide phosphate
NBME	National Board of Medical Examiners
NBOME	National Board of Osteopathic Medical Examiners
NBPME	National Board of Podiatric Medical Examiners
NE	norepinephrine
NET	norepinephrine transporter
NF	neurofibromatosis
NFAT	nuclear factor of activated T-cell
NH_3	ammonia
NH_4^+	ammonium
NK	natural killer [cells]
NK_1	neurokinin-1
N_M	nicotinic ACh receptor in neuromuscular junction
NMDA	N-methyl-d-aspartate
NMJ	neuromuscular junction
NMS	neuroleptic malignant syndrome
N_N	nicotinic ACh receptor in autonomic ganglia
NREM	non-rapid eye movement (sleep)
NRMP	National Residency Matching Program
NNRTI	non-nucleoside reverse transcriptase inhibitor
NO	nitric oxide
N_2O	nitrous oxide
NPH	neutral protamine Hagedorn, normal pressure hydrocephalus
NPV	negative predictive value
NRTI	nucleoside reverse transcriptase inhibitor
NSAID	nonsteroidal anti-inflammatory drug
NSE	neuron-specific enolase
NSTEMI	non–ST-segment elevation myocardial infarction
NTD	neural tube defect
Nu*	nucleolus
OAA	oxaloacetic acid
OCD	obsessive-compulsive disorder
OCP	oral contraceptive pill
ODC	oxygen-hemoglobin dissociation curve
OH	hydroxy
$1,25\text{-OH } D_3$	calcitriol (active form of vitamin D)
$25\text{-OH } D_3$	storage form of vitamin D
OPV	oral polio vaccine
OR	odds ratio
ori	origins of replication
OS	opening snap
OSA	obstructive sleep apnea
OTC	Ornithine transcarbamylase
OVLT	organum vasculosum of the lamina terminalis

ABBREVIATION	MEANING
P-body	processing body (cytoplasmic)
P-450	cytochrome P-450 family of enzymes
PA	posteroanterior, pulmonary artery
PABA	*para*-aminobenzoic acid
$Paco_2$	arterial Pco_2
$PAco_2$	alveolar Pco_2
PAH	*para*-aminohippuric acid
PAMP	pathogen-associated molecular patterns
PAN	polyarteritis nodosa
Pao_2	partial pressure of oxygen in arterial blood
Pao_2	partial pressure of oxygen in alveolar blood
PAP	Papanicolaou [smear], prostatic acid phosphatase, posteromedial papillary muscle
PAPPA	pregnancy-associated plasma protein A
PAS	periodic acid–Schiff
Pat*	patella
P_B	Barometric (atmospheric) pressure
PBP	penicillin-binding protein
PC	platelet count, pyruvate carboxylase
PCA	posterior cerebral artery
PCC	prothrombin complex concentrate
PCL	posterior cruciate ligament
Pco_2	partial pressure of carbon dioxide
PCom	posterior communicating [artery]
PCOS	polycystic ovarian syndrome
PCP	phencyclidine hydrochloride, *Pneumocystis jirovecii* pneumonia
PCR	polymerase chain reaction
PCT	proximal convoluted tubule
PCV13	pneumococcal conjugate vaccine
PCWP	pulmonary capillary wedge pressure
PDA	patent ductus arteriosus, posterior descending artery
PDE	phosphodiesterase
PDGF	platelet-derived growth factor
PDH	pyruvate dehydrogenase
PE	pulmonary embolism
PECAM	platelet–endothelial cell adhesion molecule
$Peco_2$	expired air Pco_2
PEP	phosphoenolpyruvate
PF	platelet factor
PFK	phosphofructokinase
PFK-2	phosphofructokinase-2
PFT	pulmonary function test
PG	phosphoglycerate
P_{H_2O}	water pressure
P_i	plasma interstitial osmotic pressure, inorganic phosphate
PICA	posterior inferior cerebellar artery
PID	pelvic inflammatory disease
Pio_2	Po_2 in inspired air
PIP	proximal interphalangeal [joint]
PIP_2	phosphatidylinositol 4,5-bisphosphate
PIP_3	phosphatidylinositol 3,4,5-bisphosphate
PKD	polycystic kidney disease
PKR	interferon-α–induced protein kinase
PKU	phenylketonuria

*Image abbreviation only

ABBREVIATION	MEANING
PLAP	placental alkaline phosphatase
PLP	pyridoxal phosphate
PML	progressive multifocal leukoencephalopathy
PMN	polymorphonuclear [leukocyte]
P_{net}	net filtration pressure
PNET	primitive neuroectodermal tumor
PNS	peripheral nervous system
P_{O_2}	partial pressure of oxygen
PO_4^{3-}	phosphate
POMC	proopiomelanocortin
Pop*	popliteal artery
Pop a*	popliteal artery
Post*	posterior
PPAR	peroxisome proliferator-activated receptor
PPD	purified protein derivative
PPI	proton pump inhibitor
PPM	parts per million
PPSV23	pneumococcal polysaccharide vaccine
PPV	positive predictive value
PR3-ANCA/ c-ANCA	cytoplasmic antineutrophil cytoplasmic antibody
PrP	prion protein
PrP^C	cellular prion protein
PrP^{SC}	scrapie isoform of the prion protein
PRPP	phosphoribosylpyrophosphate
PSA	prostate-specific antigen
PSS	progressive systemic sclerosis
PT	prothrombin time, proximal tubule
PTEN	phosphatase and tensin homolog
PTH	parathyroid hormone
PTHrP	parathyroid hormone–related protein
PTSD	post-traumatic stress disorder
PTT	partial thromboplastin time
PV	plasma volume, venous pressure, portal vein
pv*	pulmonary vein
PVC	polyvinyl chloride
PVR	pulmonary vascular resistance
PYR	pyrrolidonyl aminopeptidase
R	correlation coefficient, right, R variable [group]
R_3	Registration, Ranking, & Results [system]
RA	right atrium, right atrial
RAAS	renin-angiotensin-aldosterone system
RANK-L	receptor activator of nuclear factor-κ B ligand
RAS	reticular activating system
RBF	renal blood flow
RCA	right coronary artery
REM	rapid eye movement
RER	rough endoplasmic reticulum
Rh	*rhesus* antigen
RLL*	right lower lobe (of lungs)
RLQ	right lower quadrant
RML*	right middle lobe (of lung)
RNA	ribonucleic acid
RNP	ribonucleoprotein

ABBREVIATION	MEANING
ROS	reactive oxygen species
RPF	renal plasma flow
RPGN	rapidly progressive glomerulonephritis
RPR	rapid plasma reagin
RR	relative risk, respiratory rate
rRNA	ribosomal ribonucleic acid
RS	Reed-Sternberg [cells]
RSC*	right subclavian artery
RSV	respiratory syncytial virus
RTA	renal tubular acidosis
RUL*	right upper lobe (of lung)
RUQ	right upper quadrant
RV	residual volume, right ventricle, right ventricular
RVH	right ventricular hypertrophy
[S]	substrate concentration
SA	sinoatrial
SAA	serum amyloid–associated [protein]
SAM	S-adenosylmethionine
SARS	severe acute respiratory syndrome
SARS-CoV-2	severe acute respiratory syndrome coronavirus 2
SCC	squamous cell carcinoma
SCD	sudden cardiac death
SCID	severe combined immunodeficiency disease
SCJ	squamocolumnar junction
SCM	sternocleidomastoid muscle
SCN	suprachiasmatic nucleus
SD	standard deviation
SE	standard error [of the mean]
SEP	Spoken English Proficiency
SER	smooth endoplasmic reticulum
SERM	selective estrogen receptor modulator
SERT	serotonin transporter
SGLT	sodium-glucose transporter
SHBG	sex hormone–binding globulin
SIADH	syndrome of inappropriate [secretion of] antidiuretic hormone
SIDS	sudden infant death syndrome
SJS	Stevens-Johnson syndrome
SLD	steatotic liver disease
SLE	systemic lupus erythematosus
SLL	small lymphocytic lymphoma
SLT	Shiga-like toxin
SMA	superior mesenteric artery
SMX	sulfamethoxazole
SNARE	soluble NSF attachment protein receptor
SNc	substantia nigra pars compacta
SNP	single nucleotide polymorphism
SNr	substantia nigra pars reticulata
SNRI	serotonin and norepinephrine receptor inhibitor
snRNA	small nuclear RNA
snRNP	small nuclear ribonucleoprotein
SO	superior oblique [muscle]
SOAP	Supplemental Offer and Acceptance Program
Sp*	spleen

*Image abbreviation only

ABBREVIATION	MEANING
spp	species
SR	superior rectus [muscle]
SRP	signal recognition particle
SS	single stranded
ssDNA	single-stranded deoxyribonucleic acid
SSPE	subacute sclerosing panencephalitis
SSRI	selective serotonin reuptake inhibitor
ssRNA	single-stranded ribonucleic acid
St*	stomach
ST	Shiga toxin
StAR	steroidogenic acute regulatory protein
STEMI	ST-segment elevation myocardial infarction
STI	sexually transmitted infection
STN	subthalamic nucleus
SV	splenic vein, stroke volume
SVC	superior vena cava
SVR	systemic vascular resistance
SVT	supraventricular tachycardia
T*	thalamus, trachea
$t_{1/2}$	half-life
T_3	triiodothyronine
T_4	thyroxine
TAA	thoracic aortic aneurysm
TAPVR	total anomalous pulmonary venous return
TB	tuberculosis
TBG	thyroxine-binding globulin
TBV	total blood volume
3TC	dideoxythiacytidine [lamivudine]
TCA	tricarboxylic acid [cycle], tricyclic antidepressant
Tc cell	cytotoxic T cell
TCR	T-cell receptor
TDF	tenofovir disoproxil fumarate
TdT	terminal deoxynucleotidyl transferase
TE	tracheoesophageal
TFT	thyroid function test
TG	triglyceride
TGA	transposition of great arteries
TGF	transforming growth factor
Th cell	helper T cell
THF	tetrahydrofolic acid
TI	therapeutic index
TIA	transient ischemic attack
Tib*	tibia
TIBC	total iron-binding capacity
TIPS	transjugular intrahepatic portosystemic shunt
TLC	total lung capacity
TLR	toll-like receptors
T_m	maximum rate of transport
TMP	trimethoprim
TN	true negative
TNF	tumor necrosis factor
TNM	tumor, node, metastases [staging]
TOP	topoisomerase
ToRCHeS	*Toxoplasma gondii*, rubella, CMV, HIV, HSV-2, syphilis
TP	true positive
tPA	tissue plasminogen activator
TPO	thyroid peroxidase, thrombopoietin

*Image abbreviation only

ABBREVIATION	MEANING
TPP	thiamine pyrophosphate
TPPA	*Treponema pallidum* particle agglutination assay
TPR	total peripheral resistance
TR	tricuspid regurgitation
TRAP	tartrate-resistant acid phosphatase
TRECs	T-cell receptor excision circles
TRH	thyrotropin-releasing hormone
tRNA	transfer ribonucleic acid
TSH	thyroid-stimulating hormone
TSI	triple sugar iron
TSS	toxic shock syndrome
TSST	toxic shock syndrome toxin
TTP	thrombotic thrombocytopenic purpura
TTR	transthyretin
TXA_2	thromboxane A_2
UDP	uridine diphosphate
UMN	upper motor neuron
UMP	uridine monophosphate
UPD	uniparental disomy
URI	upper respiratory infection
USMLE	United States Medical Licensing Examination
UTI	urinary tract infection
UTP	uridine triphosphate
UV	ultraviolet
V_1, V_2	vasopressin receptors
V_A	alveolar ventilation
VC	vital capacity
V_d	volume of distribution
V_D	physiologic dead space
V(D)J	variable, (diversity), joining gene segments rearranged to form Ig genes
VDRL	Venereal Disease Research Laboratory
V_E	minute ventilation
VEGF	vascular endothelial growth factor
V_H	variable region, heavy chain [antibody]
VHL	von Hippel-Lindau [disease]
VIP	vasoactive intestinal peptide
VIPoma	vasoactive intestinal polypeptide-secreting tumor
VJ	light-chain hypervariable region [antibody]
V_L	variable region, light chain [antibody]
VLCFA	very-long-chain fatty acids
VLDL	very low density lipoprotein
VMA	vanillylmandelic acid
VMAT	vesicular monoamine transporter
V_{max}	maximum velocity
VPL	ventral posterior nucleus, lateral
VPM	ventral posterior nucleus, medial
VPN	vancomycin, polymyxin, nystatin [media]
V̇/Q̇	ventilation/perfusion [ratio]
VRE	vancomycin-resistant enterococcus
VSD	ventricular septal defect
V_T	tidal volume
VTE	venous thromboembolism
vWF	von Willebrand factor
VZV	varicella-zoster virus
XLA	X-linked agammaglobulinemia
XR	X-linked recessive
XX/XY	normal complement of sex chromosomes for female/male
ZDV	zidovudine [formerly AZT]

Image Acknowledgments

In this edition, in collaboration with MedIQ Learning, LLC, and a variety of other partners, we are pleased to include the following clinical images and diagrams for the benefit of integrative student learning.

Portions of this book identified with the symbol ℞ are copyright © USMLE-Rx.com (MedIQ Learning, LLC).

Portions of this book identified with the symbol ℞Ⓤ are copyright © Dr. Richard Usatine and are provided under license through MedIQ Learning, LLC.

Portions of this book identified with the symbol ✳ are listed below by page number.

This symbol ⓒⓔ refers to material that is available in the public domain.

This symbol ⓒⓔ refers to the Creative Commons Attribution license, full text at http://creativecommons.org/licenses/by/4.0/.

This symbol ⓒⓔⓢ refers to the Creative Commons Attribution-Share Alike license, full text at: http://creativecommons.org/licenses/by-sa/4.0/.

Original images may have been modified by cropping and/or labeling. Where appropriate, all rights to the derivative work by MedIQ Learning, LLC are reserved.

Biochemistry

32 **Chromatin structure.** Electron micrograph showing heterochromatin, euchromatin, and nucleolus. ⓒⓔⓢ Roller RA, Rickett JD, Stickle WB. The hypobranchial gland of the estuarine snail *Stramonita haemastoma canaliculata* (Gray) (Prosobranchia: Muricidae): a light and electron microscopical study. *Am Malac Bull.* 1995;11(2):177-190. Available at https://archive.org/details/americanm101119931994amer.

47 **Cilia structure: Image A.** Cross section of Chlamydomonas flagella with the membrane removed. ⓒⓔ Bui KH, Pigino G, Ishikawa T. Three-dimensional structural analysis of eukaryotic flagella/cilia by electron cryo-tomography. *J Synchrotron Radiat.* 2011 Jan;18(1):2-5. DOI: 10.1107/S0909049510036812.

47 **Cilia structure: Image B.** Cilia structure of basal body. ⓒⓔ Riparbelli MG, Cabrera OA, Callaini G, et al. Unique properties of *Drosophila* spermatocyte primary cilia. *Biol Open.* 2013 Nov 15;2(11):1137–1147. DOI: 10.1242/bio.20135355.

47 **Primary ciliary dyskinesia.** Dextrocardia. ⓒⓔ Oluwadare O, Ayoka AO, Akomolafe RO, et al. The role of electrocardiogram in the diagnosis of dextrocardia with mirror image atrial arrangement and ventricular position in a young adult Nigerian in Ile-Ife: a case report. *J Med Case Rep.* 2015;9:222. DOI: 10.1186/s13256-015-0695-4.

49 **Osteogenesis imperfecta: Image A.** Skeletal deformities in upper extremity of child. ⓒⓔ Vanakker OM, Hemelsoet D, De Paepe. Hereditary connective tissue diseases in young adult stroke: a comprehensive synthesis. *Stroke Res Treat.* 2011;712903. DOI: 10.4061/2011/712903.

49 **Osteogenesis imperfecta: Image B.** Blue sclera. ⓒⓔ Herbert L. Fred, MD, Hendrik A. van Dijk. Images of Memorable Cases: Cases 40, 41 & 42. OpenStax CNX. Dec 3, 2008. Download for free at http://cnx.org/contents/fe89fbf7-c641-4ad8-8871-80017adfd2cf@3.

49 **Ehlers-Danlos syndrome: Images A and B.** Hyperextensibility of skin (A) and DIP joint (B). ⓒⓔ Whitaker JK, Alexander, P, Chau DYS, et al. Severe conjunctivochalasis in association with classic type Ehlers-Danlos syndrome. *BMC Ophthalmol.* 2012;2:47. DOI: 10.1186/1471-2415-12-47.

53 **Karyotyping.** ⓒⓔ Paar C, Herber G, Voskova, et al. available under: A case of acute myeloid leukemia (AML) with an unreported combination of chromosomal abnormalities: gain of isochromosome 5p, tetrasomy 8 and unbalanced translocation der(19)t(17;19) (q23;p13). *Mol Cytogenet.* 2013;6:40. DOI: 10.1186/1755-8166-6-40.

53 **Fluorescence in situ hybridization.** ⓒⓔ Paar C, Herber G, Voskova D, et al. A case of acute myeloid leukemia (AML) with an unreported combination of chromosomal abnormalities: gain of isochromosome 5p, tetrasomy 8 and unbalanced translocation der(19)t(17;19)(q23;p13). *Mol Cytogenet.* 2013 Sep 30;6(1):40. DOI: 10.1186/1755-8166-6-40.

55 **Genetic terms.** Café-au-lait spots. ⓒⓔ Dumitrescu CE and Collins MT. McCune-Albright syndrome. *Orphanet J Rare Dis.* 2008;3:12. DOI: 10.1186/1750-1172-3-12.

59 **Muscular dystrophies.** Fibrofatty replacement of muscle. ⓒⓔ The US Department of Health and Human Services and Dr. Edwin P. Ewing, Jr.

64 **Vitamin A.** Bitot spots on conjunctiva. ⓒⓔ The US Department of Health and Human Services and Dr. J. Justin Older.

65 **Vitamin B₂.** Angular cheilitis. ⓒⓔ Shetti A, Gupta I, Charantimath SM. Oral candidiasis: aiding in the diagnosis of HIV-A case report. *Case Rep Dent.* 2011:929616. DOI: 10.1155/2011/929616.

65 **Vitamin B₃.** Pellagra. ⓒⓔ van Dijk HA, Fred H. Images of memorable cases: case 2. Connexions Web site. Dec 4, 2008. Available at: http://cnx.org/contents/3d3dcb2e-8e98-496f-91c2-fe94e93428a1@3@3/.

68 **Vitamin D.** X-ray of lower extremity in child with rickets. ⓒⓔ Linglart A, Biosse-Duplan M, Briot K, et al. Therapeutic management of hypophosphatemic rickets from infancy to adulthood. *Endocr Connect.* 2014 Mar 14;3(1):R13-30. DOI: 10.1530/EC-13-0103.

69 **Protein-energy malnutrition: Image A.** Child with kwashiorkor. ⓒⓔ The US Department of Health and Human Services and Dr. Lyle Conrad.

69 **Protein-energy malnutrition: Image B.** Child with marasmus. ⓒⓔ The US Department of Health and Human Services and Don Eddins.

82 **Alkaptonuria.** Ochronotic pigment on the sclera of the eyes of the patient. ⓒⓔ Wilke A, Steverding D. Ochronosis as an unusual cause of valvular defect: a case report. *J Med Case Reports.* 2009;3:9302. DOI: 10.1186/1752-1947-3-9302.

86 **Lysosomal storage diseases: Image A.** "Cherry-red" spot on macula in Tay-Sachs disease. ⓒⓔ Dr. Jonathan Trobe.

86 **Lysosomal storage diseases: Image B.** Angiokeratomas. ⓒⓔ Burlina AP, Sims KB, Politei JM, et al. Early diagnosis of peripheral nervous system involvement in Fabry disease and treatment of neuropathic pain: the report of an expert panel. *BMC Neurol.* 2011;11:61. DOI: 10.1186/1471-2377-11-61.

86 **Lysosomal storage diseases: Image C.** Gaucher cells in Gaucher disease. ⊚⓪ Mohindroo S. Type-3 Gaucher disease with bilateral necrosis of the neck of femur: a case report. *Cases J.* 2009; 9380. DOI: 10.1186/1757-1626-2-9380.

86 **Lysosomal storage diseases: Image D.** Foam cells in Niemann-Pick disease. ⊚⓪ Degtyareva, A, Mikhailova, S, Zakharova, Y, et al. Visceral symptoms as a key diagnostic sign for the early infantile form of Niemann–Pick disease type C in a Russian patient: a case report. *J Med Case Reports.* 2016;10:143. DOI: 10.1186/s13256-016-0925-4.

92 **Abetalipoproteinemia.** Small bowel mucosa shows clear enterocytes. ⊚⓪ Najah M, Youssef SM, Yahia HM, et al. Molecular characterization of Tunisian families with abetalipoproteinemia and identification of a novel mutation in MTTP gene. *Diagn Pathol.* 2013 Apr 4;8:54. DOI: 10.1186/1746-1596-8-54.

Immunology

94 **Lymph node: Image A.** Lymph node histology. ⊚ The US Department of Health and Human Services and Dr. Edwin P. Ewing, Jr.

96 **Thymus.** "Sail sign" on x-ray of normal thymus in neonate. ⊚⓪ Di Serafino M, Esposito F, Severino R, et al. Think thymus, think well: the chest x-ray thymic signs. *J Pediatr Moth Care.* 2016;1(2):108-109. DOI: 10.19104/japm.2016.108.

105 **Complement disorders.** Urine discoloration in paroxysmal nocturnal hemoglobinuria. ⊚⓪ Nakamura N, Sugawara T, Shirato K, et al. Paroxysmal nocturnal hemoglobinuria in systemic lupus erythematosus: a case report. *J Med Case Reports.* 2011;5:550. DOI: 10.1186/1752-1947-5-550

115 **Immunodeficiencies: Image A.** Telangiectases on face. ⊚⓪ Scarano V, De Santis D, Suppressa P, et al. Hypogonadotropic hypogonadism associated with hereditary hemorrhagic telangiectasia. *Case Reports in Endo.* 2013;vol 2013. DOI: 10.1155/2013/520284.

115 **Immunodeficiencies: Image B.** Giant granules in granulocytes in Chédiak-Higashi syndrome. ⊚⓪ Morrone K, Wang Y, Huizing M, et al. Two Novel Mutations Identified in an African-American Child with Chediak-Higashi Syndrome. *Case Rep Med.* 2010;2010:967535. vol. 2010, Article ID 967535, 4 pages, 2010.DOI: 10.1155/2010/967535.

Microbiology

123 **Stains: Image A.** *Trypanosoma lewisi* on Giemsa stain. ⊚ The US Department of Health and Human Services and Dr. Mae Melvin.

123 **Stains: Image B.** Foamy macrophages containing the characteristic rod-shaped inclusion bodies of Whipple disease. ⊚⓪ Tran HA. Reversible hypothyroidism and Whipple's disease. *BMC Endocr Disord.* 2006 May 10;6:3. DOI: 10.1186/1472-6823-6-3.

123 **Stains: Image C.** *Mycobacterium tuberculosis* on Ziehl-Neelsen stain. ⊚ The US Department of Health and Human Services and Dr. George P. Kubica.

123 **Stains: Image D.** *Cryptococcus neoformans* on India ink stain. ⊚ The US Department of Health and Human Services.

123 **Stains: Image E.** *Coccidioides immitis* on silver stain. ⊚ The US Department of Health and Human Services and Dr. Edwin P. Ewing, Jr.

125 **Encapsulated bacteria.** Capsular swelling of *Streptococcus pneumoniae* using the Neufeld-Quellung test. ⊚ The US Department of Health and Human Services.

126 **Catalase-positive organisms.** Oxygen bubbles released during catalase reaction. ⊚ The US Department of Health and Human Services and Annie L. Vestal.

133 **Hemolytic bacteria.** α- and β-hemolysis. ⊚ The US Department of Health and Human Services and Richard R. Facklam, Ph.D.

133 **Staphylococcus aureus.** ⊚ The US Department of Health and Human Services and Dr. Richard Facklam.

134 **Streptococcus pneumoniae.** ⊚ The US Department of Health and Human Services and Dr. Mike Miller.

134 **Streptococcus pyogenes (group A streptococci).** ⊚ The US Department of Health and Human Services and Dr. Mike Miller.

135 **Bacillus anthracis.** Ulcer with black eschar in cutaneous anthrax. ⊚ The US Department of Health and Human Services and James H. Steele.

136 **Clostridioides difficile.** Pseudomembranous enterocolitis on colonoscopy. ⊚⓪ Abe I, Kawamura YJ, Sasaki J, Konishi F. Acute fulminant pseudomembranous colitis which developed after ileostomy closure and required emergent total colectomy: a case report. *J Med Case Rep.* 2012 May 14;6:130. DOI: 10.1186/1752-1947-6-130.

136 **Clostridia: Image A.** Gas gangrene due to *Clostridium perfringens*. ⊚⓪ Schröpfer E, Rauthe S, Meyer T. Diagnosis and misdiagnosis of necrotizing soft tissue infections: three case reports. *Cases J.* 2008;1:252. DOI: 10.1186/1757-1626-1-252.

137 **Corynebacterium diphtheriae.** Endoscopic findings of epiglottis and larynx. ⊚⓪ Tagini F, Pillonel T, Croxatto A, et al. Distinct genomic features characterize two clades of *Corynebacterium diphtheriae*: proposal of *Corynebacterium diphtheriae* Subsp. diphtheriae Subsp. nov. and *Corynebacterium diphtheriae* Subsp. lausannense Subsp. nov. *Front. Microbiol.* 2018;9. DOI: 10.3389/fmicb.2018.01743.

137 **Listeria monocytogenes.** Actin rockets. ⊚⓪ Schuppler M, Loessner MJ. The opportunistic pathogen *Listeria monocytogenes*: pathogenicity and interaction with the mucosal immune system. *Int J Inflamm.* 2010;2010:704321. DOI: 10.4061/2010/704321.

137 **Nocardia vs Actinomyces: Image A.** *Nocardia* on acid-fast stain. ⊚⓪ Venkataramana K. Human *Nocardia* infections: a review of pulmonary nocardiosis. *Cereus.* 2015;7(8):e304. DOI: 10.7759/cureus.304.

137 **Nocardia vs Actinomyces: Image B.** *Actinomyces israelii* on Gram stain. ⊚ The US Department of Health and Human Services.

138 **Mycobacteria.** Acid-fast stain. ⊚ The US Department of Health and Human Services and Dr. George P. Kubica

139 **Leprosy: Image B.** Tuberculoid lesion. ⊚ The US Department of Health and Human Services and Dr. Robert Fass, Ohio State Dept. of Medicine.

140 **Neisseria: Image A.** Intracellular N *gonorrhoeae*. ⊚ The US Department of Health and Human Services and Bill Schwartz.

141 **Legionella pneumophila.** Lung findings of unilateral and lobar infiltrate. ⊚⓪ Robbins NM, Kumar A, Blair BM. *Legionella pneumophila* infection presenting as headache, confusion and dysarthria in a human immunodeficiency virus-1 (HIV-1) positive patient: case report. *BMC Infect Dis.* 2012;12:225. DOI: 10.1186/1471-2334-12-225.

141 **Pseudomonas aeruginosa: Image A.** ⊚⓪ Gormley M, Aspray T, Kelly D, et al. Pathogen cross-transmission via building sanitary plumbing systems in a full scale pilot test-rig. *PLOS ONE.* 2017;12(2):e0171556.DOI: 10.1371/journal.pone.0171556.

141 **Pseudomonas aeruginosa: Image B.** Ecthyma gangrenosum. ⊚⓪ Gençer S, Ozer S, Ege Gül A, et al. Ecthyma gangrenosum without bacteremia in a previously healthy man: a case report. *J Med Case Rep.* 2008 Jan 22;2:14. DOI: 10.1186/1752-1947-2-14.

143 **Klebsiella.** ⊚ The US Department of Health and Human Services.

143 **Campylobacter jejuni.** ⊚ The US Department of Health and Human Services.

144 **Vibrio cholerae.** ⊚⓪ Phetsouvanh R, Nakatsu M, Arakawa E, et al. Fatal bacteremia due to immotile *Vibrio cholerae* serogroup O21 in Vientiane, Laos—a case report. *Ann Clin Microbiol Antimicrob.* 2008;7:10. DOI: 10.1186/1476-0711-7-10.

144 **Helicobacter pylori.** ⊚ The US Department of Health and Human Services, Dr. Patricia Fields, and Dr. Collette Fitzgerald.

144 Spirochetes. Appearance on darkfield microscopy. ⊚ The US Department of Health and Human Services.

144 Lyme disease: Image A. *Ixodes* tick. ⊚ The US Department of Health and Human Services and Dr. Michael L. Levin.

144 Lyme disease: Image B. Erythema migrans. ⊚ The US Department of Health and Human Services and James Gathany.

145 Syphilis: Image A. Treponeme on darkfield microscopy. ⊚ The US Department of Health and Human Services and Renelle Woodall.

145 Syphilis: Image B. Whole-body maculopapular rash in secondary syphilis. ⊚ The US Department of Health and Human Services and Susan Lindsley.

145 Syphilis: Image C, left. Maculopapular rash on palms in secondary syphilis. ⊚ The US Department of Health and Human Services.

145 Syphilis: Image C, right. Maculopapular rash on palms in secondary syphilis. ⊚ Drahansky M, Dolezel M, Urbanek J, et al. Influence of skin diseases on fingerprint recognition. *J Biomed Biotechnol.* 2012;2012:626148. DOI: 10.1155/2012/626148.

145 Syphilis: Image D. Condyloma lata. ⊚ The US Department of Health and Human Services and Susan Lindsley.

145 Syphilis: Image E. Gumma. ⊚ Chakir K, Benchikhi H. Granulome centro-facial révélant une syphilis tertiaire. *Pan Afr Med J.* 2013;15:82. DOI: 10.11604/pamj.2013.15.82.3011.

145 Syphilis: Image F. Snuffles and rhagades in congenital syphilis. ⊚ The US Department of Health and Human Services and Susan Lindsley.

145 Syphilis: Image G. Hutchinson teeth in congenital syphilis. ⊚ The US Department of Health and Human Services and Susan Lindsley.

147 *Gardnerella vaginalis.* ⊚ The US Department of Health and Human Services and M. Rein.

148 Rickettsial diseases and vector-borne illnesses: Image A. Rash of Rocky Mountain spotted fever. ⊚ The US Department of Health and Human Services.

148 Rickettsial diseases and vector-borne illnesses: Image B. *Ehrlichia* morulae. ⊚ Williams CV, Van Steenhouse JL, Bradley JM, et al. Naturally occurring *Ehrlichia chaffeensis* infection in two prosimian primate species: ring-tailed lemurs (*Lemur catta*) and ruffed lemurs (*Varecia variegata*). *Emerg Infect Dis.* 2002;8(12):1497-1500. DOI: 10.3201/eid0812.020085.

148 Rickettsial diseases and vector-borne illnesses: Image C. *Anaplasma phagocytophilium* in neutrophil. Courtesy of Dr. Bobbi Pritt.

148 *Mycoplasma pneumoniae.* ⊚ Rottem S, Kosower ND, Kornspan JD. Contamination of tissue cultures by *Mycoplasma.* In: Ceccherini-Nelli L, ed: Biomedical tissue culture. 2016. DOI: 10.5772/51518.

149 Systemic mycoses: Image A. *Histoplasma.* ⊚ The US Department of Health and Human Services and Dr. D.T. McClenan.

149 Systemic mycoses: Image B. *Blastomyces dermatitidis* undergoing broad-base budding. ⊚ The US Department of Health and Human Services and Dr. Libero Ajello.

149 Systemic mycoses: Image C. Lesions of blastomycosis. ⊚ The US Department of Health and Human Services and Dr. Lucille K. Georg.

149 Systemic mycoses: Image D. Endospheres in coccidiomycosis. ⊚ The US Department of Health and Human Services.

149 Systemic mycoses: Image E. "Captain's wheel" shape of *Paracoccidioides.* ⊚ The US Department of Health and Human Services and Dr. Lucille K. Georg.

150 Opportunistic fungal infections: Image A. Budding yeast of *Candida albicans.* ⊚ The US Department of Health and Human Services and Dr. Gordon Roberstad.

150 Opportunistic fungal infections: Image B. Germ tubes of *Candida albicans.* ⊚ The US Department of Health and Human Services and Dr. Hardin.

150 Opportunistic fungal infections: Image C. Oral thrush. ⊚ The US Department of Health and Human Services and Dr. Sol Silverman, Jr.

150 Opportunistic fungal infections: Image E. Aspergilloma in left lung. ⊚ Souilamas R, Souilamas JI, Alkhamees K, et al. Extra corporal membrane oxygenation in general thoracic surgery: a new single veno-venous cannulation. *J Cardiothorac Surg.* 2011;6:52. DOI: 10.1186/1749-8090-6-52.

150 Opportunistic fungal infections: Image F. *Cryptococcus neoformans* on India ink stain. ⊚ The US Department of Health and Human Services and Dr. Leanor Haley.

150 Opportunistic fungal infections: Image G. *Cryptococcus neoformans* on mucicarmine stain. ⊚ The US Department of Health and Human Services and Dr. Leanor Haley.

150 Opportunistic fungal infections: Image H. Mucor. ⊚ The US Department of Health and Human Services and Dr. Lucille K. Georg.

150 Opportunistic fungal infections: Image I. Mucormycosis. ⊚ Jiang N, Zhao G, Yang S, et al. A retrospective analysis of eleven cases of invasive rhino-orbito-cerebral mucormycosis presented with orbital apex syndrome initially. *BMC Ophthalmol.* 2016;16:10. DOI: 10.1186/s12886-016-0189-1.

151 *Pneumocystis jirovecii*: Image A. Interstitial opacities in lung. ⊚ Chuang C, Zhanhong X, Yinyin G, et al. Unsuspected *Pneumocystis* pneumonia in an HIV-seronegative patient with untreated lung cancer: circa case report. *J Med Case Rep.* 2007;1:15. DOI: 10.1186/1752-1947-1-115.

151 *Pneumocystis jirovecii*: Image B. CT of lung. ⊚ Oikonomou A, Prassopoulos P. Mimics in chest disease: interstitial opacities. *Insights Imaging.* 2013 Feb;4(1):9-27. DOI: 10.1007/s13244-012-0207-7.

151 *Pneumocystis jirovecii*: Image C. Disc-shaped yeast. ⊚ Kirby S, Satoskar A, Brodsky S, et al. Histological spectrum of pulmonary manifestations in kidney transplant recipients on sirolimus inclusive immunosuppressive regimens. *Diagn Pathol.* 2012;7:25. DOI: 10.1186/1746-1596-7-25.

151 *Sporothrix schenckii.* Subcutaneous mycosis. ⊚ Govender NP, Maphanga TG, Zulu TG, et al. An outbreak of lymphocutaneous sporotrichosis among mine-workers in South Africa. *PLoS Negl Trop Dis.* 2015 Sep;9(9):e0004096. DOI: 10.1371/journal.pntd.0004096.

152 Protozoa—gastrointestinal infections: Image A. *Giardia lamblia* trophozoite. ⊚ The US Department of Health and Human Services and Dr. Stan Erlandsen.

152 Protozoa—gastrointestinal infections: Image B. *Giardia lamblia* cyst. ⊚ The US Department of Health and Human Services.

152 Protozoa—gastrointestinal infections: Image C. Flask-shaped ulcers in colon in *Entamoeba histolytica* infection. ⊚ The US Department of Health and Human Services and Dr. Mae Melvin.

152 Protozoa—gastrointestinal infections: Image D. *Entamoeba histolytica* trophozoites. ⊚ The US Department of Health and Human Services.

152 Protozoa—gastrointestinal infections: Image E. *Entamoeba histolytica* cyst. ⊚ The US Department of Health and Human Services.

152 Protozoa—gastrointestinal infections: Image F. *Cryptosporidium* oocysts. ⊚ The US Department of Health and Human Services.

153 Protozoa—CNS infections: Image A. Ring-enhancing lesion in brain due to *Toxoplasma gondii.* ⊚ Rabhi S, Amrani K, Maaroufi M, et al. Hemichorea-hemiballismus as an initial manifestation in a Moroccan patient with acquired immunodeficiency syndrome and toxoplasma infection: a case report and review of the literature. *Pan Afr Med J.* 2011;10:9. DOI: 10.4314/pamj.v10i0.72216.

153 **Protozoa—CNS infections: Image B.** *Toxoplasma gondii* tachyzoite. ⬛ The US Department of Health and Human Services and Dr. L.L. Moore, Jr.

153 **Protozoa—CNS infections: Image C.** Primary amebic meningoencephalitis. ⬛ The US Department of Health and Human Services and Dr. Govinda S. Visvesvara.

153 **Protozoa—CNS infections: Image D.** *Trypanosoma brucei gambiense.* ⬛ The US Department of Health and Human Services and Dr. Mae Melvin.

154 **Protozoa—hematologic infections: Image A.** *Plasmodium* trophozoite ring form. ⬛ The US Department of Health and Human Services and Steven Glenn.

154 **Protozoa—hematologic infections: Image B.** *Plasmodium* with trophozoite ring. ⬛ The US Department of Health and Human Services and Mae Melvin.

154 **Protozoa—hematologic infections: Image C.** Gametocyte of *Plasmodium falciparum* in RBC membrane. ⬛ The US Department of Health and Human Services.

154 **Protozoa—hematologic infections: Image D.** *Babesia* with ring form and with "Maltese cross" form. ⬛ The US Department of Health and Human Services.

155 **Protozoa—others: Image A.** *Trypanosoma cruzi.* ⬛ The US Department of Health and Human Services and Dr. Mae Melvin.

155 **Protozoa—others: Image B.** Cutaneous leishmaniasis. ⬛ Sikorska K, Gesing M, Olszański R, et al. Misdiagnosis and inappropriate treatment of cutaneous leishmaniasis: a case report. *Trop Dis Travel Med Vaccines.* 2022 Aug 1;8(1):18. DOI: 10.1186/s40794-022-00175-5.

155 **Protozoa—others: Image C.** Macrophage with amastigotes. ⬛ The US Department of Health and Human Services and Dr. Francis W. Chandler.

155 **Protozoa—others: Image D.** *Trichomonas vaginalis.* ⬛ The US Department of Health and Human Services.

156 **Nematodes (roundworms): Image A.** *Enterobius vermicularis* egg. ⬛ The US Department of Health and Human Services, B.G. Partin, and Dr. Moore.

156 **Nematodes (roundworms): Image B.** *Ascaris lumbricoides* egg. ⬛ The US Department of Health and Human Services.

156 **Nematodes (roundworms): Image C.** Cutaneous larva migrans. ⬛ Benbella I, Khalki H, Lahmadi K, et al. Syndrome de larva migrans cutanée sur pied malformé (à propos d'un cas). *Pan Afr Med J.* 2016;23;50. DOI: 10.11604/pamj.2016.23.50.8696.

156 **Nematodes (roundworms): Image D.** *Trichinella spiralis* cysts in muscle. ⬛ Franssen FFJ, Fonville M, Takumi K, et al. *Vet Res.* Antibody response against *Trichinella spiralis* in experimentally infected rats is dose dependent. 2011;42(1):113. DOI: 10.1186/1297-9716-42-113.

156 **Nematodes (roundworms): Image E.** Elephantiasis. ⬛ The US Department of Health and Human Services.

157 **Cestodes (tapeworms): Image A.** *Taenia solium.* ⬛ The US Department of Health and Human Services Robert J. Galindo.

157 **Cestodes (tapeworms): Image B.** Neurocysticercosis. ⬛ Sonhaye L, Tchaou M, Amadou A, et al. Valeur diagnostique de la tomodensitométrie dans la cysticercose cérébrale à Lomé. *Pan Afr Med J.* 2015;20:67. DOI: 10.11604/pamj.2015.20.67.6085.

157 **Cestodes (tapeworms): Image C.** *Echinococcus granulosus.* ⬛ The US Department of Health and Human Services.

157 **Cestodes (tapeworms): Image D.** Hyatid cyst of *Echinococcus granulosus.* ⬛ The US Department of Health and Human Services and Dr. I. Kagan.

157 **Cestodes (tapeworms): Image E.** *Echinococcus granulosus* cyst in liver. ⬛ Ma Z, Yang W, Yao Y, et al. The adventitia resection in treatment of liver hydatid cyst: a case report of a 15-year-old boy. *Case Rep Surg.* 2014;2014:123149. DOI: 10.1155/2014/123149.

157 **Trematodes (flukes): Image A.** *Schistosoma mansoni* egg with lateral spine. ⬛ The US Department of Health and Human Services and Dr. D. S. Martin.

157 **Trematodes (flukes): Image B.** *Schistosoma haematobium* egg with terminal spine. ⬛ The US Department of Health and Human Services.

158 **Ectoparasites: Image A.** Scabies. ⬛ Siegfried EC, Hebert AA. Diagnosis of atopic dermatitis: mimics, overlaps, and complications. *Clin Med.* 2015 May;4(5):884–917. DOI: 10.3390/jcm4050884.

158 **Ectoparasites: Image B.** Nit of a louse. ⬛ Turgut B, Kurt J, Çatak O, et al. Phthriasis palpebrarum mimicking lid eczema and blepharitis. *J Ophthalmol.* 2009;803951. DOI: 10.1155/2009/803951.

161 **DNA viruses: Image B.** Febrile pharyngitis. ⬛ Balfour HH Jr, Dunmire SK, Hogquist KA. *Clin Transl Immunology.* 2015;4(2):e33. DOI: 10.1038/cti.2015.1.

163 **Herpesviruses: Image A.** Keratoconjunctivitis in HSV-1 infection. ⬛ Yang HK, Han YK, Wee WR, et al. Bilateral herpetic keratitis presenting with unilateral neurotrophic keratitis in pemphigus foliaceus: a case report. *J Med Case Rep.* 2011;5:328. DOI: 10.1186/1752-1947-5-328.

163 **Herpesviruses: Image B.** Herpes labialis. ⬛ The US Department of Health and Human Services and Dr. Herrmann.

163 **Herpesviruses: Image C.** Neonatal herpes. ⬛ The US Department of Health and Human Services.

163 **Herpesviruses: Image D.** Varicella zoster rash. ⬛ The US Department of Health and Human Services and Dr. John Noble, Jr.

163 **Herpesviruses: Image F.** Hepatosplenomegaly due to EBV infection. ⬛ Gow NJ, Davidson RN, Ticehurst R, et al. Case report: no response to liposomal daunorubicin in a patient with drug-resistant HIV-associated visceral leishmaniasis. *PLoS Negl Trop Dis.* 2015 Aug;9(8):e0003983. DOI: 10.1371/journal.pntd.0003983.

163 **Herpesviruses: Image G.** Atypical lymphocytes in Epstein-Barr virus infection. ⬛ Takahashi T, Maruyama Y, Saitoh M, et al. Fatal Epstein-Barr virus reactivation in an acquired aplastic anemia patient treated with rabbit antithymocyte globulin and cyclosporine A. *Case Rep Hematol.* 2015;2015:926874. DOI: 10.1155/2015/926874.

163 **Herpesviruses: Image I.** Roseola vaccinia. ⬛ The US Department of Health and Human Services.

163 **Herpesviruses: Image J.** Kaposi sarcoma. ⬛ The US Department of Health and Human Services and Dr. Steve Kraus.

163 **HSV identification.** Positive Tzanck smear in HSV-2 infection. ⬛ The US Department of Health and Human Services and Joe Miller.

165 **Rotavirus.** ⬛ The US Department of Health and Human Services and Erskine Palmer.

166 **Rubella virus.** Rubella rash. ⬛ The US Department of Health and Human Services.

167 **Acute laryngotracheobronchitis.** Steeple sign. Reproduced, with permission, from Dr. Frank Gaillard and www.radiopaedia.org.

167 **Measles (rubeola) virus.** Koplik spots. ⬛ The US Department of Health and Human Services.

167 **Mumps virus.** Swollen neck and parotid glands. ⬛ The US Department of Health and Human Services.

168 **Zika virus.** Noncontrast-enhanced CT scan showing cerebellar hypoplasia. Petribu NCL, Fernandes ACV, Abath MB, et al. Common findings on head computed tomography in neonates with confirmed congenital Zika syndrome. *Radiol Bras.* 2018 Nov-Dec;51(6):366-371. DOI: 10.1590/0100-3984.2017.0119.

169 **Rabies virus: Image A.** Transmission electron micrograph. The US Department of Health and Human Services Dr. Fred Murphy, and Sylvia Whitfield.

169 **Rabies virus: Image B.** Negri bodies. The US Department of Health and Human Services and Dr. Daniel P. Perl.

169 **Ebola virus.** The US Department of Health and Human Services and Cynthia Goldsmith.

170 **Hepatitis viruses.** Mild lobular activity and a Councilman body. Sedej K, Toplak N, Praprotnik M, et al. Autoimmune hepatitis as a presenting manifestation of mixed connective tissue disease in a child. Case report and review of the literature. *Pediatr Rheumatol Online J.* 2015 Nov 10;13(1):47. DOI: 10.1186/s12969-015-0046-4.

176 **Osteomyelitis.** X-ray (left) and MRI (right) views. Huang P-Y, Wu P-K, Chen C-F, et al. Osteomyelitis of the femur mimicking bone tumors: a review of 10 cases. *World J Surg Oncol.* 2013;11:283. DOI: 10.1186/1477-7819-11-283.

177 **Red rashes of childhood: Image B.** Rash of measles. The US Department of Health and Human Services.

177 **Red rashes of childhood: Image D.** Sandpaperlike rash of scarlet fever. The US Department of Health and Human Services.

177 **Red rashes of childhood: Image E.** Chicken pox. The US Department of Health and Human Services and Dr. J.D. Millar.

178 **Common vaginal infections: Image B.** *Trichomonas* vaginitis. The US Department of Health and Human Services and Jim Pledger.

178 **Common vaginal infections: Image C.** Motile trichomonads. Joe Miller.

178 **Common vaginal infections: Image D.** *Candida* vulvovaginitis. The US Department of Health and Human Services, Dr. N.J. Fiumara, and Dr. Gavin Hart.

179 **Sexually transmitted infections: Image A.** Chancroid. The US Department of Health and Human Services and Dr. Greg Hammond.

179 **Sexually transmitted infections: Image B.** Condylomata acuminata. The US Department of Health and Human Services and Susan Lindsley.

179 **Sexually transmitted infections: Image D.** Donovanosis. The US Department of Health and Human Services and Dr. Pinozzi.

179 **Sexually transmitted infections: Image E.** Buboes of lymphogranuloma venereum. The US Department of Health and Human Services and O.T. Chambers.

179 **Sexually transmitted infections: Image F.** Chancre of primary syphilis. The US Department of Health and Human Services and Susan Lindsley.

180 **TORCH infections: Image A.** "Blueberry muffin" rash. Benmiloud S, Elhaddou G, Belghiti ZA, et al. Blueberry muffin syndrome. *Pan Afr Med J.* 2012;13:23.

180 **TORCH infections: Image B.** Cataract in infant with contenital rubella. The US Department of Health and Human Services.

180 **TORCH infections: Image C.** Periventricular calcifications in congenital cytomegalovirus infection. Bonthius D, Perlman S. Congenital viral infections of the brain: lessons learned from lymphocytic choriomeningitis virus in the neonatal rat. *PLoS Pathog.* 2007;3:e149. DOI: 10.1371/journal.ppat.0030149.

181 **Pelvic inflammatory disease: Image A.** Purulent cervical discharge. The US Department of Health and Human Services and Dr. Lourdes Fraw and Jim Pledger.

181 **Pelvic inflammatory disease: Image B.** Adhesions in Fitz-Hugh-Curtis syndrome. Grigoriadis G, Green J, Amin A, et al. Fitz-Hugh-Curtis syndrome: an incidental diagnostic finding during laparoscopic sterilization. *Cureus* 12(9):e1030 4. DOI: 10.7759/cureus.10304.

186 **Vancomycin.** Red man syndrome. O'Meara P, Borici-Mazi R, Morton R, et al. DRESS with delayed onset acute interstitial nephritis and profound refractory eosinophilia secondary to vancomycin. *Allergy Asthma Clin Immunol.* 2011;7:16. DOI: 10.1186/1710-1492-7-16.

Pathology

205 **Necrosis: Image A.** Coagulative necrosis. The US Department of Health and Human Services and Dr. Steven Rosenberg.

205 **Necrosis: Image B.** Liquefactive necrosis. Ghaly R, Candido K, Knezevic N. Perioperative fatal embolic cerebrovascular accident after radical prostatectomy. *Surg Neurol Int.* 2010;1:26. DOI: 10.4103/2152-7806.65055.

205 **Necrosis: Image C.** Caseous necrosis. Szaluś-Jordanow O, Augustynowicz-Kopeć E, Czopowicz M, et al. Intracardiac tuberculomas caused by Mycobacterium tuberculosis in a dog. *BMC Vet Res.* 2016 Jun 14;12(1):109. DOI: 10.1186/s12917-016-0731-7.

205 **Necrosis: Image D.** Fat necrosis. Chee C. Panniculitis in a patient presenting with a pancreatic tumour and polyarthritis: a case report. *J Med Case Rep.* 2009 Jul 6;3:7331. DOI: 10.4076/1752-1947-3-7331.

205 **Necrosis: Image E.** Fibrinoid necrosis. Ahmed S, Kitchen J, Hamilton S, et al. A case of polyarteritis nodosa limited to the right calf muscles, fascia, and skin: a case report. *J Med Case Rep.* 2011 Sep 12;5:450. DOI: 10.1186/1752-1947-5-450.

205 **Necrosis: Image F.** Acral gangrene. The US Department of Health and Human Services and William Archibald.

206 **Ischemia.** Van Assche LM, Kim HW, Jensen CJ, et al. A new CMR protocol for non-destructive, high resolution, ex-vivo assessment of the area at risk simultaneous with infarction: validation with histopathology. *J Cardiovasc Magn Reson.* 2012;14(Suppl 1):O7. DOI: 10.1186/1532-429X-14-S1-O7.

206 **Types of infarcts: Image B.** Pale infarct. Hanes DW, Wong ML, Jenny Chang CW, et al. Embolization of the first diagonal branch of the left anterior descending coronary artery as a porcine model of chronic trans-mural myocardial infarction. *J Transl Med.* 2015 Jun 6;13:187. DOI: 10.1186/s12967-015-0547-4.

207 **Types of calcification.** Dystrophic calcification. Adapted from da Silva RMS, de Mello RJV. Fat deposition in the left ventricle: descriptive and observacional study in autopsy. *Lipids Health Dis.* 2017 May 2;16(1):86. DOI: 10.1186/s12944-017-0475-9.

207 **Psammoma bodies.** Wang C, Chen Y, Zhang L, et al. Thoracic psammomatous meningioma with osseous metaplasia: a controversial diagnosis of a case report and literature review. *World J Surg Oncol.* 2019 Aug 24;17(1):150. doi: 10.1186/s12957-019-1694-5.

208 **Amyloidosis: Image A.** Gastric amyloid deposits on Congo red stain. Desport E, Bridoux F, Sirac C, et al. Centre national de référence pour l'amylose AL et les autres maladies par dépôts d'immunoglobulines monoclonales. Al amyloidosis. *Orphanet J Rare Dis.* 2012 Aug 21;7:54. doi: 10.1186/1750-1172-7-54.

208 **Amyloidosis: Image B.** Gastric amyloid deposits on Congo stain viewed under polarized light. Desport E, Bridoux F, Sirac C, et al. Centre national de référence pour l'amylose AL et les autres maladies par dépôts d'immunoglobulines monoclonales. Al amyloidosis. *Orphanet J Rare Dis.* 2012 Aug 21;7:54. doi: 10.1186/1750-1172-7-54.

210 **Acute inflammation.** Pericardium with severe inflammation, neutrophilic infiltration and fibrin with entrapped clusters of bacteria. Ajili F, Souissi A, Bougrine F, et al. Coexistence of pyoderma gangrenosum and sweet's syndrome in a patient with ulcerative colitis. *Pan Afr Med J.* 2015;21:151. DOI: 10.11604/pamj.2015.21.151.6364.

213 **Granulomatous inflammation.** Granuloma. Guirado E, Schlesinger LS. Modeling the Mycobacterium tuberculosis granuloma: the critical battlefield in host immunity and disease. *Front. Immunol.* 2013;4:98. DOI: 10.3389/fimmu.2013.00098.

214 **Scar formation: Image A.** Hypertrophic scar. Baker R, Urso-Baiarda F, Linge C, et al. Cutaneous scarring: a clinical review. *Dermatol Res Pract.* 2009;2009:625376. DOI: 10.1155/2009/625376.

214 **Scar formation: Image B.** Keloid scar. Tirgan MH. Neck keloids: evaluation of risk factors and recommendation for keloid staging system. *F1000Res.* 2016 Jun 28;5:1528. DOI: 10.12688/f1000research.9086.2.

219 **Common metastases: Image A.** Multiple foci of low signal intensity of the bone marrow. Oprea-Lager DE, Cysouw MCF, Boellaard R, et al. Bone metastases are measurable: the role of whole-body MRI and positron emission tomography. *Front. Oncol.* 2021;11:772530. DOI: 10.3389/fonc.2021.772530

219 **Common metastases: Image B.** Right liver lobe with a metastatic tumor and a satellite focus. Paschke L, Juszczak M, Slupski M. Surgical treatment of recurrent urachal carcinoma with liver metastasis: a case report and literature review. *World J Surg Oncol.* 2016 Nov 28;14(1):296. DOI: 10.1186/s12957-016-1057-4.

225 **Lipofuscin.** Bae Y, Ito T, Iida T, et al. Intracellular propionibacterium acnes infection in glandular epithelium and stromal macrophages of the prostate with or without cancer. *PLoS One.* 2014 Feb 28;9(2):e90324. DOI: 10.1371/journal.pone.0090324.

Cardiovascular

288 **Heart anatomy: Image A.** MRI showing normal cardiac anatomy. Zhang J, Chen L, Wang X, et al. Compounding local invariant features and global deformable geometry for medical image registration. *PLoS One.* 2014;9(8):e105815. DOI: 10.1371/journal.pone.0105815.

302 **Congenital heart diseases: Image B.** Tetralogy of Fallot. Rashid AKM: Heart diseases in Down syndrome. In: Dey S, ed: Down syndrome. DOI: 10.5772/46009.

303 **Congenital heart diseases: Image D.** Atrial septal defect. Teo KSL, Dundon BK, Molaee P, et al. Percutaneous closure of atrial septal defects leads to normalisation of atrial and ventricular volumes. *J Cardiovasc Magn Reson.* 2008;10(1):55. DOI: 10.1186/1532-429X-10-55.

303 **Congenital heart diseases: Image E.** Patent ductus arteriosus. Henjes CR, Nolte I, Wesfaedt P. Multidetector-row computed tomography of thoracic aortic anomalies in dogs and cats: patent ductus arteriosus and vascular rings. *BMC Vet Res.* 2011;7:57. DOI: 10.1186/1746-6148-7-57.

304 **Coarction of the aorta.** MRI showing coarctation of the aorta. Parissis, H, Al-Alao, B, Soo, A,. et al. Single stage repair of a complex pathology: end stage ischaemic cardiomyopathy, ascending aortic aneurysm and thoracic coarctation. *J Cardiothorac Surg.* 2011;6:152. DOI: 10.1186/1749-8090-6-152.

304 **Hypertension.** "String of beads" appearance of renal artery in fibromuscular dysplasia. Plouin PF, Perdu J, LaBatide-Alanore A, et al. Fibromuscular dysplasia. *Orphanet J Rare Dis.* 2007;7:28. DOI: 10.1186/1750-1172-2-28.

305 **Hyperlipidemia signs: Image C.** Tendinous xanthoma. Huri G, Joachim N. An unusual case of hand xanthomatosis. *Case Rep Orthop.* 2013;2013:183018. DOI: 10.1155/2013/183018.

306 **Cholesterol emboli syndrome.** Cholesterol emboli. Yamaguchi S, Kakazu M, Osamu A. Intestinal cholesterol embolism resulting from intra-aortic balloon pumping: a case report. *J Med Case Rep.* 2014 Jun 20;8:213. DOI: 10.1186/1752-1947-8-213.

306 **Arteriosclerosis: Image A.** Hyaline type. Sostaric-Zuckermann IC, Borel N, Kaiser C, et al. Chlamydia in canine or feline coronary arteriosclerotic lesions. *BMC Res Notes.* 2011 Sep 9;4:350. DOI: 10.1186/1756-0500-4-350.

306 **Arteriosclerosis: Image B.** Hyperplastic type. Huang J, Han SS, Qin DD, et al. Renal interstitial arteriosclerotic lesions in lupus nephritis patients: a cohort study from China. *PLoS One.* 2015 Nov 6;10(11):e0141547. DOI: 10.1371/journal.pone.0141547.

307 **Aortic dissection.** Qi Y, Ma X, Li G, et al. Three-dimensional visualization and imaging of the entry tear and intimal flap of aortic dissection using CT virtual intravascular endoscopy. *PLoS One.* 2016;11(10) e0164750. DOI: 10.1371/journal.pone.0164750.

309 **Evolution of myocardial infarction: Images A and B.** Heart tissue at 0-24 hours (image A) and 1-3 days (image B) after myocardial infarction. Chang J, Nair V, Luk A, et al. Pathology of myocardial infarction. *Diagn Histopath.* 2013;19:7-12. DOI: 10.1016/j.mpdhp.2012.11.001.

309 **Evolution of myocardial infarction: Image C.** Heart tissue 3-14 days after myocardial infarction. Diarmid AK, Pellicori P, Cleland JG, et al. Taxonomy of segmental myocardial systolic dysfunction. *Eur Heart J.* 2017 Apr 1;38(13):942–954. DOI: 10.1093/eurheartj/ehw140.

309 **Evolution of myocardial infarction: Image D.** Heart tissue after myocardial infarction showing dense fibrous scar replacing myocyte loss. Michaud K, Basso C, d'Amati G, et al on behalf of the Association for European Cardiovascular Pathology. Diagnosis of myocardial infarction at autopsy: AECVP reappraisal in the light of the current clinical classification. *Virchows Arch.* 2020;476:179–194.

314 **Myocardial infarction complications: Image A.** Papillary muscle rupture. Routy B, Huynh T, Fraser R, et al. Vascular endothelial cell function in catastrophic antiphospholipid syndrome: a case report and review of the literature. *Case Rep Hematol.* 2013;2013:710365. DOI: 10.1155/2013/710365.

314 **Myocardial infarction complications: Image B.** Free wall rupture of left ventricle. Zacarias ML, da Trindade H, Tsutsu J, et al. Left ventricular free wall impeding rupture in post-myocardial infarction period diagnosed by myocardial contrast echocardiography: case report. *Cardiovasc Ultrasound.* 2006;4:7. DOI: 10.1186/1476-7120-4-7.

315 **Cardiomyopathies: Image A.** Dilated cardiomyopathy. Gho JMIH, van Es R, Stathonikos N, et al. High resolution systematic digital histological quantification of cardiac fibrosis and adipose tissue in phospholamban p.Arg14del mutation associated cardiomyopathy. *PLoS One.* 2014;9:e94820. DOI: 10.1371/journal.pone.0094820.

315 **Cardiomyopathies: Image B.** Hypertrophic obstructive cardiomyopathy. Benetti MA, Belo Nunes RA, Benvenuti LA. Case 2/2016 - 76-year-old male with hypertensive heart disease, renal tumor and shock. *Arq Bras Cardiol.* 2016 May; 106(5): 439–446. DOI: 10.5935/abc.20160067.

316 **Heart failure.** Pitting edema. Ong HS, Sze CW, Koh TW, Coppack SW. How 40 kilograms of fluid retention can be overlooked: two case reports. *Cases J.* 2009;2(1):33. DOI: 10.1186/1757-1626-2-33.

317 **Cardiac tamponade: Image A.** Echocardiogram showing cardiac tamponade. Maharaj SS, Chang SM. Cardiac tamponade as the initial presentation of systemic lupus erythematosus: a case report and review of the literature. *Pediatr Rheumatol Online J.* 2015;13: 9. DOI: 10.1186/s12969-015-0005-0.

318 **Infective endocarditis: Image A.** Vegetations on heart valves. The US Department of Health and Human Services and Dr. Edwin P. Ewing, Jr.

318 **Infective endocarditis: Image C.** Osler nodes. Yang ML, Chen YH, Lin WR, et al. Case report: infective endocarditis caused by *Brevundimonas vesicularis. BMC Infect Dis.* 2006;6:179. DOI: 10.1186/1471-2334-6-179.

319 **Acute pericarditis.** Bogaert J, Francone M. Cardiovascular magnetic resonance in pericardial diseases. *J Cardiovasc Magn Reson.* 2009;11:14. DOI: 10.1186/1532-429X-11-14.

320 **Hereditary hemorrhagic telangiectasia.** Telangiectasias on the tongue and hard palate. Kiyeng JC, Siika A, Koech C, et al. Definite hereditary hemorrhagic telangiectasia in a 60-year-old black Kenyan woman: a case report. *J Med Case Rep.* 2016 May 25;10(1):126. DOI: 10.1186/s13256-016-0909-4.

Endocrine

330 **Thyroid development: Image A.** Thyroglossal duct cyst. Kartini D, Panigoro S, Harahap A. Sistrunk procedure on malignant thyroglossal duct cyst. *Case Rep Oncol Med.* 2020 Jan 16;2020:6985746. DOI: 10.1155/2020/6985746.

344 **Hypothyroidism vs hyperthyroidism: Image A.** Onycholysis. Gallouj S, Mernissi FZ. Leuconychie transversale induite par la manucurie: y a-t-il un apport de la dermoscopie? [Transverse leuconychia induced by manicure: is there a contribution from dermoscopy?]. *Pan Afr Med J.* 2014;18:39. Published 2014 May 10. DOI: 10.11604/pamj.2014.18.39.3761.

344 **Hypothyroidism vs hyperthyroidism: Image B.** Pretibial myxedema. Fred H, van Dijk HA. Images of memorable cases: case 144. Connexions Web site. Dec 8, 2008. Available at: https://cnx.org/contents/SCJeD6JM@3/Images-of-Memorable-Cases-Case-144.

344 **Hypothyroidism vs hyperthyroidism: Image C.** Periorbital edema. Dandekar F, Camacho M, Valerio J, et al. *Case Rep Ophthalmol Med.* 2015;2015:126501. DOI: 10.1155/2015/126501.

345 **Hypothyroidism: Image B.** Florid Hashimoto's thyroiditis histology. Oruci M, Ito Y, Buta M, et al. Right thyroid hemiagenesis with adenoma and hyperplasia of parathyroid glands -case report. *BMC Endocr Disord.* 2012 Nov 13;12:29. DOI: 10.1186/1472-6823-12-29.

345 **Hypothyroidism: Image C.** Mazza E, Quaglino F, Suriani A, et al. Thyroidectomy for painful thyroiditis resistant to steroid treatment: three new cases with review of the literature. *Case Rep Endocrinol.* 2015;2015:138327. DOI: 10.1155/2015/138327.

345 **Hypothyroidism: Image E.** Before and after treatment of congenital hypothyroidism. Bailey P. The thyroid gland in medicine. *Popular Science Monthly* August 1897;481-489. Available at https://archive.org/details/popularsciencemo51newy/page/486/mode/2up.

345 **Hypothyroidism: Image F.** Congenital hypothyroidism. Rastogi MV, LaFranchi SH. Congenital hypothyroidism. *Orphanet J Rare Dis.* 2010 Jun 10;5:17. DOI: 10.1186/1750-1172-5-17.

346 **Hyperthyroidism: Image B.** Graves disease histology. LiVolsi VA, Baloch ZW. The pathology of hyperthyroidism. *Front Endocrinol (Lausanne).* 2018 Dec 3;9:737. DOI: 10.3389/fendo.2018.00737.

346 **Thyroid adenoma.** Terada T. Brain metastasis from thyroid adenomatous nodules or an encapsulated thyroid follicular tumor without capsular and vascular invasion: a case report. *Cases J.* 2009;2:7180. DOI: 10.4076/1757-1626-2-7180.

348 **Hypoparathyroidism.** Shortened 4th and 5th digits. Ferrario C, Gastaldi G, Portmann L, et al. Bariatric surgery in an obese patient with Albright hereditary osteodystrophy: a case report. *J Med Case Rep.* 2013;7:111. DOI: 10.1186/1752-1947-7-111.

349 **Hyperparathyroidism.** Multiple lytic lesions. Khaoula BA, Kaouther BA, Ines C, et al. An unusual presentation of primary hyperparathyroidism: pathological fracture. *Case Rep Orthop.* 2011;2011:521578. DOI: 10.1155/2011/521578.

353 **Adrenal insufficiency.** Mucosal hyperpigmentation in primary adrenal insufficiency. Wina Dharmesti NW, Saraswati MR, Suastika K, et al. Challenging Diagnosis of Addison's Disease Presenting with Adrenal Crisis. *Case Rep Endocrinol.* 2021 Oct 11;2021:7137950. DOI: 10.1155/2021/7137950.

355 **Pheochromocytoma.** Muneer T, Tariq A, Siddiqui A H, et al. Malignant pheochromocytoma with widespread bony and pulmonary metastases. *Cureus.* 10(9):e3348. DOI: 10.7759/cureus.3348.

356 **Multiple endocrine neoplasias.** Mucosal neuroma. Martucciello G, Lerone M, Bricco L, et al. Multiple endocrine neoplasias type 2B and RET proto-oncogene. *Ital J Pediatr.* 2012;38:9. DOI: 10.1186/1824-7288-38-9.

357 **Carcinoid tumors.** Katsuyoshi F, Hidenobu K, Masayuki O, et al. Gastric Carcinoid with Hypergastrinemia: Report of Three Cases. *Case Reports in Medicine.* 2010;348761. DOI: 10.1155/2010/348761.

Gastrointestinal

365 **Ventral wall defects: Image A.** Gastroschisis. Bhat V, Moront M, Bhandari V. Gastroschisis: a state-of-the-art review. *Children (Basel).* 2020 Dec 17;7(12):302. DOI: 10.3390/children7120302.

365 **Ventral wall defects: Image B.** Omphalocele. Lamquami S, Mamouni N, Errarhay S, et al. Antenatal diagnosis of isolated omphalocele. *Pan Afr Med J.* 2015 Jul 31;21:233. doi: 10.11604/pamj.2015.21.233.7151.

365 **Ventral wall defects: Image C.** Congenital diaphragmatic hernia. Rastogi MV, LaFranchi SH. Congenital hypothyroidism. *Orphanet J Rare Dis.* 2010;5:17. DOI: 10.1186/1750-1172-5-17.

366 **Intestinal atresia.** Saha M. Alimentary tract atresias associated with anorectal malformations: 10 years' experience. *J Neonatal Surg.* 2016 Oct-Dec;5(4):43. DOI: 10.21699/jns.v5i4.449.

367 **Pancreas and spleen embryology.** Annular pancreas. Mahdi B, Selim S, Hassen T, et al. A rare cause of proximal intestinal obstruction in adults—annular pancreas: a case report. *Pan Afr Med J.* 2011;10:56.

367 **Retroperitoneal structures.** Sammut J, Ahiaku E, Williams DT. Complete regression of renal tumour following ligation of an accessory renal artery during repair of an abdominal aortic aneurysm. *Ann R Coll Surg Engl.* 2012 Sep;94(6):e198–e200. DOI: 10.1308/003588412 X13373405384972.

369 **Digestive tract anatomy.** Transverse histologic section of the normal oesophageal wall. Wei Y, Wu S, Shi D, et al. Oesophageal carcinoma: comparison of ex vivo high-resolution 3.0 T MR imaging with histopathological findings. *Sci Rep.* 2016 Oct 11;6:35109. DOI: 10.1038/srep35109.

369 **Digestive tract histology: Image A.** Sato Y, Fujino T, Kasagawa A, et al. Twelve-year natural history of a gastric adenocarcinoma of fundic gland type. *Clin J Gastroenterol.* 2016 Dec;9(6):345-351. DOI: 10.1007/s12328-016-0680-5.

369 **Digestive tract histology: Image B.** Jejunum. Non-neoplastic parietal cells. Chen J, Tellez G, Richards JD, Escobar J. Identification of Potential Biomarkers for Gut Barrier Failure in Broiler Chickens. *Front Vet Sci.* 2015 May 26;2:14. DOI: 10.3389/fvets.2015.00014.

374 **Liver tissue architecture.** Portal triad. Liver development. In: Zorn AM. Stem book. Cambridge: Harvard Stem Cell Institute, 2008. Available at www.stembook.org/node/512.

375 **Biliary structures.** Gallstones. Issa H, Al-Salem AH. Hepatobiliary manifestations of sickle cell anemia. *Gastroenterology Res.* 2010 Feb;3(1):1-8. DOI: 10.4021/gr2010.01.

377 **Hernias: Image A.** Congenital diaphragmatic hernia. Tovar J. Congenital diaphragmatic hernia. *Orphanet J Rare Dis.* 2012;7:1. DOI: 10.1186/1750-1172-7-1.

381 **Peyer patches.** Kapoor K, Singh O. Ileal and jejunal Peyer's patches in buffalo calves: Histomorphological comparison. *Vet World.* 2015 Nov;8(11):1273-8. DOI: 10.14202/vetworld.2015.1.

383 **Oral pathologies: Image A.** Apthous ulcer. Peterson DE, O'Shaughnessy JA, Rugo HS, et al. Oral mucosal injury caused by mammalian target of rapamycin inhibitors: emerging perspectives on pathobiology and impact on clinical practice. *Cancer Med.* 2016 Aug;5(8):1897–1907. DOI: 10.1002/cam4.761.

383 **Oral pathologies: Image B.** Leukoplakia of tongue. The US Department of Health and Human Services and J.S. Greenspan, B.D.S., University of California, San Francisco; Sol Silverman, Jr., D.D.S.

383 **Oral pathologies: Image C.** Sialolithiasis. Pastor-Ramos V, Cuervo-Diaz A, Aracil-Kessler L. Sialolithiasis. Proposal for a new minimally invasive procedure: piezoelectric surgery. *J Clin Exp Dent.* 2014 Jul;6(3):e295–e298. DOI: 10.4317/jced.51253.

383 **Oral pathologies: Image D.** Pleomorphic adenoma histology. Genelhu MC, Cardoso SV, Gobbi H, Cassali GD. A comparative study between mixed-type tumours from human salivary and canine mammary glands. *BMC Cancer.* 2007 Nov;28;7:218. DOI: 10.1186/1471-2407-7-218.

383 **Achalasia.** Agrusa A, Romano G, Frazzetta G, et al. Achalasia secondary to submucosal invasion by poorly differentiated adenocarcinoma of the cardia, siewert II: consideration on preoperative workup. *Case Rep Surg.* 2014;2014:654917. DOI: 10.1155/2014/654917.

384 **Other esophageal pathologies: Image A.** White pseudomembrane of *Candida* infection in esophagitis. Takahashi Y, Nagata N, Shimbo T. Long-term trends in esophageal candidiasis prevalence and associated risk factors with or without HIV infection: lessons from an endoscopic study of 80,219 patients. *PLoS One.* 2015; 10(7):e0133589. DOI: 10.1371/journal.pone.0133589.

384 **Other esophageal pathologies: Image B.** Esophageal varices on endoscopy. Costaguta A, Alvarez F. Etiology and management of hemorrhagic complications of portal hypertension in children. *Int J Hepatol.* 2012;2012:879163. DOI: 10.1155/2012/879163.

384 **Other esophageal pathologies: Image C.** Pneumomediastinum. Bakhshaee M, Jokar MH, Mirfeizi Z, et al. Subcutaneous emphysema, pneumomediastinum and pneumothorax in a patient with dermatomyositis. *Iran J Otorhinolaryngol.* 2017 Mar;29(91):113-116.

385 **Barrett esophagus: Image A.** Endoscopy image. Japan Esophageal Society. Japanese classification of esophageal cancer, 11th edition: part I. *Esophagus.* 2017;14(1):1–36. DOI: 10.1007/s10388-016-0551-7.

386 **Ménétrier disease.** Chung M, Pittenger J, Flomenhoft D, et al. Atypical clinical and diagnostic features in Ménétrier's disease in a child. *Case Rep Gastrointest Med.* 2011;2011:480610. DOI: 10.1155/2011/480610.

386 **Gastric cancer.** Tan Y, Fu J, Li X. A minor (<50%) signet-ring cell component associated with poor prognosis in colorectal cancer patients: a 26-year retrospective study in China. *PLoS One.* 2015;10(3):e0121944. DOI: 10.1371/journal.pone.0121944.

387 **Ulcer complications.** Free air under diaphragm in perforated ulcer. Reproduced, with permission, from Dr. Frank Gaillard and www.radiopaedia.org.

388 **Malabsorption syndromes: Image A.** Celiac disease. Celiac disease. Sedda S, Caruso R, Marafini I, et al. Pyoderma gangrenosum in refractory celiac disease: a case report. *BMC Gastroenterol.* 2013;13:162. DOI: 10.1186/1471-230X-13-162.

388 **Malabsorption syndromes: Image B.** *Tropheryma whipplei* on PAS stain. Tran HA. Reversible hypothyroidism and Whipple's disease. *BMC Endocr Disord.* 2006;6:3. DOI: 10.1186/1472-6823-6-3.

389 **Inflammatory bowel diseases: Image A.** Wall thickening in Crohn disease. Imširović, Bilal & Zerem, Enver & Guso, Emir. (2021). Role of Imaging in Small Bowel Crohn's Disease. 10.5772/intechopen.96098.

389 **Inflammatory bowel diseases: Images B and C.** Normal mucosa (B) and punched-out ulcers (C) in ulcerative colitis. Ishikawa D, Ando T, Watanabe O, et al. Images of colonic real-time tissue sonoelastography correlate with those of colonoscopy and may predict response to therapy in patients with ulcerative colitis. *BMC Gastroenterol.* 2011;11:29. DOI: 10.1186/1471-230X-11-29.

390 **Appendicitis.** Ali M, Iqbal J, Sayani R. Accuracy of computed tomography in differentiating perforated from nonperforated appendicitis, taking histopathology as the gold standard. *Cureus.* 2018 Dec 15;10(12):e3735. DOI: 10.7759/cureus.3735.

390 **Diverticula of the gastrointestinal tract: Image B.** Diverticulosis. Sartelli M, Moore FA, Ansaloni L, et al. A proposal for a CT driven classification of left colon acute diverticulitis. *World J Emerg Surg.* 2015;10:3. DOI: 10.1186/1749-7922-10-3.

390 **Diverticula of the gastrointestinal tract: Image C.** Diverticulitis. Hupfeld L, Burcharth J, Pommergaard HC, Rosenberg J. The best choice of treatment for acute colonic diverticulitis with purulent peritonitis is uncertain. *Biomed Res Int.* 2014;2014:380607. DOI: 10.1155/2014/380607.

391 **Zenker diverticulum.** Dionigi G, Sessa F, Rovera F, et al. Ten year survival after excision of squamous cell cancer in Zenker's diverticulum: report of a case. *World J Surg Oncol.* 2006 Mar 28;4:17. DOI: 10.1186/1477-7819-4-17.

392 **Intussusception.** Ultrasound showing target sign. Christianakis E, Sakelaropoulos A, Papantzimas C, et al. Pelvic plastron secondary to acute appendicitis in a child presented as appendiceal intussusception. a case report. *Cases J.* 2008;1:135. DOI: 10.1186/1757-1626-1-135.

392 **Volvulus.** Coffee bean sign. Yigit M, Turkdogan KA. Coffee bean sign, whirl sign and bird's beak sign in the diagnosis of sigmoid volvulus. *Pan Afr Med J.* 1014;19:56. DOI: 10.11604/pamj.2014.19.56.5142.

393 **Other intestinal disorders: Image A.** Necrosis due to occlusion of SMA. Van De Winkel N, Cheragwandi A, Nieboer K, et al. Superior mesenteric arterial branch occlusion causing partial jejunal ischemia: a case report. *J Med Case Rep.* 2012;6:48. DOI: 10.1186/1752-1947-6-48.

393 **Other intestinal disorders: Image B.** Loops of dilated bowel suggestive of small bowel obstruction. Welte FJ, Crosso M. Left-sided appendicitis in a patient with congenital gastrointestinal malrotation: a case report. *J Med Case Rep.* 2007;1:92. DOI: 10.1186/1752-1947-1-92.

393 **Other intestinal disorders: Image C.** Pneumatosis intestinalis. Pelizzo G, Nakib G, Goruppi I, et al. Isolated colon ischemia with norovirus infection in preterm babies: a case series. *J Med Case Rep.* 2013;7:108. DOI: 10.1186/1752-1947-7-108.

394 **Colonic polyps: Image A.** Shussman N, Wexner SD. Colorectal polyps and polyposis syndromes. *Gastroenterol Rep (Oxf).* 2014 Feb;2(1):1-15. doi: 10.1093/gastro/got041.

394 **Colonic polyps: Image B.** Peutz-Jeghers syndrome. Gondak RO, et al. Oral pigmented lesions: Clinicopathologic features and review of the literature. *Med Oral Patol Oral Cir Bucal.* 2012 Nov 1;17(6):e919-24.

394 **Colonic polyps: Image D.** Adenomatous polyps in villous adenoma. Rehani B, Chasen RM, Dowdy Y, et al. Advanced adenoma diagnosis with FDG PET in a visibly normal mucosa: a case report. *J Med Case Reports.* 2007;1:99. DOI: 10.1186/1752-1947-1-99.

395 **Colorectal cancer: Image A.** Polyp. 🅾 Takiyama A, Nozawa H, Ishihara S, et al. Secondary metastasis in the lymph node of the bowel invaded by colon cancer: a report of three cases. *World J Surg Oncol.* 2016;14:273. DOI: 10.1186/s12957-016-1026-y.

396 **Cirrhosis and portal hypertension.** Liver abnormalities in cirrhosis. 🅾 Blackburn PR, Hickey RD, Nace RA, et al. Silent tyrosinemia type I without elevated tyrosine or succinylacetone associated with liver cirrhosis and hepatocellular carcinoma. *Hum Mutat.* 2016 Oct;37(10):1097–1105. DOI: 10.1002/humu.23047.

398 **Alcoholic liver disease: Image B.** Mallory bodies. 🅾 The US Department of Health and Human Services and Dr. Edwin P. Ewing, Jr.

398 **Alcoholic liver disease: Image C.** 🅾 Miranda-Mendez A, Lugo-Baruqui A, Armendariz-Borunda J. Molecular basis and current treatment for alcoholic liver disease. *Int J Environ Res Public Health.* 2010 May;7(5):1872-88. DOI: 10.3390/ijerph7051872.

399 **Liver tumors: Image A.** Cavernous liver hemangioma. 🅾 Yano T, Kobayashi T, Kuroda S, et al. Obstructive jaundice caused by a giant liver hemangioma with Kasabach-Merritt syndrome: a case report. *Surg Case Rep.* 2015 Dec;1(1):93. DOI: 10.1186/s40792-015-0095-4.

399 **Liver tumors: Image B.** Hepatocellular carcinoma/hepatoma. Reproduced, with permission, from Jean-Christophe Fournet and Humpath.

400 **α₁-antitrypsin deficiency.** Liver histology. 🅾 Dettmer M, Cathomas G, Willi N. Alpha 1-antitrypsin retention in an ectopic liver. *Diagn Pathol.* 2011 Feb 28;6:16. DOI: 10.1186/1746-1596-6-16.

402 **Wilson disease.** Kayser-Fleischer rings. 🅾 Herbert L. Fred, MD, Hendrik A. van Dijk. Images of Memorable Cases: 50 Years at the Bedside. OpenStax CNX. Dec 8, 2008. Download for free at http://cnx.org/contents/e7b71f2c-a51e-4c9f-8db2-066a4c3643e4@7.2.

402 **Hemochromatosis.** Hemosiderin deposits. 🅾 Mathew J, Leong MY, Morley N, et al. A liver fibrosis cocktail? Psoriasis, methotrexate and genetic hemochromatosis. *BMC Dermatol.* 2005;5:12. DOI: 10.1186/1471-5945-5-12.

402 **Biliary tract disease.** Endoscopic retrograde cholangiopancreatography shows "beading" of bile ducts in primary sclerosing cholangitis. 🅾 Law S-T, Lee W-K, Li MK-K, et al. A gentleman with anemia and cholestasis. *Case Rep Med.* 2010;2010:536207. DOI: 10.1155/2010/536207.

403 **Cholelithiasis and related pathologies: Image B.** Large gallstone. 🅾 Spangler R, Van Pham T, Khoujah D, et al. Abdominal emergencies in the geriatric patient. *Int J Emerg Med.* 2014;7:43. DOI: 10.1186/s12245-014-0043-2.

403 **Cholelithiasis and related pathologies: Image C.** Porcelain gallbladder. 🅾 Fred H, van Dijk H. Images of memorable cases: case 19. Connexions Web site. December 4, 2008. Available at: http://cnx.org/content/m14939/1.3/.

404 **Pancreatitis: Image A.** Diffuse peripancreatic stranding. 🅾 Landa E, Ganim I, Vigandt E, et al. Meloxicam-induced pancreatitis. *Cureus.* 2021 Jan 28;13(1):e12976. DOI: 10.7759/cureus.12976.

404 **Pancreatitis: Image B.** Pancreatic pseudocyst. 🅾 Cawich SO, Murphy T, Shah S, et al. Endoscopic transmural drainage of pancreatic pseudocysts: technical challenges in the resource poor setting. *Case Rep Gastrointest Med.* 2013;2013:942832. DOI: 10.1155/2013/942832.

404 **Pancreatitis: Image C.** Chronic pancreatitis. 🅾 Sommer CA, Wilcox CM. Pancreatico-pericardial fistula as a complication of chronic pancreatitis. *F1000Res.* 2014 Jan 29;3:31. DOI: 10.12688/f1000research.3-31.v1.

405 **Pancreatic adenocarcinoma: Image A.** Histology. 🅾 Zapata M, Cohen C, Siddiqui MT. Immunohistochemical expression of SMAD4, CK19, and CA19-9 in fine needle aspiration samples of pancreatic adenocarcinoma: Utility and potential role. *Cytojournal.* 2007 Jun 22;4:13. DOI: 10.1186/1742-6413-4-13.

Hematology and Oncology

412 **Neutrophils: Image A.** 🅾 The US Department of Health and Human Services and Dr. F. Gilbert.

412 **Neutrophils: Image B.** Dohle bodies. 🅾 Modabbernia MJ, Mirsafa AR, Modabbernia A, et al. Catatonic syndrome associated with lead intoxication: a case report. *Cases J.* 2009 Aug 11;2:8722. DOI: 10.4076/1757-1626-2-8722.

413 **Erythrocytes.** 🅾 The US Department of Health and Human Services and Drs. Noguchi, Rodgers, and Schechter.

413 **Thrombocytes (platelets).** 🅾 The US Department of Health and Human Services and Dr. F. Gilbert.

413 **Monocytes.** 🅾 The US Department of Health and Human Services and Dr. Mae Melvin.

413 **Macrophages.** 🅾 De Tommasi AS, Otranto D, Furlanello T, et al. Evaluation of blood and bone marrow in selected canine vector-borne diseases. *Parasit Vectors.* 2014;7:534. DOI: 10.1186/s13071-014-0534-2.

414 **Dendritic cells.** 🅾 Cheng J-H, Lee S-Y, Lien Y-Y, et al. Immunomodulating activity of *Nymphaea rubra* roxb. extracts: activation of rat dendritic cells and improvement of the TH1 immune response. *Int J Mol Sci.* 2012;13:10722-10735. DOI: 10.3390/ijms130910722.

414 **Mast cells.** 🅾 Borelli V, Martinelli M, Luppi S, et al. Mast cells in peritoneal fluid from women with endometriosis and their possible role in modulating sperm function. *Front. Physiol.* 2020;10:1543. DOI: 10.3389/fphys.2019.01543.

415 **Plasma cells.** 🅾 The US Department of Health and Human Services and Dr. Francis W. Chandler.

420 **RBC morphology: Image J.** Sickle cell. 🅾 The US Department of Health and Human Services and the Sickle Cell Foundation of Georgia, Jackie George, and Beverly Sinclair.

421 **RBC inclusions: Image A.** Ringed sideroblast. 🅾 Invernizzi R, Quaglia F, Porta MG. Importance of classical morphology in the diagnosis of myelodysplastic syndrome. *Mediterr J Hematol Infect Dis.* 2015 May 1;7(1):e2015035. DOI: 10.4084/MJHID.2015.035.

421 **RBC inclusions: Image B.** Basophilic stippling. 🅾 Herbert L. Fred, MD, and Hendrik A. van Dijk. Images of Memorable Cases: Case 81. *OpenStax CNX.* Dec 3, 2008.

421 **RBC inclusions: Image C.** Howell-Jolly bodies. 🅾 Vives-Corrons J-I. The rare anaemias. 2019. DOI: 10.5772/intechopen.86986.

425 **Microcytic, hypochromic anemias: Image A.** 🅾 Bock F, Borucki K, Vorwerk P, et al. A two-and-a-half-year-old breastfed toddler presenting with anemia: a case report. *BMC Res Notes.* 2014;7:917. DOI: 10.1186/1756-0500-7-917.

425 **Microcytic, hypochromic anemias: Image D.** "Hair-on-end" appearance and thinning of the outer table of the skull. 🅾 Sunil A, Sivarajakumar B, Kumari V. Beta-thalassemia presenting as moyamoya syndrome with a review of skeletal manifestations. *Cureus.* 15(5):e38372. DOI: 10.7759/cureus.38372.

425 **Microcytic, hypochromic anemia: Image E.** Lead lines in lead poisoning. Reproduced, with permission, from Dr. Frank Gaillard and www.radiopaedia.org.

428 **Intrinsic hemolytic anemias.** 🅾 El Ariss AB, Younes M, Matar J. Prevalence of sickle cell trait in the southern suburb of Beirut, Lebanon. *Mediterr J Hematol Infect Dis.* 2016;8(1):e2016015. DOI: 10.4084/MJHID.2016.015.

430 **Heme synthesis, porphyrias, and lead poisoning: Image A.** Basophilic stippling in lead poisoning. 🅾 van Dijk HA, Fred HL. Images of memorable cases: case 81. Connexions Web site. December 3, 2008. Available at https://cnx.org/contents/MZa_Ph4e@4/Images-of-Memorable-Cases-Case-81.

430 **Heme synthesis, porphyrias, and lead poisoning: Image B.** Porphyria cutanea tarda. Bovenschen HJ, Vissers WHPM. Primary hemochromatosis presented by porphyria cutanea tarda: a case report. *Cases J.* 2009;2:7246. DOI: 10.4076/1757-1626-2-7246.

431 **Coagulation disorders.** Hemarthrosis. Lakjiri S, Mernissi FZ. Tabetic arthropathy revealing neurosyphilis: a new observation. *Pan Afr Med J.* 2014;18:198. DOI: 10.11604/pamj.2014.18.198.4893.

434 **Hodgkin lymphoma.** Reed-Sternberg cells. Knecht H, Righolt C, Mai S. Genomic instability: the driving force behind refractory/relapsing Hodgkin's lymphoma. *Cancers (Basel).* 2013 Jun;5(2):714–725. DOI: 10.3390/cancers5020714.

435 **Non-Hodgkin lymphoma: Image B.** Jaw lesion in Burkitt lymphoma. Bi CF, Tang Y, Zhang WY, et al. Sporadic Burkitt lymphomas of children and adolescents in Chinese: a clinicopathological study of 43 cases. *Diagn Pathol.* 2012;7:72. DOI:10.1186/1746-1596-7-72.

435 **Non-Hodgkin lymphoma: Image C.** Primary CNS lymphoma. Mansour A, Qandeel M, Abdel-Razeq H, et al. MR imaging features of intracranial primary CNS lymphoma in immune competent patients. *Cancer Imaging.* 2014;14(1):22. DOI: 10.1186/1470-7330-14-22.

435 **Non-Hodgkin lymphoma: Image D.** Mycosis fungoides/Sézary syndrome. Chaudhary S, Bansal C, Ranga U, et al. Erythrodermic mycosis fungoides with hypereosinophilic syndrome: a rare presentation. *Ecancermedicalscience.* 2013;7:337. DOI:10.3332/ecancer.2013.337

436 **Plasma cell dyscrasias: Image C.** Multiple plasma cells in multiple myeloma. Mehrotra R, Singh M, Singh PA, et al. Should fine needle aspiration biopsy be the first pathological investigation in the diagnosis of a bone lesion? An algorithmic approach with review of literature. *Cytojournal.* 2007;4:9. DOI: 10.1186/1742-6413-4-9.

436 **Myelodysplastic syndromes.** Neutrophil with bilobed nuclei. Ali SF, Sonu RJ, Dwyre DM, et al. Translocation (6;15)(q12;q15): a novel mutation in a patient with therapy-related myelodysplastic syndrome. *Case Rep Hematol.* 2015;2015:318545. DOI: 10.1155/2015/318545.

437 **Leukemias: Image A.** Chiaretti S, Zini G, Bassan R. Diagnosis and subclassification of acute lymphoblastic leukemia. *Mediterr J Hematol Infect Dis.* 2014;6(1):e2014073. DOI: 10.4084/MJHID.2014.073.

437 **Leukemias: Image C.** Hairy cell leukemia. Chan SM, George T, Cherry AM, et al. Complete remission of primary plasma cell leukemia with bortezomib, doxorubicin, and dexamethasone: a case report. *Cases J.* 2009;2:121. DOI: 10.1186/1757-1626-2-121.

438 **Myeloproliferative neoplasms: Image A.** Erythromelalgia in polycythemia vera. Fred H, van Dijk H. Images of memorable cases: case 151. Connexions Web site. December 4, 2008. Available at http://cnx.org/content/m14932/1.3/.

439 **Langerhans cell histiocytosis: Image A.** Birbeck granules. Bubolz A, Weissinger SE, Stenzinger A, et al. Potential clinical implications of *BRAF* mutations in histiocytic proliferations. *Oncotarget.* 2014;5:4060-4070.

441 **Warfarin.** Bakoyiannis C, Karaolanis G, Patelis N. Dabigatran in the treatment of warfarin-induced skin necrosis: A new hope. *Case Rep Dermatol Med.* 2016;2016:3121469. DOI: 10.1155/2016/3121469.

Musculoskeletal, Skin, and Connective Tissue

451 **Rotator cuff muscles.** Glenohumeral instability. Koike Y, Sano H, Imamura I, et al. Changes with time in skin temperature of the shoulders in healthy controls and a patient with shoulder-hand syndrome. *Ups J Med Sci* 2010;115:260-265. DOI: 10.3109/03009734.2010.503354.

452 **Brachial plexus lesions: Image A.** Cervical rib. Dahlin LB, Backman C, Duppe H, et al. Compression of the lower trunk of the brachial plexus by a cervical rib in two adolescent girls: case reports and surgical treatment. *J Brachial Plex Peripher Nerve Inj.* 2009;4:14. DOI: 10.1186/1749-7221-4-14.

452 **Brachial plexus lesions: Image B.** Winged scapula. Boukhris J, Boussouga M, Jaafar A, et al. Stabilisation dynamique d'un winging scapula (à propos d'un cas avec revue de la littérature). *Pan Afr Med J.* 2014;19:331. DOI: 10.11604/pamj.2014.19.331.3429.

453 **Wrist region: Image B.** Anatomic snuff box. Rhemrev SJ, Ootes D, Beeres FJP, et al. Current methods of diagnosis and treatment of scaphoid fractures. *Int J Emerg Med.* 2011;4:4. DOI: 10.1186/1865-1380-4-4.

459 **Motoneuron action potential to muscle contraction.** Two muscle sarcomeres in parallel. Ottenheijm CAC, Heunks LMA, Dekhuijzen RPN. Diaphragm adaptations in patients with COPD. *Respir Res.* 2008;9(1):12. DOI: 10.1186/1465-9921-9-12.

463 **Clavicle fractures.** X-ray of clavicle fracture. Tagliapietra J, Belluzzi E, Biz C, et al. Midshaft clavicle fractures treated nonoperatively using figure-of-eight bandage: are fracture type, shortening, and displacement radiographic predictors of failure? *Diagnostics (Basel).* 2020 Oct 5;10(10):788. DOI: 10.3390/diagnostics10100788.

463 **Wrist and hand injuries.** Metacarpal neck fracture. Bohr S, Pallua N. Early functional treatment and modern cast making for indications in hand surgery. *Adv Orthop.* 2016;2016:5726979. DOI: 10.1155/2016/5726979.

463 **Psoas abscess.** Destruction of sacroiliac joint. Kramer L, Geib V, Evison J, et al. Tuberculous sacroiliitis with secondary psoas abscess in an older patient: a case report. *J Med Case Reports.* 2018;12:237. DOI: 10.1186/s13256-018-1754-4.

464 **Common knee conditions: Image A.** ACL tear. Chang MJ, Chang CB, Choi J-Y, et al. Can magnetic resonance imaging findings predict the degree of knee joint laxity in patients undergoing anterior cruciate ligament reconstruction? *BMC Musculoskelet Disord.* 2014;15:214. DOI: 10.1186/1471-2474-15-214.

464 **Common knee conditions: Images B and C.** Prepatellar bursitis (B) and Baker cyst (C). Hirji Z, Hunhun JS, Choudur HN. Imaging of the bursae. *J Clin Imaging Sci.* 2011;1:22. DOI: 10.4103/2156-7514.80374.

466 **Childhood musculoskeletal conditions.** Slipped capital femoral epiphysis. Marquez D, Harb E, Vilchis H. Slipped capital femoral epiphysis and hypothyroidism in a young adult: a case report. *J Med Case Rep.* 2014;8(1):336. DOI: 10.1186/1752-1947-8-336.

467 **Common pediatric fractures: Image A.** Greenstick fracture. Randsborg PH, Sivertsen EA. Classification of distal radius fractures in children: good inter- and intraobserver reliability, which improves with clinical experience. *BMC Musculoskelet Disord.* 2013;13:6. DOI: 10.1186/1471-2474-13-6.

467 **Common pediatric fractures: Image B.** Torus (buckle) fracture. Aksel Seyahi, et al. Tibial torus and toddler's fractures misdiagnosed as transient synovitis: a case series. *J Med Case Reports.* 2011;5:305. DOI: 10.1186/1752-1947-5-305.

467 **Osteoporosis.** Vertebral compression fractures of spine. Luo Y, Jiang T, Guo H, et al. Osteoporotic vertebral compression fracture accompanied with thoracolumbar fascial injury: risk factors and the association with residual pain after percutaneous vertebroplasty. *BMC Musculoskelet Disord.* 2022 Apr 11;23(1):343. DOI: 10.1186/s12891-022-05308-7.

468 **Osteopetrosis.** Kant P, Sharda N, Bhowate RR. Clinical and radiological findings of autosomal dominant osteopetrosis type II: a case report. *Case Rep Dent.* 2013;2013:707343. DOI: 10.1155/2013/707343.

468 **Osteomalacia/rickets: Image A.** Clinical photo and x-ray of leg deformity in rickets. ⊙⊙ Linglart A, Biosse-Duplan M, Briot K, et al. Therapeutic management of hypophosphatemic rickets from infancy to adulthood. *Endocr Connect.* 2014;3:R13-R30. DOI: 10.1530/EC-13-0103.

468 **Osteomalacia/rickets: Image B.** Rachitic rosary on chest x-ray. ⊙⊙ Ayadi ID, Hamida EB, Rebeh RB, et al. Perinatal lethal type II osteogenesis imperfecta: a case report. *Pan Afr Med J.* 2015;21:11. DOI: 10.11604/pamj.2015.21.11.6834.

468 **Osteitis deformans.** Thickened calvarium. ⊙⊙ Pons Escoda A., Naval Baudin P, Mora P, et al. Imaging of skull vault tumors in adults. *Insights Imaging.* 2020;11, 23. DOI: 10.1186/s13244-019-0820-9.

469 **Avascular necrosis of bone.** Bilateral necrosis of femoral head. ⊙⊙ Ding H, Chen S-B, Lin S, et al. The effect of postoperative corticosteroid administration on free vascularized fibular grafting for treating osteonecrosis of the femoral head. *Sci World J.* 2013;708014. DOI: 10.1155/2013/708014.

471 **Primary bone tumors: Image B.** Osteoid osteoma. ⊙⊙ Iwai T, Oebisu N, Hoshi M, et al. Finite element analysis could predict and prevent a pathological femoral shaft fracture after en bloc resection of a large osteoid osteoma. *Children (Basel).* 2022 Jan 26;9(2):158. DOI: 10.3390/children9020158.

471 **Primary bone tumors: Image C.** Giant cell tumor. Reproduced, with permission, from Dr. Frank Gaillard and www.radiopaedia.org.

471 **Primary bone tumors: Image D.** Codman triangle in osteosarcoma. ⊙⊙ Xu SF, Yu XC, Zu M, et al. Limb function and quality of life after various reconstruction methods according to tumor location following resection of osteosarcoma in distal femur. *BMC Musculoskelet Disord.* 2014;15:453. DOI: 10.1186/1471-2474-15-453.

471 **Primary bone tumors: Image E.** Starburst pattern in osteosarcoma. ⊙⊙ Ding H, Yu G, Tu Q, et al. Computer-aided resection and endoprosthesis design for the management of malignant bone tumors around the knee: outcomes of 12 cases. *BMC Musculoskelet Disord.* 2013;14:331. DOI: 10.1186/1471-2474-14-331.

472 **Osteoarthritis vs rheumatoid arthritis: Image A.** Osteoarthritis. ⊙⊙ Visser J, Busch VJJF, de Kievit-van der Heijden IM, et al. Non-Hodgkin's lymphoma of the synovium discovered in total knee arthroplasty: a case report. *BMC Res Notes.* 2012;5:449. DOI: 10.1186/1756-0500-5-449.

472 **Osteoarthritis vs rheumatoid arthritis: Image B.** Rheumatoid arthritis. ⊙⊙ Clement ND, Breusch SJ, Biant LC. Lower limb joint replacement in rheumatoid arthritis. *J Orthop Surg Res.* 2012;7:27. DOI: 10.1186/1749-799X-7-27.

472 **Osteoarthritis vs rheumatoid arthritis: Image C.** Histology of rheumatoid nodule. ⊙⊙ Gomez-Rivera F, El-Naggar AK, Guha-Thakurta N, et al. Rheumatoid arthritis mimicking metastatic squamous cell carcinoma. *Head Neck Oncol.* 2011;3:26. DOI: 10.1186/1758-3284-3-26.

473 **Gout: Image A.** Uric acid crystals under polarized light. ⊙⊙ Zhang Y, Lee SY, Zhang Y, et al. Wide-field imaging of birefringent synovial fluid crystals using lens-free polarized microscopy for gout diagnosis. *Sci Rep.* 2016;Jun 30. DOI:10.1038/srep28793.

473 **Gout: Image B.** Podagra. ⊙⊙ Roddy E. Revisiting the pathogenesis of podagra: why does gout target the foot? *J Foot Ankle Res.* 2011;4:13. DOI: 10.1186/1757-1146-4-13.

473 **Calcium pyrophosphate deposition disease.** Calcium phosphate crystals. ⊙⊙ Reproduced with permission from The National Aeronautics and Space Administration.

474 **Sjögren syndrome.** Dry tongue. ⊙⊙ Negrato CA, Tarzia O. Buccal alterations in diabetes mellitus. *Diabetol Metab Syndr.* 2010;2:3. DOI: 10.1186/1758-5996-2-3.

474 **Septic arthritis.** Redness and swelling of skin localizing to the sternoclavicular joint. ⊙⊙ Tanaka Y, Kato H, Shirai K, et al. Sternoclavicular joint septic arthritis with chest wall abscess in a healthy adult: a case report. *J Med Case Rep.* 2016 Mar 26;10:69. DOI: 10.1186/s13256-016-0856-0.

475 **Seronegative spondyloarthropathies: Image C.** Bamboo spine. ⊙⊙ Manoj E, Ragunathan M. Disease flare of ankylosing spondylitis presenting as reactive arthritis with seropositivity: a case report. *J Med Case Rep.* 2012;6:60. DOI: 10.1186/1752-1947-6-60.

477 **Polymyositis/dermatomyositis: Image A.** Groton papules of dermatomyositis. ⊙⊙ Lamquami S, Errarhay S, Mamouni N, et al. Dermatomyositis revealing breast cancer: report of a case. *Pan Afr Med J.* 2015;21:89. DOI: 10.11604/pamj.2015.21.89.6971.

477 **Polymyositis/dermatomyositis: Image D.** Thickening and cracking of skin in dermatomyositis. ⊙⊙ Sohara E, Saraya T, Sato S, et al. Mechanic's hands revisited: is this sign still useful for diagnosis in patients with lung involvement of collagen vascular diseases? *BMC Res Notes.* 2014;7:303. DOI: 10.1186/1756-0500-7-303.

479 **Vasculitides: Image A.** Arthritic swelling in right knee. ⊙⊙ Guardado, K, Sergent, S. Pediatric unilateral knee swelling: a case report of a complicated differential diagnosis and often overlooked cause. *Journal of Osteopathic Medicine.* 2022;122:2;105-109. DOI: 10.1515/jom-2020-0332.

479 **Vasculitides: Image D.** Strawberry tongue in patient with Kawasaki disease. ⊙⊙ The Department of Health and Human Services.

479 **Vasculitides: Image E.** Coronary artery aneurysm in Kawasaki disease. ⊙⊙ Kawamura Y, Miura H, Matsumoto Y, et al. A case of Epstein-Barr virus-associated hemophagocytic lymphohistiocytosis with severe cardiac complications. *BMC Pediatr.* 2016 Oct 28;16(1):172. DOI: 10.1186/s12887-016-0718-3.

479 **Vasculitides: Image F.** Polyarteritis nodosa. Reproduced, with permission, from Dr. Frank Gaillard and www.radiopaedia.org.

479 **Vasculitides: Image G.** Panda R, Krieger T, Hopf L, et al. Neutrophil extracellular traps contain selected antigens of anti-neutrophil cytoplasmic antibodies. *Front Immunol.* 2017 Apr 13;8:439. DOI: 10.3389/fimmu.2017.00439.

479 **Vasculitides: Image H.** Churg-Strauss syndrome histology. ⊙⊙ Helliwell TR. Non-infectious inflammatory lesions of the sinonasal tract. *Head Neck Pathol.* 2016 Mar;10(1):32-39. DOI: 10.1007/s12105-016-0689-6.

479 **Vasculitides: Image I.** Granulomatosis with polyangiitis and PR3-ANCA/c-ANCA. ⊙⊙ Panda R, Krieger T, Hopf L, et al. Neutrophil extracellular traps contain selected antigens of anti-neutrophil cytoplasmic antibodies. *Front Immunol.* 2017 Apr 13;8:439. DOI: 10.3389/fimmu.2017.00439.

479 **Vasculitides: Image J.** Henoch-Schönlein purpura. ⊙⊙ Oshikata C, Tsurikisawa N, Takigawa M, et al. An adult patient with Henoch-Schönlein purpura and non-occlusive mesenteric ischemia. *BMC Res Notes.* 2013 Jan 23;6:26. DOI: 10.1186/1756-0500-6-26.

480 **Raynaud phenomenon.** ⊙⊙ Dixit S, Kalkur C, Sattur AP, et al. Scleroderma and dentistry: two case reports. *J Med Case Rep.* 2016 Oct 24;10(1):297. DOI: 10.1186/s13256-016-1086-1.

482 **Epithelial cell junctions: Image A.** Tight junction. ⊙⊙ Tang VW. Proteomic and bioinformatic analysis of epithelial tight junction reveals an unexpected cluster of synaptic molecules. *Biol Direct.* 2006;1:37. DOI: 10.1186/1745-6150-1-37.

482 **Epithelial cell junctions: Image B.** Large, electron-dense actin structures within adherens junction. ⊙⊙ Taylor RR, Jagger DJ, Saeed SR, et al. Characterizing human vestibular sensory epithelia for experimental studies: new hair bundles on old tissue and implications for therapeutic interventions in ageing. *Neurobiol Aging.* 2015 Jun;36(6):2068–2084. DOI: 10.1016/j.neurobiolaging.2015.02.013.

482 **Epithelial cell junctions: Image C.** Desmosome. Massa F, Devader C, Lacas-Gervais S, et al. Impairement of HT29 cancer cells cohesion by the soluble form of neurotensin receptor-3. *Genes Cancer.* 2014 Jul;5(7-8):240–249. DOI: 10.18632/genesandcancer.22.

482 **Epithelial cell junctions: Image D.** Gap junction. Shu X, Lev-Ram V, Deerinck TJ. A genetically encoded tag for correlated light and electron microscopy of intact cells, tissues, and organisms. *PLoS Biol.* 2011 Apr;9(4):e1001041. DOI: 10.1371/journal.pbio.1001041.

482 **Epithelial cell junctions: Image E.** Hemidesmosome. Nguyen NM, Pulkkinen L, Schlueter JA, et al. Lung development in laminin gamma2 deficiency: abnormal tracheal hemidesmosomes with normal branching morphogenesis and epithelial differentiation. *Respir Res.* 2006 Feb 16;7:28. DOI: 10.1186/1465-9921-7-28.

484 **Seborrheic dermatitis.** Savoia P, Cavaliere G, Zavattaro E, et al. Inflammatory cutaneous diseases in renal transplant recipients. *Int J Mol Sci.* 2016 Aug 19;17(8):1362. DOI: 10.3390/ijms17081362.

485 **Common skin disorders: Image F.** Keratosis pilaris. Siegfried EC, Hebert AA. Diagnosis of atopic dermatitis: mimics, overlaps, and complications. *J. Clin. Med.* 2015;4(5):884-917.

485 **Common skin disorders: Image O.** Urticaria. Cugno M, Tedeschi A, Borghi A, et al. Activation of blood coagulation in two prototypic autoimmune skin diseases: a possible link with thrombotic risk. *PLoS One.* 2015 Jun 9;10(6):e0129456. DOI: 10.1371/journal.pone.0129456.

486 **Vascular tumors of skin: Image C.** Glomus tumor under fingernail. Suzuki R, Hashimoto H, Okamoto O. Solitary subungual neurofibroma with glomus tumor-like appearance: a case report. *Case Reports Plast Surg Hand Surg.* 2020 Apr 14;7(1):43-45. DOI: 10.1080/23320885.2020.1750018.

487 **Skin infections: Image C.** Erysipelas. The US Department of Health and Human Services and Dr. Thomas F. Sellers.

488 **Cutaneous mycoses: Image G.** Pityriasis. The US Department of Health and Human Services and Dr. Gavin Hart.

489 **Autoimmune blistering skin disorders: Image D.** Bullous pemphigoid on immunofluorescence. Si X, Ge L, Xin H, et al. Erythrodermic psoriasis with bullous pemphigoid: combination treatment with methotrexate and compound glycyrrhizin. *Diagn Pathol.* 2014;9;102. https://doi.org/10.1186/1746-1596-9-102.

491 **Cutaneous ulcers: Image B.** Arterial ulcer. Kalinchenko S, Zemlyanoy A, Gooren L. Improvement of the diabetic foot upon testosterone administration to hypogonadal men with peripheral arterial disease. Report of three cases. *Cardiovasc Diabetol.* 2009;8;19. DOI: 10.1186/1475-2840-8-19.

492 **Miscellaneous skin disorders: Image G.** Pityriasis rosea, herald patch. The US Department of Health and Human Services and Dr. Gavin Hart.

493 **Estimation of body surface area: Images A and B.** 18 hours (A) 11 days (B) after inhalational injury. Bai C, Huang H, Yao X, et al. Application of flexible bronchoscopy in inhalation lung injury. *Diagn Pathol.* 2013;8:174. DOI: 10.1186/1746-1596-8-174.

Neurology and Special Senses

501 **Brain malformations: Image A.** Holoprosencephaly. Pallangyo P, Lyimo F, Nicholaus P, et al. Semilobar holoprosencephaly in a 12-month-old baby boy born to a primigravida patient with type 1 diabetes mellitus: a case report. *J Med Case Rep.* 2016;10:358. https://doi.org/10.1186/s13256-016-1141-y.

501 **Brain malformations: Image B.** Lissencephaly. Tian G, Cristancho AG, Dubbs HA, et al. A patient with lissencephaly, developmental delay, and infantile spasms, due to de novo heterozygous mutation of KIF2A. *Mol Genet Genomic Med.* 2016 Nov;4(6):599–603. DOI: 10.1002/mgg3.236.

502 **Posterior fossa malformations: Image A.** Chiari I malformation. Toldo I, De Carlo D, Mardari R, et al. Short lasting activity-related headaches with sudden onset in children: a case-based reasoning on classification and diagnosis. *J Headache Pain.* 2013;14(1):3. DOI: 10.1186/1129-2377-14-3.

502 **Posterior fossa malformations: Image B.** Dandy-Walker malformation. Krupa K, Bekiesinska-Figatowska M. Congenital and acquired abnormalities of the corpus callosum: a pictorial essay. *Biomed Res Int.* 2013;2013:265619. DOI: 10.1155/2013/265619.

502 **Syringomyelia.** Reproduced, with permission, from Dr. Frank Gaillard and www.radiopaedia.org.

509 **Limbic system.** Schopf V, Fischmeister FP, Windischberger C, et al. Effects of individual glucose levels on the neuronal correlates of emotions. *Front Hum Neurosci.* 2013 May 21;7:212. DOI: 10.3389/fnhum.2013.00212.

510 **Cerebellum.** Jarius S, Wandinger KP, Horn S, et al. A new Purkinje cell antibody (anti-Ca) associated with subacute cerebellar ataxia: immunological characterization. *J Neuroinflammation.* 2010;7:21. DOI: 10.1186/1742-2094-7-21.

511 **Basal ganglia.** Rudger P, Jaunmuktane Z, Adlard P, et al. Iatrogenic CJD due to pituitary-derived growth hormone with genetically determined incubation times of up to 40 years. *Brain.* 2015 Nov;138(11):3386–3399. DOI: 10.1093/brain/awv235.

513 **Cerebral arteries—cortical distribution.** Cortical watershed areas. Isabel C, Lecler A, Turc G, et al. Relationship between watershed infarcts and recent intra plaque haemorrhage in carotid atherosclerotic plaque. *PLoS One.* 2014;9(10):e108712. DOI: 10.1371/journal.pone.0108712.

514 **Dural venous sinuses.** Cikla U, Aagaard-Kienitz B, Turski PA, et al. Familial perimesencephalic subarachnoid hemorrhage: two case reports. *J Med Case Rep.* 2014;8:380. DOI: 10.1186/1752-1947-8-380.

525 **Cerebral edema: Image A.** Vasogenic edema. Ahmad A, Ginnebaugh KR, Sethi S, et al. miR-20b is up-regulated in brain metastases from primary breast cancers. *Oncotarget.* 2015 May 20;6(14):12188-95. DOI: 10.18632/oncotarget.3664.

527 **Effects of strokes: Image A.** Large abnormality of the left middle cerebral artery territory. Hakimelahi R, Yoo AJ, He J, et al. Rapid identification of a major diffusion/perfusion mismatch in distal internal carotid artery or middle cerebral artery ischemic stroke. *BMC Neurol.* 2012 Nov 5;12:132. DOI: 10.1186/1471-2377-12-132.

527 **Effects of strokes: Image B.** Lacunar infarct of lenticulostriate artery. Zhou L, Ni J, Yao M, et al. High-resolution MRI findings in patients with capsular warning syndrome. *BMC Neurol.* 2014;14:16. DOI: 10.1186/1471-2377-14-16.

527 **Effects of strokes: Image C.** Infarction of posterior cerebellar artery. Nouh A, Remke J, Ruland S. Ischemic posterior circulation stroke: a review of anatomy, clinical presentations, diagnosis, and current management. *Front Neurol.* 2014 Apr 7;5:30. DOI: 10.3389/fneur.2014.00030.

527 **Effects of strokes: Image D.** MRI showing hyperintensity in various brain areas consistent with an acute stroke in the left medullary restiform body and left cerebellar hemisphere. Alsaad AA, Austin CO, Robinson MT, Phillips MB. Pacemaker placement in patients with stroke-mediated autonomic dysregulation. *Case Rep Med.* 2017;2017:6301430. DOI: 10.1155/2017/6301430.

528 **Intracranial hemorrhage: Images A and B.** Epidural hematoma. Al-Mahfoudh R, Clark S, Kandasamy J, May P. A neurosurgical golf injury. *Clin Med Case Rep.* 2008 May 22;1:77-9. DOI: 10.4137/ccrep.s736.

528 **Intracranial hemorrhage: Image C.** Fronto-temporal subdural haematoma over the left hemisphere. Rasmussen M, Björk Werner J, Dolk M, Christensson B. Lactococcus garvieae endocarditis presenting with subdural haematoma. *BMC Cardiovasc Disord.* 2014;14:13. DOI: 10.1186/1471-2261-14-13.

528 **Intracranial hemorrhage: Image E.** Subarachnoid hemorrhage. Hakan T, Turk CC, Celik H. Intra-operative real time intracranial subarachnoid haemorrhage during glial tumour resection: a case report. *Cases J.* 2008;1:306. DOI: 10.1186/1757-1626-1-306.

529 **Diffuse axonal injury.** Moenninghoff C, Kraff O, Maderwald S, et al. Diffuse axonal injury at ultra-high field MRI. *PLoS One.* 2015;10(3):e0122329. DOI: 10.1371/journal.pone.0122329.

530 **Aneurysms.** Saccular aneurysm. Dolati P, Pittman D, Morrish W F, et al. The Frequency of Subarachnoid Hemorrhage from Very Small Cerebral Aneurysms (< 5 mm): A Population-Based Study. *Cureus.* 2015.7(6): DOI:10.7759/cureus.279.

534 **Neurodegenerative movement disorders: Image A.** Melanized dopaminergic neurons of the substantia nigra. Mazzio EA, Close F, Soliman KF. The biochemical and cellular basis for nutraceutical strategies to attenuate neurodegeneration in Parkinson's disease. *Int J Mol Sci.* 2011 Jan 17;12(1):506-69. DOI: 10.3390/ijms12010506.

534 **Neurodegenerative movement disorders: Image B.** Lewy body in substantia nigra. Werner CJ, Heyny-von Haussen R, Mall G, et al. Parkinson's disease. *Proteome Sci.* 2008;6:8. DOI: 10.1186/1477-5956-6-8.

535 **Dementia: Image C.** Pick bodies in frontotemporal dementia. Neumann M. Molecular neuropathology of TDP-43 proteinopathies. *Int J Mol Sci.* 2009 Jan;10(1):232–246. DOI: 10.3390/ijms10010232.

535 **Dementia: Image D.** Leukoencephalopathy and encephalomalacia foci in vascular dementia. Wang R, Chen Z, Fu Y, et al. Plasma Cystatin C and high-density lipoprotein are important biomarkers of Alzheimer's disease and vascular dementia: A cross-sectional study. *Front Aging Neurosci.* 2017;9:26. Published 2017 Feb 7. DOI:10.3389/fnagi.2017.00026.

535 **Dementia: Image E.** Spongiform changes in brain in Creutzfeld-Jacob disease. The US Department of Health and Human Services and Sherif Zaki; MD; PhD; Wun-Ju Shieh; MD; PhD; MPH.

536 **Hydrocephalus: Image B.** Communicating hydrocephalus. Torres-Martin M, Pena-Granero C, Carceller F, et al. Homozygous deletion of *TNFRSF4*, *TP73*, *PPAP2B* and *DPYD* at 1p and *PDCD5* at 19q identified by multiplex ligation-dependent probe amplification (MLPA) analysis in pediatric anaplastic glioma with questionable oligodendroglial component. *Mol Cytogenet.* 2014;7:1. DOI: 10.1186/1755-8166-7-1.

536 **Hydrocephalus: Image C.** Ex vacuo ventriculomegaly. Ghetti B, Oblak AL, Boeve BF, et al. Frontotemporal dementia caused by microtubule-associated protein tau gene (*MAPT*) mutations: a chameleon for neuropathology and neuroimaging. *Neuropathol Appl Neurobiol.* 2015 Feb;41(1):24-46. DOI: 10.1111/nan.12213.

537 **Multiple sclerosis.** Periventricular plaques. Dooley MC, Foroozan R. Optic neuritis. *J Ophthalmic Vis Res.* 2010 Jul;5(3):182–187.

538 **Other demyelinated and dysmyelinating disorders: Image A.** Central pontine myelinolysis. Chang KY, Lee IH, Kim GJ, et al. Plasma exchange successfully treats central pontine myelinolysis after acute hypernatremia from intravenous sodium bicarbonate therapy. *BMC Nephrol.* 2014 Apr 4;15:56. DOI: 10.1186/1471-2369-15-56.

538 **Other demyelinating and dysmyelinating disorders: Image B.** Progressive multifocal leukoencephalopathy. Garrote H, de la Fuente A, Ona R, et al. Long-term survival in a patient with progressive multifocal leukoencephalopathy after therapy with rituximab, fludarabine and cyclophosphamide for chronic lymphocytic leukemia. *Exp Hematol Oncol.* 2015;4:8. DOI: 10.1186/s40164-015-0003-4.

539 **Neurocutaneous disorders: Image A.** Port wine stain in Sturge-Weber syndrome. Babaji P, Bansal A, Krishna G, et al. Sturge-Weber syndrome with osteohypertrophy of maxilla. *Case Rep Pediatr.* May 2013;964596. DOI: 10.1155/2013/964596.

539 **Neurocutaneous disorders: Image B.** Leptomeningeal angioma in Sturge-Weber syndrome. Reproduced, with permission, from Dr. Frank Gaillard and www.radiopaedia.org.

539 **Neurocutaneous disorders: Image C.** Angiomas in tuberous sclerosis. Fred H, van Dijk H. Images of memorable cases: case 143. Connexions Web site. December 4, 2008. Available at: http://cnx.org/content/m14923/1.3/.

539 **Neurocutaneous disorders: Image D.** Ash leaf spots in tuberous sclerosis. Falsafi P, Taghavi-Zenouz A, Khorshidi-Khiyavi R, et al A case of tuberous sclerosis without multiorgan involvement. *Glob J Health Sci.* 2015 Feb 24;7(5):124-31. DOI: 10.5539/gjhs.v7n5p124.

539 **Neurocutaneous disorders: Image E.** Angiomyolipoma in tuberous sclerosis. Coskuner ER, Ozkan B, Yalcin V. The role of partial nephrectomy without arterial embolization in giant renal angiomyolipoma. *Case Rep Med.* 2012;2012:365762. DOI: 10.1155/2012/365762.

539 **Neurocutaneous disorders: Image F.** Café-au-lait spots in neurofibromatosis type I. Nishi T, Kawabata Y, Hari Y, et al. A case of pancreatic neuroendocrine tumor in a patient with neurofibromatosis-1. *World J Surg Oncol.* 2012 Jul 23;10:153. DOI: 10.1186/1477-7819-10-153.

539 **Neurocutaneous disorders: Image H.** Cutaneous neurofibromas in neurofibromatosis type I. Kim BK, Choi YS, Gwoo S, et al. Neurofibromatosis type 1 associated with papillary thyroid carcinoma incidentally detected by thyroid ultrasonography: a case report. *J Med Case Rep.* 2012;6:179. DOI: 10.1186/1752-1947-6-179.

539 **Neurocutaneous disorders: Image I.** Zywicke H, Palmer C, Vaphiades M, et al. Optic nerve hemangioblastoma: a case report. *Case Rep Pathol.* 2012;2012:915408. DOI:10.1155/2012/915408.

539 **Neurocutaneous disorders: Image J.** Brainstem and spinal cord hemangioblastomas in von Hippel-Lindau disease. Park DM, Zhuang Z, Chen L, et al. von Hippel-Lindau disease-associated hemangioblastomas are derived from embryologic multipotent cells. *PLoS Med.* 2007 Feb;4(2):e60. DOI: 10.1371/journal.pmed.0040060.

541 **Adult primary brain tumors: Image A.** Butterfly glioma. Rossmeisl JH, Clapp K, Pancotto TE. Canine butterfly glioblastomas: A neuroradiological review. *Front Vet Sci.* 2016;3:40. DOI: 10.3389/fvets.2016.00040.

541 **Adult primary brain tumors: Image B.** Classical histologic findings of glioblastoma. Lim SM, Choi J, Chang JH, et al. Lack of *ROS1* gene rearrangement in glioblastoma multiforme. *PLoS One.* 2015;10(9):e0137678. DOI: 10.1371/journal.pone.0137678.

541 **Adult primary brain tumors: Image C.** Left frontal astrocytoma grade II. Smits A, Zetterling M, Lundin M, et al. Neurological impairment linked with cortico-subcortical infiltration of diffuse low-grade gliomas at initial diagnosis supports early brain plasticity. *Front Neurol.* 2015;6:137. DOI: 10.3389/fneur.2015.00137.

541 **Adult primary brain tumors: Image E.** Meningioma with dural tail. Hunt CM, Thomas V, Alexander J. Glioblastoma multiforme survivor with radiation-induced consequences: a case report. *Cureus.* 2022;4(9):e29397. DOI:10.7759/cureus.29397.

541 **Adult primary brain tumors: Image G.** Cerebellar hemangioblastoma. Park DM, Zhengping Z, Chen L, et al. von Hippel-Lindau disease-associated hemangioblastomas are derived from embryologic multipotent cells. *PLoS Med.* 2007 Feb;4(2):e60. DOI: 10.1371/journal.pmed.0040060.

541 **Adult primary brain tumors: Image H.** Lipidized stromal cells. Zywicke H, Palmer CA, Vaphiades MS, Riley KO. Optic nerve hemangioblastoma: a case report. *Case Rep Pathol.* 2012;2012:915408. DOI: 10.1155/2012/915408.

541 **Adult primary brain tumors: Image J.** Prolactinoma. Wang CS, Yeh TC, Wu TC, et al. Pituitary macroadenoma co-existent with supraclinoid internal carotid artery cerebral aneurysm: a case report and review of the literature. *Cases J.* 2009;2:6459. DOI: 10.4076/1757-1626-2-6459.

542 **Childhood primary brain tumors: Image A.** MRI of pilocytic astrocytoma. Hafez RFA. Stereotaxic gamma knife surgery in treatment of critically located pilocytic astrocytoma: preliminary result. *World J Surg Oncol.* 2007;5:39. DOI: 10.1186/1477-7819-5-39.

542 **Childhood primary brain tumors: Image B.** Rosenthal fibers in pilocytic astrocytoma. Pećina-Šlaus N, Gotovac K, Kafka A, et al. Genetic changes observed in a case of adult pilocytic astrocytoma revealed by array CGH analysis. *Mol Cytogenet.* 2014;7:95. DOI: 10.1186/s13039-014-0095-2.

542 **Childhood primary brain tumors: Image C.** CT of medulloblastoma. Łastowska M, Jurkiewicz E, Trubicka J, et al. Contrast enhancement pattern predicts poor survival for patients with non-WNT/SHH medulloblastoma tumours. *J Neurooncol.* 2015;123:65–73. DOI: 10.1007/s11060-015-1779-0.

542 **Childhood primary brain tumors: Image E.** MRI of ependymoma. Nobori C, Kimura K, Ohira G, et al. Giant duodenal ulcers after neurosurgery for brainstem tumors that required reoperation for gastric disconnection: a report of two cases. *BMC Surg.* 2016 Nov 17;16(1):75. DOI: 10.1186/s12893-016-0189-3.

542 **Childhood primary brain tumors: Image F.** Ependymoma histology. Bettegowda C, Agrawal N, Jiao Y, et al. Exomic Sequencing of Four Rare Central Nervous System Tumor Types. *Oncotarget.* 2013;4: 572-583. DOI: 10.18632/oncotarget.964.

542 **Childhood primary brain tumors: Image G.** CT of craniopharyngioma. Garnet MR, Puget S, Grill J, et al. Craniopharyngioma. *Orphanet J Rare Dis.* 2007;2:18. DOI: 10.1186/1750-1172-2-18.

542 **Childhood primary brain tumors: Image H.** Craniopharyngioma histology. El-Bilbeisi H, Ghannam M, Nimri CF, Ahmad AT. Craniopharyngioma in a patient with acromegaly due to a pituitary macroadenoma. *Ann Saudi Med.* 2010 Nov-Dec;30(6):485-8. DOI: 10.4103/0256-4947.70581.

545 **Friedreich ataxia.** Kyphoscoliosis. Axelrod FB, Gold-von Simson. Hereditary sensory and autonomic neuropathies: types II, III, and IV. *Orphanet J Rare Dis.* 2007;2:39. DOI: 10.1186/1750-1172-2-39.

546 **Facial nerve lesions.** Facial nerve palsy. Socolovsky M, Paez MD, Di Masi G, et al. Bell's palsy and partial hypoglossal to facial nerve transfer: Case presentation and literature review. *Surg Neurol Int.* 2012;3:46. DOI: 10.4103/2152-7806.95391.

547 **Otitis externa.** Discharge. Alizadeh Taheri P, Rostami S, Sadeghi M. External otitis: an unusual presentation in neonates. *Case Rep Infect Dis.* 2016;2016:7381564. DOI: 10.1155/2016/7381564.

547 **Otitis media.** Erythematous tympanic membrane. Kuruvilla A, Shaikh N, Hoberman A, et al. Automated diagnosis of otitis media: vocabulary and grammar. *Int J Biomed Imaging.* 2013;2013:327515. DOI: 10.1155/2013/327515.

548 **Cholesteatoma.** Kuo CL, Shiao AS, Yung M, et al. Updates and knowledge gaps in cholesteatoma research. *Biomed Res Int.* 2015;2015:854024. DOI: 10.1155/2015/854024.

550 **Lens disorders.** Juvenile cataract. Chen C, Yang J, Zhang X, et al. A case report of Werner's syndrome with bilateral juvenile cataracts. *BMC Ophthalmol.* 2018;18:199. DOI: 10.1186/s12886-018-0873-4.

551 **Glaucoma: Image C.** Acute angle closure glaucoma. Kaushik S, Sachdev N, Pandav S, et al. Bilateral acute angle closure glaucoma as a presentation of isolated microspherophakia in an adult: case report. *BMC Ophthalmol.* 2006;6:29. DOI: 10.1186/1471-2415-6-29.

553 **Retinal disorders: Image B.** Diabetic retinopathy. Sundling V, Gulbrandsen P, Straand J. Sensitivity and specificity of Norwegian optometrists' evaluation of diabetic retinopathy in single-field retinal images – a cross-sectional experimental study. *BMC Health Services Res.* 2013;13:17. DOI: 10.1186/1472-6963-13-17.

553 **Retinal disorders: Image C.** Hypertensive retinopathy. Diallo JW, Méda N, Tougouma SJB, et al. Intérêts de l'examen du fond d'œil en pratique de ville: bilan de 438 cas. *Pan Afr Med J.* 2015;20:363. DOI: 10.11604/pamj.2015.20.363.6629.

553 **Retinal disorders: Image E.** Retinal vein occlusion. Alasil T, Rauser ME. Intravitreal bevacizumab in the treatment of neovascular glaucoma secondary to central retinal vein occlusion: a case report. *Cases J.* 2009;2:176. DOI: 10.1186/1757-1626-2-176.

553 **Retinal disorders: Image F.** Retinal detchment. Courtesy of EyeRounds.

553 **Retinal disorders: Image G.** Retinitis pigmentosa. Courtesy of EyeRounds.

553 **Retinal disorders: Image H.** Retinoblasoma. Aerts I, Lumbroso-Le Rouic L, Gauthier-Villars M, et al. Retinoblastoma. *Orphanet J Rare Dis.* 2006 Aug 25;1:31. DOI: 10.1186/1750-1172-1-31.

553 **Papilledema.** Kanonidou E, Chatziralli I, Kanonidou C, et al. Unilateral optic disc edema in a paediatric patient: diagnostic dilemmas and management. *Case Rep Med.* 2010;2010:529081. DOI: 10.1155/2010/529081.

553 **Leukocoria.** Aerts I, Lumbroso-Le Rouic L, Gauthier-Villars M, et al. Retinoblastoma. *Orphanet J Rare Dis.* 2006 Aug 25;1:31. DOI: 10.1186/1750-1172-1-31.

553 **Uveitis.** Weber AC, Levison AL, Srivastava, et al. A case of *Listeria monocytogenes* endophthalmitis with recurrent inflammation and novel management. *J Ophthalmic Inflamm Infect.* 2015;5(1):28. DOI: 10.1186/s12348-015-0058-8.

555 **Ocular motility.** Blowout fracture of orbit with entrapment of superior rectus muscle. Kozakiewicz M, Szymor P. Comparison of pre-bent titanium mesh versus polyethylene implants in patient specific orbital reconstructions. *Head Face Med.* 2013;9:32. DOI:10.1186/1746-160X-9-32.

Psychiatry

580 **Trichotillomania.** Zhao X, Wang S, Hong X, et al. A case of trichotillomania with binge eating disorder: combined with N-acetylcysteine synergistic therapy. *Ann Gen Psychiatry.* 2021 Sep 25;20(1):46. DOI: 10.1186/s12991-021-00369-9.

Renal

597 **Horseshoe kidney.** Rispoli P, Destefanis P, Garneri P, et al. Inferior vena cava prosthetic replacement in a patient with horseshoe kidney and metastatic testicular tumor: technical considerations and review of the literature. *BMC Urol.* 2014;14:40. DOI: 10.1186/1471-2490-14-40.

599 **Course of ureters.** Vaidyanathan S, Soni BM, Oo T, et al. Infection of Brindley sacral anterior root stimulator by Pseudomonas aeruginosa requiring removal of the implant: long-term deleterious effects on bowel and urinary bladder function in a spinal cord injury patient with tetraplegia: a case report. *Cases J.* 2009 Dec 21;2:9364. DOI: 10.1186/1757-1626-2-9364.

599 **Glomerular filtration barrier.** Feng J, Wei H, Sun Y, et al. Regulation of podocalyxin expression in the kidney of streptozotocin-induced diabetic rats with Chinese herbs (Yishen capsule). *BMC Complement Altern Med.* 2013;13:76. DOI: 10.1186/1472-6882-13-76.

612 **Casts in urine: Image C.** Fatty casts. Li S, Wang ZJ, Chang TT. Temperature oscillation modulated self-assembly of periodic concentric layered magnesium carbonate microparticles. *PLoS One.* 2014;9(2):e88648. DOI:10.1371/journal.pone.0088648.

612   **Casts in urine: Image D.** Hyaline casts. Chu-Su Y, Shukuya K, Yokoyama T, et al. Enhancing the detection of dysmorphic red blood cells and renal tubular epithelial cells with a modified urinalysis protocol. *Sci Rep.* 2017;7:40521. DOI: 10.1038/srep40521.

615   **Nephritic syndrome: Image A.** Histology of acute poststreptococcal glomerulonephritis. Miquelestorena-Standley E, Jaulerry C, Machet MC, et al. Clinicopathologic features of infection-related glomerulonephritis with IgA deposits: a French Nationwide study. *Diagn Pathol.* 2020 May 27;15(1):62. DOI: 10.1186/s13000-020-00980-6.

615   **Nephritic syndrome: Image B.** Immunofluorescence of acute poststreptococcal glomerulonephritis. Immunofluorescence of acute poststreptococcal glomerulonephritis. Oda T, Yoshizawa N, Yamakami K, et al. The role of nephritis-associated plasmin receptor (naplr) in glomerulonephritis associated with streptococcal infection. *Biomed Biotechnol.* 2012;2012:417675. DOI 10.1155/2012/417675.

615   **Nephritic syndrome: Image C.** Histology of rapidly progressive glomerulonephritis. Mayer U, Schmitz J, Bräsen JH, Pape L. Crescentic glomerulonephritis in children. *Pediatr Nephrol.* 2020 May;35(5):829-842. DOI: 10.1007/s00467-019-04436-y.

615   **Nephritic syndrome: Image D.** Lupus nephritis with wire loop appearance in glomerular capillary wall. Kiremitci S, Ensari A. Classifying lupus nephritis: an ongoing story. *Scientific World J.* 2014;2014:580620. DOI: 10.1155/2014/580620.

615   **Nephritic syndrome: Image E.** "Tram tracks" appearance in membranoproliverative glomerulonephritis. Wu CK, Leu J-G, Yang A-H, et al. Simultaneous occurrence of fibrillary glomerulonephritis and renal lesions in nonmalignant monoclonal IgM gammopathy. *BMC Nephrol.* 2016;17:17. DOI: 10.1186/s12882-015-0198-y.

616   **Nephrotic syndrome: Image A.** Effacement of podocyte foot processes in minimal change disease. Teoh DCY, El-Modir A. Managing a locally advanced malignant thymoma complicated by nephrotic syndrome: a case report. *J Med Case Reports.* 2008;2:89. DOI: 10.1186/1752-1947-2-89.

618   **Nephrotic syndrome: Image B.** Histology of focal segmental glomerulosclerosis. Asinobi AO, Ademola AD, Okolo CA, Yaria JO. Trends in the histopathology of childhood nephrotic syndrome in Ibadan Nigeria: preponderance of idiopathic focal segmental glomerulosclerosis. *BMC Nephrol.* 2015 Dec 15;16:213. DOI: 10.1186/s12882-015-0208-0.

616   **Nephrotic syndrome: Image D.** Diabetic glomerulosclerosis with Kimmelstiel-Wilson lesions. The US Department of Health and Human Services and Dr. Edwin P. Ewing, Jr.

617   **Kidney stones: Image A.** Calcium kidney stones. Nair S, George J, Kumar S, et al. Acute oxalate nephropathy following ingestion of *Averrhoa bilimbi* juice. *Case Rep Nephrol.* 2014;2014. DOI: 10.1155/2014/240936.

617   **Kidney stones: Image D.** Cysteine kidney stones. Cayla Devine.

618   **Hydronephrosis.** Hydronephrosis on ultrasound. Ucar AK, Kurugoglu S. Urinary ultrasound and other imaging for ureteropelvic junction type hydronephrosis (UPJHN). *Front. Pediatr.* 2020;8:546. DOI: 10.3389/fped.2020.00546.

619   **Pyelonephritis: Image A.** Acute pyelonephritis with neutrophilic infiltration. Isling LK, Aalbaek B, Schrøder M, Leifsson PS. Pyelonephritis in slaughter pigs and sows: morphological characterization and aspects of pathogenesis and aetiology. *Acta Vet Scand.* 2010 Aug 12;52(1):48. DOI: 10.1186/1751-0147-52-48.

623   **Renal cell carcinoma: Image A.** Fúnez R, Pereda T, Rodrigo I, et al. Simultaneous chromophobe renal cell carcinoma and squamous renal cell carcinoma. *Diagn Pathol.* 2007 Aug 21;2:30. DOI: 10.1186/1746-1596-2-30.

623   **Renal cell carcinoma: Image B.** The US Department of Health and Human Services and Dr. Edwin P. Ewing, Jr.

623   **Renal cell carcinoma: Image C.** CT scan. Behnes CL, Schlegel C, Shoukier M, et al. Hereditary papillary renal cell carcinoma primarily diagnosed in a cervical lymph node: a case report of a 30-year-old woman with multiple metastases. *BMC Urol.* 2013;13:3. DOI: 10.1186/1471-2490-13-3.

624   **Renal oncocytoma: Image A.** CT abdomen. Qu J, Zhang Q, Song X, et al. CT differentiation of the oncocytoma and renal cell carcinoma based on peripheral tumor parenchyma and central hypodense area characterisation. *BMC Med Imaging.* 2023;23:16.

624   **Renal oncocytoma: Image B.** Gross specimen. Maiers TJ, Wang DC, Houjaij AH, Darwish OM. Renal oncocytoma and retroperitoneal ancient schwannoma: a benign mimic of metastatic renal cell carcinoma. *Case Rep Urol.* 2019 Feb 20;2019:2561289. DOI: 10.1155/2019/2561289.

624   **Renal oncocytoma: Image C.** Histology. Algaba F. Renal adenomas: pathological differential diagnosis with malignant tumors. *Adv Urol.* 2008;2008:974848. DOI: 10.1155/2008/974848.

624   **Nephroblastoma.** Dumba M, Jawad N, McHugh K. Neuroblastoma and nephroblastoma: a radiological review. *Cancer Imaging.* 2015 Apr 8;15(1):5. DOI: 10.1186/s40644-015-0040-6.

624   **Urothelial carcinoma of the bladder: Image A.** Geavlete B, Stanescu F, Moldoveanu C, et al. NBI cystoscopy and bipolar electrosurgery in NMIBC management—an overview of daily practice. *J Med Life.* 2013;6:140-145.

624   **Urothelial carcinoma of the bladder: Image B.** Transitional cell carcinoma. Tanaka T, Miyazawa K, Tsukamoto T, et al. Pathobiology and chemoprevention of bladder cancer. *J Oncol.* 2011;2011:528353. DOI: 10.1155/2011/528353.

Reproductive

636   **Umbilical cord: Image A.** Meckel diverticulum. Mathur P, Gupta R, Simlot A, et al. Congenital pouch colon with double Meckel's diverticulae. *J Neonatal Surg.* 2013 Oct-Dec;2(4):48.

640   **Uterine (Müllerian) duct anomalies: Images A and B.** Septate uterus (A), bicornuate uterus (B). Jayaprakasan K, Ojha K. Diagnosis of Congenital Uterine Abnormalities: Practical Considerations. *Journal of Clin Med.* 2022; 11(5):1251. DOI:10.3390/jcm11051251.

655   **Sex chromosome disorders: Image A.** Klinefelter syndrome showing gynecomastia. Singer-Granick CJ, Reisler T, Granick M. Gynecomastia and Klinefelter syndrome. *Eplasty.* 2015;15:ic61. PMID: 26715949. PMCID: PMC4684628.

655   **Sex chromosome disorders: Image B.** Turner syndrome. Mehri I. Surgical correction of the webbed neck: an alternative lateral approach.*GMS Interdiscip Plastic Reconstr. Surg.* DGPW. 2017; 2;6:Doc04. DOI:10.3205/iprs000106.

657   **Placental disorders.** Placenta previa percreta. Tikkanen M, Stefanovic V, Paavone J. Placenta previa percreta left in situ - management by delayed hysterectomy: a case report. *J Med Case Rep.* 2011;5:418. DOI: 10.1186/1752-1947-5-418.

659   **Ectopic pregnancy.** Li W, Wang G, Lin T, et al. Misdiagnosis of bilateral tubal pregnancy: a case report. *J Med Case Rep.* 2014;8:342. DOI: 10.1186/1752-1947-8-342.

659   **Hydatidiform mole: Image A.** Cluster of cluster of grapes appearance in complete hydatidiform mole. DiBartola K, Smith D, Rood K, et al. Management of Complete Hydatidiform Mole with Co-existing Fetus. *Obstet Gynecol Cases Rev.* 2020; 7:173. DOI: 10.23937/2377-9004/1410173.

660 Choriocarcinoma: Image B. "Cannonball" metastases. Lekanidi K, Vlachou PA, Morgan B, et al. Spontaneous regression of metastatic renal cell carcinoma: case report. *J Med Case Rep.* 2007;1:89. DOI: 10.1186/1752-1947-1-89.

661 Vulvar pathology: Image A. Bartholin cyst. The US Department of Health and Human Services and Susan Lindsley.

661 Vulvar pathology: Image B. Lichen sclerosis. Lambert J. Pruritus in female patients. *Biomed Res Int.* 2014;2014:541867. DOI: 10.1155/2014/541867.

661 Vulvar pathology: Image C. Vulvar carcinoma. Ramli I, Hassam B. Carcinome épidermoïde vulvaire: pourquoi surveiller un lichen scléro-atrophique. *Pan Afr Med J.* 2015;21:48. DOI: 10.11604/pamj.2015.21.48.6018.

661 Vulvar pathology: Image D. Extramallary Paget disease. Wang X, Yang W, Yang J. Extramammary Paget's disease with the appearance of a nodule: a case report. *BMC Cancer.* 2010;10:405. DOI: 10.1186/1471-2407-10-405.

662 Polycystic ovary syndrome. Goncharenko V, Beniuk V, Kalenska, O.V. et al. Predictive diagnosis of endometrial hyperplasia and personalized therapeutic strategy in women of fertile age. *EPMA Journal.* 2013;4:24. DOI: 10.1186/1878-5085-4-24.

665 Ovarian tumors: Image A. Mucinous cystadenoma. Kamel RM. A massive ovarian mucinous cystadenoma: a case report. *Reprod Biol Endocrinol.* 2010:8;24. https://doi.org/10.1186/1477-7827-8-24.

665 Ovarian tumors: Image C. Struma ovarii. Li Z, Wang J. & Chen Q. Struma ovarii and peritoneal strumosis during pregnancy. *BMC Pregnancy Childbirth.* 2021;21:347. https://doi.org/10.1186/s12884-021-03815-4.

665 Ovarian tumors: Image D. Dysgerminoma. Montesinos L, Acien P, Martinez-Beltran M, et al. Ovarian dysgerminoma and synchronic contralateral tubal pregnancy followed by normal intra-uterine gestation: a case report. *J Med Rep.* 2012;6:399. DOI: 10.1186/1752-1947-6-399.

665 Ovarian tumors: Image E. Alami M, Janane A, Abbar M, et al. La tumeur testiculaire du sac vitellin: une entité rare chez l'adulte [Testicular yolk sac tumor: a rare entity in adults]. *Pan Afr Med J.* 2014 May 24;18:80. French. DOI: 10.11604/pamj.2014.

665 Ovarian tumors: Image F. Call-Exner bodies. Katoh T, Yasuda M, Hasegawa K, et al. Estrogen-producing endometrioid adenocarcinoma resembling sex cord-stromal tumor of the ovary: a review of four postmenopausal cases. *Diagn Pathol.* 2012;7:164. DOI: 10.1186/1746-1596-7-164.

666 Uterine conditions: Image A. Endometriosis lesion. Hastings JM, Fazleabas AT. A baboon model for endometriosis: implications for fertility. *Reprod Biol Endocrinol.* 2006;4(suppl 1):S7. DOI: 10.1186/1477-7827-4-S1-S7.

666 Uterine conditions: Image B. Endometritis with inflammation of the endometrium. Montesinos L, Acien P, Martinez-Beltran M, et al. Ovarian dysgerminoma and synchronic contralateral tubal pregnancy followed by normal intra-uterine gestation: a case report. *J Med Rep.* 2012;6:399. DOI: 10.1186/1752-1947-6-399.

666 Uterine conditions: Image C. Leiomyoma (fibroid), gross specimen Soliman AA., ElSabaa B, Hassan N, et al. Degenerated huge retroperitoneal leiomyoma presenting with sonographic features mimicking a large uterine leiomyoma in an infertile woman with a history of myomectomy: a case report. *J Med Case Rep.* 2011;5:578. https://doi.org/10.1186/1752-1947-5-578

666 Uterine conditions: Image D. Leiomyoma (fibroid) histology. Londero AP, Perego P, Mangioni C, et al. Locally relapsed and metastatic uterine leiomyoma: a case report. *J Med Case Rep.* 2008;2:308. DOI: 10.1186/1752-1947-2-308.

666 Uterine conditions: Image E. Endometrial carcinoma. Izadi-Mood N, Yarmohammadi M, Ahmadi SA, et al. Reproducibility determination of WHO classification of endometrial hyperplasia/well differentiated adenocarcinoma and comparison with computerized morphometric data in curettage specimens in Iran. *Diagn Pathol.* 2009;4:10. DOI:10.1186/1746-1596-4-10.

667 Benign breast diseases. Phyllodes cyst on ultrasound. Crenshaw, S, Roller, M, Chapman, J. Immediate breast reconstruction with a saline implant and AlloDerm, following removal of a Phyllodes tumor. *World J Surg Onc.* 2011;9:34. DOI:10.1186/1477-7819-9-34.

668 Breast cancer: Image A. Mammography of breast cancer. Molino C, Mocerino C, Braucci A, et al. Pancreatic solitary and synchronous metastasis from breast cancer: a case report and systematic review of controversies in diagnosis and treatment. *World J Surg Oncol.* 2014;12:2. DOI:10.1186/1477-7819-12-2

668 Breast cancer: Image D. Invasive lobular carcinoma. Franceschini G, Manno A, Mule A, et al. Gastro-intestinal symptoms as clinical manifestation of peritoneal and retroperitoneal spread of an invasive lobular breast cancer: report of a case and review of the literature. *BMC Cancer.* 2006;6:193. DOI:10.1186/1471-2407-6-193.

668 Breast cancer: Image E. Peau d'orange of inflammatory breast cancer. Levine PH, Zolfaghari L, Young H, et al. What is inflammatory breast cancer? Revisiting the case definition. *Cancers (Basel).* 2010 Mar 3;2(1):143-52. DOI: 10.3390/cancers2010143.

669 Penile pathology: Image A. Peyronie disease. Tran VQ, Kim DH, Lesser TF, et al. Review of the surgical approaches for Peyronie's disease: corporeal plication and plaque incision with grafting. *Adv Urol.* Sept 2008;263450. DOI: 10.1155/2008/263450.

669 Cryptorchidism. Pandey A, Gangopadhyay AN, Kumar V. High anorectal malformation in a five-month-old boy: a case report. *J Med Case Reports.* 2010;4:296. DOI: 10.1186/1752-1947-4-296.

669 Varicocele. Mak CW, Tzeng WS. Sonography of the scrotum. Available at https://www.intechopen.com/chapters/27883.

670 Benign scrotal lesions. Transillumination of hydrocele. Bryson D. Transillumination of testicular hydrocele. *Clin Med Img Lib.* 2017;3:075. DOI: 10.23937/2474-3682/1510075

671 Testicular tumors. Seminoma. Thorvaldsen TE, Nødtvedt A, Grotmol T, et al. Morphological and immunohistochemical characterisation of seminomas in Norwegian dogs. *Acta Vet Scand.* 2012;54:52. https://doi.org/10.1186/1751-0147-54-52.

Respiratory

679 Alveolar cell types: Image A. Electron micrograph of type II pneumocyte. Fehrenbach H, Tews S, Fehrenbach A, et al. Improved lung preservation relates to an increase in tubular myelin-associated surfactant protein A. *Respir Res.* 2005 Jun 21;6:60. DOI: 10.1186/1465-9921-6-60.

679 Alveolar cell types: Image B. Micrograph of type II pneumocyte. Dr. Thomas Caceci.

679 Neonatal respiratory distress syndrome. Bogdanović R, Minić P, Marković-Lipkovski J, et al. Pulmonary renal syndrome in a child with coexistence of anti-neutrophil cytoplasmic antibodies and anti-glomerular basement membrane disease: case report and literature review. *BMC Nephrol.* 2013 Mar 22;14:66. DOI: 10.1186/1471-2369-14-66.

681 Lung anatomy: Image A. X-ray of normal lung. Namkoong H, Fujiwara H, Ishii M, et al. Immune reconstitution inflammatory syndrome due to *Mycobacterium avium* complex successfully followed up using 18 F-fluorodeoxyglucose positron emission tomography-computed tomography in a patient with human immunodeficiency virus infection: A case report. *BMC Med Imaging.* 2015;15:24. DOI 10.1186/s12880-015-0063-2.

681 Lung anatomy: Image B. CT scan of the chest. Wang JF, Wang B, Jansen JA, et al. Primary squamous cell carcinoma of lung in a 13-year-old boy: a case report. *Cases J.* 2008 Aug 22;1(1):123. DOI: 10.1186/1757-1626-1-123.

689 Cyanide vs carbon monoxide poisoning. MRI of presumed carbon monoxide poisoning. Dekeyzer S, De Kock I, Nikoubashman O, et al. "Unforgettable": a pictorial essay on anatomy and pathology of the hippocampus. *Insights Imaging.* 2017 Apr;8(2):199-212. DOI: 10.1007/s13244-016-0541-2.

690 Rhinosinusitis. Strek P, Zagolski O, Sktadzien J. Fatty tissue within the maxillary sinus: a rare finding. *Head Face Med.* 2006;2:28. DOI: 10.1186/1746-160X-2-28.

691 Pulmonary emboli: Image B. CT scan. Lee K, Rincon F. Pulmonary complications in patients with severe brain injury. *Crit Care Res Pract.* 2012;2012:207247. DOI: 10.1155/2012/207247.

693 Obstructive lung diseases: Image A. Barrel-shaped chest in emphysema. Solazzo A, D'Auria V, Moccia LG, et al. Posterior mediastinal extramedullary hematopoiesis secondary to hypoxia. *Transl Med UniSa.* 2016 May 16;14:1-4.

693 Obstructive lung diseases: Image B. Emphysema histology. Cheng SL, Wang HC, Yu CJ, et al. Prevention of elastase-induced emphysema in placenta growth factor knock-out mice. *Respir Res.* 2009 Nov 23;10(1):115. DOI: 10.1186/1465-9921-10-115.

693 Obstructive lung diseases: Image C. Centrilobular emphysema. The US Department of Health and Human Services and Dr. Edwin P. Ewing, Jr.

693 Obstructive lung diseases: Image D. CT of centriacinar emphysema. Zhu D, Qiao C, Dai H, et al. Diagnostic efficacy of visual subtypes and low attenuation area based on HRCT in the diagnosis of COPD. *BMC Pulm Med.* 2022 Mar 6;22(1):81. DOI: 10.1186/s12890-022-01875-6.

693 Obstructive lung diseases: Image E. Mucus plugs in asthma. Song L, Liu D, Wu C, et al. Antibody to mCLCA3 suppresses symptoms in a mouse model of asthma. *PLoS One.* 2013 Dec 9;8(12):e82367. DOI: 10.1371/journal.pone.0082367.

693 Obstructive lung diseases: Image F. Curschmann spirals. Alvarado A. Bronchial mucus: basic research and clinical application. *Clin Res Trials.* 2020;6. DOI: 10.15761/CRT.1000316.

693 Obstructive lung diseases: Image G. Charcot-Leyden crystals on bronchalverolar lavage. Gholamnejad M, Rezaie N. Unusual presentation of chronic eosinophilic pneumonia with "reversed halo sign": a case report. *Iran J Radiol.* 2014 May;11(2):e7891. DOI: 10.5812/iranjradiol.7891.

693 Obstructive lung diseases: Image H. Bronchiectasis in cystic fibrosis. Alvarado A. Bronchial mucus: basic research and clinical application. *Clin Res Trials* 2020;6. DOI: 10.15761/CRT.1000316.

695 Sarcoidosis: Image A. Kajal B, Harvey J, Alowami S. Melkerrson-Rosenthal Syndrome, a rare case report of chronic eyelid swelling. *Diagn Pathol.* 2013;8:188. DOI: 10.1186/1746-1596-8-188.

695 Sarcoidosis: Images B and C. X-ray (B) and CT (C) of the chest. Lønborg J, Ward M, Gill A, et al. Utility of cardiac magnetic resonance in assessing right-sided heart failure in sarcoidosis. *BMC Med Imaging.* 2013;13:2. DOI: 10.1186/1471-2342-13-2.

696 Pneumoconioses: Image A. CT scan of asbestosis. Miles SE, Sandrini A, Johnson AR, et al. Clinical consequences of asbestos-related diffuse pleural thickening: a review. *J Occup Med Toxicol.* 2008;3:20. DOI: 10.1186/1745-6673-3-20.

696 Pneumoconioses: Image B. Ferruginous bodies in asbestosis. The Department of Health and Human Services and Dr. Edwin P Ewing, Jr.

696 Pneumoconioses: Image C. Noncaseating granuloma. Rajebi MR, Shahrokni A, Chaisson M. Uncommon osseous involvement in multisystemic sarcoidosis. *Ann Saudi Med.* 2009 Nov-Dec;29(6):485-486. DOI: 10.4103/0256-4947.57175.

697 Acute respiratory distress syndrome: Image A. Alveolar fluid. Pires-Neto RC, Del Carlo Bernardi F, de Araujo PA. The expression of water and ion channels in diffuse alveolar damage is not dependent on DAD etiology. *PLoS One.* 2016;11(11):e0166184. DOI: 10.1371/journal.pone.0166184.

697 Acute respiratory distress syndrome: Image B. Bilateral lung opacities. Imanaka H, Takahara B, Yamaguchi H, et al. Chest computed tomography of a patient revealing severe hypoxia due to amniotic fluid embolism: a case report. *J Med Case Reports.* 2010;4:55. DOI: 10.1186/1752-1947-4-55.

699 Atelectasis. Kayal D, Minkara S, Tleiss F. Early diagnosis of left pulmonary artery sling during first week of life in a term baby boy: a case report. *Cureus.* 2020 Feb 5;12(2):e6889. DOI: 10.7759/cureus.6889.

699 Pleural effusions: Images A and B. Before (A) and after (B) treatment. Toshikazu A, Takeoka H, Nishioka K, et al. Successful management of refractory pleural effusion due to systemic immunoglobulin light chain amyloidosis by vincristine adriamycin dexamethasone chemotherapy: a case report. *Med Case Rep.* 2010;4:322. DOI: 10.1186/1752-1947-4-322.

700 Pneumothorax: Image A. CT scan. Miura K, Kondo R, Kurai M, et al. Birt-Hogg-Dubé syndrome detected incidentally by asymptomatic bilateral pneumothorax in health screening: a case of a young Japanese woman. *Surg Case Rep.* 2015 Dec;1:17. DOI: 10.1186/s40792-015-0014-8.

700 Pneumothorax: Image B. Tension pneumothorax. Rosat A, Díaz C. Reexpansion pulmonary edema after drainage of tension pneumothorax. *Pan Afr Med J.* 2015;22:143. DOI: 10.11604/pamj.2015.22.143.8097.

701 Pneumonia: Image A. Lobar pneumonia. Yoon BW, Song YG, Lee SH. Severe community-acquired adenovirus pneumonia treated with oral ribavirin: a case report. *BMC Res Notes.* 2017;10:47. DOI: 10.1186/s13104-016-2370-2.

701 Pneumonia: Image B. Interstitial pneumonia x-ray. Abro S, Bikeyeva V, Naqvi WA, et al. Clopidogrel-associated interstitial lung disease: a case report and literature review. *Cureus.* 2022 Aug 25;14(8):e28394. DOI: 10.7759/cureus.28394.

702 Lung abscess. Gross pathology. Futami S, Takimoto T, Nakagami F, et al. A lung abscess caused by secondary syphilis—the utility of polymerase chain reaction techniques in transbronchial biopsy: a case report. *BMC Infect Dis.* 2019;19:598. https://doi.org/10.1186/s12879-019-4236-4.

703 Lung cancer: Image B. Adenocarcinoma histology. Wang JF, Wang B, Jansen JA, et al. Primary squamous cell carcinoma of lung in a 13-year-old boy: a case report. *Cases J.* 2008 Aug 22;1(1):123. doi: 10.1186/1757-1626-1-123.

703 Lung cancer: Image C. Squamous cell carcinoma. Chisenga R, Adenwala T, Kim W, et al. Squamous cell carcinoma of the lung presenting as a fungating ulcerated skin lesion: a case report. *J Med Case Rep.* 2022 Apr 26;16(1):172. DOI: 10.1186/s13256-022-03352-4.

703   **Lung cancer: Image E.** Large cell lung cancer. ◉◉ Jala VR, Radde BN, Haribabu B, et al. Enhanced expression of G-protein coupled estrogen receptor (GPER/GPR30) in lung cancer. *BMC Cancer.* 2012;12:624. DOI: 10.1186/1471-2407-12-624.

704   **Pancoast tumor.** ◉◉ Manenti G, Raguso M, D'Onofrio S, et al. Pancoast tumor: the role of magnetic resonance imaging. *Case Rep Radiol.* 2013;2013:479120. DOI: 10.1155/2013/479120.

704   **Superior vena cava syndrome: Images A and B.** Blanching of skin with pressure (A) and CT of chest (B) in superior vena cava syndrome. ◉◉ Shaikh I, Berg K, Kman N. Thrombogenic catheter-associated superior vena cava syndrome. *Case Rep Emerg Med.* 2013;2013:793054. DOI 10.1155/2013/793054.

Index

▶ NOTES

▶ NOTES

▶ NOTES

About the Editors

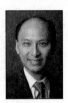

Tao Le, MD, MHS

Tao developed a passion for medical education as a medical student. He has edited more than 15 titles in the *First Aid* series. In addition, he is Founder and Chief Education Officer of USMLE-Rx for exam preparation and ScholarRx for sustainable, global medical education. As a medical student, he was editor-in-chief of the University of California, San Francisco (UCSF) *Synapse*, a university newspaper with a weekly circulation of 9000. Tao earned his medical degree from UCSF in 1996 and completed his residency training in internal medicine at Yale University and fellowship training at Johns Hopkins University. Tao subsequently went on to cofound Medsn, a medical education technology venture, and served as its chief medical officer. He is currently chief of adult allergy and immunology at the University of Louisville.

Vikas Bhushan, MD

Vikas is a writer, editor, entrepreneur, and retired teleradiologist. In 1990 he conceived and authored the original *First Aid for the USMLE Step 1*. His entrepreneurial endeavors included a student-focused medical publisher (S2S), an e-learning company (medschool.com), and an ER teleradiology practice (24/7 Radiology). Trained on the Left Coast, Vikas completed a bachelor's degree at the University of California Berkeley; an MD with thesis at UCSF; and a diagnostic radiology residency at UCLA. His eclectic interests include cryptoeconomics, information design, and avoiding a day job. Always finding the long shortcut, Vikas is an adventurer, knowledge seeker, and occasional innovator. He and his spouse, Jinky, are avid kiteboarders and worldschoolers, striving to raise their three children as global citizens.

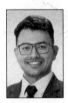

Anup Chalise, MBBS, MS, MRCSEd

Anup is a Registrar working in General Surgery at North Middlesex University Hospital, London. He is also currently working on projects with ScholarRx, including Flash Facts and Qmax. In his free time, he likes to travel for photography. He is currently looking to pursue training to integrate AI in medical education, and further his surgical training simultaneously.

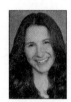

Jaimie Rogner, MD, MPH

Jaimie is a second-year psychiatry resident at NewYork-Presbyterian/Weill Cornell Medical Center. She attended Northeastern University as an undergraduate and earned her Master of Public Health at the State University of New York (SUNY) Downstate Medical University and medical degree at SUNY Upstate Medical University. After two years of an Internal Medicine/Pediatrics residency at the University of Rochester, she made a pivot to psychiatry. Her hope is to work with individuals in the correctional system as well as refugees and immigrants. Outside of medicine, she likes to indulge in nature, podcasts, live music, and cheering on her favorite athletes and sports teams.

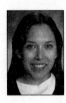

Carolina Caban Rivera

Carolina is an MD/PhD student at the Lewis Katz School of Medicine at Temple University. She completed her doctoral dissertation in neuroscience in May 2023 and is interested in pursuing a residency in dermatology. Carolina is an advocate for immigrant health, and outside of medicine, she enjoys yoga, candle-making, and rollerblading.

Caroline Coleman, MD

Caroline is an academic hospitalist at the Atlanta Veterans Affairs Medical Center and an adjunct professor of medicine at Emory University School of Medicine. She earned her undergraduate degree in Economics at the University of Georgia and her medical degree at Emory University School of Medicine, and completed her internal medicine residency training at the J. Willis Hurst Internal Medicine Residency Program at Emory University School of Medicine in 2023. Her clinical duties include teaching teams on the wards as well as rotating on the inpatient POCUS and procedure service.

Kimberly Kallianos, MD

Originally from Atlanta, Kimberly graduated from the University of North Carolina at Chapel Hill in 2006 and from Harvard Medical School in 2011. She completed her radiology residency and fellowship at UCSF and is currently an Assistant Professor of Clinical Radiology at UCSF in the cardiac and pulmonary imaging section.

Sean Evans, MD

Sean is a second-year internal medicine resident at Emory University School of Medicine. He earned his undergraduate degree at the University of Georgia and spent two years at the National Institutes of Health as a research fellow before earning his medical degree at Emory. He is interested in pursuing a career in medical oncology, and outside of medicine enjoys running, reading, and yoga.